SPORTS PHYSICAL THERAPY

SPORTS PHYSICAL THERAPY

Editor

Barbara Sanders, MS, PT, SCS
Associate Professor and Program Director
Physical Therapy
Southwest Texas State University
San Marcos, Texas

APPLETON & LANGE
Norwalk, Connecticut/San Mateo, California

0-8385-8652-X

Notice: Our knowledge in clinical sciences is constantly changing. As new information becomes available, changes in treatment and in the use of drugs become necessary. The authors and the publisher of this volume have taken care to make certain that the doses of drugs and schedules of treatment are correct and compatible with the standards generally accepted at the time of publication. The reader is advised to consult carefully the instruction and information material included in the package insert of each drug or therapeutic agent before administration. This advice is especially important when using new or infrequently used drugs.

Copyright © 1990 by Appleton & Lange
A Publishing Division of Prentice Hall

90 91 92 93 94 / 10 9 8 7 6 5 4 3 2 1

Prentice Hall International (UK) Limited, *London*
Prentice Hall of Australia Pty. Limited, *Sydney*
Prentice Hall Canada, Inc., *Toronto*
Prentice Hall Hispanoamericana, S.A., *Mexico*
Prentice Hall of India Private Limited, *New Delhi*
Prentice Hall of Japan, Inc., *Tokyo*
Simon & Schuster Asia Pte. Ltd., *Singapore*
Editora Prentice Hall do Brasil Ltda., *Rio de Janeiro*
Prentice Hall, *Englewood Cliffs, New Jersey*

Library of Congress Cataloging-in-Publication Data

Sports physical therapy / [edited by] Barbara Sanders.
     p. cm.
   ISBN 0-8385-8652-X
   1. Sports physical therapy.   I. Sanders, Barbara.
   [DNLM: 1. Physical Therapy.   2. Sports Medicine. QT 260
S7857651]
   RD97.S75   1990
   617.1'027—dc20
   DNLM/DLC
   for Library of Congress   90-8
                                                              CIP
Acquisitions Editors: Jamie Mount Sokol and William R. Schmitt
Production Editor: Sandra K. Huggard
Designer: Janice Barsevich

PRINTED IN THE UNITED STATES OF AMERICA

To my parents, Nick and Emily Furnish, who raised, nurtured, and guided me, and most of all to my family and best friends, my husband, Michael, and my daughter, Whitney.

BRS

Contributors

Arnold T. Bell, PhD, PT, ATC
Assistant Professor
Physical Therapy
Florida A & M University
Tallahassee, Florida

William S. Case, PT, SCS
Director of Physical Therapy
Rehabilitation Services of Houston
Houston, Texas

Steve Dickoff, MS, PT, ATC, SCS
Director of Sportsmedicine
North Hills Sportsmedicine Center
Pittsburgh, Pennsylvania

Michael J. Dreibelbeis, ATC, PT, SCS
Sports Medicine Centre
Iowa Methodist Medical Center
Granger, Iowa

John Eggart, MS, PT, ATC, SCS
Chief Physical Therapist
Student Health Center
University of Wisconsin-LaCrosse
LaCrosse, Wisconsin

Perry S. Esterson, MS, PT, ATC, SCS
Vienna Physical Therapy Associates, PC
Vienna, Virginia

Jeffrey E. Falkel, PhD, PT
Associate Professor
School of Physical Therapy
Ohio University
Athens, Ohio

Gary Alan Green, MD
Division of Family Medicine
UCLA School of Medicine
Los Angeles, California

Timothy Heckman, PT, ATC
Associate Director, Rehabilitation
Sports Physical Therapy Services
Cincinnati, Ohio

Walt Jenkins, MS, PT, ATC
Director of Sports Physical Therapy
Instructor
Department of Physical Therapy
Kansas University Medical Center
Kansas City, Kansas

Sam Kegerreis, MS, PT, ATC
Assistant Professor
Krannert Graduate School of Physical Therapy
University of Indianapolis
Indianapolis, Indiana

Karen A. Knortz, MS, PT, ATC, SCS
Sports Physical Therapist/Instructor
Lincoln Physical Therapy Associates
University of Nebraska-Lincoln
Lincoln, Nebraska

Susan D. Lambert, PT, ATC, SCS
Sports Physical Therapist, Athletic Trainer
Kinetix Physical Therapy
Norfolk, Virginia

Terry Malone, EdD, PT, ATC
Executive Director of Sports Medicine
Associate Professor of Physical Therapy
Duke University
Durham, North Carolina

Robert Mangine, MS, PT, ATC
Director
Sports Physical Therapy Services
Cincinnati, Ohio

Tyrone McSorley, PT, ATC,
Director and Co-owner
Sports Therapy Arthritis Rehabilitation (STAR)
Las Vegas, Nevada

A. Lynn Millar, PhD
Assistant Professor
Physical Therapy
Southwest Texas State University
San Marcos, Texas

Joseph M. Murphy, PT
Sports Orthopedics and Rehabilitative Physical
  Therapy
Gap, Pennsylvania

Tinker D. Murray, PhD
Assistant Professor
Health, Physical Education, and Recreation
Southwest Texas State University
San Marcos, Texas

Millicent Owens, MA, RD
Consulting Dietitian
Division of Graduate Nutrition
University of Texas at Austin
Austin, Texas

John A. Romero, MA, PT, ATC, SCS
President
Sports & Orthopaedic Therapy Services
Silver Springs, Maryland

Kenneth Rusche, MEd, PT, ATC, SCS
Director
Wellington Sports Medicine and Rehabilitation
  Center
Cincinnati, Ohio

Barbara Sanders, MS, PT, SCS
Associate Professor and Program Director
Physical Therapy
Southwest Texas State University
San Marcos, Texas

Michael T. Sanders, EdD
Associate Head Track Coach
University of Texas at Austin
Austin, Texas

Dallas A. Simons, PT, ATC, SCS
Vienna Physical Therapy Associates, PC
Vienna, Virginia

Diane Slaughter, MS, PT, ATC
Director, Physical Therapy
University of Kentucky Sports Medicine Center
Lexington, Kentucky

Steven R. Tippett, PT, ATC, SCS
Director, Sports Medicine
Center for Sports Medicine and Health Fitness
Peoria, Illinois

Michael Voight, MEd, PT, ATC, SCS
Instructor, School of Medicine
Orthopaedics and Rehabilitation,
  Division of Physical Therapy
University of Miami
Miami, Florida

James E. Zachazewski, MS, PT, ATC
Director, Athletic Training and Rehabilitation
UCLA Department of Athletics
Los Angeles, California

Peter Zulia, PT, ATC
Assistant Director
Wellington Sports Medicine and Rehabilitation
Cincinnati, Ohio

Contents

Preface

Sports physical therapy has developed at a rapid pace in the past 15 years. This book was spurred by the development of the specialty process and the advanced clinical competencies identified through that process.

The goal of this book is to provide information relevant to the needs of the practicing physical therapist who intends to work with the athletic population; thus the major emphasis has been directed at the needs of the practicing physical therapist.

Sports physical therapy has been an important part of my career since I first met George Davies in 1976. He is responsible for "grabbing" my interest and nurturing my professional development. I thank him for that. My many colleagues in the sports physical therapy section have encouraged and guided me, have given me support, and quite often have challenged me. I am especially appreciative of them; Sandy Quillen, who recommended me for this project; Tab Blackburn, Lynn Wallace, Bob Mangine, Gary Derscheid, Jim Gould and Terry Malone, who provided advice, consultation, and assistance; and Kathy Johnson, who continually gave me encouragement that I could accomplish this undertaking.

I would be remiss not to acknowledge the help and support I have received from the Southwest Texas State University Physical Therapy faculty and staff, Diana Hunter, Lynn Millar, Julie Caroselli, Barb Melzer, Elizabeth Cole, and Mark Pape; from my University of Texas graduate school colleagues, Leona Fields and Mary Rubright; and all of my other friends and colleagues who have knowingly or unknowingly helped me with this book. Thanks too to Bill Schmitt and Jamie Mount Sokol for their patience and guidance in working with a neophyte author and editor.

Finally thank you to all the gifted clinicians, educators, and specialists who have taken their time to share their contributions with us. My most important thanks to my most important support—my family, Mike and Whitney Sanders.

Barbara Sanders, MS, PT, SCS
San Marcos, Texas

1 Sports Physical Therapy and the Role of the Physical Therapist

Barbara Sanders and Terry Malone

INTRODUCTION

Sports physical therapy was officially recognized as a special interest group by the American Physical Therapy Association (APTA) when Section status was granted by the APTA House of Delegates in 1973. The founders consisted of physical therapists who felt that there was a common body of knowledge related to the physical therapy care of the athlete. They were interested in providing opportunities for education, communication, and consultation in the area that we know as sports medicine. The original name was the Sports Medicine Section of the APTA and was changed during the 1980s to reflect more accurately the membership of the group.

Other professional groups have organized to facilitate their interest in sports medicine practice. These include the National Athletic Trainers Association (NATA), the American College of Sports Medicine (ACSM), the American Osteopathic Academy of Sports Medicine, the Canadian Academy of Sports Medicine, the American Orthopaedic Society for Sports Medicine (AOSSM), the International Federation of Sports Medicine (FIMS), the American Medical Association–Committee on Medical Aspects of Sports, and others.

Although there is no single definition of sports medicine, sources agree that sports medicine is a multidisciplinary activity related both to the clinical and training aspects of exercise and sports participation. The first modern definition of sports medicine was provided by the Institute for Cardiology and Sports Medicine in Cologne in 1958: "Sports medicine includes those theoretical and practical branches of medicine which investigate the influence of exercise, training and sport on healthy and ill people, as well as the effects of lack of exercise, to produce useful results for prevention, therapy, rehabilitation and the athlete." This definition was adopted by the FIMS Scientific Commission in 1977.[1]

The ACSM defines sports medicine as

the study of the physiological, biomechanical, psychosocial, and pathological phenomena associated with exercise and athletics and clinical application of the knowledge gained from the study to the improvement and maintenance of functional capacities for physical labor, exercise and athletics and to the prevention and treatment of disease and injuries related to exercise and athletics.[2]

Another definition states that sports medicine

is the application of medical art and science to the practice of agonistic sport and of physical activities in general, in order to take advantage of the preventive and therapeutic possibilities of sport to maintain the state of health and to avoid any damage connected with excess or lack of physical exercise.[3]

The Sports Physical Therapy Section defines sports physical therapy as "the practice of sports physical therapy involving injury prevention, performance enhancement, recognition, and management of acute athletic injuries, treatment and rehabilitation of athletic injuries, protection or athletic injury, education and research."[4]

As is obvious from these various definitions, the primary goal of professionals involved in the care of athletes is to prevent as many injuries and illnesses as possible and to treat injuries and illnesses that do occur with prompt and complete rehabilitation to allow the person's return to sports activities.[5] The consensus is that the treatment of athletes is different from the care of other patients because athletes impose higher demands on the cardiovascular, respiratory, and musculoskeletal system. Athletes are generally healthy and well motivated; thus any injury may be perceived to be a serious handicap. Treatment of the athlete must be tailored to the athlete's individual needs. Rest does not mean complete rest from all activities, but rather the continuation of exercise within one's threshold for pain

and soreness. Certainly the level of rest and activity depends on the sport and can include continuing the activity with changes in equipment, stroke, or level of participation. Rehabilitation must be both physical and psychological because the athlete must be prepared to return to the same forces that caused the injury. Flexibility and strength must be greater than the "clinical" normal. Education of the athlete is critical in the successful rehabilitation and prevention of further injury.

Sports medicine, however, is not just for the athletic population. Recreational sports and athletic participation have become quite popular because of the health and performance benefits. Research indicates that sports are important throughout our lives. Therefore, sports medicine has emerged as an important area of medicine. Today's approach to sports medicine includes a highly organized and qualified team to provide comprehensive medical care. Team members encompass all medical specialties—biomechanical, psychological, nutritional, environmental, pathological, and physiological.[1] Sports medicine is a growing and dynamic field, with increasing numbers of professional groups with subspecialties contributing to the literature, research, and education.

Because this book is on sports physical therapy, the remainder of this chapter is devoted to a discussion of the role of the sports physical therapist in organizing and delivering quality care for the sports physical therapy patient population.

The sports physical therapist needs a variety of specific skills as well as a sound base of traditional physical therapy basic science. The understanding of sports and the demands placed upon each athlete in every position, skill, and circumstance inherent to the specific sport is vital. Such an understanding of sports mechanics allows for easier diagnosis, treatment, protection, and prevention of injury.[6] The scope of care provided by the sports physical therapist includes injury assessment, injury treatment, injury prevention, research, education, and administration.[4]

Assessment

Injury assessment starts with the basic approach that all physical therapists have learned, which includes a statement of the problem, collection of data regarding the problem, and creation of a solution to resolve the problem. The sports physical therapist is normally assisted by other health care professionals in making these determinations but is often the primary care provider at a practice or competition site. The assessment is different from traditional physical therapy due to the immediate sequelae of acute injury (muscle spasm, ligament laxity, pain, unconsciousness, etc.) or possible life-threatening events upon which extraneous circumstances are imposed (e.g., equipment, weather,

crowds). Therefore a variety of special assessment skills are required:

- Primary assessment—establish status of respiration, circulation, and level of consciousness.
- Secondary assessment—evaluate acute neurological, musculoskeletal, internal organs, genitourinary, ocular, or integumentary injury.

Although the type of patient differs from the traditional physical therapy patient, the assessment tools still include the history, objective findings via observation, palpation, and testing. These skills and specific assessment procedures will be discussed in other chapters in this text.

Treatment

Treatment of injuries includes the ongoing evaluation, management, care and rehabilitation of acute, subacute and chronic athletic injuries. Treatment is an obvious function of the sports physical therapist but may vary from treating the general patient with a musculoskeletal injury. The proper management of an athletic injury is essential in order to restore the athlete to the greatest possible level of function in the shortest time possible. A thorough understanding of the specific sport is essential in order to accomplish this goal.

Specific treatments will be discussed in individual chapters of this book. Treatment must be based on the initial assessment, however, and may need to be geared toward life-threatening situations. Thus, the sports physical therapist must have emergency medical training and treatment skills, including cardiopulmonary resuscitation, advanced first aid, familiarity with emergency equipment, and awareness of a preplanned and organized emergency management/transportation system.

Treatment goals in non-life-threatening injuries include proper stabilization and support, prevention/limitation of swelling, and decreasing pain. The acronym PRICE is used to characterize the most often used treatment for musculoskeletal injury—protection, rest, ice, compression, and elevation.

The treatment of the athlete in subacute situations does not vary significantly from the treatment of traditional physical therapy patients. One should be mindful of several key points when caring for the athlete. Specific treatment goals are to restore full pain-free range of motion and flexibility, strength, endurance, and to restore the athlete to a functional level which allows the return to athletic participation. Demands on the athlete are different from those placed on the traditional physical therapy patient; treatment must reflect this fact. The SAID principle (specific adaptation to imposed demands) is vital to a comprehensive rehabilitation program. Demands vary from sport to sport and

from athlete to athlete. Functional progression bridges the gap between a player who is ready to return to competition and an athlete who is competition ready. Functional progression is a series of fundamental movement patterns specific to a sport that are provided in an orderly fashion based on the tolerance and performance of the athlete, and offers both physical and psychological benefits to the athlete.[6,7]

Treatment of the entire athlete is critical to successful rehabilitation and includes more than just rehabilitation of the injury. Many times additional steps such as taping, splinting, or special padding may be required as well as education of the athlete, parents and coaching staff.

Prevention

Prevention involves not only the sports physical therapist and the athlete, but also interaction with other health care personnel, coaches, equipment managers, athletic trainers, parents, administrators, and so forth. Some of the important aspects of injury prevention are preparticipation physical examinations, proper taping techniques, equipment fitting, splinting, padding or immobilization techniques, and off-season conditioning programs. A key to preventing injuries is to have a good working relationship with the entire team—open and honest communication and trust of all members will strengthen the athletic program.

Research

As in all health care, pertinent, basic, scientific research is required to assure the most effective and efficient means of care for the athlete. The sports physical therapist can help promote the growth of the practice of sports physical therapy through research. Suitable areas include the treatment, management, and prevention of injuries. Many current practices are based on research conducted by sports physical therapists and include competition criteria, rule changes, protective equipment standards, and utilization of equipment and implements.

Education

With the rapid advances in sports care, the need to stay current is imperative and is the responsibility of each individual providing services to the athlete. Formal and informal education must be an ongoing commitment for every sports physical therapist. The sports physical therapist is a vital source of information for the athletes, coaches, parents, athletic trainers, medical, and other health care personnel. Sports physical therapists are frequently required to provide information regarding the assessment, management, and prevention of injuries. They should also be ready to discuss nutrition, hygiene, ergogenic aids, and drugs.

Administration

Administration can be a vital aspect of sports physical therapy. Record keeping is just as important in sports physical therapy as for traditional physical therapists. Referral and treatment records must reflect current treatment and progress; supplies and equipment must be purchased, serviced, and maintained; third-party reimbursement requirements must be met; supportive personnel must be appropriately supervised; and the sports physical therapist must communicate with the team members—physician, coach, athlete, parent, athletic trainer, and others intimately involved in the quality care of the athlete.

Sports physical therapy is a growing specialty within physical therapy. Because of the growth of sports medicine, there is overlap in the role of the sports physical therapist with the athletic trainer, physician, emergency medical care personnel, and strength coach, among others. The obvious niche of the sports physical therapist is the ongoing assessment and rehabilitation of the injured athlete and determining methodologies of injury prevention.

SPORTS CARE FACILITIES AND ORGANIZATION

Sports physical therapy settings are varied and thus reflect an array of responsibilities, staffing, and financial arrangements. A basic premise of the sports physical therapy delivery system is that the well-designed delivery system focuses on providing comprehensive, continuous, and coordinated care. A single individual should be designated to coordinate care and should be a well-trained professional—physical therapist, athletic trainer, or physician.[8]

The system must have a clearly described mission or philosophy upon which to build the operational goals for the unit. The philosophy and goals will be directly related to the needs of the community, setting, or organization in which the sports care unit is located. In any of the settings, the organization and administration of the sports physical therapy services must be solidly based in fiscal and management practices. Therefore, any service should have established required policies and procedures that are designed to provide the athletes with the most effective health care. A plan for the management of accurate and detailed records for injury and treatment must be developed, along with the selection, purchase, and maintenance of equipment. Other members of the care delivery team must be instructed and supervised.

The size and scope of the service will depend on the locale, the available facilities and resources, and the age and number of athletes. Proper care is depen-

dent upon prevention programs such as preparticipation screening, conditioning, evaluation and management of equipment and environment, prompt evaluation and treatment of injuries; referral when necessary, and rehabilitation and record keeping for insurance purposes, injury reporting, and treatment records.

Sports physical therapy is practiced in many settings such as colleges and universities, professional athletic organizations, high schools, clinics, and hospitals. The role of the sports physical therapist in each of these settings is varied.

Many physical therapists are employed at the *university* level to treat the enrolled athletes. These physical therapists are often certified trainers (PT/ATC). The PT/ATC and the team physician coordinate the management of the sports-medicine care. The therapist is paid a salary and has specific year-round duties that are directed toward the care of university athletic teams—male, female, or coeducational (Figs 1–1 and 1–2). If the physical therapist is functioning as an athletic trainer, responsibilities may include

- Traveling with the athletic teams
- Budgeting for team needs for the season

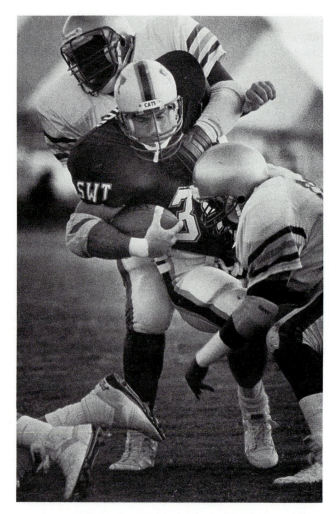

Figure 1-2. Varsity university football.

- Scheduling other staff members, students, volunteers
- Assessing athletic injuries
- Managing injuries/illnesses
- Other duties (prn)

In this setting the physical therapist may have such additional responsibilities as teaching in physical therapy, athletic training, physical education, or other programs/departments. The physical therapist may also work in the student health center, university-based hospital physical therapy department, private practice, or other areas. Research opportunities are abundant for the sports physical therapist employed in such a setting.

Smaller colleges may have a contract with a physical therapist to treat athletes or to work closely with the athletic trainer and team physician to provide quality care for the athletes. The sports physical therapist in this setting may have little or no participation in site/game coverage.

As in the collegiate and university setting, most physical therapists employed at the *professional* level are also certified athletic trainers. Many professional

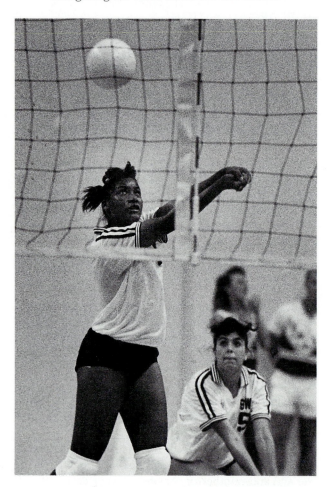

Figure 1-1. Varsity university women's volleyball.

teams, however, employ physical therapists who serve strictly as rehabilitation specialists and have little or no involvement in actual game/participation coverage. In the professional setting, sports physical therapists are either employed by the team or are affiliated with private or hospital-based clinics or physician groups who treat the professional athletes. Nearly all of the professional football, basketball, hockey, baseball, and soccer teams have a strong affiliation with a sports physical therapist.

Many physical therapists consult with professional teams during the off-season to establish preparticipation evaluation programs. Some of the touring professionals in individual sports have a traveling trainer who may also be a physical therapist (i.e., golf, tennis, rodeo).

Although the need for a sports physical therapist is greatest at the *high school* level, there are not many physical therapists involved at this level. Very few high schools presently employ athletic trainers. Thus, many athletes are participating in a variety of sports at the high school level without adequate sports medical care. In some instances, physical therapists are employees of the high school on a full- or part-time basis. Sometimes they may serve as teachers or deliver physical therapy services to the handicapped student population as well as the athletes.[8]

Most frequently high schools are served by physical therapists who are employees of private or hospital-based clinics, physician groups, or on a volunteer basis. Coverage for the high school is less than full-time, varying from game/event-only coverage to daily visits for injury assessment. This means that coverage may or may not include practices or games. The clinics often contract for services, charging a minimal fee or providing such services gratis in order to generate positive public relations and additional clientele for the clinic/hospital.

High school situations can be very rewarding:

- Services are provided for those athletes who desperately need them.
- The arrangement between the physical therapist and high school may be financially or professionally feasible.
- An opportunity is provided to work with community members and other health care professionals in a different setting.
- Coaches, athletes, parents, and school administrators are generally appreciative of the professional care provided for the athletes.
- Physical therapists are provided the opportunity to serve a "needy" population while gaining expertise in sports medicine.

The sports physical therapist in this setting is responsible for preventing and managing injuries; educating coaches, school nurses, and student trainers; developing a centralized training room; implementing policies and procedures; and establishing a medical record-keeping system. The high school setting does not require the significant resource allocation that many administrators feel is required.[8]

One effective delivery model is an arrangement between a local or team physician and physical therapist/athletic trainer. The physician provides the primary medical care, coordinates the services that are needed, seeks consultation, and provides ongoing care with the PT/ATC, thus gaining the respect and trust of the athlete, coach, trainer, and administrator. The PT/ATC works to educate the coach, athlete, student trainers, manage the training room, develop and maintain an injury surveillance system, and provide day-to-day treatments and coordination of sports injury care. The physician and PT/ATC can coordinate on-site care of athletes—emergency coverage of events, hospital arrangements, and essential consultation services. The lynchpin of the system is a well-designed record-keeping system that allows effective and efficient communication among all members of the athletic injury care team.

Sports physical therapists are increasingly being found in the *clinic setting*. The clinic may be private, hospital based, or located in a physician's office. The 1988 Physician and Sportsmedicine Directory of Sports Medicine Clinics listed 552 clinics, an increase of 277 clinics in 8 years.[9] The role of the sports physical therapist is readily apparent in this growth. Most of those clinics (75%) listed employ a physical therapist. These clinics do not always treat only sports-related injuries, but also the traditional outpatient physical therapy patients. As mentioned in the discussion on collegiate and high school settings, these clinics may also contract to provide a variety of services for athletic injury management. The clinic setting may generate sports medicine research and education. Many clinics provide public service educational programs on the prevention and management of athletic injuries, as well as provide medical coverage for community events such as 10-kilometer runs, marathons, and triathalons.

Medical center based sports medicine clinics may serve a wider population than the aforementioned clinics. Quite often the staff in these settings are simultaneously employed by the athletic department to provide ongoing sports care. In addition, these clinics provide a variety of services to the university, community, and high schools by providing a center for preventive programs, first aid and emergency care, evaluation and diagnostic services, nonsurgical and surgical treatment, referral services, rehabilitation, research, and teaching.

Community-based settings most frequently involve therapists as volunteers with specific assignments

to clubs and organizations for consultation activities. Therapists in these settings generally have a specific interest in the sport or have friends or family members participating in the activity. Some of the areas where physical therapists are involved include dance groups, gymnastics clubs, hockey, soccer and swimming organizations, and running clubs.

Other areas where sports physical therapists serve include serving as consultants to amateur sports federations and to sports rules, regulations, and equipment committees. More and more therapists are volunteering for the United States Olympic effort. In this role physicians and health care personnel volunteer for 2 weeks of work at the Olympic Training Centers in Colorado Springs or Lake Placid. They are then selected to work at USOC events such as Sports Festivals, World University Games, Pan American Games, and the Olympics.

As one can see from this overview, the opportunities for the sports physical therapist to be involved in the care of the athletic population are virtually unlimited. With proper training and experience, the sports physical therapist can play an important role.

THE SPORTS MEDICINE TEAM

The sports medicine team consists of many health care professionals at several levels. The "full-time" team members are generally the team physician, athletic trainer, and sports physical therapist. This active team may also include resident physicians, student trainers, student physical therapists, and administrators. There are numerous other consultants who should be available to the team, including medical consultants, allied health personnel, and general consultants. Medical consultants typically include allergists, cardiologists, dermatologists, dentists, oral surgeons, gynecologists, internists, neurologists, ophthalmologists, orthopaedists, otolaryngologists, general surgeons, urologists, and radiologists. Allied health personnel can include emergency medical technicians, podiatrists, lab technologists, nurses, optometrists, opticians, pharmacists, and psychologists. Other general consultants include administrators, orthotists, coaches, equipment managers, exercise physiologists, health educators, kinesiologists, attorneys, dietitians, strength coaches, and substance abuse counselors.[5] The sports medicine team is not reserved just for the physician; the success of the team depends on all of the individuals who add expertise to complete the endeavor. Traditionally, it is the physician who is the first member of the team, with the remainder of the team comprising the relevant health care personnel listed above. The active team is responsible for the primary care of the athlete. It is vital for this team to be organized through the development of policies and procedures with clear lines of authority.

Clear lines of communication must be established among the members of the team and the individual athletes, coaches, and parents.

The sports physical therapist can be described as the professional who assists the athlete to bridge the gap from the clinic to the field of play. Too often traditional medical care does not prepare the athlete for participation. This is the key element added to the team by the sports physical therapist.

SPORTS PHYSICAL THERAPY SPECIALIZATION

This chapter should provide an overview of the role of the sports physical therapist, the areas of practice where he or she might be found, and some keys to the administration of the setting. We conclude and summarize by providing the reader with an overview of the sports specialization process for the physical therapist.

In the early 1970s APTA adopted a position statement in favor of the development of advanced clinical competency testing. In 1977, a working document, *Competencies in Therapy: An Analysis of Practice*, was published describing the competencies in physical therapy.[10] This era also saw the initiation of a task force to study clinical specialization. This group proposed the *Essentials of Certification of Advanced Clinical Competencies* for establishing specialty areas and recommended the initiation of the specialization process.[11] The Essentials were adopted by the House of Delegates of the APTA, thus creating the supervisory organization titled the Board for Certification of Advanced Clinical Competencies (BCACC). This group developed the operational framework and devised the application process for interested groups to gain recognition as specialties within the physical therapy profession. In 1981, four interest groups presented petitions and were approved as specialty areas in physical therapy (cardiopulmonary, orthopaedics, pediatrics and sports). Specialty councils were selected by the BCACC, with the original Sports Council consisting of Tab Blackburn, Lynn Wallace, and Terry Malone (Chairman). In 1986, the name for the BCACC was changed to the American Board of Physical Therapy Specialties (ABPTS), which is more reflective of its function.

In the late 1970s the Sports Physical Therapy Section of the APTA began to identify competencies specific to the practice of sports physical therapy. A task force surveyed the section's membership to identify specific clinical skills and to what extent/frequency clinicians were applying those competencies in the clinical setting.[12] In 1984 a second major competency project was completed. This project examined the level of competency and the level of preparation provided by the professional education programs in physical therapy.

The results of that study further validated the competencies and the level of importance to the practice of sports physical therapy.[13] These competencies have been divided into patient care services, administrative services, educational services, and research activities. The certification examination is based on these competencies. The first certification examination in sports physical therapy was given in 1988 and 16 physical therapists were certified as Board-Certified Sports Physical Therapy Specialists.

The following list includes the 16 competencies, many of which are addressed in this book, needed by the sports physical therapist:

1. Present recommendations concerning the return of an athlete to activity.
2. Conduct on the field examination of an injured athlete.
3. Conduct preventive conditioning programs for the athlete.
4. Administer acute emergency care to the athlete.
5. Apply external bandages, dressings, and supports.
6. Be knowledgeable of arthrology as applied to the athlete.
7. Provide health status information and recommendations to coaches, parents, and physicians.
8. Administer preparticipation physical examinations.
9. Be knowledgeable of the causative factors in macro and micro trauma in sports injuries.
10. Recommend activity limitations based on environmental conditions.
11. Practice sports physical therapy practice/management skills.
12. Recommend modifications to playing environments.
13. Select, fit, and maintain athletic equipment.
14. Recognize dermatologic, infectious, and medical problems of the athlete.
15. Test and make recommendations on weight gain/loss as implicated in athletics.
16. Counsel athletes on the use of ergogenic aids.

REFERENCES

1. Hollman W. The definition and scope of sports medicine. In: Dirix A, Knuttgen HG, Tittel K, eds. *The Olympic Book of Sports Medicine.* Oxford: Blackwell Scientific Publications; 1988; 1:xi–xii.
2. Lombardo JA. Sportsmedicine: A team effort. *Phys Sportsmed.* 1985; 13(4):12–81.
3. Venerando A. Fundamental aspects of the role and organization of sports medicine. *J Sports Med.* 1975; 15:68–74.
4. Sports Physical Therapy, Brochure of the Sports Physical Therapy Section, American Physical Therapy Association, 1989.
5. Booher JM, Thibodeau GA. *Athletic Injury Assessment.* St Louis, Mo: Times Mirror/Mosby College Publishing; 1985.
6. Tippet S. *Role of the Sports Physical Therapist and Facility Organization.* Sports Physical Therapy Section, APTA, Clinical Competency Workshop Notebook; 1988
7. Kegerreis S. The construction and implementation of functional progression as a component of athletic rehabilitation. *J Orthopaed Sports Phys Ther.* 1983; 5:14–19.
8. Puffer JC. Sports medicine delivery systems for the athlete: A multi-sport model. In Grana WA, ed. *Advances in Sports Medicine and Fitness.* Chicago, Ill: Yearbook Medical Publishers; 1989: 287–294.
9. Ryan AJ. Sports medicine directory 1987. *Phys Sportsmedicine.* 1987; 13:221–238.
10. *Competencies in Therapy: An Analysis of Practice.* American Physical Therapy Association; 1977.
11. *Essentials for Certification of Advanced Clinical Competency.* American Physical Therapy Association; 1978.
12. Skovly R, Davies G, Mangine R, Mansell R. Wallace L. Results of the task analysis study—Sports Physical Therapy Section. *J Orthopaed Sports Phys Ther.* 1980; 1:229–238.
13. Krugh J. *Advanced Clinical Competencies for the Sports Physical Therapist.* University of North Carolina, Chapel Hill, 1984. Thesis.

BIBLIOGRAPHY

Arnheim DD. *Modern Principles of Athletic Training,* 6th ed. St Louis, Mo: Times Mirror/Mosby College Publishing; 1985.
Appenzeller O, ed. *Sports Medicine.* Baltimore, Md: Urban & Schwarzenberg; 1988.
Ellison AE, ed. *Athletic Training and Sports Medicine.* Chicago, IL: American Academy of Orthopaedic Surgeons; 1984.
Gould JA, Davies GJ, eds. *Orthopaedic and Sports Physical Therapy.* St Louis, Mo: C V Mosby Co; 1985.
Kuland DN: *The Injured Athlete.* Philadelphia, Pa: J B Lippincott Co; 1982.
O'Donoghue DH: *Treatment of Injuries to Athletes,* 4th ed. Philadelphia, Pa: W B Saunders Co; 1984.
Roy S, Irvin R: *Sports Medicine: Prevention, Evaluation, Management, and Rehabilitation.* Englewood Cliffs, NJ: Prentice-Hall Inc; 1983.

2 | Sports Rehabilitation Concepts

Steven R. Tippett

INTRODUCTION

As evidenced by the approximately 6000 physical therapists who are members of the Sports Physical Therapy Section of the American Physical Therapy Association (APTA), the care of injured athletes is a very popular area indeed. Physical therapists working in hospitals or private clinics, for universities, at local high schools, for professional sports teams, or sports organizations treat a wide variety of athletes on a daily basis. As the field of sports medicine grows, however, so does the confusion and controversy regarding the role of the physical therapist. Coaches, chiropractors, athletic trainers, athletic training students, and others also assist the injured athlete in a return to sport activities.

The organization and subsequent evolution of the physical therapy profession is based upon the rehabilitation of the physically impaired patient. Accreditation processes required of institutions training future physical therapists help assure that minimum educational standards are met and maintained. A sound educational background in the basic sciences along with special training in pertinent related areas make the physical therapist a rehabilitation natural. The standard physical therapy curriculum, however, does not prepare the student for competence in a given specialized area of physical therapy. Thus, although the physical therapist is a rehabilitation natural, physical therapists are not automatically sport rehabilitation specialists, simply on the basis of educational background. Taking this one step further, simply because a physical therapist may routinely treat individuals with knee ligamentous pathology, and these injuries may often occur in sport activities, does not mean that the therapist should be considered a specialist in sport rehabilitation. Numerous other factors are involved in the special area of sport physical therapy. An understanding of the basic components inherent to sport physical therapy will clarify the difference between traditional physical therapy and sport rehabilitation.

SPORT PHYSICAL THERAPY COMPETENCIES

Practicing physical therapists should possess a well-rounded background and competence in a variety of areas to provide the highest standard of care to all their athletic clientele. A brief description of these competencies will help to more fully explain the specific concepts of sport rehabilitation.

Expanded Basic Science Background

A background in the basic sciences is essential for all physical therapists. Additional knowledge of the musculoskeletal system and arthrology as it relates to the athlete is also necessary, as is a thorough understanding of exercise physiology, which is used in prescribing preventative conditioning programs. Understanding the body's response to exercise is also necessary in order for the sport physical therapist to effectively assess the effects of environmental conditions (heat, cold, atmosphere, altitude, etc.) on the athlete and athletic performance. A good working knowledge of the body's normal response to exercise is also required to extrapolate and then explain to the athlete the effects of performance-enhancing (ergogenic) aids.

Knowledge of Specific Sport Mechanics

In order for the sports physical therapist to be able to understand and subsequently explain mechanisms of injury, the therapist does not necessarily have to be a participant in a given sport. A working knowledge of a sport, however, as well as playing surface, playing rules/regulations, and physical demands of each athlete participating in a given sport is essential. The physical therapist who has a good grasp of the intricacies of a sport or activity within a sport better understands the causes of acute or overuse injuries and is thus in a better position to minimize them. Modifications to playing environments and the use of standard and specially adapted protective equipment can also be simplified

with a thorough understanding of the demands of a certain sporting activity. Hand in hand with this area is the sports physical therapist's ability to break down sport function and gear rehabilitation efforts towards specific functions required in a given sport.

Special Nontraditional Background Abilities/Skills

Skills not routinely taught and not routinely encountered in traditional physical therapy are required in sports physical therapy. The sports physical therapist must be capable of on-the-field assessment of an injured athlete in an acute, and sometimes life-threatening, situation. Once the acute assessment has been performed, special emergency care procedures may also be required of the sport physical therapist. It may be necessary for the sports physical therapist to use nontraditional medical equipment and accessories. Everyday routines can necessitate that the sport physical therapist be able to recognize and address dermatologic, infectious, and medical problems encountered by the athlete.

Strong Interpersonal/Communication Skills

As in all areas of physical therapy, a vital prerequisite for sound patient care is good communication skills. This is necessary in sport physical therapy in addressing not only the athlete but the coach, parent, physician, trainer, and others as well.

A summary of the advanced competencies that should be basic to the sport physical therapist can be found in Table 2–1. With a general understanding of the traits that a sport physical therapist should possess, I will concentrate on specific rehabilitation concepts as they relate to sport physical therapy.

SPORT REHABILITATION: THE BASICS

As is true of any rehabilitation program, a sport rehabilitation program is only as good as the initial evaluation. A sound sport rehabilitation program thus begins with a thorough evaluation. Questions that are carefully framed to elicit the nature of the problem, its severity, and most importantly the mechanism of injury are essential to this evaluation and an invaluable skill of the sport physical therapist. Appropriate methods to question the patient and good interpersonal skills to interact with the patient should be natural for the therapist. Yet before the physical therapist can know what questions to ask, a thorough understanding of common microtraumatic and macrotraumatic causative factors of sport injury is required of the sport. For example, in the subjective evaluation of a baseball pitcher with shoulder pain, the standard questions regarding onset, duration, and nature of the pain along with measures

TABLE 2-1. ADVANCED CLINICAL COMPETENCIES (SPORTS)

1. Presenting recommendations concerning the return of an athlete to activity
2. On-the-field examination of an injured athlete
3. Conducting preventative conditioning programs for the athlete
4. Administering acute emergency care to the athlete
5. Applying external bandages, dressings, and supports
6. Arthrology as applied to the athlete
7. Providing health status information and recommendations to coaches, parents, and physicians
8. Administration of preparticipation physical examinations
9. Causative factors in macrotrauma and microtrauma in sports injuries
10. Recommending activity limitations based on environmental conditions
11. Sports physical therapy practice/management skills
12. Recommending modifications to playing environments
13. Selection, fitting, and maintenance of athletic equipment
14. Recognition of dermatologic, infectious, and medical problems of the athlete
15. Testing and making recommendations on weight gain/loss as implicated in athletics
16. Counseling athletes on the use of ergogenic aids

From Zachazewski J, et al. Therapy: Advanced Clinical Competency Workshops. J Orthopae Sports Phys Ther. 1986; 8:43, with permission.

that exacerbate or temper the pain are all fine and good. In order to fully ascertain the source of the shoulder symptoms, however, the sports physical therapist should be able to take the subjective evaluation a step further. During which phase of the throwing mechanism which pain arises, which particular pitch causes most pain, how many innings can the athlete pitch prior to the onset of pain are only some of the areas that need to be addressed. A thorough understanding of the sport and the athlete's particular physical demands for that activity is necessary if the sport physical therapist is to perform a comprehensive subjective as well as objective examination.

An understanding of the intricacies of a given sport provides the sport physical therapist with knowledge of the body parts commonly injured as well as the nature of these injuries. Common acute and overuse injury patterns should be easily part of the sports therapist's diagnostic acumen. Advanced manual skills for musculoskeletal evaluation is essential for today's sport therapist, as is a working knowledge of the many therapeutic devices used for evaluation. Isokinetic strength testing devices, instrumented knee laxity measuring devices, and instruments that help in the comprehensive objective assessment of the athlete must be familiar to the therapist.

Once the carefully planned, thoroughly executed subjective and objective evaluation has been completed, rehabilitation goals should be established. The general goal of sport rehabilitation is the return of the athlete to the highest level of function in the shortest time possible. When taking into account the highest level of function, it is vital that function be addressed specifically. Efforts to rehabilitate the injured athlete should be based on the SAID principle, where SAID stands for specific adaptations to imposed demands. Simply put, the SAID principle requires that the rehabilitation program be geared towards the physical demands that the athlete will place on the injured body part when resuming preinjury activities. Hand in hand with the SAID principle are Wolff's law and Davis' law, which state that both bone and soft tissue respond to physical demands placed upon them, causing them to remodel or heal along these lines of stress. Frequently injury and reinjury occurs because the SAID principle is ignored during the rehabilitation phase. A common example is the recurrent ankle sprain. Frequently an athlete sustains a lateral ankle sprain of minor or moderate severity. Initial x-rays rule out fracture, time passes, and swelling, pain, and dysfunction disappear. If, however, rehabilitation fails to address the range of motion, strength, and proprioception demands that the athlete will face upon returning to sport, the healing ligamentous structures will be unable to assume preinjury demands.

In order for injured tissue to heal to its maximum potential, demands on the tissue must be both specific and timely. Specificity refers to specific sport function. The rehabilitation program for an ankle sprain sustained by a basketball player must be specific to the demands of basketball. The injured basketball player will not be rehabilitated in the same fashion as a gymnast who sustains the same lateral ankle sprain. Taking this a step further, in team sports, the demands upon a player may differ from position to position. An offensive lineman in football would not therefore be rehabilitated in the same manner as the team's quarterback with a comparable injury.

Another important consideration in sport rehabilitation specificity is the fact that at times what is considered normal for the traditional physical therapy patient is not normal for the athlete and vice-versa. An example is low back extension in a nonathlete versus the lumbar extension required for a female gymnast. Also, normal glenohumeral external rotation for a nonthrowing athlete is 90 degrees. Compare this with the "normal" external rotation of 130 to 140 degrees for a professional baseball pitcher.

Demands placed upon the athlete during the rehabilitation phase must be timely as well. Rehabilitation efforts must be aggressive and specific but should not be overly zealous with regard to tissue healing time constraints. In rehabilitating acute injuries as well as overuse syndromes, stresses placed upon the healing tissue should not exceed the tissue's readiness to accept these forces. Areas to consider in sport rehabilitation after athletic injury are similar to those encountered in other areas of physical therapy. Motion must be full, unrestricted, and painfree. Swelling should be managed by the judicious use of ice, compression (constant or intermittent), and elevation. Activity should be gauged as symptoms allow. If pain or swelling is present with activity or after activity, then that particular activity is too strenuous. This especially holds true in the management of overuse injury. Overuse injury is rated according to the presence of pain in relation to activity (Table 2–2). If pain is present only after activity then the condition can be monitored, play can continue and appropriate therapeutic exercise or modalities may be employed. If pain is present during activity, however, especially if the pain alters the way the athlete performs that activity, then activities should be decreased or alternate activities identified.

To summarize the basic principles of sport rehabilitation:

1. A prerequisite for efficient rehabilitation is a thorough, sport-specific evaluation.
2. Sport rehabilitation must be specific to the demands of the sport.
3. Sport rehabilitation must be performed with tissue-healing time constraints in mind.

TABLE 2–2. CLASSIFYING OVERUSE INJURIES

Staging Overuse Injury by Pain[a]

Stage 1.	Pain only after activity with no impairment of function
Stage 2.	Pain during and after activity with satisfactory level of function
Stage 3.	Prolonged pain during and after with increasing difficulty in satisfactory performance

Modified Blazina Staging[b]

Level 1.	No pain
Level 2.	Pain with extreme exertion that disappears when activity stops. No effect on sports performance
Level 3.	Pain with exertion that remains 1 to 2 hours after exertion
Level 4.	Pain during athletic activity that remains 4 to 6 hours after exertion, intensifies with activity, and negatively affects performance
Level 5.	Pain starting as soon as athletic activity begins and causes removal from that activity
Level 6.	Pain with activities of daily living, preventing participation in sports

[a]From Blazina ME, et al. Jumpers knee. *Orthopead Clin No Am. 1973; 4:669,* with permission.
[b]From Curwin S, Stanish N. Tendinitis: Its Etiology and Treatment. *Boston, Mass: D. C. Heath and Company; 1986; 101,* with permission.

4. When setting goals for the sports rehabilitation program, remember what is normal for the nonathlete may be inadequate for the athlete. Also remember what may be abnormal for the nonathlete may be normal and absolutely necessary for the athlete.

SPORTS REHABILITATION: BEYOND THE BASICS

The basic principles of sport rehabilitation are the bare essentials required of the sport physical therapist. Experience yielding strong interpersonal skills, above-average expertise in musculoskeletal acute and overuse injury, and a working knowledge of state-of-the-art rehabilitation and evaluation products will go a long way in preparing a therapist to function adequately in the field of sport physical therapy. Various advanced competencies have been previously discussed, with these skills being a prerequisite for total sports rehabilitation. We now consider the special skills that relate intimately to the rehabilitation role of the sports therapist.

To this point the discussion has involved specifics of sport rehabilitation that will not be unfamiliar to most physical therapists. This is largely due to the fact that these areas are frequently addressed in formal physical therapy training or can be attained in physical-therapy-related continuing education opportunities. The next two areas are perhaps nontraditional and more specialized, entailing skills usually possessed by the therapist who is also a certified athletic trainer or clinical specialist in sports physical therapy. These two areas, namely the use of protective padding/bracing/supports as well as the concept of functional progression, are instrumental in sports rehabilitation.

Padding, Bracing, and Supports
In light of the controversy surrounding "prophylactic" lateral knee braces as well as functional knee bracing, excessive emphasis is sometimes placed on braces and supports. In today's "quick fix" mentality, the misguided sports consumer is often led to believe that all one needs is a brace or support and an affected body part is as good as new. Adjunctive supportive padding, properly applied braces when appropriate, and other forms of external support can play an important role in sports rehabilitation. The sport physical therapist must understand the use of such devices and weed out the facts from speculation. Using, securing, and fabricating supportive bracing and padding is essential for today's sport physical therapist. Protective equipment is discussed in detail in Chapter 17.

Functional Progression
The greatest weakness of most sport rehabilitation programs is in functional progression. Sport function is a highly complex act calling for integrated, fine-tuned body-part performance. When function breaks down as a result of injury, function must be restored to its former high level. In discussing the basics of sport rehabilitation, strength, range of motion, pain control, and management of edema and dysfunction are addressed routinely. Proprioception, however, is often neglected, as is a series of events progressing the athlete from a point of full, painfree, active range of motion and adequate strength (i.e., the achievement of clinical goals) to a safe return to competition. This individualized, gradually progressive series of events prepares the athlete for a return to sport and is known as *functional progression*. Functional progression activities should be introduced into the treatment program as soon as the athlete is able to tolerate them. Skills inherent to a given sport are broken down and the athlete is advanced through these skills in an organized fashion. Activities are progressed from slow to fast, simple to complex, loaded to unloaded, and, where appropriate, shorter distances to longer distances. The athlete's performance of the skills and tolerance to the activities are carefully assessed. If pain arises, if swelling occurs, if the athlete cannot perform the task in proper form, then the athlete does not proceed to the next step.

Benefits of the functional progression program are physical as well as psychological. The former are readily apparent. Healing tissue is stressed in a graduated fashion, thus allowing for optimum healing to occur along the lines of sport and function specific stresses. Tolerance to the activities can be easily gauged. The ideal functional progression program will have the athlete perform every conceivable task in a controlled environment prior to asking him or her to perform the task in a competitive environment. In this manner the athlete's apprehension when he or she returns to play is minimized. The functional progression program can take part during practice times, which allow the rehabilitating athlete to be in the company of coaches and teammates. This minimizes the athlete's sense of alienation during the recuperation phase. Coaches and fellow teammates can see the injured athlete working to get back into action, which serves as a positive experience for all parties concerned.

As this specific area is vital in the discussion of sport rehabilitation concepts, let us look at an example to illustrate a simple functional progression program: An injured football offensive lineman is rehabilitating a second-degree medial collateral ligament sprain of the knee. Acute management has proceeded without problems and the athlete now demonstrates full active range of motion and minimal residual laxity that is not painful to valgus stressing. Strength of the quadriceps and hamstrings are within acceptable limits via isokinetic assessment. Treatment to date has consisted of motion and strengthening work. So where do we go from here?

Efforts to this point have neglected muscular endurance as well as cardiovascular aerobic endurance. Even more importantly, since football is primarily an anaerobic event, work should be devoted to anaerobic conditioning. The functional progression program can begin to stress these areas by a walk/jog program using caution around any curves or corners that need to be negotiated in the running or jogging sequence. A sufficient aerobic base must be established, but of more significance are short-duration, anaerobic activities. Initially, a stationary cycling program to improve aerobic and anaerobic conditioning should be started. As soon as weight bearing is not painful and gait deviations are absent, the walk/jog/run/sprint program can be instituted in a straight plane, preferably away from other teammates in order to avoid inadvertent contact. Activities to stress advanced weight bearing should follow. These activities will serve to stress the healing tissue, build strength, and help to facilitate proprioceptive feedback. Appropriate activities are forward–backward and side–side stepups onto a 12- to 15-inch platform. Unresisted vertical leg press or body weight–resisted squats are also appropriate activities. Stationary jumping drills—forward and backward, side to side, and diagonally—can be added; these use momentum to create greater forces to load the healing tissue. Jumping can progress to hopping on the involved leg only. The hopping and jumping can progress from level surface in an unloaded fashion to adding resistance of a weight vest or surgical tubing. These activities can then progress to being stressed on uneven surfaces first unloaded and then against resistance. Agility drills and various straight plane grass drills can be performed with the team. Straight plane activities can be replaced by multiplane drills. Gentle figure-eight running can begin at a 40-yard distance at half speed. This can be increased to three-quarter and finally full speed. Once full-speed figure-eights are performed at 40 yards, the distance is decreased to 20 yards to make the figure-eight smaller and the maneuvering area tighter. Speeds are again brought down to half speed and progressed to three-quarter and then full speed. Finally the sequence can be repeated at 10 yards. Figure-eights are then replaced by cutting drills in which the athlete is first asked to jog to a given spot, plant the involved leg, and bring the opposite leg over in front of the planted involved leg, cutting towards the involved side (crossover cut). Next, cutting is performed off the affected leg towards the uninvolved side. This straight-cut places a valgus stress on the knee, stressing the medial collateral ligament. If required, the athlete may need to perform straight cuts at 45 degrees, 60 degrees, and then finally 90 degrees. The speeds at which the athlete approaches the site where the cut is performed are increased; after full-speed 90-degree straight cutting is achieved without difficulty, speeds are again decreased and the athlete

begins the same cutting sequence upon verbal or visual command. As the athlete conquers these maneuvers, offensive line play footwork (e.g., pulling down the line in each direction, trap blocking, pass blocking) can be stressed.

To this point, all activities have been unloaded, that is, non-contact. Because football is a collision sport, efforts must now introduce contact. Half-speed, controlled blocking and tackling drills can begin first in a straight plane and one-on-one with another player. The athlete must first know the way in which resistance offered by the other player is coming. Speeds are kept low and movements are controlled. Drills are performed at faster speeds as the athlete tolerates, and then performed with the player having to react to the resistance from the other player not being known beforehand. One-on-one, full-speed contact drills in a straight plane are progressed to multiplane activities. Next two-on-one (with the injured player being double teamed as well as doing the double teaming) are begun in a controlled fashion at slower speeds in a straight plane and progressed to faster speeds and finally in multiplane movements. All of these activities must be tolerated by the athlete before he is ready to set foot on the playing field. These drills take place in conjunction with continued, formal strengthening work and with any additional support/bracing deemed appropriate.

Functional progression is sport, player position, and injury specific. Rehabilitation of the injured athlete without a comprehensive functional progression program seriously shortchanges your athletic clientele.

SUMMARY

Sport rehabilitation includes some concepts that should be familiar to most practicing physical therapists. The prevention and evaluation of sports injuries, however, requires advanced knowledge and skill. Rehabilitation of the injured athlete is no different. Treating an injured athlete in the same fashion as a nonathlete will yield far less than satisfactory results. The athlete is a unique patient with out of the ordinary physical demands. A solid sport rehabilitation program must be comprehensive, timely, and sport specific.

BIBLIOGRAPHY

Blazina M. Jumpers knee. *Orthoped Clin N Am.* 1973; 4: 669.

Curwin S, Stanish W. *Tendinitis: Its Etiology and Treatment.* Nova Scotia: EC Health and Company; 1984.

Gould J, Davies G, eds. *Orthopaedic and Sports Physical Therapy.* St Louis, Mo: C V Mosby Co; 1985.

Kegerreis S. The construction and implementation of func-

tional progression as a component of athletic rehabilitation. *J Orthopaed Sports Phys Ther.* 1983; 5:14–19.

Kegerreis S, Malone T, McCarroll J. Functional progressions, an aid to athletic rehabilitation. *Physician Sports Med.* 1984; 12:67–71.

Yaemoto S, Hartman C, Feagin J, et al. Functional rehabilitation of the knee: A preliminary study. *J Sports Med.* 1976; 3:288–291.

Zachazewski J, et al. Therapy: Advanced clinical competency workshops. *J Orthopaed Sports Phys Ther.* 1986; 8:46.

3

Preseason Athletic Participation Evaluation

John Eggart

INTRODUCTION

Why is preseason screening needed? There are many good reasons but unless the sports physical therapist understands the reasons for the long, strenuous process, the results will not be very useful. In order to custom fit the program to the situation, the therapist must know what is wanted before the program is begun. This chapter is designed to help therapists select from the following screening processes those portions that fit the situation. Therapists must tailor their programs to meet their needs and the available resources in order to maximize the results.

Many times, preseason screening for athletes is done because it is a requirement of the state high school association,[1,2] the league, or the particular school setting where the therapist is working. Many times, the preseason screening for athletes is done to show parents and administrators or both groups that legal considerations have been taken into account. Sometimes, preseason screening is done just because it provides considerable information about the athletes that was not previously available. Frequently, however, coaches, athletes, and parents feel the preseason screening is done to disqualify those athletes who have had previous injuries.

My feeling and experience is that all athletes participating in interscholastic athletics should have a preseason physical evaluation so that there is a baseline that can be referred to at a later date. This gives the medical personnel an objective base to which to return the injured athlete. To best ensure its success, the process of preseason screening should be a mutual effort of the athletes, parents, coaches, administrators, and the medical staff.

The American Academy of Pediatrics (AAP) Committee on Sports Medicine has compiled a list of disqualifying recommendations for physicians.[3] This list should be used to determine the limitations recommended to each athlete. These recommendations will vary according to the amount of stress each sport puts on the athlete's body. This list was compiled because the 1976 guidelines created by the American Medical Association (AMA) were rapidly becoming obsolete. The "Rights of the Athlete" published by the AMA in 1976, however, are still and always will be valid. Among these "rights" is that each athlete is entitled to "Adequate Health Supervision." Adequate health supervision, as defined by the AMA, includes a thorough preseason history and medical examination.[4]

Junior and senior high school athletes should have an annual medical exam by their primary physician. This is required by at least 35 states.[5] There should be an annual update of the medical history by the athlete and his or her parents. There should also be an annual orthopedic screening by qualified personnel. College and university athletes should have a thorough medical examination by the team physician, followed by constant monitoring throughout their athletic careers. The university athletic medical staff is responsible for conducting a thorough musculoskeletal screening at the beginning of the athlete's career and care for injuries as they occur throughout the athlete's career. The National Collegiate Athletic Association (NCAA) recommends this protocol but does not enforce it. The National Association of Intercollegiate Athletics (NAIA) has no official position for athletic screening in their affiliated schools.

From a medicolegal perspective, the preseason screening protocol developed by each school should show that school personnel and medical staff have, to the best of their ability, taken steps to understand the physical capabilities of each individual athlete. Such a screening should also show that personnel have followed up on each athlete with specific recommendations for the level or type of activity.

This screening should not be used as a device to disqualify an athlete but rather as an information-gathering and participation-recommendation procedure.

School personnel have the responsibility of gathering data on each athlete. They should also provide recommendations on the athlete's ability to participate based on the data collected on that athlete. If a problem is found, referral to an individual with more expertise in the problem area such as a specialist physician is not only recommended but necessary. The amount of the screening that can be done by school personnel depends on the level of medical personnel on the staff. If medical personnel is limited, the school may need to enlist outside help.

The preseason physical evaluation should be comprehensive. The medical history, medical examination, cardiorespiratory evaluation, agility testing, strength testing, dental examination, and complete musculoskeletal screening should all be included.[6-9]

The medical history should be completed by the athlete, his or her parents, and the pediatric or primary care physician. The pediatric or primary care physician should be the physician who has monitored the health of the athlete on a routine basis. The medical history should include a family history with details of cardiac, respiratory, congenital, and other family-related medical problems. It should also contain a detailed history of the athlete's allergies, congenital problems, heredity problems, chronic disorders, previous surgical procedures, and previous injuries requiring medical attention. Any report of joint or musculotendinous surgical procedure should include the surgical method, the rehabilitation procedure, and the recommendations for activity.

Preferably, the medical examination should be performed by the pediatric or primary care physician mentioned earlier. This is not always possible, however. A colleague should be able to make use of the chart notes from the primary physician if the latter is unavailable for consultation. The examining physician should be aware of problem areas as noted in the medical chart.

The cardiorespiratory evaluation must be supervised by a physician, but the testing procedure can be administered by an allied health professional. Some methods of testing the cardiorespiratory system are discussed elsewhere.

The agility, strength, coordination, and proprioceptive ability of the athlete can also be tested by an allied health professional or by members of the coaching staff. The results of the tests, however, must be reviewed by a physician and compared to the normals. There are a variety of methods and equipment available to test the capability of the athletes in these areas.[10-12]

The dental examination can be done by personnel who have knowledge of dental structures and who have been instructed by a dentist as to specific problems requiring attention. It would take an extensive dental examination, however, by a dentist to discover all defects and abnormalities.

The musculoskeletal screening should be performed by allied health personnel, with a physician evaluating the results and reevaluating any abnormalities reported.

There are many ways to design the preseason screening process. There are no ideal methods but some guidelines have been established. The junior high and high school athletes should be seen by their primary care physician at some point in the screening process; however, this medical examination alone is not adequate to evaluate all of the systems and capabilities of the athlete. Junior high and high school athletes should follow these guidelines for an ideal preseason screening:

1. Fill out a questionnaire in conjunction with their parents
2. Receive a dental examination from the family dentist
3. Receive a medical examination from their primary physician
4. Receive an orthopedic examination under the supervision of a local orthopedist
5. Receive agility and reaction tests from trainers or coaches with results reviewed by a physician
6. Receive a cardiorespiratory evaluation from a trained technician and reviewed by a physician
7. Consult with school and medical personnel involved in the screening about the results of the entire evaluation process

Collegiate athletes should also follow these guidelines and in addition receive the entire battery of screening procedures by the medical staff of their institution.

The screening process can be done in a group session or on an individual basis. The medical examination is best accomplished by the primary care physician or team physician in a quiet one-on-one setting. Many of the other procedures lend themselves to a mass screening procedure where several stations are set up and manned by allied health personnel. Each station will see each athlete for a specific battery of screening procedures. The final station is manned by a physician along with the sports physical therapist or athletic trainer to review the findings of the other stations and give recommendations to the athlete. Another alternative for designing the screening is to have several procedures done at the same setting. For example, the musculoskeletal screening can be set up alone or in conjunction with other examinations. The agility and coordination stations can often be incorporated into the first few practices by the coaches.

The screening process is ideally conducted so as to have adequate time for the recommendations that are forthcoming from the examination to be carried out.[13] For example, if an athlete is found to have weakness in a particular muscle group, the athletic trainer alone or in conjunction with a sports physical therapist would have time to get the athlete through an adequate strengthening program. Another example would be to allow the athlete to visit a specialist for further evaluation of any specific problem that was detected by the screening process. Although early screening allows adequate time for these things, it is important that the screening is not done so far in advance that the condition of the athlete might significantly change before the season begins.

There are options for when to conduct the preseason screening. A full screening just prior to each sports season is the optimal choice. Another way, which is probably the most common, is to do the physician's medical examination at the beginning of each school year and the rest of the screening at the beginning of each sports season, with emphasis on the body areas that are most often injured in that sport. A third method is to perform the entire screening for all athletes at the beginning of each school year. The NCAA recommends a one-time medical examination with a comprehensive following of that athlete until he or she leaves the institution.[5]

PERSONNEL

It is important that all personnel know their roles and the amount of responsibility they have. This may range from screening the athlete for anomalies to making recommendations to the athlete and their parents for level and type of activity to recording information at a specific station. The number and qualification of help available will be a strong determining factor in the type of screening selected and the amount of detail this screening will involve. The first place to look for help is within an organization for people who are already associated with the sports program. This comprises the therapist, the coaches, managers, athletic department administrators, athletes, and their parents. The next place to look for personnel is the medical community. At the high school level there will be medical personnel in the community. On the collegiate and university level there will also be medical personnel within the institution. Students in allied health training programs at the local community college, a nearby university, or a community hospital should not be overlooked, nor should students who are managers, student trainers, and those enrolled in health and first-aid classes. Most communities will have some form of first responders or other emergency personnel that can prove helpful to

the screening process. Involve the physicians in the community as much as possible.[13]

Therapists should enlist the help of others to make the evaluations they personally do, go much faster by having someone record the findings as they do the screening. It is important to get the athletic administrators involved in this recruiting process. One can also involve the booster club in recruiting volunteers for the screening.

The ideal situation is to have the athlete's primary physician perform the medical portion of the examination in his or her office. Ideally, the athlete will have had a dental checkup within the past year. It is also important for parents to be involved, especially in the medical history and in the conference on activity level recommendations.

MEDICAL HISTORY AND EXAMINATION

The medical evaluation of athletes is essential before participating in athletic competition. It should be completed by the school or family physician (Fig 3–1) Prior to the examination, the athlete and his or her parents should complete a thorough medical history form (Fig 3–2), which includes past illnesses, operations, and immunizations. The athlete should then present this form to the physician at the time of the medical examination.

The examination should be proceeded by measurement of height, weight, visual and auditory acuity, heart rate, and blood pressure. Urine and blood samples should also be taken. These items can be completed by a nurse, a laboratory technician, or the athletic training staff, depending on the facility.[14] The physician then undertakes a comprehensive evaluation of a variety of body systems, as discussed in the following sections.

Skin
The skin is of primary concern for infections and scars. Acute pyogenic infections should be cleared up before any athletic activity, due to their highly contagious state and ability to spread under athletic stress.[15] Scars are an indication of prior trauma or surgery.

Head
The eyes should be checked for retinal detachment and retinal blood vessel circulation.[4] The conjunctivae should be checked for hemorrhage and infection.[15] The absence of one eye and wearing of glasses or contacts should be discussed with the athlete with necessary precautions taken for competition.[16] The parents must be included in these discussions in the case of the junior high and high school athlete or any collegiate athlete who has not reached the age of majority.

I have examined _____ on _____
                         (Patient's name)   (Date)

Height _____ Weight _____ Blood pressure _____

Laboratory work _____

Physical findings _____

_____

Has this patient any of the following? (Please explain and give approximate dates)

Chronic health problem(s) _____

_____

Serious illness/injury _____

_____

_____

Surgeries _____

_____

On medication _____

_____

IMMUNIZATION DATES:

Dip.tet. _____ Tet.tax. _____ MMR _____

Polio-oral _____ TB Test _____ Chest x-ray _____

_____ NO RESTRICTION FOR ATHLETIC PARTICIPATION

_____ Participation limited to _____

Recommendation for continuing care of this student while at the University: _____

_____

                                                    M.D. Signature _____

                                                    Printed name and address _____

                                                    _____

                                                    _____

Date _____

RETURN AS SOON AS POSSIBLE TO. . . . . .   Student Health Center
                                            University of Wisconsin-LaCrosse
                                            LaCrosse, WI 54601

Reviewed by H.C. M.D.   Needs: Athletic Office Notified _____

Date _____   _____   Complete _____   _____

OK'd by _____   _____   Incomplete _____   By _____

Figure 3-1. Physician Approval Form.

ATHLETIC PARTICIPATION FORM
STUDENT HEALTH CENTER
UNIVERSITY OF WISCONSIN-LA CROSSE

PLEASE CIRCLE CORRECT ANSWER:
Y = YES   N = NO

1) Have you had a condition which required medical attention to:

Muscle.................................Y...............................N
Joint....................................Y...............................N
Tendon ....Y...............................N
Bone ....Y...............................N

Explain _____

_____

2) Do you get a rash from tape?.....................Y...................N
Do you get a rash from linament? ....Y...................N

3) Ever have an injury producing weakness or numbness of arms or legs?...............................Y.................N

Explain _____

_____

4) Ever have a skull, neck or spine fracture?...........Y............N

X-ray of any of above? ....Y ....N

Explain _____

_____

5) Have you ever been unconscious? ....Y.................N
Fainted?.................Y...................N How many times?_____

When? _____
Hospitalized for this?...............................Y ....N

Explain _____

_____

6) Have you ever had seizures or convulsions? ....Y..........N

7) Ever have a brain wave test? ....Y ....N
When? _____

8) Do you wear:
Glasses_____ Contact lens_____

Bridgework _____ Dental braces _____
Dentures _____
Date of last visit to dentist? _____

Date _____

Name _____

SSN _____

Sport(s) _____

9) Do you have loss or seriously impaired function of any paired organ? ....Y.......................................N

Eye _____ Lung _____
Kidney _____ Testicle _____

10) List surgical operations you have had and approximate date(s) _____

_____

_____

11) Have you been seen by a physician for any illness/condition lasting more than 1 week during the past year? .... Y .....N

What? _____

_____

12) Are you under a physician's care now?
Y.................................N .... For?

_____

13) Do you have, or have you ever had:

Diabetes.................................Y..N
Epilepsy.................................Y..N
Kidney Disease ....Y ....N
Abnormal bleeding tendencies.......................Y.......................N
Arthritis ....Y..N
Heart disease ....Y ....N
(Rheumatic fever, high blood pressure, heart murmur.)

Other problems _____

_____

_____

_____

Student Signature

YOUR PERSONAL PHYSICIAN MUST COMPLETE THE REVERSE SIDE BEFORE YOU WILL BE ELIGIBLE FOR ATHLETIC PARTICIPATION.

Figure 3-2. Athletic Screening Form.

The ears should be examined for previous surgery, gross hearing, deformity, and infection.[7]

The nose should be checked for deformity, inadequate airway, and chronic infection. All of these factors can affect oxygen supply and endurance.[7]

Mouth and Teeth

A quick dental examination can be performed by the physician to determine if there appears to be a need for further evaluation by a dentist. It also is used to establish any broken or missing teeth in case the athlete chips or loses a tooth in competition. The teeth should also be checked for abscesses and other conditions that could affect the general health of the athlete.[14]

Cardiovascular System

The heart rate, size of the heart, and forcefulness of beat should be examined by auscultation and percussion.[15] The heart should also be evaluated for heart murmurs, abnormal rhythms, and mitral or aortic stenosis, which can be complicated by exertion.[2] The athlete with blood pressure of greater than 140 mm Hg systolic or 90 mm Hg diastolic should continue to be re-evaluated.[2] Cardiopulmonary endurance testing is discussed later in this chapter.

Genitourinary System

The female athlete should be evaluated for cancer of the cervix and should have a pap smear performed.[4] The breasts should be examined for tenderness, hard masses, and nipple discharge.

The male athlete should be examined for undescended or absent testicles and hydrocele, which should be corrected prior to participation in contact sports.[15] In addition, male and female athletes should be checked for lesions of the genitalia.

Thoracolumbar Region

The lungs should be examined for expansion and wheezes. A chest x-ray may be performed if pulmonary disease is suspected.

The abdomen should be palpated for an enlarged spleen or liver, which could rupture in contact sports. Palpation of masses or tumors in the abdomen should be referred to a specialist for further evaluation.[15] In addition, the inguinal region should be examined for a hernia.

A rectal examination should be performed to eliminate the possibilities of hemorrhoids, polyps, ulcers, or tumors.[4]

Laboratory Tests

A blood test should be performed to establish whether the athlete has anemia, sickle cell anemia, or syphilis. A chemistry profile done on the blood sample tests for diabetes, renal disease, and electrolyte imbalance. Certain drug testing can also be done if desired or needed.[16,17]

A tuberculosis skin test should be performed. If the test is positive, the athlete should be referred for a chest x-ray.[16]

A urine analysis should be performed to test albumin and glucose levels, which indicate abnormal kidney function and diabetes, respectively.[4,17] In addition, systemic infections should be ruled out. As with blood samples, certain drug testing can also be done as desired or needed.

Upon completion of the medical examination, the physician will determine whether the athlete's health is suitable for his or her chosen athletic activity.

Neurological System

The neurological evaluation of the athlete is usually overlooked or underestimated in most athletic preseason screening evaluations. The neurological evaluation is often very short, consisting only of a brief look into the eyes and ears of the athlete.

Although a comprehensive neurological evaluation may not be necessary, a thorough examination that includes motor, reflex, and sensory tests for peripheral nerves and cerebellar dysfunction should be done. This examination will not specifically test the higher centers of the brain. The interaction of the person doing the examination and the athlete can lead to an accurate assumption that the higher centers are intact.

A satisfactory neurological evaluation can be performed in approximately 10 to 20 minutes. The evaluation should start by taking a history. Questions regarding fainting, concussions, headaches, focal weakness or numbness, tinnitus, dizziness, and bowel and bladder control are a few general ones.[18] Some of these questions should be emphasized for certain sports, but all of them should be asked of every athlete regardless of his or her sport. The medical history should be checked at this time to determine if certain areas of examination should be emphasized.

Following the history, cranial, peripheral, and spinal nerves should be checked. The cranial nerves are a very important part of the evaluation because in addition to the actual nerves many of the infratentorial structures are also tested.

Cranial Examination. Table 3–1 lists the basic functions of the cranial nerves. Further discussion of how to test each cranial nerve follows. The test for the olfactory nerve (cranial nerve I) is a very simple one. Have the athlete close one nostril. Bring a nonirritating substance, such as tobacco or coffee, up to the other nostril, then repeat. A difference between the nostrils indicates a more serious problem than if there is just a decrease in both nostrils.[18] The most common causes of

TABLE 3-1. CRANIAL NERVE FUNCTIONS

No	Name	Function
I	Olfactory	Smell
II	Optic	Sight (both eyes)
III	Oculomotor	Droopy eyelids, diverted strabismus
IV	Trochlear	Move eyes up and in
V	Trigeminal	Pain on face and forehead
VI	Abducens	Internal stabismus—squinting
VII	Facial	Muscles of expression
VIII	Acoustic	Hearing (both ears)
IX	Glossopharyngeal	Difficulty swallowing, numb soft palate
X	Vagus	Deviated uvula, Hoarseness
XI	Accessory	Torticollis—fixed twisting of the neck
XII	Hypoglossal	Paralysis of tongue

From Gilroy J, Holiday P. *Basic Neurology.* New York, NY: Macmillan Publishing Co Inc; 1982.

decreased sensation include nasal disorders, allergies, and infections. Lesions and tumors are not neurogenic but they also can decrease the sensation of smell.[18,19]

The optic nerve (cranial nerve II) can and should be tested in three ways: (1) Visual acuity must be checked for distant and near vision. Distant vision is easily checked by using the Snellen test chart.[18] Near vision may be evaluated by using one of the many reading cards that are published.[18] (2) The eye should then be examined by using the ophthalmoscope. The person doing the examination should look for and rule out papilledema, retrobulbar neuritis, and optic atrophy.[18] (3) Lastly, the visual fields are examined. All four quadrants in each eye need to be evaluated. Pathology of the optic nerve is ruled out by this test.[19]

The oculomotor, trochlear, and the abducens (cranial nerves III, IV, and VI) can be tested at the same time. The athlete is asked to look medially, superiorly, and inferiorly.[18,19] The athlete is then asked to adduct and depress his or her eyes.[19] Finally, the athlete is asked to move his or her eyes laterally. A positive finding on this test can indicate brainstem dysfunction. Some problems at or near the brainstem that could cause pathology in these nerves include brainstem trauma, encephalitis, tumor, infection, or multiple sclerosis.[19]

The trigeminal nerve (cranial nerve V) has both motor and sensory function and has two reflexes. The motor portion is evaluated by testing the muscles of mastication, specifically the masseter and the temporalis.[18,19] The sensory portion is evaluated in three places: the forehead, the cheek, and the mandible.[18,19] Finally, the reflexes that the trigeminal nerve innervates are the corneal and jaw reflexes.[18,19]

The most common disease of the fifth cranial nerve is neuralgia.[18] Although this disease occurs most often among the middle-aged and the elderly, it has been seen in younger patients, where it is usually caused by multiple sclerosis, tumor, or aneurysm.[18] The neuralgia is characterized by history of pain in the maxillary and mandibular regions.

The facial nerve (cranial nerve VII) also has both a motor and a sensory division. Both can be checked simultaneously in two ways. First, the athlete is asked to keep one eye closed as the person doing the examination tries to force the eye open. This procedure is repeated with the other eye.[18,19] The second test is to ask the athlete to show his or her teeth.[18,19] The first test is looking for weakness and the second test is to check for symmetry of the contractions.[18,19] In addition, one may test the sensory division separate from the motor division. The sensory division of the seventh cranial nerve is responsible for taste on the anterior two thirds of the tongue.[18,19] This may be tested by touching sweet, sour, and bitter substances to the anterior portion of the tongue.[18]

The most common pathologies of the seventh cranial nerve are Bell's palsy, geniculate neuralgia, and hemifacial spasms.[18] The first two have unknown etiologies, although it is believed that a viral infection is responsible.[18] The third may be caused by compression from a vessel, multiple sclerosis, a tumor, or arachnoiditis.[18]

The acoustic nerve (cranial nerve VIII) is completely sensory but has two divisions. The auditory division is responsible for hearing, whereas the vestibular division is responsible for the sense of balance and position.[18,19] These divisions can be evaluated by two different tests. The auditory division can be evaluated by using the Rinne and Weber tests; the vestibular division is tested by using the Barany Caloric test.[18] The majority of the problems of the acoustic nerve are caused by the toxic effect of drugs.[18] Many prescription drugs affect both the auditory and vestibular divisions of the nerve.[18]

The glossopharyngeal nerve (cranial nerve IX) and the vagus nerve (cranial nerve X) both have a variety of sensory and motor functions. The testing of cranial nerve IX may be done by evaluating taste sensation on the posterior one third of the tongue, whereas the motor branch is evaluated by testing the gag reflex.[18,19]

Cranial nerve X is also evaluated with two tests. The first of these tests is to examine the soft palate.[18,19] The second is to ask the patient to swallow. While the athlete swallows, the therapist looks at his or her palate and then asks the athlete how it feels.[18,19]

Cranial nerves IX and X are also very close together in the medulla. This area is known as the nucleus ambiguous.[19] The nucleus ambiguous may be compromised in several ways; tumors in the posterior fossa, infections, myasthenia gravis, and amyotrophic

lateral sclerosis are just a few. Most of these complications are uncommon among the younger population.[19]

The accessory nerve (cranial nerve XI) and hypoglossal nerve (cranial nerve XII) are both purely motor nerves. Cranial nerve XI can be easily evaluated by muscle testing the sternocleidomastoid and the trapezius muscles.[18,19] Cranial nerve XII supplies motor fibers to the tongue.[18,19] In order to evaluate this nerve, the athlete is asked to protrude his or her tongue. Look for an asymmetry or a wasting away of the muscles in the tongue.[18,19] Also note if the tongue deviates to the left or right when protruding the tongue.[18,19]

The most common causes of cranial nerve XI and cranial nerve XII pathology are trauma and surgical procedures.[18,19] Occasionally, tumors affect cranial nerve XI.[18]

Spinal Examination. Testing procedures for the remainder of the peripheral nerves are very simple and can be executed quickly. The most efficient way to test the rest of the peripheral nerves is to test the motor, reflex, and sensory divisions from superior to inferior (Table 3–2).

The spinal nerves can be easily divided into five groups. The first group consists of the nerves from C2 to C4. All these roots innervate muscles that elevate the shoulders; thus the motor test for this area is the shoulder shrug.[20] Although there are no reflexes for this first group, all three nerves are responsible for specific dermatomal regions—C2 is on top of the head and C4 covers the upper neck and supraclavicular space.[18]

The second group is C5 through T1, also known as the brachial plexus. The motor tests are as follows: C5—biceps and deltoid; C6—biceps and wrist extensors; C7—triceps, wrist flexors, and finger extensors; C8—finger flexors; and T1—interossei muscles of the hand.[21]

There are three reflexes that can be tested. The biceps reflex is a test for C5, the brachioradialis reflex for C6, and the triceps for C7.[21]

The sensory divisions for these nerve roots are as follows: C5 dermatome is the lateral part of the arm; C6 is the lateral forearm, thumb, and index finger; C7 is the middle finger; C8 is the little finger and medial forearm; and T1 is the medial arm.[18] Figure 3–3 is an upper extremity neurological examination form.

The third group is T2 through T12. This entire group of nerves branches into the accessory breathing muscles.[20] T7 through T12 innervate muscles in the abdominal region; thus they can be tested by the trunk flexors.[20] All of the T2 through T12 dermatomes run across the chest in horizontal bands from approximately the armpits to the iliac crests.[18] No reflexes are tested for this group.

The fourth group consists of L5 through S1. There is much overlap in the motor function in the lower extremity so the testing must be done very carefully. The motor division should be tested as follows: L2 and L3—the iliopsoas; L3 and L4—the quadriceps; L5—the extensor hallucus longus; and S1—the gastrocnemius.[20,21]

There are two reflex tests for this group. The first is the patellar tendon reflex, which is the test for L4, and the second is the Achilles' tendon reflex, which tests S1.[21]

TABLE 3–2. NERVE FUNCTION LEVELS

Level	Motor	Reflex	Dermatome
C1	Head/neck flexion	None	None
C2	Head/neck extension	None	Small area on upper mandible
C3	Head/neck extension	None	Ring around the collar
C2–4	Shoulder shrug	None	
C4	Breathing/diaphragm	None	Top of shoulders
C5	Shoulder abduction	Biceps	Antero-lateral arm and forearm
C6	Wrist extension	Brachio-radialis	Radial forearm, thumb, index finger
C7	Wrist flexion	Triceps	Top of middle finger to wrist
C8	Finger flexion	None	Ulnar border hand and little finger
T1	Finger abduction and adduction	None	Horizontal trunk band and medial arm
T2–T12	Breathing	None	Horizontal trunk bands
T5–T12	Trunk Flex	None	Horizontal trunk bands
L1–L3	Hip hiking	None	Groin
L2–L4	Knee Extension		Groin
L4	DF and inversion	Patellar	Anterior diagonal front of thigh
L5	Toe extension	None	Lateral knee 2,3,4 dorsal toes
S1	Foot eversion PF	Achilles	Posterior lateral thigh leg

Adapted from Hoppenfield S. Orthopedic Neurology. Philadelphia, Pa: JB Lippincott Co; 1977, and Hoppenfield S. Physical Examination of the Spine and Extremities. New York, NY: Appleton-Century-Crofts; 1976.

The dermatomes for this group are as follows: L1 is from the iliac crest and runs approximately one third of the way down the anterior thigh, L2 is the middle one third of the anterior thigh, and L3 is the inferior one third of the anterior thigh and the knee. L4 includes the medial leg and foot and the medial portion of the great toe.[18,21] L5 runs from the lateral portion of the knee, across the anterior of the leg to the second, third, fourth, and part of the fifth toes. This includes both the dorsum and the plantar surfaces of the aforementioned areas.[18,21] The S1 dermatome includes the lateral portion of the foot and the posterior lateral portion of the leg.[18] Figure 3–4 is a lower-extremity neurological evaluation chart.

The fifth and final group of nerves are S2 through S5. S2 through S4 innervate the muscles of the pelvic floor as well as the muscles of the bowel and bladder.[20] The dermatomes for the nerves are as follows: S2 is the area of the popliteal space and posterior thigh and S3 through S5 make up the region around the anus.[21]

A verbal bowel and bladder history should be quite sufficient, with the dermatome tested if questions arise.

The pathology that the examiner should seek in the lower peripheral nerves includes radiculopathy and neuropathy.[18] These are most likely caused by trauma in younger individuals, but multiple sclerosis can also cause isolated lesions to nerve roots.[18]

Cerebellar Examination

The final portion of the evaluation is the cerebellar examination. There are many tests for the cerebellum. The two that are discussed here are the finger-to-nose test and the rebound test. The former involves exactly what is said, namely, the athlete is asked to touch his or her finger to the examiner's nose and then touch his or her own nose.[18] A person with cerebellar involvement will point past or overshoot the target.[18]

The rebound test is performed by instructing the athlete to extend his or her arm. The person doing the examination then pushes down on the athlete's arm and releases it.[18] A positive test is when the arm oscillates back and forth before returning to the resting position.[18]

As mentioned earlier, tumors of the posterior fossa do occur in the younger population.[18] If an athlete tests positive to some of the tests mentioned, then further more detailed tests are needed.

The person performing the evaluation does not necessarily need to include more than one test for each structure, but each of the previously mentioned structures do need to be tested. If problems arise with the testing procedures that are administered, then alternate tests should be considered. If the alternate tests still leave doubts in the examiner's mind, then the athlete needs to be referred to a specialist for a more extensive evaluation. Remember this is not a comprehensive evaluation, only a screening; thus the person doing the screening should refer the athlete to a neurologist if a problem is found.

CARDIOPULMONARY, VASCULAR, AND FITNESS SCREENINGS

Included in preseason evaluations should be cardiopulmonary, vascular, and fitness screenings. These are used to identify cardiac, pulmonary, and vascular insufficiencies and to measure endurance and other fitness characteristics. Depending on the number of athletes to be evaluated, individual or mass screening may be chosen.

Although a variety of procedures may be used to evaluate the integrity of the vascular system, we will highlight only a few of the easier tests. In the lower leg, Homan's test checks for deep venous thrombosis.[22] In the shoulder area there are several tests that can be grouped into the "Thoracic outlet syndrome" testing procedures. These test the vascular integrity of the upper extremity. Another test for upper extremity vascular integrity is the Allen's test.[23] In addition, all pulses should be checked for irregularity and strength. Easily checked pulses are the radial and ulnar pulses at the wrist, and the posterior tibial and dorsalis pedis pulses at the ankle. Pulses that are strong and regular are a good indication of vascular integrity to the extremities. The digital vascular supply can be checked in the toes and fingers by doing a simple digital refill test.

The Valsalva maneuver can be used to check for heart murmurs and other heartbeat irregularities.[21]

There are several tests that can be used for cardiovascular endurance testing.[9] Some of these are the pulse recovery test, step test, timed run, bicycle ergometer test, and treadmill test.[1,24,25] Three of these tests are easily administered and only require a stopwatch for equipment. The pulse recovery test is used to test the athlete's endurance and ability to recover to a resting pulse fairly quickly. The step test can be used for either an endurance test or an agility test. The 12-minute run (Cooper's test)[13] is also used as a test of the athlete's endurance and cardiac capabilities. It can also be used as a continuous check of the athlete's general physical condition. The coach can easily administer the test anytime throughout the athletic season. The results of Cooper's test can be interpreted from Table 3–3.

If a bicycle ergometer or a treadmill is available, very accurate endurance tests can be performed. The Monarch protocol for the bicycle ergometer is one of the more readily used protocols for the stationary bicycle.[25] The Bruce protocol for the treadmill is one of the more widely used tests on the treadmill.[25] Endurance testing should be done at the end of the entire screening

Physical Therapy Unit   Name _____
Student Health Center   SS# _____ Birthdate _____
University of WI-LaCrosse   Telephone# _____ Sex _____
                               Classification _____

UPPER EXTREMITY NEUROLOGICAL EVALUATION FORM

Date of onset _____ Date of Initial Eval _____ Date of Neural Eval _____

Affected area _____ R or L or B

Reason for Neuro-Eval _____

Root Level	Motor Level	Reflex	Sensory
C2	Cervical flexion & rotation		C2 Top of head
C3-4	Cervical extension		C3 Occiput area/ Side of head
C5	Shoulder Abd	Biceps	Lateral arm
C6	Wrist Ex	Brachiaradialis	Lateral forearm
C7	Wrist flex & finger ext	Triceps	Middle finger
C8	Finger flex		Medial forearm
T1	Finger Abd		Medial arm
T2-T12	Intercostals		T4 Nipple line
T5-T12	Rectus Abdominus		T7 Xiphoid process
			T10 Umbilicus
			T12 Lower abdomen

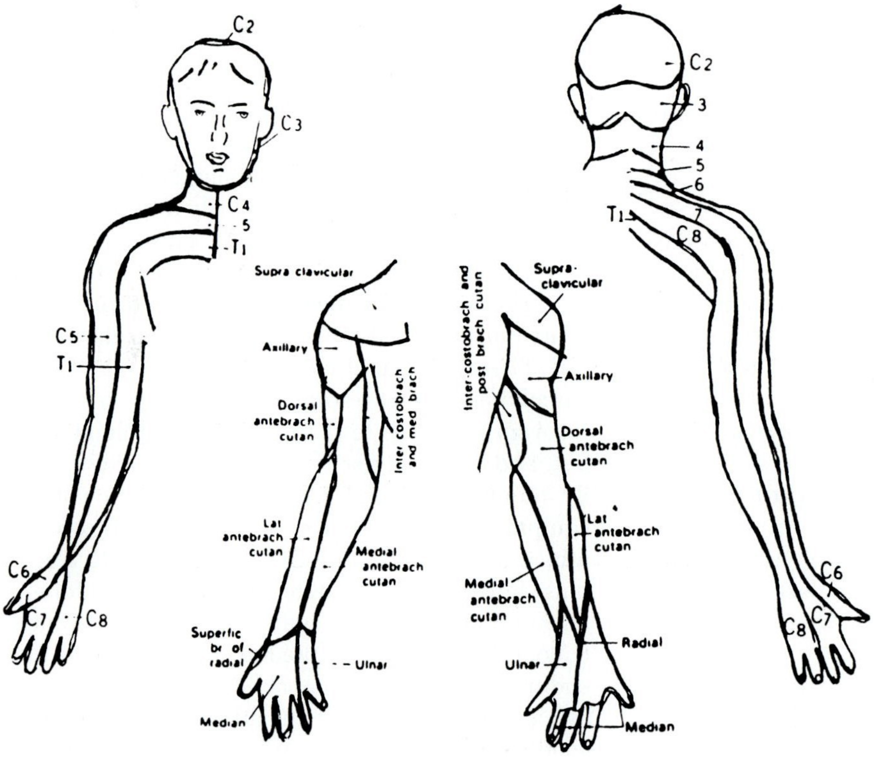

Circle affected area & explain

_____

_____

Light touch:
_____

Pin prick:
_____

Proprioception:
_____

Kinesthesia:
_____

Figure 3-3. Upper Extremity Evaluation Form.

HAND AND FINGER STRENGTH EVALUATION

Grip (Kg)   R _____   L _____

(Pt. to stand with arm straight down at side)

Pinch (Kg)

(Pt. to sit with elbow at 90° Flex. held at side and wrist neutral)

Index   R _____   L _____

Middle   R _____   L _____

Ring   R _____   L _____

Little   R _____   L _____

2 pt. Discrimination (mm)

L

_____Thumb _____

_____Index _____

_____Middle _____

_____Ring _____

_____Little _____

Pulses

At Wrist:	Radial	R	Palpable	Doppler	Absent
		L	Palpable	Doppler	Absent
	Ulnar	R	Palpable	Doppler	Absent
		L	Palpable	Doppler	Absent
At Hand:	Dorsal Metacarpal				
	1st Intermetacarpal	R		Doppler	Absent
		L		Doppler	Absent
	2nd Intermetacarpal	R		Doppler	Absent
		L		Doppler	Absent
	3rd Intermetacarpal	R		Doppler	Absent
		L		Doppler	Absent
	4th Intermetacarpal	R		Doppler	Absent
		L		Doppler	Absent

Comments: _____

_____

_____

Evaluator _____

Figure 3–3. Continued.

TABLE 3–3. FITNESS PARAMETERS

Fitness	Men	Women
Categories	Distance (mi)	Distance (mi)
Very poor	< 1.0	< 0.95
Poor	1.0–1.24	0.95–1.14
Fair	1.25–1.49	1.15–1.34
Good	1.50–1.74	1.35–1.64
Excellent	> 1.75	> 1.65

From Nichols JA. Determining fitness for participation in sports. Muscle Bone. 1981; 1(2).

process because the athlete is usually very fatigued after these tests.

Pushups, dips, and situps can also be used to measure the endurance of an athlete. The adolescent male should be able to do ten pullups.[26] The adolescent female should be able to do 15 seconds of bent arm hanging.[26] The adolescent male should be able to do 12 dips, whereas the female should be able to do at least 15 chair dips.[26] The adolescent male should be able to do 40 situps in 1 minute, whereas a female should be able to do 35.[26]

Physical Therapy Unit
Student Health Center
University of WI-LaCrosse

Name _____
SS# _____ Birthdate _____
Telephone# _____ Sex _____
Classification _____

LOWER EXTREMITY NEUROLOGICAL EVALUATION FORM

Date of onset _____ Date of Initial Eval _____ Date of Neural Eval _____

Affected area _____ R or L or B

Reason for Neuro-Eval _____

Root Level	Motor Level	Reflex	Sensory
T2-T12	Intercostal		T4 Nipple line
T5-T12	Rectus abdominus		T7 Xiphoid process
			T10 Umbilicus
			T12 Lower abdomen
L1	Paraspinals		Upper thigh
L2	Hip flex		Med thigh
L3	Quadraceps		Lower thigh
L4	Tib ant	Patellar	Medial leg and foot
L5	Toe extensors	Tib post	Lateral leg and dorsum foot
S1	Peronei	Achilles	Lateral side of foot
S2			Long strip post thigh

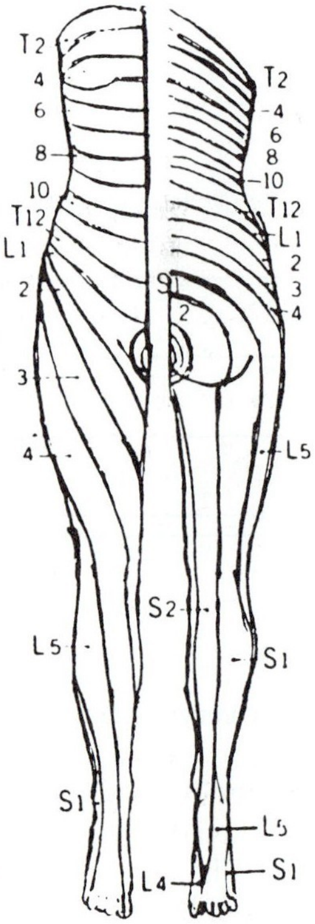

Circle affected area & explain _____

Light touch: _____

Pin prick: _____

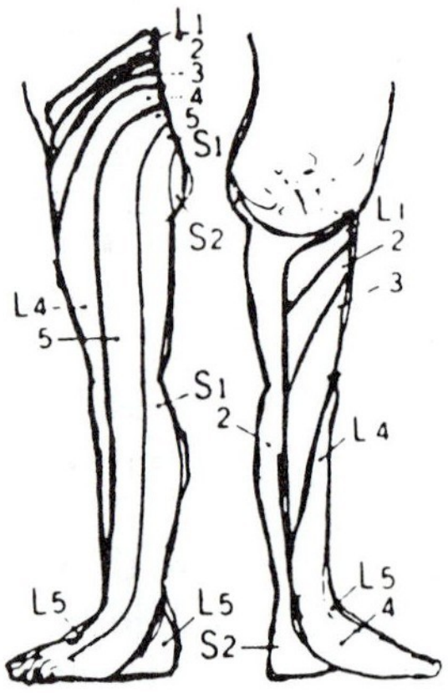

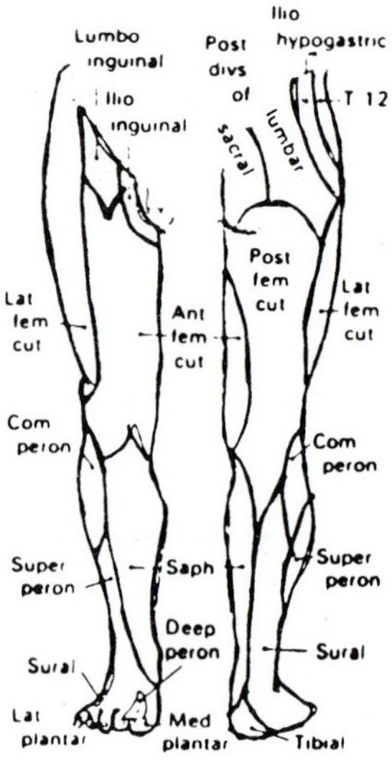

Proprioception: _____

Kinesthesia: _____

Figure 3-4. Lower Extremity.

Circulation

Post Tib	Palpable	Doppler	Absent
Dorsalis Pedis	Palpable	Doppler	Absent
Digital	Palpable	Doppler	Absent

Orthotron

Body Weight _____

Right
Quad/Ham

#3_____/_____ _____-_____%
#5_____/_____ _____-_____%
#7_____/_____ _____-_____%
#10_____/_____ _____-_____%
#( )_____/_____ _____-_____%

Right
Quad/Ham

#3_____/_____ _____-_____%
#5_____/_____ _____-_____%
#7_____/_____ _____-_____%
#10_____/_____ _____-_____%
#( )_____/_____ _____-_____%

Balance Test----------R _____ L _____

Comments: _____

_____

_____

_____

Evaluator _____

Figure 3–4. Continued.

BODY COMPOSITION

Body composition assessment is important to individuals wanting to maximize their athletic performance. The assessment reveals the percentage of body fat. Various inferences can be made from this datum, including weight losses and lean body mass increases desirable for the athlete. A desirable percentage of body fat varies from person to person depending on age, race, sex, athletic status, and personal goals.

There are two types of body composition assessment methods: laboratory techniques and anthropometric measurements. The laboratory technique is hydrostatic weighing, the standard against which all other indirect methods are usually validated.[27] This method is the most accurate and also the most time consuming in terms of personnel, training, and equipment requirements. For this reason, if mass testing is going to be performed, anthropometric techniques are preferred for efficiency and validity.

Skinfolds are more accurate predictors of body fat density than any other anthropometric variable.[28–30] The important factor is to use the correct prediction equation depending on the sex of the subject and the appropriateness of the population-specific equation or the generalized equation. The prediction equations were developed for people between the ages of 18 and 61, so that the accuracy outside of these parameters is questionable.[29] It has been shown that the prediction equations are less accurate when used with obese individuals.[29] SKyndex is an electronic body fat indicator that contains a microprocessor-based electronic caliper. This device eliminates human error and time needed for calculations. It is also convenient because it is battery operated and rechargeable. The SKyndex allows more than 100 individuals to have their percentage body fat calculated in less than 1 hour.[31,32] Recommended averages for body fat using either caliper method are listed in Table 3–4.

The prediction equations should be used with discretion when they are accompanying a training program. This is because of tissue distribution changes that have resulted from the training. In this way, training places the individual into a different population and invalidates the use of the initial prediction equations.[27] Skinfolds have a 3% to 4% error margin because of the error in the actual measurement of the skinfolds combined with individual variations in the densities of the lean body mass components, especially the bones and protein.[33]

TABLE 3-4. BODY FAT COMPOSITION

Sport	Body Fat (%)
Female	
Volleyball	15%–16%
Elite level	13%–14%
Basketball	15%–16%
Gymnastics	12%–15%
Male	
Baseball	<10%
Football	
Offensive line	<16%
Defensive line	<14%
Rest of team	<10%
Crew	<10%

From Clark M, et al. Body Composition: II Practical Considerations. Nat Strength Condit Assoc J. *1987; 9(4): 10–20.*

Bioelectric impedance is another form of assessing body composition that is easy and simple. The theory is that the body's resistance to a low-energy, high-frequency electrical signal varies with body size and composition. More studies, however, need to be done because the accuracy of the prediction equation has varied with every study done to date.[27] There are also special considerations that must be taken into account. For example, the individual must not be dehydrated; thus the individual must not drink alcohol or have exercised in a 24-hour period before the test. The individual must not eat a large meal for a period of 2 hours before the test.[27]

Bone diameters and body circumference measurements may also be used to assess body composition:

Selected body circumference measurements are substantially correlated with body density. This is especially true for the gluteal and waist circumferences for women and waist circumferences for men.[29]

Probably the most used and least accurate method of body composition assessment is the height and weight charts formulated by insurance companies. These charts do not take body frame, individual muscle mass, or other specific body components into consideration. Therefore, an individual may be "overweight" according to the chart without actually being "overfat" due to the increased muscle mass. According to one report, insurance charts "essentially have no validity." They do not consider somatotype, age, or frame size.[27]

Body fat percentages for the "normal" population should be 10% to 20% for men and 20% to 30% for women.[27] These percentages do not apply to athletes. Most athletes need to find their own "optimal-performance" levels, which are usually much lower than the levels for the "normal" population. According to doctors, there should be no specific reason for any-

one to attempt to go below 5% body fat.[27] This level has been termed the essential fat level.

Body composition is an important tool that can be used to increase athletic performance to an optimal level or to decrease fat percentages to a more healthy level. Anthropometric methods are only estimates, and it should be remembered that some error will occur simply as a result of the method.

GAIT

The gait evaluation is very important in preventing injuries. If the person performing the evaluation can detect an abnormality in the athlete's gait pattern, it can often be corrected before it can cause the athlete problems.[34]

The actual walking evaluation can be separated into eight phases. Each phase should include evaluations of the following areas—trunk, pelvis, hip, knee, ankle, and foot.[35,36] Table 3–5 lists the eight phases, with the corresponding movement of each lower extremity.

Table 3–6 lists the body areas the screener should watch during the gait evaluation. The screener should then compare the right and left side for each body area and record his or her observations. Figure 3–5 is a sample gait evaluation form.

Screeners can add comments about what they see while observing the athlete's gait. The gait evaluation can become extremely complex but athletic trainers and sports physical therapists primarily need to know that there is a problem. If the athlete is having pain or other difficulty, a podiatric referral may be in order.

TABLE 3-5. PHASES OF GAIT

Phase	Right Leg	Left Leg
Initial swing	Foot just lifting off ground	Foot firmly planted
Mid swing	Moving just ahead of left leg	Foot firmly planted
Terminal swing	Just before heel contact	Heel just lifting off
Initial contact	Heel contact	Heel just lifting off
Loading response	Foot firmly planted	Just before toe off
Mid stance	Foot firmly planted	Toe off
Terminal stance	Heel just lifting off	Just prior to heel strike
Preswing	Just prior to toe off	Foot firmly planted

From Rancho Los Amigos Hospital. Normal and Pathological Gait Syllabus. *Downey Calif: Rancho Los Amigos Hospital; 1978; 2–5.*

TABLE 3-6. GAIT CHART

Head	WNL	Tilt R	Tilt L
Shoulders	Level	Low R	Low L
Arm swing	Even	More R	More L
Hip varus		R	L
Hip valgus		R	L
Knee flexion	Equal	More R	More L
Knee extension	Equal	More R	More L
Knee recurvatum		R	L
Knee varum		R	L
Knee valgum		R	L
Knee internal rotation		R	L
Knee external rotation		R	L
Tibia varum		R	L
Tibia valgum		R	L
Calcaneal varum		R	L
Calcaneal valgum		R	L
Forefoot supination		R	L
Forefoot pronation		R	L
Toes—R _____			
—L. _____			

From Hoppenfeld. Physical Examination of the Spine and Extremities. New York, NY: Appleton-Century-Crofts; 1976.

POSTURE

Posture screening must be done with the athlete standing in his or her normal relaxed posture. The posture screening can be done in conjunction with the back, trunk, and neck screening or as a separate station. The posture screening should include observation of the body in a standing position from all angles. It should also include moving from a standing posture to the particular posture the individual uses for his or her activity, such as a three-point stance for a football offensive lineman. The athlete's ability to get in and out of his or her activity posture is often related to flexibility. Therefore, it is extremely important to check flexibility in conjunction with the posture examination or to be sure it is being tested with the other portions of the overall screening. It is also important to observe the body type of the individual athlete.[37] The screener should assess whether this body type may predispose the athlete to injury or make the activity more difficult to accomplish.

From a posterior view, screeners must look for prominences or differences from one side of the body to the other. They also need to observe a plumb line following the mid-line from the head to the floor. The line should equally bisect the head, the shoulders, the trunk, the pelvis, and the crotch. It should be equidistant to each knee and ankle.[22,37] The shoulders and pelvis should be level.[37] The carrying angles of the elbows and the body angles should be bilaterally equal, as should the space between the body and elbows.[23,38] The

screener must look for any signs of a scoliosis.[37] The screener should observe if the feet are equally pronated or supinated and if the angle of the lower Achilles is symmetrical bilaterally.[37]

The anterior view may also reveal unilateral differences. The screener should observe the level of the shoulders, the nipples on men, the body angles, the anterior superior iliac spines (ASISs), the tips of the fingers as the hands hang relaxed beside the body, and the patella.[22]

The lateral view reveals whether the athlete has any excess kyphosis, lordosis, and genu recurvatum. There should be a plumb line through the ear lobe, the tip of the shoulder, the greater trochanter, just posterior to the patella, and slightly anterior to the lateral malleolus.[39]

Leg length differences need to be noted. Are there true or apparent differences? Are there true differences in the thighs, lower legs, or feet? To answer these questions, leg length measurements need to be taken during both weight bearing and non-weight bearing.[37] Table 3-7 provides a reference for these measurements.[23]

Flexibility screening is usually done in conjunction with a posture examination but can be done with individual body area stations. Table 3-8 lists some common flexibility tests. The relationship of the inominates to each other and to the sacrum needs to be determined by visual observation and by palpation. Table 3-9 addresses this postural relationship.

Because the strength of the abdominals can have a significant effect on the relationship of the pelvis to the spine, abdominal muscle testing is necessary. Figure 3-6 is a posture evaluation form.

MUSCULOSKELETAL SCREENING

For the purpose of doing a complete and thorough screening, the body is separated into nine areas. These

TABLE 3-7. LEG LENGTH MEASUREMENTS

Measurements	
ASIS to medial malleolus	Weight bearing
ASIS to medial malleolus	Non-weight bearing
Umbilicus to floor	Weight bearing
ASIS to floor	Weight bearing
Greater trochanter to lateral malleolus	Non-weight bearing
Greater trochanter to knee joint line	Non-weight bearing
Lateral knee joint line to tip of lateral malleolus	Non-weight bearing
Medial knee joint line to tip of medial malleolus	Non-weight bearing

From Magee DJ. Orthopedic Physical Assessment. Philadelphia, Pa: W.B. Saunders Co; 1987.

Physical Therapy Unit
Student Health Center
UW-LaCrosse

Name _____

SS# _____ Birthdate _____

Telephone# _____ Sex _____

Classification _____

GAIT EVALUATION

Date of onset _____ Date of initial eval _____

Date of gait eval _____ Painful area _____ R or L or B

Reason for gait eval _____

S: Activity: Running or walking or other _____

   Duration of activity _____
   Change in (Mileage Y or N) (Intensity Y or N) (Shoes Y or N) (Surface Y or N)

   Explain Y answers and comments _____

_____

   Shoe type _____ Type of surface run on _____

O: Step length: (Equal) or (R greater than L) or (L greater than R)
   Stance ratio: (Equal) or (R greater than L) or (L greater than R)

Special Tests:	Right	Left
Hamstring tightness	_____	_____
Thomas test	_____	_____
Ober test	_____	_____
Heel cord tightness	_____	_____
Gastroc tightness	_____	_____
Soleus tightness	_____	_____
Leg length	_____	_____
Q-angle	_____	_____
Arch height	_____	_____
Femoral torsion	_____	_____
Malleolar torsion	_____	_____
Forefoot relationship (in neutral STJ)	_____	_____
Hindfoot relationship (in neutral STJ)	_____	_____
Relaxed calcaneal stance	_____	_____

Plantar Callus Lesions

Right   Left

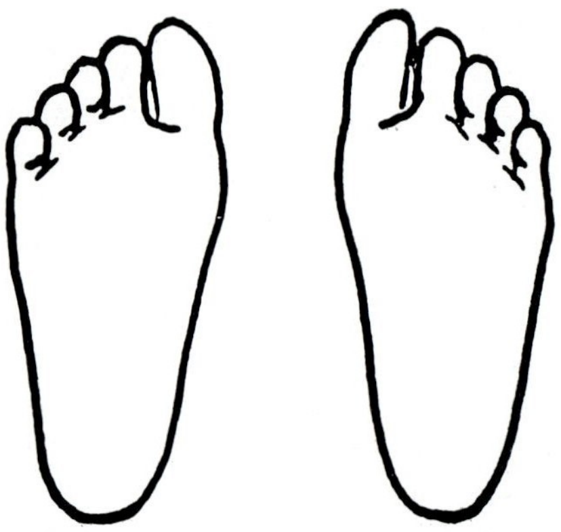

Shoe Wear Pattern

Right   Left

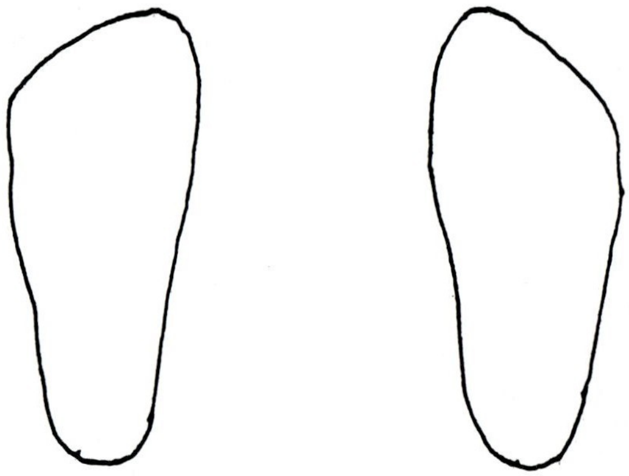

Figure 3-5. Gait Evaluation Form.

Place number of appropriate phase by description of abnormalities present in that phase (eg. Ankle: #6: excessive pronation)

INITIAL SWING	MID-SWING	TERMINAL SWING	INITIAL CONTACT	LOADING RESPONSE	MID-STANCE	TERMINAL STANCE	PRE-SWING
1	2	3	4	5	6	7	8

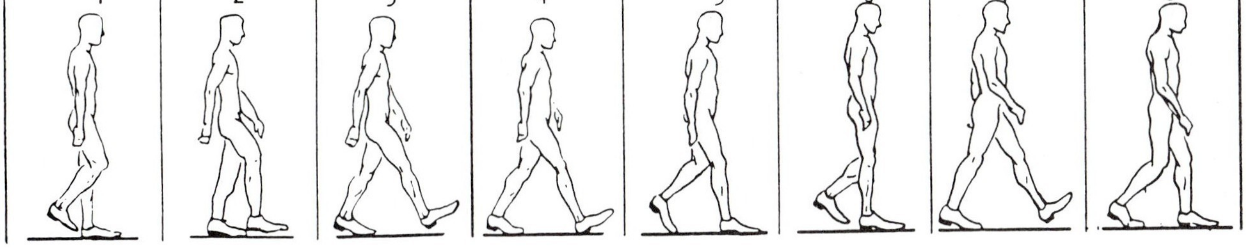

Trunk: _____

Pelvis: _____

Hip: _____

Knee: _____

Ankle: _____

Foot: _____

Note any differences between walking and running gait: _____

_____

A: _____   P: _____

_____   _____

_____   _____

Evaluator   Date   PT Supervisor   Date

Figure 3-5. Continued.

areas are the foot, the ankle and lower leg, the knee and thigh, the thigh and hip, the low back, the trunk, the cervical spine, the shoulder and shoulder girdle, the elbow, and the forearm, wrist, and hand.

Each major area of the body must be evaluated for range of motion and joint stability. It is also important to test the flexibility of the musculotendinous structures of each joint area. This is because although no limitation may be found in the range of motion, a limitation may be present with the joint in a certain position due to a musculotendinous insufficiency.[40] The normal range of motion of each joint is readily available in the literature.[41] Primary stability tests are discussed along with supplemental tests to be done if a certain primary test reveals a deficiency.

The muscles that provide certain functions at each joint must be evaluated for motor function and strength. The motor function is related to the spinal cord segments discussed in the section on the neurological assessment.[42] Information on which muscles provide certain motions at each individual joint is readily available in the literature.[20,39]

The strength of each muscle group should be tested manually.[43,44] There are many muscle groups that can be tested for strength by means of equipment. This equipment adds objectivity to the results of the screening process. The availability of this equipment, the personnel skilled in the operation of the equipment, and the time needed to use the equipment must be considered when deciding if a particular type of equipment will be used in a screening program. The easiest piece of equipment to use for muscle strength testing is a dynamometer.[12] The more complicated equipment to use includes various isokinetic testing and exercise devices.[45-49]

It is impossible to list all of the testing devices in this chapter. I do, however, point out in each section, areas where muscle testing with equipment would be desirable.

It is essential that the soft tissue of the body be inspected visually. Any abnormalities discovered must then be further evaluated by palpation and possibly using equipment, such as x-ray. There are certain areas of the body that should be routinely evaluated by palpation during the screening process. The palpations necessary for each part of the body are discussed in the appropriate section below.

Physical Therapy Unit   Name _____
Student Health Center   SS# _____ Birthdate _____
University of WI-LaCrosse   Telephone# _____ Sex _____
                                 Classification _____

POSTURE EVALUATION FORM

Date of onset _____ Date of Initial Eval _____ Date of Posture Eval _____
Affected area _____ R or L or B or Center

Reason for Posture Eval _____
Body type: Ectomorph   Endomorph   Mesomorph

Height _____ Weight _____ Handedness _____

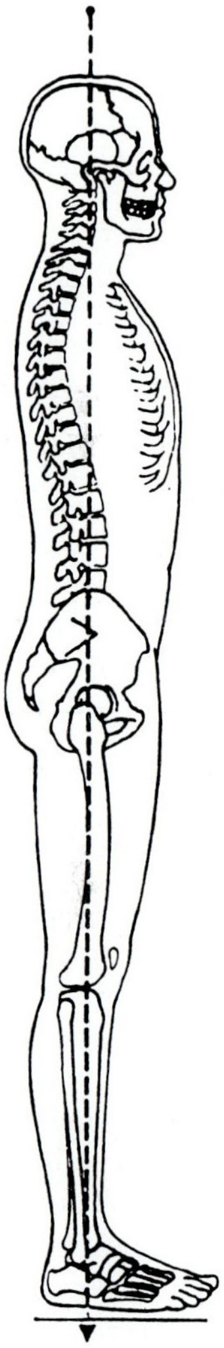

_____
Head
_____
Cervical Spine
_____
Shoulders
_____
Scapula
_____
Body Angle
_____
Thoracic Spine
_____
Lumbar Spine
_____
Pelvis
_____
Hip Joints
_____
Lower Ext
_____
Knee Joint
_____
Ankle Joint
_____
Feet

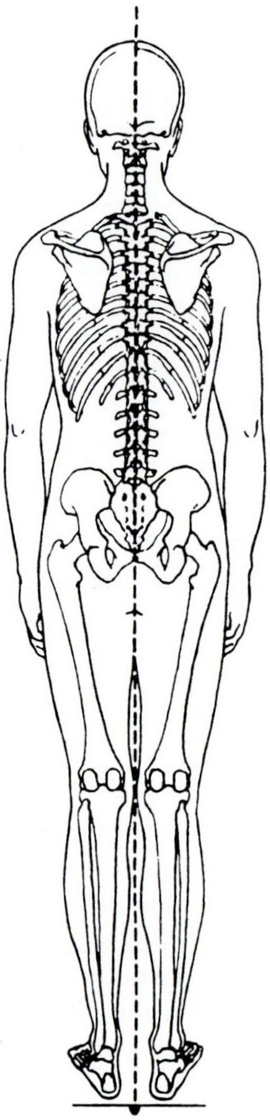

Leg Length Measurements   Supine _____
                                        to
ASIS To Med Maleolus: .   Long Sit _____
      WB R_____ L _____
                                     ASIS (R HIGH/L HIGH/LEVEL)
      NWB R_____ L _____   PSIS (R HIGH/L HIGH/LEVEL)
Umbilicus To Floor: Crests (R HIGH/L HIGH/LEVEL)
                                     ASIS (R FORW/L FORW/EQUAL)
      WB R_____ L _____
ASIS To Floor:

      WB R_____ L _____

Figure 3-6. Posture Evaluation Form.

Special Tests

Low back tightness	Neg or _____
Hip flexor tightness	Neg or _____
Hamstring tightness	Neg or _____
Trendelenburg	Neg or _____
IT band tightness	Neg or _____
Sit up	Grade _____
X-rays taken? Y OR N	Result _____

ROM
Normal
S 30-0-85
F 30-0-30
R 45-0-45

Flexibility (fingers to toes in long sitting)

_____

_____

_____

A: _____

_____

_____

S: Short term _____

_____

_____

Mid term _____

_____

_____

Long term _____

_____

_____

_____

| Evaluator | Date | Physical Therapy Supervisor | Date | Physician Review | Date |

Figure 3-6. Continued.

The Cervical Spine

The cervical spine is capable of flexion, extension, lateral flexion to both sides, and rotation to both sides. The screener should assess each vertebra using segmental spring testing for hypermobility and hypomobility. These tests are discussed in terms of their elicited symptoms in Table 3–10. The screener must observe the active motion in all directions to determine any asymmetry. At the end of the motion the screener should apply excess pressure to determine if there is pain at the end ranges and to assess for an inadequate end feel, indicating possible joint laxity.

The strength of the neck can be tested manually.

It should be tested in all six motions to determine if there is any unilateral or singular motion weaknesses.

The screener should palpate the cervical vertebrae to locate any vertebral misplacement.

Trunk

The thoracic spine is primarily checked for rotation.[11] The abdominal muscles of flexion are discussed in the following section. The trunk rotation is measured by a modified situp (hands behind the head) with trunk rotation. The screener needs to observe for symmetrical movement. When flexion of the trunk is observed it is important that one observes for a gentle smooth curve

TABLE 3-8. POSTURE EXAMINATION

Routine Test	Symptom
Cervical flexion	Cannot put chin to chest
Cervical extension	Cannot bring head to horizontal
Cervical rotation	Cannot bring chin in line with shoulder
Cervical lateral flexion	Cannot bring ear to shoulder
Apley scratch—interior rotation	Unable to touch opposite scapula behind back
Apley scratch—exterior rotation	Unable to get humerus parallel to chest with hands locked behind back
Low back tightness	Unable to arch back with legs out straight when lying supine
Hamstring tightness	Unable to reach toes with hands long sitting-tripod 90–90
Quad tightness test	Flexion of knee causes flex of hip
Hip flexor tightness (Thomas)	Femur unable to go horizontal when in supine with other knee brought up
Iliotibial band tightness (Ober's)	Side lying-top leg does not fall below horizontal
Gastroc tightness	With knee straight, 10 degree of dorsi flex not possible
Soleus tightness	With knee at 90 degree, 20 degree of doris flex not possible

Adapted from Novel Products Inc, P.O. Box 308, 80 Fairbanks Street, Addison, ILL, Hoppenfield S. Physical Examination of the Spine and Extremities. *New York, NY: Appleton-Century-Crofts; 1976, Gould JA, Davies GJ.* Orthopedic and Sports Physical Therapy, *2nd ed. St. Louis, Mo: CV Mosby Co; 1985, Kendall HO, Kendall FP, Boynton DA.* Posture and Pain. *Huntington, NY: K. E. Krieger Publishing Co Inc: 1977, and Cailliet R.* Foot and Ankle Pain. *Philadelphia, Pa: F. A. Davis Co; 1976.*

of the spine. Asymmetry of the rib cage should also be observed and noted. Routine tests for the trunk are listed in Table 3–11.

Lumbar Spine

The joint stability of the lumbar spine is extremely difficult to assess, but certain levels of instability can be determined by certain movements and by doing segmental spring testing. It is not uncommon to have one

TABLE 3-9. PELVIC OBSERVATIONS

Front view			
ASIS	level	(R) high	(L) high
Rear view			
PSIS	level	(R) high	(L) high
Illiac Crests	level	(R) high	(L) high
Ischial tuberosity	level	(R) high	(L) high
Gluteal fold	level	(R) high	(L) high
Side view			
ASIS	equal	(R) forward	(L) forward

From Saunders et al. Evaluation, Treatment and Prevention of Musculoskeletal Disorders. *Minneapolis, Minn Viking Press Inc; 1985.*

TABLE 3-10. CERVICAL TESTS

Routine Test	Symptom	Follow-up
Segmental spring (Sprillings)[23]	Pain	Quadrant[11]
	Hyper or Hypo Mobility	
Compression[23]	Pain or Neuro Sx	Quadrant
Distraction[22]	Pain or Neuro Sx	Valsalva[40]
Adson's test[40]	Lower pulse or Neuro Sx	Wrights[40]
		Adson's maneuver[40]
		Hyperabduction[40]
		Vertebral artery test[22]
		Swallow[21]
		Elevated arm[23]
		Allen maneuver[22]
		Halstead[22]

hypermobile segment and other segments that are hypomobile. Sacroiliac instability is not uncommon. The sacroiliac joint can be quickly screened by the Patrick test and the Long sit to supine test. Table 3–11 lists the symptoms the examiner might elicit.

The athlete should be able to sit on the floor with

TABLE 3-11. TRUNK TESTING

Routine Test	Symptom	Follow-up
Double leg lift[39]	Weak lower abdominals	Strengthen
Modified situp[43]	Weak upper abdominals, umbilical deviation	Strengthen
Long sit to supine[40]	SI dysfunction	Sacral push, caudal[23]
		Sacral push, cranial[23]
Patrick's[22]	SI dysfunction	SI compression
		SI distraction
		Standing flexion
		Sitting flexion
Segmental spring testing[23]	Segmental hypermobility	
	Segmental hypomobility	
SLR[22]	Pain or neurological Sx	Well leg SLR[22]
		Reverse SLR[22]
		Well leg Reverse SLR[22]
		Chin to chest[22]
		Heel slam[38]
		Bowstring[22]
		Toe walking[40]
		90–90[38]
SLR[22]	Tightness of hamstring	Stretching[39]

the legs extended and touch his or her toes. The athlete should be able to bend laterally equally to each side. The athlete should be able to bend forward and touch the tips of his or her fingers to the floor. Lower back tightness or hamstring tightness might prevent the forward flexion.

Athletes should be able to do a modified situp with their hands behind the head if they have adequate upper abdominal strength. They should be able to lift both legs, extended, about 5 cm off the plinth without arching of the low back if they have adequate lower abdominal strength. They should be able to extend with their hands behind their heads if they have adequate back extension strength.

Palpation of the paraspinal muscle will determine if the athlete has back spasms. The iliolumbar ligament area should be palpated for tenderness.

The visual inspection of the lumbar spine is primarily done during the posture screening. The screener must also observe for asymmetrical body contour and asymmetrical motion.

Hip

The hip is inherently very durable and not very susceptible to injury. Some congenital abnormalities that exist without the athlete's knowledge may be revealed during a very thorough screening. The hip joint stability can be tested by the Fabre test. This and other tests are listed in Table 3–12.

The functional action of the hip joint muscles are flexion, extension, internal rotation, external rotation, abduction, and adduction. The normal range of each of these motions is available in the literature. These can be tested by manual muscle tests but most readily lend themselves to isokinetic equipment testing. The functional activity of the hip can also be determined by testing the iliotibial band flexibility at the hip and hip

flexor tightness. Any "groin" pain needs to be further assessed by a physician to rule out various forms of hernia.[50]

Visual inspection needs to be non-weight bearing and during gait. The screener should be looking for bilateral asymmetry, visual leg length difference, and other anomalies.

The screener must be sure to palpate the trochanteric bursa, which is immediately posterior and superior to where one palpates the greater trochanter.[50] Palpation of the anterior thigh for myositis ossificans is also extremely important in anyone who has previously participated in any contact sports or had a thigh injury.

Knee and Thigh

The knee is a joint that is very susceptible to injury. For this reason additional time and care should be taken when evaluating the knee. Although the knee is considered a hinge joint, it also has a rotatory component. Any significant instability should be further evaluated by an orthopedist. Any muscle weakness or imbalance must be rehabilitated by an athletic trainer or sports physical therapist. The flexibility of the hamstrings, the quadriceps, the iliotibial band, and the adductors must be checked.[11]

The person doing the screening can test the general stability of the knee by doing a few simple primary tests. If any of these tests show significant laxity, a more thorough stability examination will be needed. If the primary tests reveal problems other than laxity, then these problems also need to be further evaluated. The more extensive evaluations need to be done by an athletic trainer, sports physical therapist, or physician. They should be done when the person doing the evaluation can spend more time with the athlete.

Doing the Lachman's, valgus and varus, McMurray's, and posterior sag tests will give the person who is doing the screening a quick and accurate indication of the overall stability of the ligaments of the knee. The person doing the screening must also do the apprehension, patellar grinding, and patellar ballottment tests to check for patellar–femoral problems and joint effusion. The "Q" angle should be noted, especially when evaluating runners. This and other tests are listed in Table 3–13.

The motor function of the knee can be tested by having the athlete extend the knee while sitting and flex the knee while in a prone position. The hamstrings should be tested for flexibility. This can be done by, again, having the athlete extend the knee in a sitting position. The iliotibial band should also be tested for flexibility.

The strength of the quadriceps and the hamstrings can be tested very easily by isokinetic devices. These devices also provide a graphic printout that may aid in determining where and to what extent deficits exist.

TABLE 3–12. HIP TESTING

Routine Test	Symptom	Follow-up
Ober test[21,22]	Tight iliotibia	Proximal iliotibial friction Palpate trochanteric bursa[38]
Fabre test[21]	Painful hip	Axial compression of the femur with external rotation and abduction,[21] then internal rotation and adduction[21]
Thomas test[21]	Tight hip flexors	Stretching[39]
SLR[22]	Hamstring tightness	90–90 test[38]
Visual inspection of leg length[21]	Visual leg length difference	Measure leg length[21]

TABLE 3-13. KNEE TESTS

Routine Test	Symptom	Follow-Up
Lachman's[68]	Anterior laxity	Anterior drawer[37] Slocum rotary[22] Pivot shift[37] Losse[22]
Posterior sag[22]	Posterior laxity	Posterior drawer[37] Slocum rotary[22] Pivot shift[37] Losse[22]
McMurray (valgus—exterior rotation)[22]	Medial laxity	Valgus stress (20-degree flexion)[22] Valgus stress (0-degree flexion)[22] Anterior drawer[37] Slocum rotary[22] Pivot shift[37] Losse[22]
	Clunk or pain	Squat[50] Duck walk[50]
McMurray (varus—interior rotation)[22]	Lateral laxity	Varus stress (20-degree flexion)[22] Varus stress (0-degree flexion)[22] Anterior drawer[37] Slocum rotary[22]
	Clunk or pain	Squat[50] Duck walk[50]
Patellar grinding[21]	Crepitus—Pain	Stutter[42] Resisted Quad set[22]
Apprehension[21]	Involuntary quad set	
Ballottment[21]	Effusion	Bounce Home[21] Circumference measurement[37]
90–90[21]	Unable to extend knee	SLR[37] Knee range[22]
Ober's[22]	Iliotibial-band tightness and pain	
"Q" angle[22]	Excess of 15 degrees in men Excess of 20 degrees in women	

Visual inspection of the knee is a quick method of determining knee joint effusion, quadriceps atrophy, or bony abnormalities. Atrophy of the vastus medialis or vastus medialis obliquus is quite common following any injury to this area. Enlargement of the tibial tuberosity is common following an episode of Osgood–Schlater's disease.[22]

Palpation of the knee should include checking for tenderness on the joint line, along the collateral ligaments, and over the infrapatellar tendon. Tenderness of the facets of the patella and the patellar femoral groove should be assessed. The quadricep attachment to the patella and the posterior part of the knee should also be checked for tenderness. The quadricep needs to be palpated because this is a frequent site for calcium deposits after injuries.[51]

Table 3–13 is a list of the primary and followup tests that should be done during a routine preseason screening evaluation of the knee.

Foot, Ankle, and Lower Leg

The inversion ankle sprain is one of the most common injuries to athletes.[52] This fact exemplifies the need to evaluate the stability of the ankle thoroughly. If the athlete has a history of ankle injuries or the person screening the athlete discovers ankle instability, it is essential that the athlete be put on a comprehensive ankle rehabilitation program.

Lateral ankle stability is tested by the anterior drawer test and the calcaneal fibular ligament test (talar tilt test). Medial ankle stability is tested by an eversion stress test. The ankle mortise stability is tested if there is any lateral or medial laxity discovered or if the athlete has a history of ankle injuries. The test for the stability of the ankle mortise is the side-to-side test. Table 3–14 provides an overview of ankle and lower leg tests.

The athlete's ability to invert, evert, dorsiflex, and plantarflex the ankle determines the level of motor function of the ankle. The motor function of the foot is tested by the amount of active flexion and extension the athlete has in the toes. The athlete should be able to walk on the toes, heels, lateral side of the foot, and the

TABLE 3-14. ANKLE AND LOWER LEG TESTS

Routine Test	Symptom	Follow-up
Anterior drawer[22]	Anterior laxity	Side to side[37]
Lateral stability[21]	Lateral laxity	Side to side[37]
Medial stability[21]	Medial laxity	Side to side[37]
Toe rise[22]	Unable to rise	Thompson[22]
Walk on heels, toes, lateral or medial border of foot[22]	Unable to do	Ankle dorsiflexion test (knee 0 degrees)[21] Ankle dorsiflexion test (knee 90 degrees)[21] Objective strength testing of plantarflexor dorsiflexor inverter everter muscle groups[22]
Balance test	Less than 20 seconds Asymmetrical	Objective proprioceptive testing[69]

medial side of the foot. If the athlete is unable to do these tests, more specific range of motion and flexibility tests need to be administered.

The strength of the ankle invertors, evertors, dorsiflexors, plantarflexors, and toe flexors and extensors can be manually tested. Ankle plantarflexors and dorsiflexors can be readily tested by isokinetic devices.

Proprioceptive testing should be done if there is any history of injury. This can be done by using a stopwatch to time one-foot standing balance and comparing it to the bilateral test. There are also some commercially available electronic balance boards available for testing.[10,53,54]

The visual inspection is primarily for comparing the right and the left sides for asymmetry. The person screening the athlete should look for any lateral ankle edema.[55] The person screening the athlete should also routinely note such things as hallux valgus (bunion), pes planus, pes cavus, hammer toes, athletes' foot, and any other anomalia.[56]

Palpation of the ankle should include but is not limited to the lateral ankle ligaments, the anterior deltoid ligament, and the anterior inferior tibial fibular ligament. On the foot the person screening the athlete should palpate the medial calcaneal tubercle, the plantar surface of the foot between the third and fourth metatarsal heads, the posterior section of the calcaneus for pain and the dorsal pedal and posterior tibial pulses. The posterior middle one third of the tibial crest must also be palpated for tenderness.

Table 3–14 lists the routine and subsequent follow-up tests that are commonly used during a preseason screening of the ankle and lower leg.

Shoulder and Shoulder Girdle

The shoulder girdle is connected to the body primarily via muscular attachments. There is a bony attachment at the sternoclavicular joint but this is only a butt joint. Because of this loose connection to the body, the shoulder girdle has considerable movement alone and in conjunction with the glenohumeral joint. The glenohumeral joint does not have a strong static stabilization. This again allows considerable movement. This does, however, lead to problems when certain external forces are applied in certain ways.[57] The shoulder area sometimes manifests certain symptoms that in actuality are cervical problems.

The glenohumeral joint in conjunction with the shoulder girdle is capable of considerable range and motion. The glenohumeral joint flexes, extends, abducts, and adducts. It also allows for internal and external rotation. Horizontal abduction and adduction may also take place. The glenohumeral joint is capable of total circumduction. The shoulder girdle also has considerable movement on the thoracic wall. Scapular elevation, depression, protraction, and retraction are primarily shoulder girdle movements. Normal values are readily available in the literature. When the athlete is taken through the ranges it is important to observe the smoothness of the motion so as to detect painful arcs or blockage of certain movements.[58] Winging of the scapula indicates muscle weakness.[44] General assessment tests with their respective symptoms are listed in Table 3–15. The shoulder muscle complex can be tested manually fairly quickly and effectively. Machine testing can be done primarily in singular planes but is very time consuming and cumbersome. Certain motions may be tested objectively on isokinetic equipment in the particular sports in which athletes have high shoulder usage.

The shoulder complex has several joints and other structures that must be palpated for tenderness. The acromioclavicular joint and sternoclavicular joints are at either end of the clavicle and are very superficial. The glenohumeral joint is more difficult to palpate, but it is important to attempt to locate the joint line for palpation. If one palpates up under the deltoid anteriorly and posteriorly much of the glenohumeral joint line is palpable. The coracoid process needs to be palpated for tenderness as its tenderness is an indication of possible acromioclavicular joint problems and bicep problems. The tendinous insertions of the rotator cuff as well as the supraspinatus musculotendinous junction need to be palpated to help rule out rotator cuff problems.[58] This is especially important in sports that require considerable upper extremity usage.

TABLE 3–15. SHOULDER TESTS

Routine Test	Symptom	Follow-up
Apley scratch— abduction and exterior Rotation[21]	Decreased motion	ROM measure[37] Anterior apprehension[22] Quadrant[22] Locking[22] Posterior apprehension[22]
Apley scratch— adduction and interior rotation[21]	Decreased motion	ROM measure[37] Anterior apprehension[22] Quadrant[22] Locking[22] Posterior apprehension[22]
Drop arm[21]	Pain Weakness	Empty can[22] Impingement[11]
Yergason[22] Test[22]	Pain	Speed's
	Biceps tendon subluxation	
A-C traction[37]	Laxity	Clavicular movement[40]
Wall pushup[23]	Scapular winging	MMT serratus[43]

Elbow

The medial and lateral stability of the elbow is relatively easy to test with the simple varus and valgus stresses listed in Table 3–16. The elbow is capable of flexion and extension. Supination and pronation of the forearm is often considered as part of the elbow as the radial head turns at the elbow. The testing of elbow flexion and extension strength is most easily performed manually. The medial and lateral epicondyles must be palpated, as they are often inflamed from tennis, golf, throwing, or other upper extremity activities. It is important to check the tinel sign at the elbow to rule out ulnar nerve pathology.

Wrist, Hand, and Fingers

When evaluating the wrist, hand, and fingers, there are a few areas to which the screener should pay particularly close attention (Table 3–17). Any pain in the snuffbox area needs to be further evaluated with x-ray.[59] The metacarpal phalangeal (MCP) joint of the thumbs must be tested for ulnar collateral stability, as it is a very common area of injury.[15] Any deformities or other abnormalities of the fingers and thumb should be evaluated by an orthopedic physician. Signs of carpal tunnel syndrome should be referred to an orthopedic physician. It is extremely important to observe the function of the entire hand and wrist area, with extensive follow-up in deficient areas.

The fingers flex, extend, abduct, and adduct. The thumb flexes, extends, abducts, and opposes. The wrist is capable of flexion, extension, radial deviation, ulnar deviation, and a combination of these motions. A quick method of wrist function testing is to have the patient actively circumduct both wrists. If their movement is bilaterally equal and within normal limits (WNLs) this should be adequate for the screening unless specific injuries or complaints exist. The forearm needs to be tested for pronation and supination. Normal joint ranges are readily available in the literature.

The strength of the finger, hand, wrist, and forearm muscles is easily tested manually but some relatively simple devices are available for more objective testing. A hand dynamometer for testing grip strength is relatively easy to use.[37] The important thing is to test the wrists using a standard protocol so the test can be

TABLE 3–16. ELBOW TESTS

Routine Test	Symptom	Follow-up
Valgus stress[22]	Laxity Pain	Tennis elbow test[23]
Varus stress[22]	Laxity Pain	Tennis elbow test[23]
Tinel[22]	Neurological Sx Pain	Neurological referral

TABLE 3–17. WRIST AND HAND TESTS

Routine Test	Symptom	Follow-up
Palpate snuffbox[21]	Pain	X-ray
Radial stress thumb MTP[37]	Pain Laxity	X-ray
Ulnar stress thumb MTP[37]	Pain Laxity	X-ray
Tinel (at the wrist)[22]	Pain Neurological symptoms	Neurological referral

repeated. We have used the position of having the arm and hand down to the athlete's side. The gripping motion should be a slow steady one rather than a quick grasp. A pinch gauge can be used to test the strength of opposition between the thumb and fingers.[37] Again, a standard protocol with careful attention to positioning should be developed and followed.[26] Supination and pronation are difficult to test but can be done manually.[22] Figure 3–7 is a hand and wrist strength evaluation form. Figure 3–8 is a form for doing the entire musculoskeletal screening.

FUNCTIONAL TESTING

The athlete should be put through a series of functional tests to determine his or her ability to receive and react to external stimuli. This ability is important in almost all sports, but some sports require individual task performance. When possible, the screener should use functional tests that are similar to the task that the athlete is required to accomplish.[26]

Any injury suffered by an athlete will reduce their proprioceptive ability. This ability can often be restored but it takes time and dedication on the athlete's part.

Testing the athlete's standing balance on one leg at a time will determine if the athlete has the ability to balance equally on both legs. The inability to balance equally is usually a good indication of a previous lower extremity injury. The athlete's balance can be tested by simply using a stop watch to time them or by using force detection platform.[53,54,60]

Athletes who have to move their legs and feet very quickly in different directions can be tested with shuttle runs, cariokas, and figures-of-eight. These can be run for speed and for accuracy.[1,24,61–64]

There are devices that test the reaction time and ability of the upper extremity.[65] This time may also be tested by having the athlete react to a moving object. Sports such as basketball, volleyball, and racket sports require quick reaction by the athlete with the upper extremities.

```
┌─────────────────────────────────────────────────────────────────────────────────┐
│  Physical Therapy Unit          Name _____     │
│  Student Health Center          SS# _____ Birthdate _____ │
│  University of WI-LaCrosse       Telephone# _____ Sex _____  │
│                                 Classification _____        │
│                                                                                   │
│  Hand and Finger Strength Evaluation                                              │
│                                                                                   │
│  Grip (Kg)        R _____    L _____                            │
│                                                                                   │
│  Pt. to stand with arm straight down at side                                      │
│                                                                                   │
│  Pinch (Kg)                                                                        │
│  Pt. to sit with elbow at 90° flex held at side and wrist neutral                 │
│                                                                                   │
│  Index      R _____      L _____                                │
│                                                                                   │
│  Middle     R _____      L _____                                │
│                                                                                   │
│  Ring       R _____      L _____                                │
│                                                                                   │
│  Little     R _____      L _____                                │
│                                                                                   │
│                                            Evaluator _____   │
└─────────────────────────────────────────────────────────────────────────────────┘
```

Figure 3–7. Hand Strength Form.

SPECIFIC SPORT CONCERNS

Each athlete is entitled to and should receive a thorough screening of all systems and body areas. There are, however, areas that warrant extra attention because of the activity in which the athlete is engaged.[17] Certain sports have inherent characteristics that lead to a high incidence of related injuries.[66] These sports may demand a more detailed evaluation of the entire athlete or just of certain areas. Some sports, due to heavy contact, high impact, and forceful collisions, are more conducive to athletic injuries. Table 3–18 lists those sports that, due to their violent nature, require the athlete to be screened with the likelihood of injury in mind. Additional time should be spent with these athletes when it comes to discussing their injury susceptibility secondary to deficiencies found in their screenings.

TABLE 3–18. HIGH-IMPACT, HEAVY-CONTACT, FORCEFUL-COLLISION SPORTS

Field Hockey
Football
Weight lifting
Wrestling
Soccer
Lacrosse
Rugby
Ice hockey
Gymnastics
Volleyball

From the American Academy of Pediatrics Policy Statement: Recommendations for participation in competitive sports. Physician Sportsmed. 1988; 16(5) and Nichols JA. Determining fitness for participation in sports. Muscle Bone. 1981; 1(2).

Table 3–19 lists some of the specific body areas that are more susceptible to injury because of the nature of the particular sport. It also shows specific injuries that are often associated with particular sports. Any athlete with a history of these injuries needs to be screened more thoroughly. Additional time must be spent with the athlete to help him or her become aware of steps that can be taken to reduce the chance of injury or reinjury.

DISSEMINATION OF INFORMATION

The information received from the evaluation is valuable for many reasons. Among its many uses are that of a data base, detector of abnormalities, a source of research data, and a determinant of proper activities for each athlete.

The data base is the most important use of the preseason screening. This is the preseason condition of the athlete's body. This includes ligament laxity, muscle strength, agility, and many other areas as presented earlier in this chapter. After an athlete sustains an injury, such as a sprained ankle, the person doing the rehabilitation with the athlete will refer to the information gathered from the screening and will attempt to return the athlete's condition to that level. The data base can also be used to determine if there is an injury present. For example, each person has a certain degree of laxity in his or her ligaments. The person doing a postinjury ligament stress test will refer to the preseason evaluation to determine if the athlete had previously had a high degree of laxity or if there is a serious injury present.

The preseason screening can also be used to detect

Physical Therapy Unit   Name _____
Student Health Center   SS# _____ Birthdate _____
University of WI-LaCrosse   Telephone# _____ Sex _____ ____
                               Classification _____

ORTHOPEDIC SCREENING FORM

Date of screening _____

Height _____ Weight _____ Balance test R _____ sec L _____ sec

Pulse recovery test: resting _____ post ex. _____ 1 min _____ 3 min _____

TRUNK—Eval by _____
    Cervical Spine _____
    _____

    Thoracic Spine _____
    _____

    Lumbar Spine _____
    _____

    Sacro Illiac _____
    _____

    Anterior Torso (sit up grade _____) _____
    _____

UPPER EXTREMITY—Eval by _____

    Pulses-Radial _____ Ulnar _____

    Reflexes- Biceps R _____ L _____, Triceps R _____ L _____
    Attach Hand & Finger Strength Eval:

    Shoulder _____
    _____

    Upper arm _____

    Elbow _____

    Forearm _____

    Wrist _____

    Hand _____

LOWER EXTREMITY—Eval by _____

    Pulses - Dorsalis pedis _____ Post tib _____

    Reflexes- Knee jerk R _____ L _____, Ankle jerk R _____ L _____
    Attach Orthotron Eval

    Hip _____

    Thigh _____

    Knee _____
    _____

    Shin _____

    Ankle _____

Figure 3–8. Orthopaedic Screening Form.

Foot _____

Gait _____

Problem areas	Recommendations

Reviewed by _____

Figure 3–8. Continued.

abnormalities in the athlete's body. If these abnormalities are serious enough, they can be corrected before they cause the athlete any problems. For example if an athlete who wishes to compete in running events has extremely pronated feet, this can cause many lower extremity problems. If the athlete is referred for a podiatric evaluation before he or she competes, these problems can be avoided.

Valuable research data can be compiled from the information gathered from the preseason evaluations. An example of this research value would be to show which sports are prone to which types of injury based upon frequency of injury occurrence. With this information, attention can be addressed to specific areas to prevent injuries.[26]

Another manner in which research can benefit is the establishment of normals. This is done by taking all of the information gathered from the evaluations and taking an average or "normal" of all the information. This "normal" can be used to determine the degree of deviance in the athlete's body. In areas such as muscle strength the normal may be used as a goal for athletes to achieve if they are deficient in a specific area.[26]

The screening can be used to recommend the sport for which a particular athlete is best suited. It should not be used to disqualify an athlete from a sport but rather to guide an athlete to a sport better suited for

him or her. For example, a student with a history of a shoulder subluxation may be better suited for a running event as opposed to playing quarterback for a football team. The shoulder subluxation does not disqualify him from playing quarterback but he may be better suited for a running sport where he would not have to put as much stress on the shoulder. In the case of the junior high and high school athlete the discussion about changes in sport or activity should include the parents.[67]

CONCLUSION

The most important aspect of preseason screening is to evaluate the athlete as thoroughly as possible with the available resources and provide the feedback to the athlete regarding his or her condition. Recommendations for follow-up and specific sport participation are often very difficult to carry out but are a vital aspect of the entire process.

The process of preseason athletic screening is quite time consuming for all of the individuals involved, from the organizer to the athlete. It is, however, worth every minute of time and every ounce of effort if one athlete is spared the agony of an injury that could and should have been prevented. Athletes spend so much

TABLE 3-19. COMMON SPORT-SPECIFIC INJURIES

Activity, Injuries	Body Area	Specific
Boxing	Hand	Fractures
Football		
Receivers	Hand	Finger injuries
Defensive back	Shoulder	Dislocation
Running backs	Knees	Sprains
	Thigh	Contusions
	Ankle	Sprains
Linemen	Neck	Pinched nerve
	Arm	Contusion
	Hand	Contusions and sprains
Wrestling	Neck	Sprains and strains
	Shoulder	Dislocation
	Low Back	Strains
Baseball		
Pitchers	Hand	Blisters
	Shoulder	Rotator cuff Strain
Catchers	Shoulder	Rotator cuff
	Hand	Finger injuries
Basketball	Ankle	Sprains
	Hand	Finger injuries
Bicycling	Back	Strain
Gymnastics	Shoulder	Sprain
	Elbow	Epycondylitis
Ice skating	Ankle	Sprain
Snow skiing	Knees	Sprain
Softball	Shoulder	Rotator cuff Strain
	Hand	Finger injuries
Handball	Ankle	Sprain
	Shoulder	Sprain
	Elbow	Epycondylitis
Racket sports	Elbow	Epicondylitis
	Wrist	Sprain
Running	Knee	Runner's knee
	Knee	Iliotibial band
	Knee	Friction
	Foot	PFPS
		Foot pain
Swimming	Shoulder	Impingement
Whip kick	Knee	MCL sprain
Golf	Back	Strain
Field weight events	Shoulder	Strain
	Upper back	Strain
High jumper	Knee	Jumper's knee

Adapted from American Academy of Pediatrics Policy Statement: Recommendations for participation in competitive sports. Phys Sportsmed. *1988; 16(5) 165–167, Committee on the Medical Aspects of Sports. Medical Evaluation of the Athlete: A guide.* Monroe Wi: American Medical Association; 1979, Stepp S, Shankman G. Fit for action: Pre-season physicals help prevent injuries. Sportscare Fitness. 1989: 2(3); 17–22, Hughston JC, Walsh WM, Puddu G, *Patellar Subluxation and Dislocation. Philadelphia, Pa: W. B. Saunders Co; 1984, Vol 5, American Academy of Orthopedic Surgeons. Athletic Training and Sports Medicine. Chicago, Ill; 1984, Brody D. Running injuries. Clin Symp. 1980; 32:4, and Zarins B, Andrews JR, Carson WG Jr.* Injuries to the throwing arm. *Philadelphia, Pa: W.B. Saunders Co; 1985.*

time and effort to reach the pinnacle of success that it is extremely hurtful when an injury takes them out of competition.

The athlete, the coach, the parents, and everyone else who is involved in the athletic program should assess the importance of proper care and prevention of athletic injuries and take the time to go about the entire process in an organized and comprehensive fashion. The excuse of not having an athletic trainer employed by the school or not having enough resources to carry out preseason screening is of little avail when an athlete sustains an injury that could have been prevented by proper screening and preparation for the athletic event. In today's atmosphere of medicolegal liability and high salaries for professional athletes, it is important that the athlete have the optimum opportunity to avoid unnecessary injuries and reach his or her potential. The first step in providing that optimum opportunity is to reduce as many injury factors as possible. It is my strong feeling that preseason screening is one very large step in the right direction.

REFERENCES

1. Fox EL, Mathews DK. *Interval Training: Conditioning for Sports and General Fitness.* London: W B Saunders Co; 1974.
2. Wisconsin Interscholastic Athletic Association. *Guide for Athletic Disqualification of Junior and Senior High Level;* 1968.
3. American Academy of Pediatrics Policy Statement: Recommendations for participation in competitive sports. *Phys Sportsmed.* 1988; 16(5).
4. Committee on the Medical Aspects of Sports. *Medical Evaluation of the Athlete: A guide.* Monroe, WI: American Medical Association; 1979.
5. Feinstein RA, Soileau ES, Daniel WA Jr. A national survey of pre-participation physical examination requirements. *Phys Sports Med.* 1988; 16(5):51–59.
6. Abdenour TH, Weir NJ. Medical assessment of the prospective student athlete. *Athlet Training.* 1986; 21(2):122,186.
7. Beranek P, Eggart JS. Pre-participation physical evaluation at University of Wisconsin–LaCrosse. *APTA Sports Med Sect Newslet.* 1976;2:1.
8. Sanders B, Eggart JS, eds. *Guidelines for Pre-season Athletic Participation Evaluation,* 2nd ed. Ad-Hoc Committee on Pre-Season Athletic Participation Evaluations.
9. Stepp S, Shankman G. Fit for action: Pre-season physicals help prevent injuries. *Sportcare Fitness* 1989; 2(3):17–22.
10. Camp International Inc, World Headquarters, Jackson Miss.

11. Novel Products Inc, P. O. Box 308, 80 Fairbanks Street, Addison, Ill.

12. Preston, J A Corp, Back-Leg-Chest Dynamometer, 60 Page Road, Clifton, NJ.

13. Nichols JA. Determining fitness for participation in sports. *Muscle Bone.* 1981:1(2).

14. Allman FL, Garrick JG, Marshall JL, et al. The pre-participation physical examination. *Phys Sportsmed.* 1974; 2(8):26–27,29.

15. Ryan AJ: *Medical Care of the Athlete.* Academic Press New York, NY 1962:36–40.

16. Roundtable: The office examination of the athlete. *Phys Sportsmed.* 1976;4(10):90–91,99.

17. Bonci CM, Ryan R. Pre-participation screening in intercollegiate athletics. Postgrad *Adv Sports Med.* 1988:3–6.

18. Gilroy J, Holiday P. *Basic Neurology.* New York, NY: Macmillan Publishing Co Inc; 1982.

19. Simpson J, Magee K. *Clinical Evaluation of the Nervous System.* Boston, Mass: Little, Brown, and Co; 1973.

20. Hollingshead WH, Jenkins DB. *Functional Anatomy of the Limbs and Back*, 5th ed. Philadelphia, Pa: W B Saunders Co; 1981.

21. Hoppenfeld S. *Physical Examination of the Spine and Extremities.* New York, NY: Appleton-Century-Crofts; 1976.

22. Magee DJ. *Orthopedic Physical Assessment.* Philadelphia, Pa: W B Saunders Co; 1987.

23. Wadsworth C: *Manual Examination and Treatment of the Spine and Extremities.* Baltimore, Md: Williams & Wilkins; 1988.

24. DeVries HA. *Physiology of Exercise for Physical Education and Athletics.* Dubuque, Ia: William C Brown Group; 1968.

25. Noble BJ. *Physiology of Exercise and Sport.* St. Louis, Mo: Times Mirror/Mosby College Publishing; 1986:95–150, 229–250.

26. Hunter SC. Getting the most out of the preseason physical exam. *J Musculoskeletal Med.* 1985; 2(8):13–21.

27. Doxey GE, Fairbanks B, Housch T, et al. Body composition: I. Scientific considerations. *Nat Strength Condit Assoc J.* 1987; 9(3):12–26.

28. Basccardin J, Schneider H, Shapiro R, et al. Human body composition measurement: A skin fold method. *Sports Care Fitness.* 1988; 1(5):11–13.

29. Jackson AS, Pollock M. Practical assessment of body composition. *Phys Sports Med.* 1985; 13(5):76–89.

30. Johnson BL, Nelson JK. *Practical Measurements for Evaluation in Physical Education.* Minneapolis, Minn: Burgess Publishing Co; 1979.

31. Cramer Products Inc, P.O. Box 1001, Gardner, Ks.

32. SKyndex: A measure of fitness. *First Aider.* 1982; 51(8):1–6.

33. Clark M, Stanforth P, Leduc D. et al. Body composition: II. Practical considerations. *Natl Strength Condit Assoc J.* 1987; 9(4):10–20.

34. Subotnik SI: *Cures for Common Running Injuries.* Mountain View, Calif: World Publications Inc; 1979.

35. Blake RL, Ross AS, Volmassy RL. Biomechanic gait evaluation. *Podiatr Sports Med.* 1981; 71:6.

36. Rancho Los Amigos Hospital. *Normal and Pathological Gait Syllabus.* Downey, Calif: Rancho Los Amigos Hospital; 1978; 2–5.

37. Roy S, Irvin R. *Sports Medicine: Prevention, Evaluation, Management, and Rehabilitation.* Englewood Cliffs, NJ: Prentice-Hall Inc; 1983.

38. Gould JA, Davies GJ. *Orthopedic and Sports Physical Therapy*, 2nd ed. St. Louis, Mo: C V Mosby Co; 1985.

39. Kendall HO, Kendall FP, Boynton DA: Posture and Pain. Huntington, NY: K E Krieger Publishing Co Inc; 1977.

40. Saunders DH. *Evaluation, Treatment, and Prevention of Musculoskeletal Disorders.* Minneapolis, Minn: Viking Press Inc; 1985.

41. American Academy of Orthopedic Surgeons; *Joint Motion: Method of Measuring and Recording*, Chicago, Ill: 1965.

42. Hughston JC, Walsh WM, Puddu G. *Patellar Subluxation and Dislocation.* Philadelphia, Pa: W B Saunders Co; 1984, vol 5.

43. Daniels L. Worthingham C. Muscle Testing: Techniques of Manual Examination, 5th ed. Philadelphia, Pa: W B Saunders Co; 1986.

44. Kendall FP, McCreary EK: *Muscles: Testing and Functions*, 3rd ed. Baltimore, Md: Williams & Wilkins; 1983.

45. Biodex Corp, 32 Chichester Avenue, P.O. Box 656, Center Moriches, NY.

46. Chattecx Corporation, Kin-Com, 101 Memorial Drive, P.O. Box 4287, Chattanooga, Tenn.

47. Lumex Inc, Cybex Division. *Cybex II Testing Protocol.* Bay Shore, NY: Lumex Inc; 1975.

48. Mini-Gym Inc. *Isokinetic Exerciser by Mini-Gym: Operation Manual for Models.* Independence, Mo: Mini-Gym Inc; 1979; 101:180–500.

49. Portable Isokinetics, 3522 Lousma Drive Southeast, Grand Rapids, Mich.

50. Birnbaum J. *The Musculoskeletal Manual.* New York, NY: Academic Press Inc; 1982.

51. Kulund DN. *The Injured Athlete.* Philadelphia, Pa: J B Lippincott Co; 1982.

52. Kimura IF, Navoczenski D, Epier M, Owen M. Effect of the air stirrup in controlling ankle inversion stress. *J Orthopaed Sports Phys Ther.* 1987; 9(5):190–193.

53. ExerDyn, P.O. Box 1144, Rockford, Ill.

54. Regency Medical Co, 2847 North 74th Avenue, Elmwood Park, Ill.

55. McRae R. *Clinical Orthopedic Examination.* New York, NY: Churchill Livingstone; 1976.

56. Cailliet R. *Foot and Ankle Pain.* Philadelphia, Pa: F A Davis Co; 1976.

57. Zarins B, Andrews JR, Carson WG Jr. *Injuries to the Throwing Arm.* Philadelphia, Pa: WB Saunders Co.; 1985.

58. Cyriax J. *Textbook of Orthopedic Medicine: Treatment by Manipulation, Massage, and Injection.* 8th ed. Baltimore, Mo: Williams & Wilkins Co; 1974.

59. Booker JM, Thibodeau GA. *Athletic Injury Assessment.* St. Louis, Mo: Times Mirror/Mosby College Publishing; 1985.

60. Cailliet R. *Scoliosis Diagnosis and Management.* Philadelphia, Pa: F A Davis Co; 1975.

61. Appenzeller O, Atkinson R. *Sports Medicine: Fitness-*

Training-Injuries, 2nd ed. Baltimore, Md: Urban and Schwarzenberg; 1983.

62. Dunnam LO, Hunter GR, Willions BP, et al. Comprehensive evaluation of the University of Alabama at Birmingham women's volleyball training program. *Nat Strength Condit Assoc J* 1988; 19(1):43–49.

63. Pate RR. A new definition of youth fitness. *Phys Sportsmed.* 1983; 11:77–83.

64. Wilmore JH. Athletic Training and Physical Fitness. Boston, Mass: Allyn and Bacon Inc; 1978.

65. AcuVision Systems Inc, 355 Lexington Avenue, Suite 200, New York, NY.

66. D'Ambrosia RD. *Prevention and Treatment of Running Injuries.* Thorofare, NJ. Charles B Slack Inc; 1982.

67. Baxter JA. A comprehensive pre-participation program. *First Aider* 1986; 56(1):1–5.

68. Knight KL. Testing anterior cruciate ligaments. *Phys Sportsmed.* 1980; 8(5):37–42.

69. Carr JH, Shepard RB. *Physiotherapy in Disorders of the Brain.* London: William Heinemann Medical Books; 1980.

4

Emergency Care and on-the-Field Management

Michael Voight

INTRODUCTION

During the past decade, there has been a sharp rise in the number of people participating in sporting activities. This is in part due to the increased public awareness of health issues and the benefits of regular physical fitness. With increased sports participation and more strenuous competition come an increased incidence of sports injuries. Fortunately, most injuries occurring in sport are not characterized as emergency situations requiring immediate decision making. Improvements in both training techniques and equipment as well as increased awareness as to the inherent risks of athletic participation have helped to reduce the number of emergency situations. Life-threatening emergencies, however, can and do happen in athletics and the medical staff must be prepared to deal with this situation when it arises. No amount of preparation can completely eliminate the possibility of a life-threatening injury from occurring.

When an athlete becomes injured, the initial on-the-field and sideline evaluation is an extremely important step in the overall management of the injury. Although most physical therapists are comfortable dealing with musculoskeletal disorders on a regular basis, it is important that they also become proficient in dealing with life-threatening conditions in the event they are faced with an emergency situation. The severity of a life-threatening emergency can be reduced considerably if the possibility of such an occurrence is anticipated. Prompt recognition of an emergency situation and appropriate initial treatment maximizes the athlete's chance for recovery. Prior knowledge of what to do and proper preparation by the medical staff will result in prompt and effective care.

It must always be kept in mind that the ultimate goal of injury management is the return of the injured athlete to action as soon and as safely as possible. This requires early recognition and an accurate diagnosis. The most important step in providing emergency care to the injured athlete is the initial evaluation of the injury. Emergency care revolves around the maintenance of cardiovascular function because failure within this system can lead to death. Due to the seriousness of cardiovascular injury, the evaluation must be performed as swiftly and accurately as possible to ensure prompt delivery of aid. Further injury or death can result if immediate evaluation and delivery of care are delayed.

When injury occurs and the medical staff is called to the scene, it is important to determine the mechanism of the injury. Certain injuries are considered common to various situations because they are the injuries most often produced. Always remember that for every obvious injury there may be a number of hidden injuries. Obvious injuries do not always present as a life-threatening situation, whereas hidden injuries can quickly become fatal if they go undetected. Emergency care that is based only on the observation and treatment of obvious injuries is dangerous. Consider the situation in which a basketball player has just fallen to the floor, striking his head. The only obvious injury at this time is a bleeding laceration on the forehead. The sports physical therapist rushes to the athlete to dress and bandage what appears to be a serious head injury. In treating the laceration, however, the therapist turns the athlete's head to one side, causing broken vertebral segments to impinge on and sever the spinal cord. Due to a hurried approach and obvious neglect of screening for hidden injury, the athlete is now confined to a wheelchair for the remainder of his life. If the sports therapist had realized that the forehead laceration was not a life-threatening condition and taken a few additional minutes to properly evaluate the athlete, this situation could have been avoided. Therefore, following injury, the athlete should be evaluated right where

the injury occurred. If serious injury is suspected, the examination should be conducted without moving the athlete.

EMERGENCY EVALUATION

Emergency evaluation of the injured athlete centers around prompt and accurate recognition of the site and severity of the injury. This initial assessment of the athlete not only establishes the type and severity of the injury, but also helps formulate the initial plan of care. It is imperative that the initial evaluation be made at the time of injury before the signs and symptoms become masked due to pain and swelling. To accurately evaluate the injured athlete, the sports physical therapist must have a good working knowledge of the anatomy in the injured region. A comprehensive assessment involves the isolation and evaluation of each anatomic structure suspected of being at fault. By having a good understanding of the underlying anatomic structures, the sports physical therapist can develop an organized and systematic sequence of evaluation that will reduce the chance of error in the examination.

To a great extent, successful emergency care is also dependent upon the evaluation of the athlete's vital signs and overall injury. The examiner's ability to recognize basic physiological vital signs is imperative when dealing with life-threatening conditions. The vital signs measure the ability of the body to support essential bodily functions. Interpreting the signs and symptoms correctly is the basis for differentiating life-threatening from non-life-threatening conditions.

Diagnostic Signs and Symptoms

It is extremely important that the sports physical therapist be able to recognize the basic physiological signs and symptoms of an injury: breathing/respiration, pulse, blood pressure, body temperature, skin color, pupil diameter, and the ability to move (Table 4–1).

Breathing/Respiration. The rate at which a person breathes in and out can be indicative of an injury. The normal respiration rate in adults is 12 breaths per minute. In children it is approximately 20 to 25 breaths per minute. Normal respirations should be painfree and

TABLE 4-1. DIAGNOSTIC SIGNS AND SYMPTOMS

Breathing
Pulse
Blood pressure
Temperature
Skin color
Pupil diameter
Ability to move

without effort. It is important to observe the pattern of breathing to determine possible pathology. Shallow breathing can indicate shock whereas irregular gasping for air could indicate cardiovascular impairment.

Pulse. The normal pulse rate for adults ranges between 60 and 80 beats per minute, and in children is 80 to 100 beats per minute. The highly trained athlete will usually have a lower pulse rate than normal, however.

An alteration in the pulse rate may indicate the presence of injury. When palpating a pulse, note the following: rhythm, strength, and rate. Possible findings can include a rapid weak pulse, which is indicative of shock or heat exhaustion. A rapid strong pulse could mean heatstroke whereas no pulse means cardiac arrest.

Blood Pressure. Blood pressure is an index of the efficiency of the complete cardiovascular system. Blood pressure normally varies with the age and sex of the individual. The usual guideline for systolic pressure in men is 100 plus the individual's age up to 140 to 150 mm Hg. Normal diastolic pressure in men is 60 to 90 mm Hg. Both the systolic and diastolic pressures are approximately 10 mm Hg lower in women. A lowered blood pressure can indicate possible shock or heart attack. Hypertension will produce higher than normal pressure readings.

Temperature. Changes in body temperature should alert the sports therapist to possible injury or illness. An athlete whose temperature is low may be suffering from shock or hypothermia. A high temperature can be indicative of illness with fever or heat illness.

Skin temperature will rise when the blood vessels lying near the skin dilate. When the blood vessels constrict, the temperature will fall. High environmental temperatures cause the vessels to dilate, whereas shock will cause them to constrict. Therefore, hot, dry skin is indicative of excessive body heat whereas cold, damp skin is present with shock.

Skin Color. The color of the skin reflects the circulation immediately underlying the skin as well as the oxygen saturation of the blood. In lightly pigmented individuals, skin color is a very good indicator of health. The colors red, white, and blue are commonly associated with medical emergencies. A red skin color indicates a lack of oxygen and is associated with heat stroke and high blood pressure. Pale, white skin indicates insufficient circulation and is associated with shock, hemorrhage, and heat exhaustion. A bluish tint to the skin is indicative of poorly oxygenated circulating blood. This can be present with airway obstruction or heart attack.

In the case of darkly pigmented individuals, color changes will not be readily evident in the skin but may be assessed by examining the fingernail beds, the mucous membranes of the eyes, or the tissue beneath the tongue. A healthy black athlete should normally display a pinkish color in the nailbeds, lips, and mucous membranes around the mouth. This same individual in shock from the lack of oxygen will not exhibit the same color changes as the white athlete. The skin surrounding the nose and mouth will display a gray cast. The mucous membranes will be blue and the nailbeds and lips will also have a blue tinge. If the shock is due to bleeding, the mucous membranes in the mouth and tongue will not appear blue but will have a pale, grayish, waxy pallor.

Pupils. The pupils of the eyes are sensitive to changes within the nervous system. Normally, the pupils are round, regular in outline, equal, and reactive to light. Dilation of the pupils occur with unconsciousness, pain, deficient oxygen in the blood, brain injury, cardiac arrest, shock, and with the use of certain medications. Although unequal pupil diameter is present in approximately 3% of the population, athletes who have sustained a head injury may have unequal pupil size due to swelling of the brain tissues. A constricted pupil should alert the sports therapist to the fact that the athlete may be using drugs or medications that act on the central nervous system.

Ability to Move. The ability or inability to move a body segment can be indicative of a serious central nervous system injury. Paralysis can occur with spinal injuries. Cerebrospinal accident or head injury can cause the inability to move one side of the body.

PRIMARY SURVEY

The evaluation of the injured athlete can be broken down into two separate mini-assessments—the primary and secondary surveys.

The primary survey is the evaluation of the basic life support mechanisms—airway, breathing, and circulation (Table 4–2). These three mechanisms are usually referred to as the ABCs of life support. Insufficiency of any of the ABCs is potentially a life-threatening situation. The primary survey should be completed swiftly, in many cases before reaching the scene of the injured athlete. If the athlete is conscious

TABLE 4–2. PRIMARY SURVEY

Airway
Breathing
Circulation

and talking, it can safely be assumed that adequate breathing and circulation are present. If the athlete is unconscious, the primary assessment must be conducted swiftly. Decision making on the field should be conducted rapidly following the assessment of respiration and pulse (Fig 4–1).

The unconscious athlete is the most difficult problem facing the sports physical therapist. Due to the inability to communicate with the athlete, this presents an unusual situation that requires an accurate sequence of evaluation. The most common cause of unconsciousness is traumatic head injury. Other medical conditions such as heat stroke and diabetes can also lead to unconsciousness (Figs 4–2, 4–3). Because the exact nature of the problem will not be apparent initially, it is imperative that a systematic approach be employed. Signs and symptoms need to be quickly evaluated so that emergency care can be initiated immediately. In addition to the suspected head injury, the unconscious athlete should always be suspected of having cervical pathology until proven otherwise.

The airway can be obstructed by anything that blocks the passage of air into the lungs. Although foreign objects such as gum or tobacco can block the airway, the most common obstruction is the tongue in the unconscious athlete. The muscles that control the lower jaw and tongue relax. With forward flexion of the neck the mandible will sag. As the tongue is attached to the mandible, it drops against the back of the pharynx and blocks the opening to the trachea (Fig 4–4). Because oxygen is the fuel for all cells within the body, restoration of an adequate airway is a priority. Cells of the brain and nervous system may die within 4 to 6 minutes after being deprived of oxygen.

Restoration of the airway can be accomplished by moving the mandible forward, thereby lifting the tongue away from the back of the pharynx. There are methods that will create a forward motion of the mandible:

1. *Head tilt–neck lift.* This is the most common method for opening an airway. The neck is lifted with one hand while the forehead is pressed downward with the other. This maneuver will extend the neck and lift the tongue from the back of the pharynx (Fig 4–5).
2. *Head tilt–chin lift.* This maneuver is similar to the neck lift; however, instead of lifting the neck, the therapist brings the mandible forward with the tips of his or her fingers (Fig 4–6).
3. *Jaw thrust without head tilt.* Whenever a cervical injury is suspected, movement of the cervical spine must be avoided. The jaw thrust can be accomplished by placing the fingers of each hand behind the angles of the athlete's lower

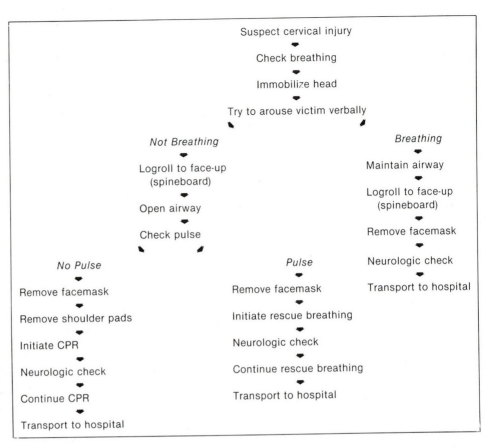

Figure 4–1. Field decision making—Head and neck injuries (unconscious athlete). *(From Torg Joseph S. Athletic Injuries to the Head Neck and Face. Philadelphia, Pa: Lea & Febiger; 1982, with permission.)*

jaw. The mandible should be brought forward without tilting the head back (Fig 4–7).

Once the tongue has been lifted away from the pharynx, the athlete may begin spontaneous breathing again. If no air exchange is noted following proper airway positioning, the rescuer should attempt to force four quick breaths into the athlete's mouth. Lack of air exchange now will indicate an occluded airway. If the object is visible, the airway can be cleared with a finger sweep. If this fails to open the airway, the American Heart Association (AHA) method of back blows and chest thrusts should be used until the airway is cleared. If spontaneous breathing does not resume, immediate steps to ventilate the athlete's lungs artificially must be undertaken.

There are many techniques of artificial ventilation, including mouth-to-mouth, mouth-to-nose, and mouth-to-adjunct ventilation or ventilation with a mechanical device. After the four initial quick breaths, the athlete's breathing and pulse should be observed. If he or she is still not breathing, but there is a pulse present, provide one breath every 5 seconds (approximately 12 per minute). Observe the athlete's chest rise and fall with each ventilation as well as listen and feel the air escape during passive exhalation.

There are a few sports (i.e., football) in which the athletes wear helmets with face masks. Because the face mask will interfere with the administration of artificial ventilation, a special plan of action should be available and practiced to deal with the situation. The helmet should not be removed until cervical spine injury has been completely ruled out. Face mask removal depends on the type of face mask used. If the helmet has a hinged face mask, a sharp knife can be used to cut the plastic mounts, thereby releasing the mask. In many cases, the face mask is permanently fixed to the helmet. In this situation, a pair of bolt cutters is required to cut through the mask (Fig 4–8). These should therefore always be available on the sidelines in the event of an emergency.

A more common respiratory emergency in athletes is difficult or labored breathing, called dyspnea. This is most often the result of hyperventilation or breathing that is deeper or more rapid than normal. Hyperventilation can be a psychological response to fear, pain, and trauma. The hyperventilating athlete may become terrified at the inability to get sufficient air into the lungs. The skin does not appear cyanotic, as would be expected with respiratory distress. Instead, the skin appears a healthy pink due to over-oxygenation. Hyperventilation flushes the carbon dioxide (CO_2) from the lungs, which will reduce the CO_2 circulating in the blood. Eventually the decrease of CO_2 and the increase of oxygen (O_2) reaching the respiratory control center causes the breathing process to slow down and stop if the O_2–CO_2 balance is not restored. The athlete may feel dizziness, faint feelings, chest pains, and numbness

Category	Problem	Cause	Pathophysiology	Management
General	Loss of consciousness	Injury or disease	Shock, head injury, other injuries, diabetes, arteriosclerosis	Need for CPR, triage
Diseases	Diabetic coma	Hyperglycemia and acidosis	Inadequate use of sugar, acidosis	Complex treatment for acidosis
	Insulin shock	Hypoglycemia	Excess insulin	Sugar
	Myocardial infarct	Damaged myocardium	Insufficient cardiac output	O_2, CPR, transport
	Stroke	Damaged brain	Loss of arterial supply to brain or hemorrhage within brain	Support, gentle transport
Injury	Hemorrhagic shock	Bleeding	Hypovolemia	Control external bleeding, recognize internal bleeding, CPR, transport
	Respiratory shock	Insufficient O_2	Paralysis, chest damage, airway obstruction	Clear airway, supplemental O_2, CPR, transport
	Anaphylactic shock	Acute contact with agent to which patient is sensitive	Allergic reaction	Intramuscular, epinephrine, support, CPR, transport
	Cerebral contusion, concussion or hematoma	Blunt head injury	Bleeding into or around brain, concussive effect	Airway, supplemental O_2, CPR, careful monitoring, transport
Emotions	Psychogenic shock	Emotional reaction	Sudden drop in cerebral blood flow	Place supine, make comfortable, observe for injuries
Environment	Heatstroke	Excessive heat, inability to sweat	Brain damage from heat	Immediate cooling, support, CPR, transport
	Electric shock	Contact with electric current	Cardiac abnormalities, fibrillation	CPR, transport, do not treat until current controlled
	Systemic hypothermia	Prolonged exposure to cold	Diminished cerebral function, cardiac arrhythmias	CPR, rapid transport, warming at hospital
	Drowning	O_2, CO_2, breath holding, H_2O	Cerebral damage	CPR, transport
	Air embolism	Intravascular air	Obstruction to arterial blood flow by nitrogen bubbles	CPR, recompression
	Decompression sickness ("bends")	Intravascular nitrogen	Obstruction to arterial blood flow by nitrogen bubbles	CPR, recompression
Injected or ingested agents	Alcohol	Excess intake	Cerebral depression	Support, CPR, transport
	Drugs	Excess intake	Cerebral depression	Support, CPR, transport (bring drug)
	Plant poisons	Contact, ingestion	Direct cerebral or other toxic effect	Support, recognition, CPR, identify plant, local wound care, transport
	Animal poisons	Contact, ingestion, injection	Direct cerebral or other toxic effect	Recognition, support, CPR, identify agent, local wound care, transport
Neurological	Epilepsy	Brain injury, scar, genetic predisposition, disease	Excitable focus of motor activity in brain	Support, protect patient transport in status epilepticus

Figure 4-2. Causes of unconsciousness in the athlete. (*From AAOS. Athletic Training and Sports Medicine. AAOS: Chicago, Ill; 1985, with permission.*)

Functional Signs	Selected Conditions						
	Fainting	Concussion	Grand Mal Epilepsy	Brain Compression and Injury	Sunstroke	Diabetic Coma	Shock
Onset	Usually sudden	Usually sudden	Sudden	Usually gradual	Gradual or sudden	Gradual	Gradual
Mental	Complete unconsciousness	Confusion or unconsciousness	Unconsciousness	Unconsciousness gradually deepening	Delirium or unconsciousness	Drowsiness, later unconsciousness	Listlessness, later unconsciousness
Pulse	Feeble and fast	Feeble and irregular	Fast	Gradually slower	Fast and feeble	Fast and feeble	Fast and very feeble
Respiration	Quick and shallow	Shallow and irregular	Noisy, later deep and slow	Slow and noisy	Difficult	Deep and sighing	Rapid and shallow with occasional deep sigh
Skin	Pale, cold and clammy	Pale and cold	Livid, later pale	Hot and flushed	Very hot and dry	Livid, later pale	Pale, cold, and clammy
Pupils	Equal and dilated	Equal	Equal and dilated	Unequal	Equal	Equal	Equal and dilated
Paralysis	None	None	None	May be present in leg and/or arm	None	None	None
Convulsions	None	None	None	Present in some cases	Present in some cases	None	None
Breath	N/A	N/A	N/A	N/A	N/A	Acetone smell	N/A
Special features	Giddiness and sway before collapse	Signs of head injury, vomiting on recovery	Bites tongue, voids urine and feces, may injure self on falling	Signs of head injury, delayed onset of symptoms	Vomiting in some cases	In early stages, headache, restlessness, and nausea	May vomit, early stages shivering, thirst, defective vision, and ear noises

Figure 4-3. Evaluating the unconscious athlete. (*From Arnheim, Daniel D.* Modern Principles of Athletic Training, *ed. 7. St. Louis, Mo: Times Mirror/Mosby College Publishing, with permission.) (Modified from International medical guide for ships, World Health Organization, Geneva, Switzerland.)*

and tingling into the extremities. The athlete should be treated in a calm manner and encouraged to relax and slow the breathing pattern. To help increase the CO_2 level in the bloodstream, the athlete should breathe into a paper bag. The bag should be positioned over the athlete's mouth and nose so that only expired air is breathed into the bag. The additional CO_2 in the trapped air will enter the bloodstream and stimulate the respiratory control center, thereby restoring a normal pattern of breathing.

An obstructed airway can quickly lead to respiratory arrest. This condition in turn will lead to cardiac arrest and certain death if proper first aid measures are not initiated immediately. Cardiac function and sys-

temic circulation can be evaluated by palpating a pulse. When cardiac arrest occurs, blood pressure cannot be measured nor can a pulse be felt. The carotid artery in the neck is the most commonly used artery to check for a pulse in an emergency situation. If the athlete does not exhibit a pulse, appropriate emergency techniques of artificial circulation should be initiated immediately by one or two rescuers. If respiratory arrest was not the cause of the cardiac arrest, respirations will stop within 15 to 30 seconds. The pupils begin to dilate 30 to 40 seconds after the cessation of circulation, and within 2 minutes become completely dilated. The brain cells begin to die, and generally within 10 minutes biologic death occurs if cardiopulmonary resuscita-

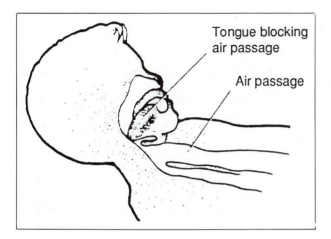

Figure 4-4. Blocked passageway. When the neck is in flexion (chin down on chest) the tongue falls back into the throat and obstructs the airway. *(From AAOS.* Athletic Training and Sports Medicine. *AAOS: Chicago, Ill; 1985, with permission.)*

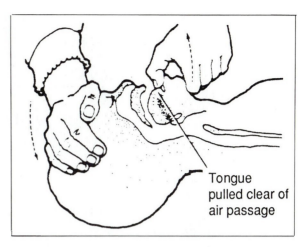

Figure 4-6. Head tilt–chin lift. While tilting the head backward with one hand, lift the chin forward with the fingers of the other. *(From AAOS.* Athletic Training and Sports Medicine. *AAOS: Chicago, Ill; 1985, with permission.)*

tion (CPR) measures are not initiated. Therefore, it is essential that every sports physical therapist have an excellent working knowledge of CPR techniques.

Shock

Within the medical profession, the term shock is used to describe the failure of the cardiovascular system to provide sufficient circulation and perfusion of blood. Shock occurs when there is a reduced amount of fluid available to the circulatory system. The result of this reduction in fluid is a relative loss of oxygen carrying blood cells.

Shock can be caused in three ways: (1) the heart is damaged so that it fails to perform properly; (2) blood loss via hemorrhage will result in a decreased volume of fluid within the system; and (3) blood vessel dilation causes the blood to pool in the now larger vessels, so that although there is enough volume of blood present, it does not circulate throughout the cardiovascular system. The net results of shock are the same regardless of

the cause: there is a reduced amount of fluid available within the cardiovascular system. This results in poor or inadequate oxygen perfusion through the body's tissues.

There are several different types of shock, all of which are related to one of the three major causes. The following are the most common types of shock:

1. *Hypovolemic shock.* Hypovolemic shock is due to blood loss. There are a number of causes, including both internal and external bleeding, crushing injuries to the blood vessel, and burns, all of which allow large amounts of plasma to escape. A decrease in the volume results in poor circulation and shock.
2. *Respiratory shock.* If breathing becomes impaired, shock can be produced because the amount of oxygen in the blood is insufficient. With this type of shock, both the volume of blood and the function of the heart are normal,

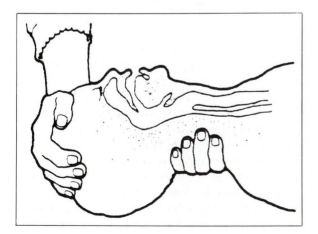

Figure 4-5. Head tilt–neck lift, further opening the airway. *(From AAOS.* Athletic Training and Sports Medicine. *AAOS: Chicago, Ill; 1985, with permission.)*

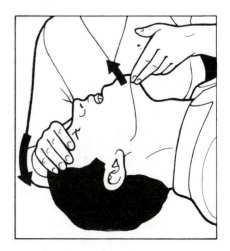

Figure 4-7. Jaw-thrust maneuver. *(From the American Red Cross, CPR manual. 1988, with permission.)*

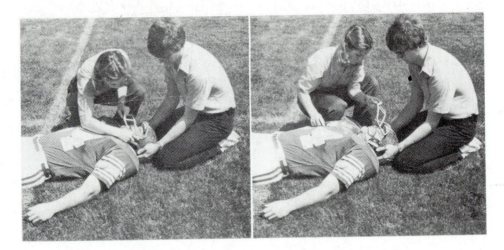

Figure 4–8. Removal of face mask. *(From Booher JM, Thibodeau GA.* Athletic Injury Assessment. *St. Louis, Mo: Times Mirror/Mosby College Publishing; 1985, with permission.)*

but the oxygen exchange in the lungs is poor and results in poorly oxygenated blood.

3. *Neurogenic shock.* Loss of the nervous system control of the blood vessels can result in shock due to increased dilation of the relaxed vessels. When this happens, the available fluid no longer can fill the system and failure results.

4. *Psychogenic shock.* This type of shock is the result of a sudden reaction of the nervous system with momentary vascular dilation. This results in a momentary interruption of blood to the brain and fainting ensues. Once the individual collapses and becomes supine, circulation to the brain is restored and the athlete recovers. Fainting can usually be prevented by lowering the head before loss of consciousness. Sitting the athlete down and placing the head between the knees will lower the head sufficiently.

5. *Cardiogenic shock.* Cardiogenic shock is caused by an inadequate functioning heart. When the heart can no longer develop the pressure required to move the blood to all parts of the body, circulation becomes impaired and shock results.

6. *Metabolic shock.* In athletes with severe illness that results in fluid loss from vomiting, diarrhea, and excessive urination, shock occurs as a result of the loss of body fluids and resultant changes in body chemistry. Metabolic shock is rarely encountered and is usually present in the end stages of chronic illness.

7. *Anaphylactic shock.* Anaphylactic shock occurs when individuals come in contact with something to which they are extremely allergic. It is the most severe form of allergic reaction. The most common causes of anaphylactic shock are insect stings, which produce rapid and severe reaction, ingested substances, which produce a slower but severe reaction, inhalation of sub-

stances, and injected substances such as anti-toxins or drugs.

Unless quickly recognized and treated, shock can lead to death. The most important indication of the possibility of shock is the presence of severe injury. Shock can develop rapidly or over the course of several hours. The progression of shock follows a continuous cycle (Fig 4–9) producing various signs and symptoms:

1. Weak and rapid pulse
2. Pale, moist, and cool skin
3. Shallow and rapid respirations
4. Profuse sweating
5. Nausea or vomiting
6. Dilated pupils in dull, lackluster eyes
7. A marked decrease in blood pressure

As soon as the sports physical therapist recognizes the signs and symptoms of shock, treatment must be started right away. The treatment of shock takes priority over all other emergency care, with the exception of the ABCs and control of profuse bleeding. If recognized quickly and treated appropriately, shock can be reversed. Recognizing the probable cause of shock allows the treatment to be appropriately directed. The steps to be taken when controlling shock are as follows:

1. Ensure adequate breathing: A secure clear airway must be maintained to allow passage of oxygen.
2. Control bleeding: Control all obvious bleeding using direct pressure over the site. We must prevent blood loss.
3. Elevate the lower extremities: Raising the lower extremities by 12 to 18 inches can improve circulation. Do not raise the feet in cases of head, spinal, or abdominal injury because this will lead to increased pressure in those areas, which is undesirable. If there is

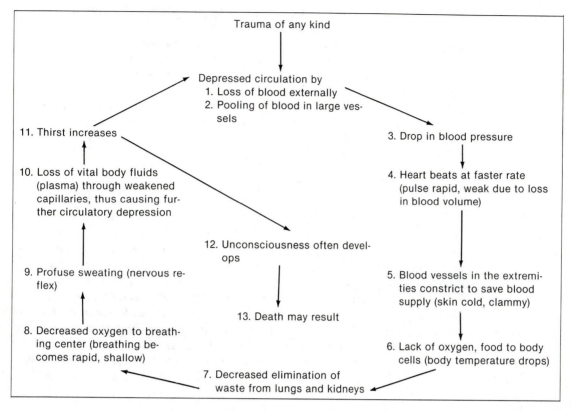

Figure 4-9. Cycle of traumatic shock. *(From Brennan WT, Ludwig DJ. Guide to Problems and Practices in First-Aid and Emergency Care, 3rd ed. Dubuque, Ia; W C Brown Co; 1976, with permission.)*

doubt as to the best position, leave the athlete lying flat.

4. Keep the athlete lying down. This will minimize stress to the circulatory system.
5. Splint fractures. This will slow down the bleeding and reduce the pain and discomfort, both of which aggravate shock.
6. Loosen or remove any pieces of clothing/uniform that may interfere with breathing or circulation.
7. Prevent loss of body heat. Keep the athlete warm but prevent overheating.
8. Avoid rough and excessive handling.
9. Give nothing by mouth.
10. Administer oxygen.
11. Record information: initial vital signs and at 5-minute intervals until emergency personnel arrive or upon reaching medical facility.

Anaphylactic shock occurs within minutes following contact with the allergic substance and should be considered as a life-threatening condition. The most reliable information concerning anaphylactic shock will come from the athlete. The following are the major signs of anaphylactic reaction:

1. Flushed skin that has an itching or burning sensation

2. Cyanosis about the lips
3. Tightness about the chest with difficulty in breathing
4. A rapid drop in blood pressure
5. A weak or imperceptible pulse
6. Dizziness
7. Fainting and coma

Anaphylactic shock is a true medical emergency because it requires the immediate subcutaneous, intramuscular (IM), or intravenous (IV) injection of medication to combat the allergic response. The injection of 0.5 to 1.0 mL of 1:1000 epinephrine will usually alleviate the anaphylactic response. In many cases, the athlete will already be aware of his or her allergy and have available an anaphylactic kit with preloaded syringes with epinephrine. Assist the athlete in administering the injection and be ready to repeat the injection should the symptoms recur and the athlete's condition worsen. The athlete should be immediately transported to a medical facility for complete checkup and continued treatment.

SECONDARY SURVEY

Once all basic life support systems have been screened and stabilized, the secondary survey should be initi-

ated. This is the portion of the examination that attempts to recognize and define all remaining injuries that may be present. When dealing with sports-related injuries, the secondary survey usually takes up the greatest portion of the total examination because life-threatening conditions are rare. Throughout the secondary survey the exact nature, location, and severity of the athletic injury is assessed. Athletes with musculoskeletal lesions will usually have complaints of both pain and dysfunction. Immediately postinjury is a "golden" period for examination because muscle spasm that would limit stress testing has not yet occurred. In addition, intraarticular effusion which may limit motion is not yet present.

The secondary survey consists of six basic components: history, observation, palpation, neurological testing, movement testing, and stress testing (Table 4–3). The type of injury will determine which components of the secondary survey to include in the examination. The severity of the injury will dictate if the examination is made at the initial site of injury or after the athlete has been removed from the field of play. In all likelihood, a quick screening will be performed at the site of injury looking for obvious injury and then a more thorough examination conducted on the sidelines once the athlete has been moved from the playing field.

History

The subjective portion of the secondary survey is the information gained from the athlete about what happened. The examiner must find out as much detailed information as possible about the mechanism of injury. This information will provide valuable clues as to the possible structures injured and serve to guide the remaining objective evaluation.

When conducting the history it is important to keep the line of questioning simple and concise. Most athletes when confronted with an injury are frightened and not willing to carry on a long conversation concerning their condition. By asking one directed question at a time, meaningful information can be obtained. Clarify the information that is gathered and then ask questions that will provide further essential information. It is important that the examiner remain calm and reassuring towards the athlete. Because each injury situation is different, it is very important that the sports physical therapist develop good history-taking skills and questions that can be used in the many different situations.

The key information to be obtained in the history portion of the examination centers around the athlete's primary or chief complaint. Where does it hurt? How did the injury occur? The examiner should try to recreate the mechanism of the injury and visualize the position of the injured region at the time of injury. Location of the pain is important in determining the possible structures involved. Be as exact as possible when determining the anatomic location. Once the anatomic location has been determined, the examiner should formulate in his or her mind the structures lying under the skin and other structures that can possibly refer pain to this region. The location of pain merely indicates the segment within which the examiner must look for the lesion.

Observation

The observation portion of the examination begins with the examiner's first contact with the injured athlete and will continue throughout the entire evaluation process. The examiner attempts to gather clues as to the nature of the injury. The entire scene surrounding the athlete should be screened. What was the position of the athlete upon arrival? Look for obvious signs of trauma such as bleeding, deformity, or swelling.

After a general survey of the athlete has been completed, the injured region is then inspected. Quite often this step occurs simultaneously with the history-taking process. Clothing and equipment that cover the injured region must be removed to allow for adequate visualization. Look for signs of trauma or deformity when compared to the uninjured side.

It is also important to observe the athlete's face throughout the examination process. This may give further clues as to the severity of the injury. Many athletes will attempt to minimize their injury in order to be allowed to remain in the game. The athlete's facial expression may disclose more pain than he or she is willing to admit.

Palpation

After information from the athlete's history has been gathered, and integrated into the observation of the injured region, further information can be gained through palpation. Palpation of the injured athlete should begin at a site away from the injury. Assessment for deformity or lack of contour is conducted. Although many injuries may seem obvious, some will present only with careful palpation. The corresponding uninjured side should also be palpated to serve as a baseline for normal contour. Intensity should begin with light pressure and increase progressively depending on the severity and type of injury. As palpation moves closer to the site of injury, the examiner again should be noting the anatomic structures that lie under the fingers.

TABLE 4–3. SECONDARY SURVEY

History
Observation
Palpation
Neurological screening
Movement testing
Stress testing

Localized point tenderness is a good indicator of the injury site. A thorough understanding of the anatomic structures lying under the site of point tenderness or greatest pain will reveal valuable information.

Other signs of injury that can be identified via palpation are swelling, temperature changes, muscle spasm, and abnormal motion or sensation. Swelling about the injured region can be due to either acute bleeding secondary to trauma or the accumulation of fluid as the result of the inflammatory response. With such an inflammatory reaction taking place, the skin temperature could also be elevated. Decreased skin temperature would serve as clue to inadequate circulation. Gross circulation should always be assessed by establishing a distal pulse. If no pulse is present distal to the site of injury, a severe medical emergency exists.

The examiner should remember that the body's mechanism to protect itself from further injury and pain is splinting or muscle guarding. The muscles surrounding the injured site reflexively contract to prevent movement that will cause pain. Therefore, it is very important that the athlete be as relaxed as possible prior to the palpation process.

Neurological Screening

Neurological screening is used to assess the integrity and nervous innervation to the soft tissues surrounding the injured site. Sensory function can be evaluated as an extension of the palpation portion of the examination. Increased or decreased sensation should be noted and compared to the contralateral uninjured site. Should sensory differences be noted, the site of altered sensation should be accurately determined and compared to dermatomal charts (Fig 4–10).

Neurology of the Upper Extremity

Disc	Root	Reflex	Muscles	Sensation
C4–C5	C5	Biceps Reflex	Deltoid Biceps	*Lateral Arm* Axillary nerve
C5–C6	C6	Brachioradialis Reflex (Biceps Reflex)	Wrist Extension Biceps	*Lateral Forearm* Musculocutaneous nerve
C6–C7	C7	Triceps Reflex	Wrist Flexors Finger Extension Triceps	*Middle Finger*
C7–T1	C8	—	Finger Flexion Hand Intrinsics	*Medial Forearm* Med. Ant. Brach. Cutaneous nerve
T1–T2	T1	—	Hand Intrinsics	*Medial Arm* Med. Brach. Cutaneous nerve

The Major Peripheral Nerves

Nerve	Motor Test	Sensation Test
Radial Nerve	Wrist Extension Thumb Extension	Dorsal web space between thumb and index finger
Ulnar Nerve	Abduction—little finger	Distal ulnar aspect—little finger
Median Nerve	Thumb pinch Opposition of thumb Abduction of thumb	Distal radial aspect—index finger
Axillary Nerve	Deltoid	Lateral Arm—Deltoid patch on upper arm
Musculocutaneous Nerve	Biceps	Lateral Forearm

Neurology of the Lower Extremity

Disc	Root	Reflex	Muscles	Sensation
L3–L4	L4	Patellar reflex	Anterior tibialis	Medial leg and medial foot
L4–L5	L5	None	Extensor hallucis longus	Lateral leg & dorsum of foot
L5–S1	S1	Achilles reflex	Peroneus longus & brevis	Lateral foot

Figure 4–10. Neurology charts. *(From Hoppenfeld S. Physical Examination of the Spine and Extremities. New York, NY: Appleton-Century-Crofts; 1976, with permission.)*

Active resisted isometric muscle contractions can be used to further assess neurological status. Motor nerve root integrity or myotomes can be evaluated with a series of isometric muscle contractions (Fig 4–10). The examiner should note any weakness that may be present. It is important to remember that pain with isometric muscle contraction also implicates the contractile elements surrounding a joint. The examiner must differentiate weakness due to pain from weakness due to neurological involvement.

Movement Testing—Selective Tissue Tension Testing

This portion of the examination consists of specific active, passive, and resistive movement tests designed to assess the status of each of the component tissues surrounding the injured region. With proper interpretation, these tests can yield very specific information relating to both the nature and extent of the injury.

Active Movement Testing. Active movement testing will only yield general information about the athlete's functional status. It provides information concerning the athlete's willingness to move the injured part. Active movements allow the examiner to assess the athlete's ability to perform common functional tasks related to the demands of the particular sport.

Both contractile and inert tissues are involved or moved during active movements. When active movements occur, one or more of the rigid structures (bones) move, and therefore all the structures attached to the bones move as well. The contractile tissues may have tension placed on them by stretching or contracting (muscle, tendon, bony insertion) whereas inert structures can have tension placed on them by stretching or pinching (joint capsule, ligaments, bursae, blood vessels, nerves, cartilage, dura mater).

When testing active movements, note and document the following:

1. When and where in the movement the onset of pain occurs
2. Whether or not movement increases the intensity or quality of pain
3. The range through which the patient is able to move the part
4. The presence of crepitus

Passive Movement Testing. In passive movement testing the joint is put through a range of motion (ROM) with the athlete relaxed. Although the movement must be gentle, the examiner must determine whether there is any limitation or excess of range, and, if so, whether it is painful. The examiner should attempt to determine the cause of range limitation. Very specific information concerning both the nature and

the extent of the injury can be obtained by assessing the total ROM that is present.

If there is a restriction in the movement of the joint, the examiner should try to determine the quality of the end feel of each passive movement. The end feel is the quality of the resistance to further movement that the examiner feels at the end of the passive movement. End feels may be normal or pathological depending upon the particular point at which they occur in the ROM. The following end feels are generally accepted as being normal:

1. *Capsular.* This is a firm "leathery" type of movement with slight give at the end. This is the most common type of end feel. (Example: external rotation at the shoulder.)
2. *Bone to bone.* This is a hard, unyielding sensation that is also painless. (Example: elbow extension.)
3. *Soft-tissue approximation.* There is a yielding compression that stops further movement. (Example: knee/elbow flexion.)

The following end feels are generally accepted as pathological:

1. *Muscle spasm.* Movement is stopped fairly abruptly due to the muscles contracting reflexively to prevent further movement. It usually accompanies pain felt at the point of restriction.
2. *Capsular.* Same as above, but does not occur where it would be expected. There is a decrease in the ROM.
3. *Springy block.* A springy rebound at the end of the joint movement, occurring where it would not be expected. It tends to be found in joints that have menisci. It is indicative of internal derangement or mechanical blockage.
4. *Empty.* The examiner feels no restriction to further movement, but movement is stopped at the insistence of the athlete due to extreme pain. No real mechanical resistance is felt by the examiner.

Resisted Isometric Movements. Resisted isometric movements are tested last in the examination of the joints. This type of movement consists of a strong, static voluntary muscle contraction. Resisted isometric testing is designed to assess the status of the contractile structures. An isometric type contraction is employed to minimize the amount of joint movement. If movement is allowed to occur at the joint, inert tissues around the joint will also move. If pain is felt, it will not be clear which structure is at fault. Therefore the joint is placed into a neutral or resting position to minimize the tension that is placed on the inert tissues. We

cannot completely eliminate joint movement, but if the joint is placed in this position, any movement that may occur will be minimized.

If there is a problem with the contractile structures, we would expect to find both the active and resisted isometric testing positive. Passive movements are usually full and painfree, with the possible exception of pain occurring at the end ROM when the muscle is stretched.

Stress Testing

The final step in the secondary survey is specific stress testing of the structures surrounding the injured site. The sports physical therapist must examine all structures from which pain might arise by gently applying "appropriate and specific stress" to each structure. Stress testing consists of passive joint play movement and stress application that tests the integrity of the non-contractile or inert structures. The information that is gained from stress testing is very valuable in establishing a working diagnosis. The passive stress tests often reproduce the biomechanical forces at the time of injury and provide clues as to the structures possibly at fault.

When performing stress tests, it is important to test the uninvolved normal extremity first. This will help to establish a baseline of information as well as demonstrate to the athlete what to expect with testing. The application of stress should be repeated several times with increasing intensity to produce the maximum amount of laxity without causing pain and muscle spasm. Remember, it is not only the amount of laxity or opening present, but also the quality of the end feel. If the inert structures or ligaments about the joint are intact, an abrupt stop or end feel will be present when the ligament is under stress. If the ligament under stress has been torn, a soft mushy end feel will be present.

Prior to stress testing, the examiner must have some understanding as to the nature of the athlete's condition. An athlete with suspected fracture or dislocation would not undergo stress testing, as it would expose him or her to further trauma and possible serious injury secondary to the initial onset.

IMMEDIATE CARE OF MUSCULOSKELETAL INJURIES

In order to provide the proper care for athletic injuries, the sports physical therapist must first have a good working knowledge of the body's physiological response to injury. This information is crucial in not only the initial injury assessment but also the subsequent management of the injury. Regardless of the type and location of the injury, the body's reaction to the injury is

the same. This reaction is known as the inflammatory response. The purpose of the inflammatory response is to heal the injured structures. The inflammatory response can be subdivided into three phases: (1) reaction or inflammatory phase, (2) regeneration or repair phase, and (3) remodeling phase.

Reaction Phase

The reaction phase begins immediately after the onset of injury. The initial stages of this response are characterized by vascular changes. This nonspecific response is designed to be the body's mechanism of defense against further trauma and to begin ridding the injured area of damaged cells in preparation for healing and repair.

Immediately following injury there is a brief period of vasoconstriction that lasts between 5 and 10 minutes. During this period, the process of coagulation begins to seal off the damaged blood vessels. The tissue spaces in the inflamed area are blocked by fibrinogen clots. This results in decreased blood flow and allows the white blood cells (WBC) to move to the periphery of the vessel walls in a process called margination. Upon reaching the damaged region the WBCs adhere to the capillary walls, with few escaping through the wall of the capillaries by ameboid action known as diapedesis. Once outside the vessel wall, the WBCs migrate to the site of the injury. Because blood flow is decreased to the traumatized region, the amount of oxygen and nutrients to the region adjacent to the injured tissue is also reduced. This can lead to further injury to the cells adjacent to those initially injured. Those cells that undergo secondary damage and death add to the debris caused by the initial injury.

The vasoconstriction is followed by a period of vasodilation and increased blood flow to the damaged region. The change to vasodilation is attributed to chemical mediators released at the site of injury. When damaged cells degenerate and die, they release substances capable of producing vascular changes. The best known chemicals are histamine and serotonin, which serve to increase the permeability of the capillary walls. The endothelial cells in the vessel wall contract and pull away from each other, thereby leaving gaps through which plasma and plasma proteins can escape into the interstitial spaces. This contributes to the amount of fluid or swelling at the site of injury. The amount of fluid (edema) in the injured region is directly proportional to the extent of the damaged vessels and the permeability of the intact vessels.

The primary goal of the acute inflammatory phase is ridding the injured area of waste products in preparation for healing. The exudate in the damaged region is rich in WBCs. These invade the damaged area and begin to concentrate at the injured site in a process known as chemotaxis. When the WBCs reach the site

of the injury, they remove the waste materials by a process of phagocytosis. The waste material is engulfed by the leukocytes (neutrophils and monocytes) and digested. The monocytes are powerful macrophages that phagocytize the cellular debris and red blood cells (RBCs), thereby clearing the way for repair to occur. After the debris has been removed by the leukocytes, the acute inflammatory process is complete and repair can begin. In most cases of injury not contaminated with bacteria or large amounts of cellular debris, the acute inflammatory response lasts 3 to 4 days and evolves into the regeneration or repair phase.

Regeneration Phase

As the cellular debris and noxious stimuli are removed from the damaged region, a dense network of capillaries is formed throughout the region. Stimulated by a lack of oxygen in the damaged area, capillary buds begin to generate in the walls of the adjacent endothelial cell walls. This proliferation of capillary buds forms a loose network of immature vessels that eventually go on to create a new capillary system. These capillaries bring oxygen and nutrients into the damaged region. Once there is sufficient oxygen at the cellular level, fibroblasts become active and collagen production is initiated. Significant amounts of collagen are laid down by the fourth or fifth day after injury. Defects in the damaged tissue are closed by a loose mesh of fibrous connective tissue. Fibroblastic proliferation and collagen production continues for 4 to 6 weeks following injury. During this time the vascularity of the new tissue is progressively decreased and the tensile strength increased. When a sufficient amount of collagen has been produced, the number of fibroblasts in the injured region decreases. The disappearance of these fibroblasts marks the beginning of the maturation and remodeling phase.

Remodeling

During the last phase of the inflammatory–healing response, changes begin to occur within the newly formed collagen fibers. Initially the collagen fibrils form a very irregular disorganized matrix. As stress is applied to the maturing fibrils, they begin to position themselves along the parallel lines of stress. The tensile strength of these fibrils continues to increase as they arrange into an organized pattern.

It is important that the physical therapist have a good understanding of the scientific basis of the inflammatory response in order to maximize the treatment response. The inflammatory response must be localized to promote the normal healing response. In addition, undue stress that might rupture the newly formed immature fibrils must be avoided.

TABLE 4-4. IMMEDIATE CARE OF MUSCULOSKELETAL INJURIES

R—Rest
I —Ice
C—Compression
E —Elevation

Rest

Resting the injured region is essential with musculoskeletal injuries to allow the body a chance to control the effects of the initial onset. (Table 4–4) Rest is best defined as the absence of abuse, not the absence of activity. Therefore in the total treatment scheme, rest is relative to the condition. Stress on the damaged structures must be controlled to prevent further injury. In general, if an activity causes pain to the point that the athlete cannot perform the activity properly, rest from that activity should take place. An athlete who attempts to continue playing on an injured area may increase the amount of initial structural damage as well as secondary injury as the result of increased hemorrhage. These both will result in a prolongation of the recovery period. Although weight-bearing activities may be contraindicated, the action of the surrounding musculature, serving as "muscle pumps" to rid the area of swelling, should not be forgotten.

Ice

Cold application to an injury site will slow down and minimize the effects of the inflammatory response. Reduction of the inflammatory reaction will in turn diminish pain and muscle spasm. Application of cold reduces the temperature level of the tissue and induces a vasoconstriction of the capillaries. Capillary permeability is reduced and the blood becomes more viscous. The increased viscosity of the blood results in decreased clotting time and rate of flow into the damaged region. Reduction of the temperature of the tissues surrounding the damage region will lower the metabolic demands and chemical reactions, in turn reducing the amount of cellular debris and helping the tissue cells to increase their survival rate during the period of relative hypoxia.

Compression

Immediate compression applied to an injured region is a valuable adjunct to the application of cold. The primary purpose of compression is to help control the swelling and provide support to the injured structures. A compression dressing will help to reduce the accumulation of fluids in the injured area. Increasing the intracellular pressure outside of the blood vessels will reduce seepage from the vessels.

Elevation

Elevation combined with cold and compression aids in the reduction of internal bleeding. Fluid pooling in the damage region is reduced, and elevating the injured part above the level of the heart will encourage venous return. The volume of fluid seeping out of the damaged capillaries is reduced with elevation because the hydrostatic pressure is decreased.

The chief purpose of the initial treatment plan is to reduce or minimize the effects of the injury at an early stage, thereby creating a sound environment for healing to occur.

SUMMARY

When an injury occurs and the sports physical therapist is called onto the field of play, he or she must remain calm and appear confident. Upon reaching the injury scene, attempt to calm the athlete. The actions of the sports therapist should not reflect panic. It is very difficult to evaluate an athlete who is excited and nervous about an injury. There is no substitute for a well-structured and thorough evaluation of the injured athlete.

Assessment of injuries also requires the sports physical therapist to use sound judgment. The pressure to allow an athlete to return to play is great at all levels of athletics. Following an injury, the athlete wants to know not only what is wrong but also when he or she can return to activity. It is important to remember that the athlete is strongly motivated to return to play. The coach, parents, and fans can also contribute to this pressure by trying to hurry the examination and subsequent return to activity. This is where sound judgment and common sense on the part of the sports physical therapist are important. When in doubt, keep the athlete out! If the therapist is unsure of the nature or severity of the athlete's injury, it is better to err on the side of being overly conservative than to allow the athlete to return to play and risk further injury.

It is extremely important that the sports physical therapist practice emergency procedures. There is no substitute for actual experience. To become proficient in dealing with acute injury assessment, the sports physical therapist should practice these skills repeatedly so that they become second nature.

It is important that a logical plan of action be established long before the actual athletic event takes place. Emergency procedures should be planned in advance so that in the event they are needed, the procedures can be carried out as easily and as efficiently as possible. Knowledge of how to obtain additional professional assistance such as hospital transportation should be reviewed on a regular basis and phone numbers readily accessible. Emergency equipment should be on hand and the operation routinely reviewed.

In summary, the sports physical therapist should plan for the worst and hope for the best. Prior planning for a medical emergency can help to ensure that the injured athlete receives the highest quality care.

SUGGESTED READINGS

American Academy of Orthopedic Surgeons. *Athletic Training and Sports Medicine*. Chicago, Ill: The Association; 1985.

American Academy of Orthopedic Surgeons. *Emergency Care and Transportation of the Sick and Injured*. 3rd ed. Chicago, Ill: The Academy; 1981.

American Heart Association. *A Manual for Instructors of Basic Life Support*. Dallas, Tex: The Association; 1977.

Arnheim, DD. *Modern Principles of Athletic Training*. 6th ed. St. Louis, Mo: C V Mosby Co; 1985.

Booher JM, Thibodeau GA. *Athletic Injury Assessment*. St. Louis, Mo: C V Mosby Co; 1985.

Bernhardt DB. Triage. In: *Clinics in Physical Therapy*. New York, NY: Churchill Livingstone; 1986; 135–153.

Clinics in Sportsmedicine. *Emergency Treatment of the Injured Athlete*. B:(1) Philadelphia, Penn: WB Saunders Co; 1989.

Grant HD, Murray R. *Emergency Care*, ed. 3, Bowie, Md: Robert J. Brady Co; 1983.

Hafen BQ, Karren KJ. *Prehospital Emergency Care & Crisis Intervention*. Denver, Co: Morton Publishing Co; 1981.

Miller RH, Cantrell JR. *Textbook of Basic Emergency Medicine*. 2nd ed. St. Louis, Mo: C V Mosby Co; 1980.

Parcel G. *Basic Emergency Care of the Sick and Injured*. 2nd ed. St. Louis, Mo: C V Mosby Co; 1982.

Roy S, Irvin R. *Sports Medicine*. Englewood Cliffs, NJ: Prentice-Hall; 1983.

Torg J. *Athletic Injuries to the Head, Neck, and Face*. Philadelphia, Penn: Lea & Febiger; 1982.

5 Environmental Conditions

Susan D. Lambert

INTRODUCTION

Athletes practice and compete in a wide variety of settings. The environment can play a significant role in athletic ability. Although not all factors can be controlled, it is important to provide athletes with the optimal environment available for good health, maximum safety, and best performance levels. Extreme conditions may require changes in event schedules and preparation and response to exercise. It is the responsibility of the sports physical therapist to be knowledgeable of environmental conditions and their effects, to inform coaches, managers and athletes of precautionary measures, and to be competent in the treatment of those athletes who become adversely affected by the environment.

LIGHT

Artificial lighting of a gymnasium or outdoor field can affect an athlete's performance to a larger degree than one might think. Lighting that is too dim can cause an athlete's eyes to become overstrained and fatigued, decreasing visual acuity. A lighting system that is too bright can also cause these same problems, in addition to creating glare on reflective surfaces. Becoming friendly with the maintenance staff and informing them of the cause and effect relationships of lighting problems can help to eliminate an often overlooked environmental problem.

Eye shields attached to football helmets have now been developed, both to minimize accidental injury as well as improve vision. Amber shields are used to enhance contrast on overcast days, smoke shields to reduce glare on bright days, and rose shields to improve contrast and diminish glare when artificial lighting is used.[1]

It should be mentioned that outdoor athletic activities may be sharply affected when executed at daybreak or dusk. These time periods represent significant and rapid change in natural lighting that is sometimes not obvious to athletes. As the relationship between recruitment of optic rods and cones is changing, visual capabilities may be diminished. Activities such as distance running and walking require caution during these hours, especially near high traffic areas.

Sun and Snow Blindness

Sun and snow blindness are problems an athlete can encounter when proper precautions are not taken with regard to light exposure. In both of these cases, the cause is overexposure to harmful ultraviolet rays, creating inflammation of the cornea and conjunctiva of the eyes. The athlete experiences a feeling of roughness, edema, and pain, and, upon visual examination, the eyes are red and watery. He or she will probably squint in effort to protect the eyes and may require hand-lead guidance, due to temporary "blindness."

Treatment for sun and snow blindness involves wearing sunglasses with blinders attached to the lens. This effect is achieved by placing cardboard shields with pinhole openings within the sunglass rims. Holes should be just large enough for the athlete to see ahead. Ointment or eye drops may be prescribed by a physician to relax ocular muscles. These conditions usually last 2 to 4 days with no long-term effects.

To prevent sun and snow blindness, close-fitting, dark sunglasses with lateral shielding protectors are useful. Precautions should be taken with all athletes whose sports require bright, direct, or indirect eye-to-sun exposure. Water sports, snow sports, and sports such as baseball and tennis will allow large amounts of ultraviolet exposure within the eyes unless they are adequately protected. Recently, athletes have found mirrored lenses and lenses coated with ultraviolet blocking agents to be helpful.[2]

Solar Radiation

Skin exposure to natural light, or solar radiation, is most pronounced at high altitudes and during summer months. Athletes must undergo gradual exposure to the sun's light, avoiding harmful sunburn. Sunscreen lotions with ultraviolet-ray blocking agents can aid in the acclimatization process. The face, chest, and shoulders are particularly sensitive to the sun. Sunvisors and shirts with sleeves are recommended for athletes who are fair and light-complected.

Should an athlete become sunburned, it is important that the sports physical therapist know the varying degrees of burns and appropriate corresponding treatment. During early phases, burn severity may be difficult to discern.

A *first-degree burn* is denoted by a pink or slightly reddened tone of the skin. Epidermal damage is superficial and generally heals spontaneously within 2 to 3 days. A *second-degree burn* is characterized by small, visible blisters on the skin's surface, in addition to increased redness of the skin. It is not advisable to deliberately open blisters, as this increases the risk of infection before the skin is fully healed. If a blister should burst, a sterile dressing should be applied. Blistered areas that may come into contact with athletic equipment or clothing should also be covered with an antiseptic ointment to reduce friction. A physician's evaluation is necessary if a second-degree burn encompasses a surface skin area greater than 2 in^2 (10 cm^2). Large-area second-degree burns may include associated symptoms of chills and nausea.

Third-degree burns are considered medical emergencies. All of the epidermal layers are compromised. Permanent damage often requires plastic surgery. It is rare that an athlete advances to this stage of sunburn, as the symptoms of pain, chills, and nausea generally alert him or her to seek shelter from the sun.[2]

Jet Lag

Athletic performance can be gravely affected by the light changes experienced when athletes travel through several time zones. This is often required of athletes who are participating in national and international competitions.

Jet lag is the term for mental and physical symptoms that occur from disruption of the body's internal time clock. This clock, commonly referred to as circadian rhythm, controls autonomic functions such as heart rate, digestion, excretion, breathing, and hormonal balances. Changes in eating, sleeping, and practice schedules may alter these functions, creating physical and mental problems that, in turn, reduce optimal athletic performance levels.

Because daily activities are governed by the light and dark cycles of a 24-hour day, much research has gone into making transitions between time zones less physically and mentally taxing. The earth has a total of 24 time zones, with a 1-hour time difference between each time zone. It is not uncommon for an athlete to pass through three time zones, as when traveling from coast to coast within the United States. International travel may require the traversal of as many as 14 to 17 time zones, as did the American athletes for the 1988 Summer Olympics in Seoul, South Korea.

In addition to time zone changing, studies have shown that performance can also be affected by an athlete's preference for early or late time schedules. "Larks" is the term given to those individuals who seem to be the most productive in the early morning hours, fatiguing at about 2:00 or 3:00 PM. "Owls," on the other hand, are people who feel they are at their best performance levels in the mid-to-late afternoon. They are generally late morning risers and do not mind staying active late into the evening.

Because mental and physical performance is usually best at the time of peak body temperature, it is important to know differences between body temperature trends in larks and owls. Larks peak at approximately 11:00 AM and plummet at 2:00 PM. Owls' highest temperatures are at about 4:00 PM and lows at 4:00 AM. This information can be useful when planning travel and event schedules.

Some athletes may be apprehensive about sleeping quarters and the cultural differences of foreign countries. This type of psychological and emotional stress contributes to fatigue associated with jet lag. It is interesting to note that owls often travel better when going east to west, whereas larks are more at ease with west to east travel. Extroverted, outgoing athletes can attribute their quick adjustment to their comfort with social contact and increased alertness due to new mental and visual stimuli.

There are also environmental factors, particular to jet flying, that contribute to jet lag. Dry, high altitudes and low cabin air humidity draw moisture from passengers' bodies. Dehydration can occur if these atmospheric conditions are ignored. High altitude flying, coupled with inhalation of others' cigarette smoke, can cause oxygen deficiency—another performance degrader.

The sports physical therapist can play a vital role in helping athletes combat jet lag. Before travel, diet should alternate heavy and light meals to promote fresh glycogen stores for the energy used when changing time zones. Preadjusting athletes' circadian rhythms to the new time zone may also be advantageous. When the athlete is traveling west, this can be done by rising and retiring 1 hour later for the same number of days as time zones to be crossed. Traveling east calls for rising and retiring 1 hour earlier for each time zone to be tra-

versed. Making arrangements for athletes to sit as far away from cigarette smoke as possible will help to minimize the chance of oxygen deficiency.

Time of departure and arrival can be critical. Avoidance of sleep deprivation, with arrival time well in advance of competition date, is important. It is estimated that the adjustment period is 1 day for each time zone crossed.

Several measures can be taken in-flight to promote easy time zone transition. Have athletes set their watches for the new time zone just after boarding the plane. Encourage increased fluid intake, avoiding alcoholic and caffeinated beverages. Bring along snacks rich in fiber to help avoid symptoms of constipation from dehydration. Instruct athletes to move about when possible. This can assist in reducing stiffness and fatigue by improving circulation. An easy isometric program can be carried out while seated. Sleep should be based on final destination arrival time. If it will be morning, encourage sleeping on the plane. If it will be evening, sleep should be avoided while in transit.

After arrival, athletes should attempt to accept the local time for all scheduled activities—training, sleeping, and eating. Initial training sessions should begin with light activities. Difficult or strenuous skills may not be well performed due to the mental and physiological adjustments taking place soon after arrival. Failure can create loss of confidence and increase emotional stress.

Quiet, dark, and temperature-regulated sleeping environments can ease the discomfort of retiring in unfamiliar surroundings. Naps should be avoided until time zone adjustment is fully achieved. If insomnia occurs, instruct athletes in relaxation exercises and recommend a high carbohydrate snack before bedtime. Carbohydrates are known to facilitate drowsiness by increasing brain serotonin levels. In efforts to avoid gastrointestinal problems, the diet should remain as familiar as possible. Discourage sampling of new cuisines prior to competition.[3]

PLAYING SURFACES

Natural Turf

There is presently no conclusive evidence to support the notion that natural turf is, overall, any more or less likely to cause athletic injury than artificial surfaces.[4,5] Addressing some of the problems incurred on grass (not for the purpose of comparison), however, may help the sports physical therapist with injury prevention and management.

Because grass surfaces change with use and weather, it becomes important for those individuals involved with on-the-field coverage to examine playing areas closely prior to the commencement of game or practice. Slippery, muddy areas or divots and holes should be reported to coaches, referees, and athletes. In addition, grounds maintenance crews should be alerted as soon as possible to allow prompt correction of these potentially injurious areas. Playing fields should be visually scanned for sharp objects, such as broken equipment parts or trash left by passers-by.

No two natural turf surfaces are identical. Variations occur with growing season, grass-types, maintenance, and usage. Inspection of unfamiliar fields can assist players in proper mental preparation and shoe/cleat selection.

Other considerations for natural surfaces include hard and rough terrain. Earth that is dry and rocky requires a shoe with high shock absorbency and thick tread. This is particularly important for mountain climbing and dry summer preseason training camps. "Shin splints" appears to be a common complaint of athletes who do not heed to the recommendation of a more supportive shoe under these conditions.

Artificial Turf

In 1966, artificial turf made its debut in the Houston Astrodome under the trade name Astroturf. The surface was originally manufactured in response to an effort to provide inner city children with a more optimal environment to develop physical skills and growth patterns. Since that time, Superturf, Tartan Turf, and Polyturf have been developed; the latter two have been discontinued, although some stadiums still house these surfaces.[5]

There are limited data available concerning the differences among artificial surfaces. Most reports have generalized the guidelines for athletic participation of all artificial turf types as being similar.

Wear of synthetic turf has been closely observed by Bowers and Martin. Results of their testing indicate that older surfaces demonstrate significantly less impact absorbency than newer surfaces. Surprisingly, Astroturf was similar to (but not equivalent to) shock absorption on natural Kentucky bluegrass.[6]

Another problem particular to use is the creation of airborne "grass" fibers. This green dust can impede athletic performance by interfering with respiratory function, in similar fashion to other types of air pollution. Also, just as with grass fields, surface irregularities in artificial turf occur based on brand, age, climate, maintenance, and use.

Torg et al. were among the first to recognize the need of a modified shoe for proper shoe–turf interface.[7] A molded sole shoe with fifteen $\frac{3}{8}$-in-long, $\frac{1}{2}$-in-diameter cleats may be the safest shoe for all surfaces and conditions.[7]

Although some studies have supported the safety

of both natural and artificial surfaces, it is generally agreed that the incidence of "turf-toe" is increased on artificial turf. The mechanism of injury is forced hyperextension or hyperflexion of the first metatarsophalangeal joint. This may reveal the flaws of a more flexible shoe sole, or perhaps a difference in playing surface that has not yet been revealed. Further research will help to recognize the cause and allow additional improvements in artificial surface manufacturing and athletic shoe design.

Player-to-player impact injuries can be, in part, correlated to speed upon contact. Many athletes will report a faster game on synthetic surfaces. Running, as well as ball travel, seems quicker. These factors may need to be considered when evaluating injury potential on artificial turf.[8]

The following guidelines for artificial turf are helpful:

1. Familiarization of athletes to new field surfaces promotes better concentration on the game. When possible, recommend early arrival time for athletes to become accustomed to the turf. A light game of touch football or volleyball 1 day before the game can help athletes adapt to the change.
2. Insist that athletes wear the proper shoes.
3. Educate players in proper foot care. This includes cutting toenails, trimming callouses, lubricating high friction areas, wearing proper socks, and providing first aid for blisters.
4. Teach proper care of abrasions. Abrasions should be dressed with antiseptics for 2 to 3 days.
5. If the field is wetted to cool surface temperatures, assure uniformity of wetting so athletes do not experience irregularity while running.
6. Fibers become thinned and matted down with use and age. Check that the field is properly maintained, including vacuuming of "grass" fiber dust and replacement of pile showing reduced shock absorbency.[9]

ATMOSPHERIC CONDITIONS

Exercise at High Altitudes

It is well known that physiological function and work capacity are depressed with work at high altitudes. A well-trained athlete, however, can complete activities with greater ease than the untrained individual, due to the fact that the trained athlete will use a smaller percentage of his or her maximum aerobic capacity.

High altitude is considered to be 3048 to 5486 ft (929 to 1673 m). Air density, or barometric pressure, progressively decreases at this range as compared to sea level. Oxygen is driven into the bloodstream, due to the decrease in density of oxygen molecules as one ascends. Oxygen is then less available for muscle performance. Increased respiratory rate and decreased cardiac output yield decreased aerobic capacity at high altitudes. Although anerobic activities remain uncompromised, recovery time is usually longer as compared to recovery at sea level.

Oxygen equipment is necessary for climbs to altitudes of 5000 ft (1524 m). In 1978, Rienhold Messner climbed Mount Everest without any oxygen equipment. This, unfortunately, prompted "no-oxygen" climbing to gain popularity. The result has been a considerable number of deaths and instances of permanent damage to the central nervous system. When Messner's climb was analyzed, it was found that ideal seasonal, lunar, tidal, and equatorial factors had contributed to his success. Because these conditions would be difficult to duplicate, oxygen equipment for high elevation climbing should be advocated.[10]

Acute Mountain Sickness. Table 5–1 depicts the body's immediate and long-term adjustments to altitude hypoxia, or lack of oxygen. *Acute mountain sickness* is experienced by most climbers and skiers at high altitudes. Symptoms begin 6 hours to 4 days after arrival and usually present in the form of headache, fatigue, insomnia, dyspnea, weakness, nausea, and vomiting. Loss of appetite can result in weight loss and cold, dry mountain air can cause moderate dehydration.[11]

High-Altitude Pulmonary Edema. *High-altitude pulmonary edema* is a more serious disorder, primarily occurring after descending and reascending. Following the symptoms of acute mountain sickness, chest pain, apnea, and production of frothy, bloody sputum is observed. Respiratory evaluation through a stethoscope reveals rales and abnormal breath sounds. When high altitude pulmonary edema exists, the athlete must be returned to lower altitude levels immediately. Oxygen is given and climbing activities are restricted until all signs and symptoms are negative.[12]

High-Altitude Cerebral Edema. Extreme heights can lead to a less common form of altitude illness known as *high-altitude cerebral edema*. Initial symptoms are those of acute mountain sickness, progressing to more bizarre characteristics such as bradycardia, mental confusion, emotional instability, forgetfulness, irrational behavior, and hallucinations. Muscle strength and coordination are reduced, followed by reflex changes. Severe swelling of the brain also causes decreased visual acuity, papilledema, and even hemorrhage within the eye. This is a medical emergency that, if left untreated, is likely to result in coma and death. High-altitude cerebral edema requires the immediate attention of a physician.

TABLE 5–1. IMMEDIATE AND LONGER TERM ADJUSTMENTS TO ALTITUDE HYPOXIA

System	Immediate	Longer Term
Pulmonary	Hyperventilation	Hyperventilation
Acid–base	Body fluids become more alkaline due to reduction in CO_2 with hyperventilation	Excretion of base via the kidneys and concomitant reduction in alkaline reserve
Cardiovascular	Increase in submaximal heart rate	Submaximal heart rate remains elevated
	Increase in submaximal cardiac output	Submaximal cardiac output falls to or below sea-level values
	Stroke volume remains the same or is slightly lowered	Stroke volume is lowered
	Maximum heart rate remains the same or is slightly lowered	Maximum heart rate is lowered
	Maximum cardiac output remains the same or is slightly lowered	Maximum cardiac output is lowered
Hematologic	—	Decrease in plasma volume
		Increased hematocrit
		Increased hemoglobin concentration
		Increase in total number of red blood cells
Local	—	Possible increased capillarization of skeletal muscle
		Increased red-blood-cell 2,3-DPG
		Increased mitochondria
		Increased aerobic enzymes

From McArdle, WD, Katch FI, Katch VL. Exercise Physiology. *Philadelphia, PA: Lea & Febiger; 1986:324, with permission.*

Altitude Acclimatization. Duration and intensity of exertion, speed of ascent, and prior physical condition all play a role in the health of athletes exercising at high elevations. Preascent strength and aerobic capacity are of the utmost importance in preventing illness and maximizing performance levels. This can be achieved by running 12 to 15 miles a day (or its equivalent) for several months prior to ascent.

Acclimatization refers to the adjustment time necessary for bodily adaptation to a rapid, extreme change in environment. In summary of the progression of acclimatization, Bill has determined that physiological adaptation to altitude occurs in four phases[13]:

1. *Acute phase* (first 30 minutes of exposure)—Maximal oxygen consumption and aerobic capacity is reduced by less than 10% of normal levels.
2. *Second phase* (1 to 3 days)—Aerobic capacity is reduced by 20% to 30%.
3. *Third phase* (several weeks)—Adaptation begins.
4. *Fourth phase* (approximately 1 year or more)—Red blood cell (RBC) volume reaches a maximum.

It should be remembered that acclimatization at mid-range elevations provides only partial adaptation for higher altitudes. Because of the specificity of exercise principles, athletes should be allowed to condition themselves before competing at high altitudes. With regard to initial workouts at high elevations, low-duration, high-intensity sessions are best, using supplemental oxygen as necessary.

At elevations of 5000 ft (1524 m) or greater, training can take several weeks to months. Although it may take years, it is conceivable to reach sea level performance levels at elevations as high as 13,200 ft (4024 m). As a rule, altitudes below 3000 ft (915 m) require no elevation acclimatization and there seems to be no advantage to high-altitude training for sea level competitions.

Eating before, but not during, travel to high altitudes will minimize gastrointestinal problems. High-carbohydrate diets with ample quantities of fresh juice and water are necessary during preliminary altitude training bouts to eliminate the incidence of symptoms associated with acute mountain sickness. Athletes who encounter difficulties with altitude adjustment should have their body weight monitored regularly.

Air Pollution

Unless heat-related, air conditions are seldom reason for event cancellation. They are, however, deterrents that can affect performance. Common types of detracting air factors are fog, smoke, haze, sulfur dioxide, carbon monoxide, and pollen.

Fog is defined as a large mass of water vapor condensed to fine particles, just above the earth's surface.

Smoke is the vaporous matter that arises from burning substances. Ash and larger dust particles may be visible. A combination of fog and smoke is called *smog*. The term *haze* is used when the vapor consists of a combination of fog, smoke, and other dusty pollutants. Haze can often take on colors, depending upon its composition. Both smog and haze are found in and around congested industrial cities.

Specific by-product pollutants include sulfur dioxide and carbon monoxide. *Sulfur dioxide* is the gaseous substance given off when sulfur is burned. Its smell is obvious when passing by an industrial plant that is emitting fumes into the air. It has a strong, unpleasant odor and causes irritation to the eyes, nose, mouth, throat, and lungs.

Carbon monoxide (produced by incomplete carbon combustion) is given off by motor vehicles. High levels can sometimes also be found in indoor ice rinks. Arenas with ice rinks should be frequently ventilated by opening windows and doors. Ice resurfacing machines should be fueled with propane and fitted with catalytic converters to minimize carbon monoxide emission. Regular tuneups (just as with automobiles) can also drastically reduce carbon monoxide levels. The sports physical therapist can assure periodic checking of carbon monoxide levels through the use of a carbon monoxide monitor. This portable, lightweight instrument is easy to calibrate and testing can be completed in 15 to 20 minutes.

Pollen is also considered an air pollutant, with levels increasing in the fall and spring. Very often television weather information will cover the pollution and pollen indexes during the daily forecast. Another source is the local Air Pollution Control Board, which can be contacted by telephone. There are a variety of over-the-counter and prescription medications that can allow safe and successful athletic participation of those who suffer from pollen-related allergies.

If one must exercise in air-polluted environments, several precautions should be taken:[14]

1. Choose early morning workout times when possible.
2. Avoid strenuous, lengthy workouts when pollution levels are high.
3. Athletes with a history of respiratory or cardiac dysfunction should avoid outdoor exercise when pollution levels exceed recommended air quality standards.
4. Avoid highways and high-traffic streets.
5. Warm up indoors.
6. Avoid exercising in indoor facilities where smoking is permitted and proper ventilation is not adequate.
7. Allow 3 hours postexposure to carbon gases before the commencement of exercise for those athletes with heart conditions.
8. Acclimatization training to high pollution areas *is not* recommended.

UNDERWATER CONDITIONS

The primary concern in recreational diving is making proper adjustments to the pressure changes that occur. Although the human body is primarily composed of water, the respiratory system, along with many cranial sinuses and cavities, is subject to significant volume and pressure changes during diving.

Table 5–2 shows the relationship of water depth to pressure and volume. As a diver increases in depth, pressure against his or her body is increased. This is due to the pressure of the column of air above the water's

TABLE 5–2. RELATIONSHIP OF DEPTH IN WATER TO PRESSURE AND VOLUME

Depth		Pressure		Hypothetical Lung Volume (mL)	Inspired Air	
(ft)	(m)	(atm)	(mm Hg)		P_{O_2}	P_{N_2}
Sea level		1	760	6000	159	600
33	10	2	1520	3000	318	1201
66	20	3	2280	2000	477	1802
100	30	4	3040	1500	636	2402
133	40	5	3800	1200	795	3003
166	50	6	4560	1000	954	3604
200	60	7	5320	857	1113	4204
300	90	10	7600	600	1590	6006
400	120	13	9880	461	2068	7808
500	150	16	12160	375	2545	9610
600	180	19	14440	316	3022	11412

From McArdle WD, Katch FI, Katch VL. Exercise Physiology. *Philadelphia, PA: Lea & Febiger; 1986; 468, with permission.*

surface (1 atm) plus the pressure of the column of water above the diver. A freshwater dive at 108 ft (33 m) is said to exert a pressure of 2 atm on the diver. This same pressure exists at a dive of 107 ft (32 m) in saltwater, due to its increased density.[11]

Boyle's law states that gas volume is inversely related to the pressure exerted on it. Therefore, as a diver descends to greater and greater depths, his or her lung volume is compressed. Upon ascending, the lung volume of air expands.

To compensate for increased external pressure against the chest cavity and to allow a diver continual air supply, *self-contained underwater breathing apparatus (scuba)* is used. The open-circuit system is used for sport diving. Steel or aluminum tanks contain 1000 to 2000 L of air compressed to approximately 2200 lb/in^2 (psi). This ratio allows one to complete a dive of about 30 minutes to 1 hour at medium depths. The regulator valve between the air tanks and the diver's mouthpiece is designed to provide air to the diver at a pressure equal to the water's pressure. Exhaled air is released into the water.

Descent Problems

Descent problems, or "squeeze injuries," can occur with improper or inadequate pressure equalization between water and diver. As the diver descends, the decreased pressure within the face mask creates a vacuum. Nasal exhalation into the mask will recreate a pressure balance. If this maneuver is not executed periodically during descent, the eyes will bulge, possibly rupturing capillaries. This is called "mask squeeze."

Another type of squeeze injury is *aerotitis*, or "middle ear squeeze." This occurs when air pressure within the eustachian tubes is not equalized. In the healthy individual, descent pressures can be normalized by pinching the nostrils closed and blowing against them. A diver with an upper respiratory infection is likely to experience aerotitis, due to mucus-plugged, swollen airways. Severe pain usually precludes the dive; however, if pain is ignored and the dive made, the eardrum can rupture. In addition to infection, those individuals with a past history of eardrum rupture or respiratory disease should be excluded from participation in diving activity. It should also be noted that earplugs are contraindicated during diving, as the vacuum effect can pull them into the ear's canal, with rupture of the eardrum likely.

Mild squeeze injuries generally do not require medical attention. When eardrum rupture is suspected, the condition should be treated as a medical emergency; the diver will require prompt attention by qualified personnel. If severe or if left untreated, hearing and balance impairment can occur. Although extremely rare, lung compression or "thoracic squeeze" can result from rapid descent without breathing. This condition is life-threatening, requiring artificial resuscitation and medical treatment.

As gas pressures increase with diving depth, a diver must stay aware of the effects that can occur. At depths of 328 to 426 ft (100 to 130 m), alterations in the central nervous system can impair a diver's judgment. This condition, termed *nitrogen narcosis*, is due to extraordinarily high levels of nitrogen at these depths. Symptoms include euphoria and giddiness, similar to alcohol intoxication. The diver's logic can be affected to such a degree that personal safety is jeopardized. It would not be surprising to see a diver take off his or her scuba gear, thinking it unnecessary. Therefore, recreational diving is usually limited to no more than 1-hour intervals at a maximal depth range of 328 ft (100 m). Should a diver be suspected of "rapture of the deep," he or she should be guided to shallower waters. Recovery is usually immediate.

As previously mentioned, sport diving uses an open-circuit scuba system. *Closed-circuit systems* use pure oxygen instead of air and are not recommended for recreational dives or dives greater than 82 ft (25 m). Breathing pure oxygen can cause oxygen toxicity. This condition is characterized by convulsions, dizziness, numbness, and muscle fasciculations. If exposure continues, bronchopneumonia and impaired central nervous system function may result. If oxygen toxicity is suspected, the treatment is to return to the surface for breathing of sea-level air.

Contaminants from highly polluted, urban areas can make their way into the air tanks of divers if tanks are filled in these areas when the pollution index is high. Carbon monoxide is a common air contaminant that, if breathed under the high pressures of scuba diving, can cause tissue hypoxia. Air tanks should be filled by qualified personnel, away from engine exhaust and other contaminants.

Malfunction of special rebreathing equipment can cause another toxic condition known as *carbon dioxide poisoning*. This gas accumulates in the diver due to inadequate reabsorption of carbon dioxide. He or she experiences apnea, headaches, and a feeling of panic. Breathing clean sea-level air eliminates these symptoms.

Defects in standard scuba equipment can cause oxygen deficiency (*hypoxia*). The diver can become unconscious and death may follow if prompt emergency medical attention is not given.

Ascent Problems

A diver's ascent is not without danger. As the pressures of internal air increase, it is imperative that air is exhaled freely. Holding one's breath while ascending can lead to a deadly problem called *air embolism*. This can occur in waters as shallow as 6 to 10 feet (remember: air within the body expands with ascent!). Lung tissue

will rupture and air bubbles are then transported through the circulatory system. A variety of symptoms may be present[15]:

1. Mottling of the skin
2. Confusion, dizziness, blurred vision
3. Difficulty speaking
4. Dyspnea
5. Chest, muscle, tendon, joint, abdominal cavity pain
6. Bloody, frothy secretions from mouth/nose
7. Vomiting
8. Coma, paralysis

These symptoms will soon be followed by death if rapid recompression is not sought. Specialized recompression chambers are designed to minimize the air bubbles' size, opening blocked blood vessels. While in transit to chambers, the victim should be kept calm and quiet, lying on the left side and with the lower extremities elevated. Oxygen should be administered.

A complication of lung tissue rupture is *pneumothorax*. In this condition an air pocket is created between the chest wall lining and the lung tissue. Further air expansion in this pocket causes lung collapse with secondary stress to the heart and abdominal organs. Lying the patient on the left side is, therefore, helpful in maintaining proper positioning of the heart via gravity assistance. Treatment of pneumothorax may include aspiration of unwanted air pockets. As previously mentioned, no one with a known respiratory disease should be allowed to dive. As a rule, ascending should be gradual, with full exhalation of air and deep inhalations avoided, especially near the surface. Simply, divers should be encouraged to breathe normally!

Decompression sickness, or caisson's disease, is yet another type of diving disorder. Associated with repetitive, or lengthy, deep dives, it is a problem rarely seen in recreational diving. Nevertheless, its potential exists and is, therefore, worthy of discussion.

Not unlike a capped bottle of soda pop, the high internal levels of nitrogen gas are under a great deal of pressure within the diver during deep dives. Should a diver stay down too deep or too long, a regular ascent causes external pressures to drop too rapidly, similar to the removal of the soda pop cap. As can be imagined, large bubbles then form in the body's tissues unless decompression stops or pauses are incorporated into the ascent.

Associated symptoms may be in the muscles, ligaments, tendons, skin, or organs. Discomfort often causes the diver to double over in pain, thus the term "the bends" has been coined as a nickname for decompression sickness. A diver with the bends may complain of itchy skin or tightness in the joints. More seriously, nitrogen bubbles, trapped in the lungs, can choke and asphyxiate; in the brain, they can block the coronary arteries. Permanent neurological disability can result. Unlike the immediate onset of symptoms associated with air embolism, these symptoms may not present themselves until hours after a dive. To minimize cerebral damage, oxygen should be administered during transport of the victim to a hyperbaric chamber. Recompression will return the nitrogen to a liquid state. Decompression should then follow, to simulate a proper ascent, allowing the nitrogen to escape from the diver's body.[16]

Prevention of all breathing-related dive injuries requires a sound knowledge of the principles of gas exchange. The use of specialized dive tables to determine appropriate ascent rates and pauses at various dive depths and durations can significantly reduce the risk of carelessness during dives. Regular equipment checks can minimize the occurrence of defective gear. Proper diver hydration can promote efficient gas exchange. Avoidance of strenuous exercise 6 hours postdive or flying 12 to 24 hours postdive can also reduce the risk of decompression sickness. It should be noted that some individuals are unusually susceptible to diving disorders. This is good reason for dives to never actually meet the time limits indicated on dive charts. Being conservative can save lives!

WEATHER CONDITIONS

Heat and Humidity

Perhaps the most widely discussed environmental hazards are those associated with heat and humidity. It is unfortunate that, although a general awareness of the topic exists, proper precautions are often ignored. Heat and humidity combined can create not only illness, but death as well. A thorough understanding of problems associated with hot, humid environments is the key in providing safe surroundings for athletic participation.

The *hypothalamus* is a mass of specialized neurons, located at the base of the brain. It functions as the body's thermostat for temperature regulation as blood flows through it. There are also peripheral thermal receptors in the skin that provide temperature input to the hypothalamus. Blood flow and thermal receptor sensitivity are especially important during strenuous exercise.

There are four ways in which the body may dissipate heat: conduction, convection, radiation, and evaporation. *Conduction* involves the exchange of heat through surface contact with another object. *Convection* is the transfer of heat via liquid to gas. *Radiation* is heat exchange by way of electromagnetic waves. *Evaporation* is the process of changing liquid to gas and is the body's primary means of cooling when the environmental temperature is higher than the body temperature.

Evaporation requires a thin film of perspiration on the skin's surface. This moisture cools blood in the epidermal capillaries. The rate of cooling is dependent upon the amount of surface area exposed, the rate of air circulation, the amount and type of clothing worn, and the relative humidity.

Relative humidity is the most critical factor with regard to evaporation efficiency. It refers to the moisture-carrying capacity of the air at a specific temperature. When relative humidity increases, evaporation of sweat decreases. This significantly reduces the body's ability to thwart excess internal heat. Although perspiration may be given off, it simply beads and rolls off the skin. This ineffective water loss can cause heat illness and dehydration.

The most comprehensive measure of heat stress is the *wet bulb–globe temperature index* (WBGT). The following formula is used:

$$WBGT = 0.1 \times DBT + 0.7 \times WBT + 0.2 \times GT$$

The *dry bulb temperature* (DBT) recorded is from a regular mercury thermometer. *Wet bulb temperature* (WBT) is the reading acquired by placing a wet wick around the thermometer bulb and swinging it through the air. These temperatures can be easily measured using a device called a *sling psychrometer* that houses a scale to calculate the difference between DBT and WBT, or relative humidity. Because the sling psychrometer is most readily available and user-friendly, it is considered to be standard equipment for all athletic events.

Globe temperature (GT) measures the sun's radiation. The thermometer used must have a black metal casing around the bulb. J. H. Botsford developed an instrument called the *wet globe thermometer* that includes measurements of heat conduction, convection, evaporation, and radiation. This instrument gives one measurement without calculations and its reading is referred to as the *Corrected Effective Temperature* (CET). This type of equipment is sophisticated and less practical for low-budget, recreational athletic events. WBGT and CET can be obtained by calling the local weather bureau. It must be remembered, however, that field conditions can vary by several degrees or more from the location used by the weather bureau. Therefore, it is best to use the sling psychrometer and conservative judgment when making recommendations to coaches and athletes.[13]

Table 5–3 gives both WBGT and WBT guidelines.[17] A quick reference can be obtained through the use of Figure 5–1 for cumulative effects of heat and humidity.[14] A corresponding flag should be mounted on the field, in easy view, to aid coaches, managers, and athletes in making appropriate activity modifications.

Electrolytes. As perspiration is the body's primary means of heat dissipation, one must understand its components for the purpose of replenishment. Water constitutes approximately 90% of its mass and contains the important minerals calcium, magnesium, phosphate, potassium, and sodium. They are called electrolytes, due to their electrical conductivity. A deficiency of electrolytes within the body can cause the electrical current necessary for nerve impulse travel to be interrupted. Abnormal physiological responses often occur with a body fluid loss of greater than 1.5 L (51 oz). Athletic performance is reduced with losses of as little as 2% to 3%; losses of 4% to 5% are considered dangerous.

There are several good ways in which to replenish

TABLE 5-3. UNIVERSAL WBGT INDEX

WBGT Index for Outdoor Activities (Wet Bulb Global Temperature)			Wet Bulb Temperature Guide	
Range	Signal Flag	Activity		
82–84.9	Green	Alert for possible increase in index	Under 60°F	No precaution necessary
			61°–65°F	Alert all participants, especially heavy weight losers
85–87.9	Yellow	Active practice curtailed (un-acclimated men)	66°–70°F	Insist that appropriate fluids be given in the field
88–89.9	Red	Active practice curtailed (all men—except most acclimated)	71°–75°F	Alter practice schedules to provide rest periods every 30 min, plus above precautions
90+		All training stopped, skull session—demonstrations	76°F and up	Practice postponed or conducted in shorts
			Whenever relative humidity is 97% or higher, great precaution should be taken.	

From Gieck J, Kulund DN, eds. The Injured Athlete. 2nd ed. Philadelphia, PA: J B Lippincott; 1988: 176, with permission.

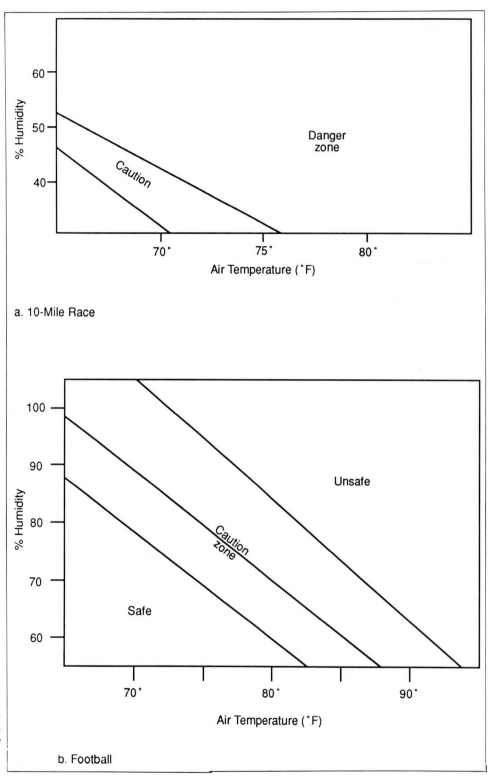

Figure 5-1. Cumulative effect of heat and high humidity on athletic activity. *(From Morris AF. Sports Medicine Handbook. Dubuque, Ia: Wm C Brown Publishers; 1984:158, with permission.)*

electrolytes through the diet. Fresh fruits and vegetables are largely composed of water and contain minerals the body needs. It is generally not necessary to use table salt or salt tablets, as most processed foods already contain more than adequate amounts of sodium. It should be noted that taking salt tablets while exercising can draw the body's fluids to the stomach and away from working muscles and organs. If sodium deficiency is suspected, laboratory work should be done to verify suspicions and help make dietary changes.

Commercial drinks are available to assist with rehydration, many of which contain various forms of artificial sweeteners or sugar. Sweeteners can actually slow gastric emptying, delaying the hydration process.

TABLE 5-4. RECOMMENDED FLUID INTAKE SCHEME

Time	Amount
2 hr before activity	1 L (34 oz)
15 min before activity	400–500 mL (13–17 oz)
Every 15–30 min during activity	400–500 mL (13–17 oz)
After activity	2–3 L (68–102 oz, 5–6 large glasses)

Adapted from Roy/Irvin. Sports Medicine: Prevention, Evaluation, Management, and Rehabilitation. *Englewood, NJ: Prentice-Hall Inc; 1983:480, with permission.*

Fluid may then take 20 to 30 minutes to reach working muscles. Because these drinks contain water, potassium, and sodium, they can be very beneficial to ingest throughout other parts of the day. There are some athletes who will not drink tasteless fluids. For these individuals, it is better that they drink some form of liquid than nothing at all. Commercial preparations on the field are worthwhile in these cases. Also useful during endurance activity in extremely hot early-acclimatization periods are drinks with low sugar content that are supplemented with moderate amounts of carbohydrates, sodium, and potassium.[18]

The single most effective means of hydration is drinking water. Athletes need to be educated in its importance and given specific guidelines for daily replenishment of fluids. Large, heavy athletes will require greater quantities and more frequent intake. The majority of heat-related deaths in American football have occurred in interior linemen, who generally have the largest muscle bulk. Those athletes who have a history of heat-related problems will also require special modifications. For average, healthy individuals, Table 5–4 suggests an appropriate daily protocol.[19]

Water must always be available during all scheduled athletic events. Cool water (4°C [39°F]) is absorbed more rapidly than warm water. Athletes should use squeeze bottles or individual cups to avoid the spread of communicable illness. They should be instructed to drink *before* actually feeling thirsty. Cold towels, showers, and the splashing of cold water over the head, neck, and trunk may assist in maintaining normal skin temperatures, but the ingestion of water is the only effective means of regulating core (inner) temperatures. Table 5–5 summarizes recommended fluid availability and intake for a strenuous 90-minute practice.[11]

Prevention. Despite the efforts of many concerned medical professionals, heat illness in athletics continues to occur, due to carelessness and ignorance among some sports participants. The American College of Sports Medicine has recognized the importance of education in this area and has published a position stand for guidelines in the prevention of thermal injuries during distance running.[20] This information is designed to educate personnel involved in the coordination of races during hot weather to take the necessary safety precautions.

Recognition of early heat-illness warning signs is

TABLE 5-5. RECOMMENDED FLUID AVAILABILITY AND INTAKE FOR A 90-MIN ATHLETIC PRACTICE (BASED ON AN 80% REPLACEMENT OF WEIGHT LOSS)

Weight Loss (lbs)	(kg)	Minutes Between Water Break	Fluid per Break (oz)	(mL)	Fluid Availability for an 11-Person Squad (gal)	(L)
8	(3.6)	No practice	—		—	
7½	(3.4)	recommended	—		—	
7	(3.2)	10	8–10	(266)	6½–8	(27.4)
6½	(3.0)	10	8–9	(251)	6½–7	(25.5)
6	(2.7)	10	8–9	(251)	6½–7	(25.5)
5½	(2.5)	15	10–12	(325)	5½–6½	(22.7)
5	(2.3)	15	10–11	(311)	5½–6	(21.8)
4½	(2.1)	15	9–10	(281)	5–5½	(19.9)
4	(1.8)	15	8–9	(251)	4½–5	(18.0)
3½	(1.6)	20	10–11	(311)	4–4½	(16.1)
3	(1.4)	20	9–10	(281)	3½–4	(14.2)
2½	(1.1)	20	7–8	(222)	3	(11.4)
2	(0.9)	30	8	(237)	2½	(9.5)
1½	(0.7)	30	6	(177)	1½	(5.7)
1	(0.5)	45	6	(177)	1	(3.8)
½	(0.2)	60	6	(177)	½	(1.9)

From McArdle WD, Katch FI, Katch VL. Exercise Physiology. *Philadelphia, Pa: Lea & Febiger; 1986:453, with permission.*

also critical in preventing more serious heat injuries. *Heat cramps* and *heat fatigue* most often present with the symptoms of heat, weakness, and fatigue. There may be involuntary muscle cramps, especially in the lower extremities. A typical sign is flushed, sweaty skin; the rectal temperature may be normal or slightly elevated. The treatment is rest and proper rehydration. Passive stretching generally helps muscle cramps.

Heat exhaustion and *heat stroke* are medical emergencies, requiring the immediate attention of trained professionals. The sports physical therapist must be able to recognize their signs and symptoms, acting quickly and judiciously to prevent potential complications such as myocardial infarction, renal or kidney failure, or cerebral edema, all of which can easily lead to death.

Table 5–6 summarizes the cause, signs, symptoms, and treatment of various heat injury types.[2,19,21,22] Mixed heat injury syndromes are not uncommon.[23] Because signs and symptoms may be confusing, the most accurate means of determining proper treatment is by obtaining rectal temperature.

Acclimatization. Athletes must be allowed adequate time for physiological adaptation to exercise in warm environments.[24] They should be instructed to begin gradual exposure prior to spring training sessions. About 7 to 21 days before scheduled practices start, athletes should begin by spending 20 to 45 minutes exercising outdoors. This acclimatization regime should gradually increase to 2 hours prior to the first day of practice.[22]

Proper hydration and activity modifications are important during individual pretraining exercise, and again during preseason practice workouts. Coaches need to arrange practices for the cooler, less humid times of day. Athletes should be allowed to wear shorts and loose-knit, light-colored cotton jerseys. Figure 5–2 plots rectal and skin temperatures with various football attire.[25] No sweatsuits or rubber suits should be permitted. Recording daily body weights of all athletes, before and after practice, can greatly assist in monitoring rehydration status. Student therapists and assistant managers can help with this task.[22]

Special Considerations. A particular sport that requires close attention of the sports physical therapist with regard to weight monitoring is wrestling. These athletes are continuously altering their diets, even using diuretics, to "make weight." The danger of electrolyte loss and dehydration is obviously great. Potassium, a vital electrolyte, can be depleted by various quick weight loss techniques. This leads to reduced muscle strength, giving opponents the competitive advantage. Proper education to coaches and athletes can promote healthy athletics.

Although age and sex do not appear to either detract from or contribute to acclimatization, obesity

TABLE 5-6. RECOGNIZING HEAT INJURY TYPES

Syndrome	Symptoms	Signs	Treatment
Heat cramps	Painful, involuntary muscle cramps–especially in the lower extremities	Normal	Hyperhydration during activity; proper rehydration techniques, local passive stretching
Heat fatigue	Hot, weak, tired	Rectal temperature of 38°–39.5°C (100.4°–103°F), flushed, sweating	Rest, fluid replenishment
Heat exhaustion	Fatigue, stupor, headache, syncope, nausea, blurred vision, cramps	Rectal temperature of 39°–40.5°C (102.2°–104.9°F), cool/ashen skin, sweating (often profuse) orthostatic hypotension/hypovolemia, rapid pulse/small pulse pressure (100–140 bpm), hypoglycemia	Intravenous fluids, cool environment, iced towels, urine output monitored for 24 hr for possible renal difficulty
Heat stroke	Confused/disoriented mental status and speech patterns, headache, extremely hot	Rectal temperature of 41°C (105.8°F) or higher, flushed warm skin, sweating often absent, unconsciousness, rapid strong or weak pulse (120–160 bpm), diastolic BP low/wide pulse pressure	Cool environment, remove clothes, iced towels, stimulated air flow, monitor vital signs, transport to ER quickly

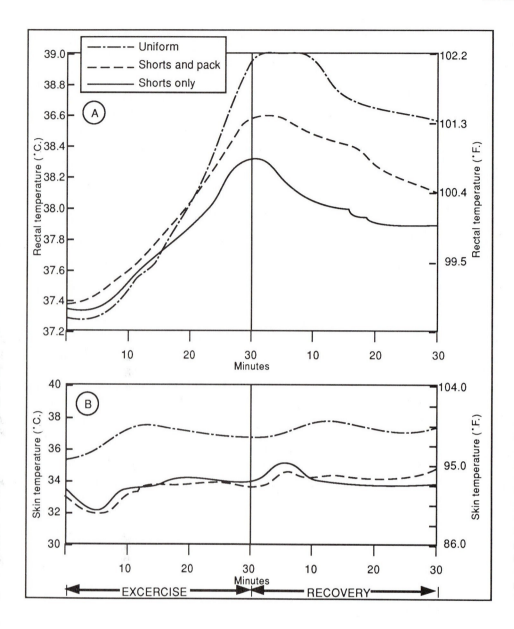

Figure 5-2. Effects of the football uniform on (A) rectal temperature and (B) skin temperature during exercise. *(From Mathews DK, Fox FL, Tanzi D. Physiological responses during exercise and recovery in a football uniform.* J Appl Physiol. *1969; 26:612, 613. Reprinted by permission in adapted form of McArdle WD, Katch FI, Katch VL. Exercise Physiology. Philadelphia, Pa: Lee & Febiger; 1981:340.)*

causes a distinct disadvantage. Fat acts as an insulator, inhibiting the shunting of internal heat to the skin's surface. Heat stroke, resulting in death, occurs over three times as often in obese exercisers as in athletes of average weight.

Malignant hyperthermia is a rare muscle disorder that causes sensitivity to anesthesia and hot environments. This disease causes muscle temperatures to increase more quickly than core temperatures. The result is frequent muscle cramps, tachycardia, and other symptoms that mimic heat stroke. The problem can be fatal to athletes with this condition who exercise in hot, humid environments. Other clues to aid in definitive diagnosis may include muscle hypertrophy, scoliosis, kyphosis, hernia, clubfoot, ptosis, joint subluxation, strabismus, and muscle weakness. Muscle-related complaints often occur following exercise and rectal temperature may remain elevated for 10 to 15 minutes.

Muscle biopsy is necessary to confirm findings. The athlete suffering from acute symptoms can be successfully treated with dantrolene. Because of the seriousness of this disease's consequences, exercise in hot, humid weather should be prohibited. Individuals with malignant hyperthermia should wear a medical alert bracelet and family members should be made aware of this familial trait.[26]

Cold Environments

As described in the section on heat and humidity, the body loses heat by means of conduction, convection, and evaporation and can absorb heat through radiation. These principles also apply when addressing heat loss in cold environments. Sports such as snow skiing, mountain climbing, hiking, kayaking, hunting, fishing, sailing, ice hockey, and ice skating are often carried out in less than comfortable environments. In these

circumstances, athletes should attempt to conserve body heat to avoid the onset of cold injury. Some cold adaptation can occur in individuals who are frequently exposed. Also body type may play a significant role in cold tolerance. Endomorphic persons seem to lose heat at a slower rate than do ectomorphs. This may be due to the endomorphs' smaller surface area exposure in relation to underlying mass, as well as increased fat tissue, a remarkable insulator.[27]

The body's average core temperature is 37°C (99°F), with skin temperature varying between 16°C (60°F) and 33°C (92°F). When an athlete becomes cold, an initial response may be to increase movement. Vigorous exercise can increase metabolic rates up to 25 to 30 times base levels. Shivering is another natural body response designed to help conserve core temperatures. In some instances, however, the body is defenseless against external conditions. This is particularly true when cold temperatures are coupled with high winds, wet environments, or both (Table 5–7).[19]

Hypothermia. *Hypothermia* refers to below-normal levels of core and shell body temperatures, due to exposure to cold environments. Predisposing factors that can increase the incidence of hypothermia include perspiration-drenched clothing, dehydration, malnutrition, alcohol consumption, and physical exhaustion.

When the body's core temperature drops below 35°C (95°F), obvious signs of hypothermia appear. Loss of coordination, lethargic behavior, and speech difficulty are present. If the temperature is allowed to drop further, blood pressure and heart sounds can no longer be heard through the body's rigid tissues. Skin takes on a waxy appearance and pupil response to light is often absent. Below body temperatures of 27° to 26°C (80° to 78°F) cardiopulmonary function shuts down.

Severe hypothermia requires prompt emergency care, with great care devoted to providing safe transport to a medical facility. Rewarming of body parts should only be attempted by skilled personnel, as improper technique can be fatal. Rewarming should not be initiated unless there is no chance of refreezing.

Finding warm, dry shelter is of primary importance. Wet clothing should be removed and replaced with dry clothes or blankets. With the vital signs being continually monitored, the victim is warmed slowly at room temperature in the head-lowered, lower-extremities-elevated position. Cardiopulmonary resuscitation (CPR) should be initiated if the pulse is or becomes absent.

In milder forms of hypothermia, the athlete may be conscious and better able to take an active role in his or her treatment. After a change to dry clothes, active movement of limbs is mandatory. A warm carbohydrate-loaded, nonalcoholic drink may be given. Body warming should be done slowly, at room temperature, with no additional blankets or local heat applied indoors, unless the athlete is truly unable to exercise. Hypothermia can occur in 3 hours or less and at air temperatures as high as 18°C (65°F) when wind chill and wetness factors are high.

Several measures can be taken to prevent hypothermia. Preactivity meals should be high in carbohydrates to assist in energy and heat expenditure. Both hot and cold drinks should be made available to athletes while exercising to assist in rehydration as well as warming bodies. Alcohol and cigarette smoking need always be prohibited, as they can cause a false sense of warming while actually restricting blood flow.

TABLE 5–7. WIND CHILL CHART

Wind (mph)	Temperature (°F)																				
Calm	40°	35°	30°	25°	20°	15°	10°	5°	0°	−5°	−10°	−15°	−20°	−25°	−30°	−35°	−40°	−45°	−50°	−55°	−60°
										Equivalent Chill Temperature											
5	35°	30°	25°	20°	15°	10°	5°	0°	−5°	−10°	−15°	−20°	−25°	−30°	−35°	−40°	−45°	−50°	−55°	−65°	−70°
10	30°	20°	15°	10°	5°	0°	−10°	−15°	−20°	−25°	−35°	−40°	−45°	−50°	−60°	−65°	−70°	−75°	−80°	−90°	−95°
15	25°	15°	10°	0°	−5°	−10°	−20°	−25°	−30°	−40°	−45°	−50°	−60°	−65°	−70°	−80°	−85°	−90°	−100°	−105°	−110°
20	20°	10°	5°	0°	−10°	−15°	−25°	−30°	−35°	−45°	−50°	−60°	−65°	−75°	−80°	−85°	−95°	−100°	−110°	−115°	−120°
25	15°	10°	0°	−5°	−15°	−20°	−30°	−35°	−45°	−50°	−60°	−65°	−75°	−80°	−90°	−95°	−105°	−110°	−120°	−125°	−135°
30	10°	5°	0°	−10°	−20°	−25°	−30°	−40°	−50°	−55°	−65°	−70°	−80°	−85°	−95°	−100°	−105°	−115°	−120°	−130°	−140°
35	10°	5°	−5°	−10°	−20°	−25°	−35°	−40°	−50°	−60°	−65°	−75°	−80°	−90°	−100°	−105°	−115°	−120°	−130°	−135°	−145°
40	10°	0°	−5°	−15°	−20°	−30°	−35°	−45°	−55°	−60°	−70°	−75°	−85°	−95°	−100°	−110°	−115°	−125°	−130°	−140°	−150°

Little danger	Increasing danger (Flesh may freeze within 1 min)	Great danger (Flesh may freeze within 30 s)

From Roy/Irvin. Sports Medicine: Prevention, Evaluation, Management, and Rehabilitation. *Englewood Cliffs, NJ: Prentice-Hall Inc; 1983:484, with permission.*

Wearing proper attire can greatly assist in prevention of hypothermia. Loosely woven materials, such as wool, will draw perspiration away from the body while maintaining warmth by trapping air. This warm, trapped air acts as an insulator. Down has much the same effect, as long as it remains dry. Various nylon combinations serve as excellent wind breakers when worn as outside layers. Because as much as 50% of the body's heat is lost through the head and neck, hats and scarves should always be mandatory. Mittens are better than gloves because the close proximity of the fingers provides greater warmth. Thermal underwear (as opposed to insulated underwear) maintains warmth while allowing evaporation of perspiration. Pantyhose also accomplishes this task. No article of clothing should be tight, as this restricts circulation. Layering clothing helps trap warm air for further insulation.

Winter sports are often played in extremely unfavorable weather. During cold winter games, sidelines should include small space heaters in sheltered bench areas. Benches can be covered with insulated materials, such as indoor–outdoor carpet. An adequate supply of towels can help to warm if wrapped around the face and neck. A white flag should be mounted to indicate WBGTs below 10°C (50°F).[2,28]

Other Cold Injuries. When the body's core temperature is maintained but the shell or outer temperature falls, frostnip, superficial or deep frostbite, chilblains, or trench foot may occur.

Frostnip. Frostnip, also called *incipient frostbite*, is often first noticed by a fellow athlete because of its gradual, painless onset. The skin is blanched in the areas of the ears, nose, cheeks, chin, fingers, or toes. The areas can be easily treated with direct pressure, warm air, or contact with warm objects. Practical means of applying these treatments include holding the body part with a warm, compressing hand, placing fingers or toes in a warm axilla, or blowing warm air onto the body part. During the thawing process, redness and tingling are likely to occur.

Superficial Frostbite. Like frostnip, *superficial frostbite* takes on a whiteness of the skin, although observation and palpation reveal a waxy firmness. A frostbitten victim will require transfer to indoor shelter for rewarming. The techniques are similar to those used with frostnip. Some edema may become visible if capillaries have been broken. Blisters may develop, along with symptoms of aching, burning, and throbbing. Pain and redness may ensue for several weeks. Frostbitten athletes should be protected from the cold until healing is complete.

Deep Frostbite. *Deep frostbite* involves both cutaneous and subcutaneous epidermal layers, often causing severe and permanent damage. The most commonly affected areas are the hands and feet. Underlying tissues are rigid. The white, cold skin becomes a darkened purple upon rewarming. Severe pain, blisters, and even gangrene may transpire over the following 24 to 48 hours. Expedient first aid care is critical in reducing or eliminating permanent damage.

Treatment of all types of frostbite includes keeping the victim warm and dry. If the condition is serious and immediate transport to a critical care unit is not feasible, warming may be initiated with warm indoor baths at 38° to 40°C (100° to 105°F). These baths must be closely monitored for temperature accuracy, with additional warm water added as the body part dissipates cold. Sterile dressings should be applied to all affected areas, being careful as to avoid body parts touching objects or each other. Any blisters should be left unbroken, as not to increase the risk of infection.[2,28]

Chilblains. *Chilblains* are edematous, red, tender areas with increased skin temperature, caused by prolonged or repeated exposure of bare skin to moderately cold conditions. This injury tends to be chronic and there is no treatment, other than protection from cold environments.

Trench Foot. The *trench foot* injury has taken on many names: immersion foot, lifeboat foot, and air-raid shelter foot. The cause is the same for all—overexposure to cold and wet conditions. The signs, symptoms, and treatment are not unlike those of other cold injuries. The cold, numb, swollen foot appears waxy and mottled. As thawing occurs, it becomes red and hot. Blisters occur and gangrene may set in. Keeping the foot warm and dry, along with maintaining healthy foot care and hygiene, will help to prevent further damage.[29]

As practical information for the sports physical therapist, only the milder forms of cold injuries, such as frostnip and superficial frostbite, should be treated on site. Using one's own body heat or the body heat of a teammate is most beneficial. Direct pressure is effective; rubbing is contraindicated. Thawing and refreezing should be avoided at all costs.

Wind Factors

Wind can take on a positive or negative role in athletics, depending upon the circumstances. On a hot, humid summer day, the increase in air circulation improves the body's surface area cooling by assisting in perspiration evaporation. Runners, cyclists, skiers, and sailors may note improved race times while traveling "with the wind."

More often, the wind is regarded as an impediment to an athlete, hindering performance. Traveling "against the wind" creates resistance that can be the difference between a qualifying or eliminating race.

Cyclists, in particular, make every effort to streamline their bodies and equipment, hoping to minimize wind resistance. Shaving body hair and wearing sleek, body-hugging clothing is done for this purpose.

Wind Chill. High wind in cold environments can chill an athlete to far greater degrees than air temperature might suggest. Table 5–7 is a chart designed to assess wind chill factor.[19] Athletes must dress and prepare accordingly, taking every precaution to avoid cold injury.

Windburn. Regardless of temperature, when winds are high, windburn can result. The most commonly affected are the face, eyes, lips, and hands. Chapping and irritation usually cause redness and burning. Treatment is simply to moisturize dry, rough areas. Mild, hypoallergenic lotion or cream can be applied to the skin. Eyedrops may soothe the eyes. Prevention includes protective clothing worn over susceptible areas. Goggles or glasses will protect the eyes. Frequent application of lip balm will protect the lips.

Precipitation

It is not uncommon to see athletes engaging in sports during inclement conditions. League games and tournaments are under the discretion of team officials and referees. These individuals will most often act conservatively with regard to athletic safety. It is the responsibility of the sports therapist, however, to advise coaches, athletes, and officials should play continue during unsafe conditions.

Rain, snow, sleet and hail significantly reduce visibility and increase the risk of injury. Any athletic event should be postponed in the event of lightning. The issue is both one of safety for the participants as well as legal coverage of the staff.

SPECIAL CONSIDERATIONS FOR SAFETY

There are a variety of man-made and indoor athletic environments where safety should be a primary concern. The sports physical therapist can significantly reduce the risk of injury to athletes through proper awareness and communication with others involved.

Gymnasiums

Floors. If concrete, floors should be sealed with a commercial floor sealer to prevent moisture from damaging mats or harboring bacteria and mold. All areas should be kept clean and free of trash.

Apparatus. Floor plates must be securely anchored in concrete. Equipment should be arranged so that athletes do not dismount looking directly into lights or window glare. Prior to use each day, all floor plates and equipment should be checked for proper setup and signs of wear. Equipment left standing during unsupervised hours should be secured from unauthorized use. Spectators should be required to stay behind a restraining barrier during all practices and competitions.

Landing pits, safety mats, and trajectory platforms should be strategically placed. Free weights, chalk trays, and other small, movable equipment should be kept and used out of the way of gymnastic floor work and mount/dismount activity.

Equipment should never be used for any activity other than that for which it was intended. Written records of a regular, comprehensive inspection and maintenance program by qualified personnel are essential. Defective equipment should be removed from use until it has been fixed to meet safety standards. Warning labels should never be removed from equipment and should be in obvious, visible locations.

Walls. Any protrusions, obstructions, or columns should be safely padded. Runways, dismount points, and high traffic areas should be kept at a sufficient distance from walls, doorways, windows, and mirrors. Stable partitions are recommended to separate concurrent sport activities taking place in the same gym. Light-colored walls best reflect light and their surfaces should be smooth at least up to 12 ft from the floor.

Ceilings. For competitive gymnastics, there should be a minimum of 9 ft (2.7 m) to the bottom of the closed ceiling, beam, or joist. For activities such as trampolining, however, a minimum ceiling height of 24 ft (7.3 m) is recommended. Air ducts, light fixtures, and pipes should also be sufficiently high for safe activity below. Safety harnesses, ropes, and spotting rigs must be properly and securely affixed to their supporting structures.

Heating, Lighting, and Plumbing Fixtures. Utility control panels should be clearly marked; their location should provide easy access. All fixtures should be routinely inspected by a contractor or engineer. If physical contact by an athlete is possible, they need to be padded or shielded. Emergency lights should always be provided.

Air, Temperature, and Light Regulation. Ventilation should aim at providing four changes of air per hour without creating drafts. Activity room temperatures should be heated to 16°C (60°F) on cold days, locker rooms to 21°C (70°F), and shower areas to 27°C (80°F). On hot days, there should be ample ventilation and a sufficient number of recessed drinking fountains, conveniently located to athletic activity.

Semidirect light is best for reducing eyestrain,

with 20 to 30 foot-candles sufficient for general activity; activities requiring preciseness may warrant a greater intensity, however.[30]

Swimming Pools

Size. A 50-m Olympic pool, 25 yd (22.9 m) wide, most safely accommodates the active or competitive swimmer. For competition, there should be eight lanes, 7 ft (2.1 m) wide with an additional 1.5 ft (45.7 cm) in the outside lanes to smooth the water and reduce the risk of contact by a swimmer.

Depth. The shallow end of the recreational pool should be 3.5 ft (1.1 m) deep. This adds safety for those who are not strong swimmers or are not comfortable in deeper waters. Diving should *never* be permitted here! Many deaths and spinal cord injuries have occurred from improper technique in waters too shallow for diving.

A diving well should be included within the complex to eliminate diving in the main pool. The ceiling should be 15 ft (4.6 m) above the highest board. The water depth should be 10 ft (3.1 m) for 1-m boards and 14 to 16 ft (4.3 to 4.9 m) for 3-m boards.

Depth markings should be located at critical points on the deck and on the face of the pool. Ladders should be recessed and located at each corner of the pool. Overflow systems are necessary for sanitation, by removing waste and debris from the water's surface.

Air, Temperature, and Lighting Regulation. There should be adequate ventilation to reduce humidity and condensation. Air intakes should be located so as not to create a draft at the water's surface. Uniformity of lighting is important to minimize glare and shadows, as well as decrease growth of algae. Fifty ft-c at the water's surface is generally accepted. Also, underwater lighting facilitates cleaning and promotes safety. Water temperature should be 27°C (80°F) for instructional classes and 23° to 24°C (74° to 76°F) for competitive swimming. Air temperature should be 3°C (5°F) warmer than the water temperature.

Water Treatment. Pool water should be circulated and filtered four times every hour. Proper control of pH balance and regular disinfection provides maximal visibility and protection against disease.

Other Concerns. Ideally, a pool should have a tiled surface for easy cleaning and to reduce the chance of an athlete slipping. Abrasive tile can be used at wall areas where competitive swimmers execute their flip-turns. An open, nonslip, dry area should be designated for strengthening, flexibility, and warmup exercises out of the water.

Circuit breakers should be located on all electrical outlets and no outlet should be located within 2.7 m (9 ft) of the water. All special devices such as starting blocks, pace clocks, kick boards, and other training equipment should be stored properly when not in use. Pool activities such as synchronized swimming, water polo, and events for the physically and mentally handicapped may require specialized safety/medical personnel and equipment.[30,31,32]

Although it may not always be possible to change the environment, astute awareness, coupled with the appropriate and available modifications, can go a long way toward improving the athlete's health and quality of exercise. The sports physical therapist has much to contribute to the safety and well-being of all who participate in athletics.

REFERENCES

1. Leader Sports Products, Inc. Lexan Polycarbonate Vision Plus Eyeshields Advertisement. New York (800) 847-2001.
2. Peterson L, Renstrom P. *Sports Injuries—Their Prevention and Treatment.* Chicago, IL: Year Book Medical Publishers Inc; 1986.
3. Davis JO, Grandjean AC, Newsom MM, Stone J, Handel PV, Voy RO. *Jet Lag and Athletic Performance.* United States Olympic Committee Sports Medicine Council; 1986.
4. Duda M. Study: More grid injuries on grass. *Physician Sportsmed.* 1988; 16(4):41.
5. Powell JW. Incidence of Injury Associated with Playing Surfaces in the National Football League 1980-1985. *Athlet Training.* Fall 1987; 202–206.
6. Bowers KD Jr, Martin RB. Impact absorption, new and old Astroturf at West Virginia University. *Med Sci Sports.* 1974; 6:217–221.
7. Torg JS. Football shoes and playing surfaces: From safe to unsafe. *Physician Sportsmed.* 1973; 1(3):51–54.
8. Hammer DA. Artificial playing surfaces. *Athlet Training.* Winter 1981; 240–242.
9. NATA Meeting and Clinical Symposium, St. Louis, Mo, June 1979: How to live with synthetic turf. *Athlet Training.* Fall 1980; 150–158.
10. White–Clergerie AM. Mountaineering without oxygen: Courting death? *Physician Sportsmed.* 1987; 15(3):38–39.
11. McArdle WD, Katch FI, Katch VL. *Exercise Physiology.* Philadelphia, Pa: Lea & Febiger; 1981.
12. Schoene RB, Bracker MD, eds. High altitude pulmonary edema: The disguised killer. *Physician Sportsmed.* 1988; 16(8):103–114.
13. deVries HA. *Physiology of Exercise.* Dubuque, Ia: Wm C Brown Publishers; 1974.
14. Morris AF. *Sports Medicine Handbook.* Dubuque, Ia: Wm C Brown Publishers; 1985.
15. Ellison AE, Boland AL Jr, DeHaven KE, Grace P, Snook GA, Calehuff H, eds. *Athletic Training and Sports Med-*

icine. Chicago, Ill: American Academy of Orthopaedic Surgeons; 1984.

16. Davis JC, Bracker MD, eds. Decompression sickness in sport scuba diving. *Physician Sportsmed.* 1988; 16(2):108–121.

17. Kulund DN. *The Injured Athlete*. Philadelphia, Pa: J B Lippincott Co; 1988.

18. Nadel ER. *Sports Science Exchange—New Ideas for Rehydration During and After Exercise in Hot Weather*. Chicago, Ill: Gatorade Sports Science Institute, 1988; 1(3).

19. Roy S, Irvin R. *Sports Medicine*. Englewood Cliffs, NJ: Prentice-Hall Inc; 1983.

20. ACSM Position Statement on prevention of thermal injuries during distance running. *MSSE.* 1987; 19(5):529–533.

21. Stoddard G, ed. Hot weather trauma—How to identify and treat heat exhaustion and heatstroke. *Mueller Sports Med Guide.* 1984; 3(2):5.

22. Murphy RJ, Kaverman D, eds. Heat illness in the athlete. *Athlet Training.* Fall 1984; 166–170.

23. Micheli LJ, Puffer JC, Yocum L. Mixed heat injury syndrome. *Sports Med Dig.* 1987; 9(7):7–8.

24. Armstrong LE, Hubbard RW, Deluca JP, Cristensen EL. Heat acclimatization during summer running in the Northeastern United States. *Med Sci Sports Exerc.* 1987; 19(2):131–136.

25. Mathews DK, Fox EL, Tanzi D. Physiological responses during exercise and recovery in a football uniform. *J Appl Phys.* 1969; 26:612, 613.

26. Hunter SL, Rosenberg H, Tuttle GH, DeWalt JL, Smodic R, Martin J. Malignant hyperthermia in a college football player. *Physician Sportsmed.* 1987; 15(12):77–81.

27. Pate RR. *Sports Science Exchange—Special Considerations for Exercise in Cold Weather*. Chicago, Ill: Gatorade Sports Science Institute 1988; 1(10).

28. Nelson WE, Gieck JH, Kolb P. Treatment and Prevention of Hypothermia and Frostbite. *Athlet Training.* Winter 1983; 330–332.

29. Steele P. Management of frostbite. *Physician Sportsmed.* 1989; 17(1):135–144.

30. Voltmer EF, Esslinger AA, McCue BF, Tillman KG. *The Organization and Administration of Physical Education*. Englewood Cliffs, NJ: Prentice-Hall Inc; 1979.

31. George GS, ed. *United States Gymnastic Federation Gymnastics Safety Manual*. Indianapolis, In: USGF Publications; 1985.

32. *Minimum Standards for Public Swimming Pools*. Alexandria, Va: National Spa and Pool Institute; 1977.

6

Ergogenic Aids

A. Lynn Millar

INTRODUCTION

Ergogenic aids have been defined as anything that helps increase work performance above levels that might be obtained under normal conditions. Ergogenic aids may be categorized by the mode in which they facilitate performance, and the typical categories include pharmacological, nutritional, physiological, psychological, and mechanical. This chapter addresses all these areas, with the exception of mechanical aids. In addition, certain topics, such as nutrition, are covered in other chapters and the reader is referred to those pertinent chapters if more specific detail is needed.

Ergogenic aids have been documented as far back as the early Greek competitions, where athletes first attempted to improve performance by eating raw meat in the hope of increasing strength, and is still prevalent today. The use of some form of ergogenic aid spans all age groups, and may often range from the seemingly innocent form of a weekend athlete who takes megadoses of vitamins to the not so innocent abuse of pharmacological substances. A disturbing fact is that many of these athletes continue to take a banned and potentially dangerous substance even while knowing the associated risks. Several surveys have found that the athletes said they would take a banned substance if it would improve their performance, even if they knew there was some risk to their health.[1,2] Unfortunately, this attitude seems to be present even among recreational athletes, who cannot expect potential financial rewards from improved performance.

Anyone involved with athletes must therefore have a knowledge of the basic advantages and disadvantages of the various types of ergogenic aids that an athlete may be considering and should be willing to act as a source of reliable information. A sports physical therapist should also be familiar with any position statements from governing bodies. For many, the decision to use or not to use an ergogenic aid becomes an ethical decision rather than a health one. Here again, some aids may be considered ethical, such as visual imagery, whereas the use of others, such as anabolic steroids, is generally considered unethical and is prohibited by most international and national amateur sport governing bodies.

PHARMACOLOGICAL AIDS

There are many drugs that are used for their performance-enhancing potential, although it should be noted that often any improvement is psychological rather than physical. This section discusses only a few drugs that are used most frequently for their ergogenic effects. Additional information regarding drugs and the athlete may be found in Chapter 7. Six types of pharmacological agents are commonly associated with sport performance. These include anabolic steroids, stimulants, barbiturates, bronchodilators, and diuretics.

Anabolic Steroids

Anabolic steroids are synthetic compounds similar to the endogenous steroid hormones, and those that are androgenic in nature (with effects similar to the male hormone testosterone) were used originally to aid recovery from malnutrition or surgery. There are several legitimate reasons for androgenic–anabolic steroid treatment; however, the use of these drugs in the sports world is not of a therapeutic nature.

Anabolic steroids may be taken orally or by injection. Some of the more common name brands and their generic names are listed in Table 6–1. The steroid is taken up by a receptor site in the cytoplasm of the muscle cells and ultimately stimulates protein synthesis.[3] Thus, the theoretical benefit of anabolic steroid usage is an increase in muscle size and strength with a resultant improvement in performance. As with most pharmacological studies, much of the original research was done in rats, which is one factor that must be considered when examining the literature regarding the effects of

TABLE 6-1. FREQUENTLY USED ANABOLIC STEROIDS

Drug	Trade Name
Oral	
Stanozolol	Winstrol
Mesterolone	Proviron
Methandrostenolone	Dianabol
Oxandrolone	Anavar
Oxymetholone	Anadrol
Methandienone	
Injectable	
Methadrostenolone	Dianabol
Stenobolone	Anatrofin
Methenolone	Primobolan
Nandrolone	
Stanozolol	

anabolic steroids. Other factors that must be examined include drug dosage, mode of administration, duration of administration, and the chemical compound taken. Factors that interact with this might be fitness level of subject, sex, nutrition, type of exercise, motivation, and so forth. Thus, research findings are often contradictory and difficult to relate to what the athlete actually may be doing.

Early research with rats found significant increases in muscular growth; Lamb,[4] however, notes that those studies that found remarkable growth either had used "sex-linked muscles" or animals with subnormal levels of androgenic steroids (usually caused by castration). In studies that looked at total muscular weight, such as that of Bauman et al,[5] the rats injected with anabolic steroids actually had a lower weight gain than the control group ($p < 0.05$). This was considered to be caused by the depressant effect that anabolic steroids may have on the appetite. It should be noted, however, that the rats were exercised in an aerobic mode, and not in the anaerobic strength-type program typically employed by athletes.

More important to this discussion is the effect of anabolic steroids on men (or women) who use them. This issue has been debated for years, and some researchers still believe that there is no conclusive evidence to support the belief that anabolic steroids will result in increased muscle size and strength. In a review of the literature, Percy notes that much of the data with humans were not true double-blind studies, and that the few that were found no improvement in the measured parameters.[6] This is a valid criticism and one that has been difficult to overcome. Freed et al found that all their subjects were able to distinguish the placebo from the real steroid, probably due to a slight sense of euphoria often caused by steroids.[7] Those who believe that steroids do increase muscle size and strength maintain that the amount of steroids given in these studies is usually substantially less (by as much as a factor of 10) than the doses reported by athletes who admitted

to steroid usage. If we examine those studies that had some type of control group, with some attempt at a double blind, the majority of the studies found increases in body weight, limb girth, and lean body mass for those subjects who had steroid treatment. Only about 50% of the studies found associated improvements in strength performance. Often the improvement is limited to a specific parameter, such as vertical jump, which thus limits the relevancy of conclusions regarding sports performance.[8]

The major argument against anabolic steroid use (ignoring the ethical one for the moment) is that of potential medical risk. Table 6–2 lists some of the side effects that have been reported either by athletes or in the medical literature. The two body systems that have been linked most with steroid abuse are the liver and reproductive systems. Kiraly studied the blood serum and skin lipid parameters of seven power athletes who had admitted to self-administration of anabolic steroids and eight power athletes who were not using any drugs.[9] He found a significant ($p < 0.05$) increase in some liver enzyme activity values for the treatment group when compared to the control group, although he noted that the impairment was considered mild. Creagh et al presented a case study of a 27-year-old body builder who died from complications following rupture of a large hepatic nodule.[10] They suggested that the potential cause of the nodule was the use of anabolic steroids, as others previously suggested. As they noted, however, convincing evidence of a cause and effect relationship between anabolic steroid use and live tumors has not been produced.

In an attempt to examine some of the physiological and pathological changes believed to be caused by anabolic steroid use, Bauman et al conducted a well-designed and controlled study with 34 male rats.[5] Two of the four groups were given anabolic steroid injections two times per week, in addition to an aerobic swimming program three times per week for a total of 5 weeks. No pathological conditions were found in the livers or other organs from any of the rats. The researchers did find that the testicular weight in the rats

TABLE 6-2. REPORTED SIDE EFFECTS OF STEROID USAGE

Physical
  Decreased testicular size
  Increased acne
  Gynecomastia
  Decreased HDL cholesterol levels
  Increased total cholesterol
  Increased incidence of musculotendinous injury
  Possible hepatic nodules, carcinomas

Psychological
  Increased aggressiveness
  Irritability
  Manic behavior

receiving steroids were significantly lower ($p < 0.001$) than those in the control group or the nonsteroidal, exercise group. This finding corroborates similar findings with human subjects, such as that of Kiraly, who found a significant ($p < 0.001$) decrease in testicular volume for the power athletes who were taking anabolic steroids.[9] It appears that these changes are reversible, but there have not been any long-term studies that have adequately addressed this question.

Recently a new area of concern has been added to the list of potential medical problems caused or linked to steroid use. Detrimental changes in blood lipid parameters have been found in athletes who use steroids, and the parameters that show a decline are directly related to risk for coronary heart disease. In 1984, Hurley et al conducted a cross-sectional study of athletes involved in several different modes of training, including a group of competitive weight-trained athletes who were admitted steroid users.[11] They found that the athletes who self-administered anabolic steroids had significant increases in blood cholesterol levels ($p < 0.05$), increases in low-density lipoprotein (LDL) levels ($p < 0.0001$), and decreases in high-density lipoprotein (HDL) levels ($p < 0.001$), thus adversely altering the lipoprotein ratios. As the authors note, both the plasma cholesterol level and the HDL to LDL ratio are considered to be good predictors for the development of coronary artery disease. Findings of reduced HDL levels were confirmed by Kantor et al in their study of ten weightlifters.[12]

The potential for an increased risk of cardiovascular disease, whether from the changes in plasma lipoprotein concentrations or from other changes in the cardiovascular system, appears to be confirmed in part by some of the case studies that are appearing in the literature. McNutt et al found serum cholesterol level of 283 mg/dL, with a LDL of 220 and a HDL of 35 mg/dL, in a 22-year-old weightlifter who was diagnosed as having had an acute myocardial infarction following admittance to the hospital for severe chest pain.[13] The athlete had no factors normally associated with an increased risk of coronary heart disease other than the abnormal blood cholesterol levels, and lipid studies on his family found all of them to have normal blood cholesterol parameters. Therefore, the elevated cholesterol levels and decreased HDL levels appeared to be directly attributable to the use of steroids and the myocardial infarction indirectly related to the use of steroids. Mochizuki and Richter reported the case of a 32-year-old bodybuilder who suffered two cerebrovascular accidents and was also found to have cardiomyopathy with associated impaired left ventricular performance.[14] The bodybuilder had used steroids intermittently for 16 years in a variety of combinations and had no other risk factors for cardiovascular problems. The authors suggested that the steroid use may have led to

the deleterious changes in the athlete's cardiovascular system, citing research that has shown impairment of left ventricular diastolic filling in weightlifters[15] and another study that documented damage to contractile elements in the myocardium in rats.[16] It should be noted however, that Salke et al found no pathological changes in an experimental study with 15 athletes on steroids, 15 nonsteroid users, and 15 control subjects.[17]

One effect of anabolic steroid use that has direct implications for physical therapists is the incidence of increased musculoskeletal injuries. Some authors had thought that the increase in injury might be related to a relatively faster increase in strength of the muscle than for the tendons and connective tissues. Wood et al, however, believe that there may actually be a change in the connective tissue structure with steroid utilization.[18] They trained 24 rats, which had been divided into four groups, two of which were given steroids. After 6 weeks, the rats were killed and the structural parameters of the Achilles' tendon were extensively examined. The authors found a significant ($p < 0.001$) change in the structure of the steroid group as compared to all of the other groups. They noted that the change in structure may make the tendon more sensitive to mechanical stress and less mechanically efficient, causing it to reach a breaking point at lower stresses.

Several potential physical risks associated with anabolic steroid use have been presented, but it is important also to consider other changes that the athlete might exhibit. Notable among these are the psychological changes that have been documented. Testimony abounds concerning "Roid rages," and a few case reports of psychiatric changes have lent some credence to testimonial evidence.[19] Pope and Katz interviewed 31 users of anabolic steroids regarding a variety of psychological traits.[20] Among these athletes, three had psychotic symptoms, four had "subthreshold" psychotic symptoms, four had evidence of manic episodes, and five had suffered major depressions. None of the subjects reported similar symptoms when not using steroids, and the authors noted that "manic-like behaviors" were typical. Tennant et al reported a case of a 23-year-old bodybuilder who exhibited clinical features consistent with opioid addiction stemming from the use of anabolic steroids.[21] Unfortunately, these psychological changes make the role of the sports physical therapist increasingly difficult, as the athlete may be less inclined to listen to evidence against steroid use.

Because of the seemingly pervasive use of anabolic steroids—some studies showing approximately 90% of surveyed health club athletes reporting steroid usage, with 74% using two or more concomitantly[1,2]—it is increasingly important that the sports physical therapist be familiar with the attributes of steroid use. The majority of the case studies presented noted that the

athletes were often using more than one steroid at a time; however, there is nothing in the literature to indicate greater risk with "stacking" than with the use of only one steroid if the total dosage is the same. The American College of Sports Medicine Position Stand concerning the use of anabolic steroids is an excellent source for additional research regarding the effects of steroid usage.[22] The five major points of the statement are as follows:

1. Anabolic–androgenic steroids in the presence of an adequate diet can contribute to increases in body weight, often in the lean mass compartment.
2. The gains in muscular strength achieved through high-intensity exercise and proper diet can be increased by the use of anabolic–androgenic steroids in some individuals.
3. Anabolic–androgenic steroids do not increase aerobic power or capacity for muscular exercise.
4. Anabolic–androgenic steroids have been associated with adverse effects on the liver, cardiovascular system, reproductive system, and psychological status in therapeutic trials and in limited research on athletes. Until further research is completed, the potential hazards of the use of the anabolic–androgenic steroids in athletes must include those found in therapeutic trials.
5. The use of anabolic–androgenic steroids by athletes is contrary to the rules and ethical principles of athletic competition as set forth by many of the sports governing bodies. The American College of Sports Medicine supports these ethical principles and deplores the use of anabolic–androgenic steroids by athletes.

Human Growth Hormone

This topic is one which has come to the forefront in the last decade, but about which the literature is dominantly medical in nature. Human growth hormone (HGH) is normally present in the healthy person and is responsible for the stimulation of growth. It is believed that HGH stimulates growth by affecting the transport of amino acids into cells. In addition, HGH accelerates fat mobilization and catabolism. Although many athletes believe this to be a steroid, it is not a steroid compound. Circulating levels vary with each individual, but it is generally agreed that the body produces what is needed. The medical literature indicates that excessive amounts of HGH result in acromegaly, an abnormal growth of some of the bones such as the jaw, long bones, and muscles, along with abnormal effects on the internal organs. Case studies of persons with acromegaly usually note an early death—50% by age 50—

due to complications such as diabetes mellitus and cardiovascular disease. It is theorized that the results of using HGH as an ergogenic aid will have the same side effects. Therefore, this is not an ergogenic aid that should be recommended, nor should it be considered lightly just because it is something which is found normally in our bodies.

Stimulants

Stimulants, such as amphetamines and caffeine, have often been thought to benefit performance, most likely due to their effect on the central nervous system. They cause an increase in the state of arousal, which, as Ivy notes, is usually perceived by the person as an increase in energy and quicker reactions, and they also stimulate the production of adrenergic hormones, presumably through the hypothalamus.[23] Interestingly, stimulants have been found to improve several types of performance, but not simple reaction time. Most of the research with amphetamines has shown significant improvements in strength, acceleration, anaerobic capacity, and time to exhaustion, even in double-blind studies.[24] Improvements in maximal oxygen consumption or in submaximal consumption have not been reported, however, when improvements in work time to exhaustion were found, thus suggesting the mechanism of improvement is an alteration of the perception of fatigue. Research findings for strength and speed are contradictory and may be related to the research design. One area in which dramatic results have been identified is that of aerobic endurance. As already noted, some of this may be a perception factor, but much of the new research suggests that the stimulant caffeine has an effect on the metabolic energy cycles that causes a rise in blood free fatty acids and the utilization of these for energy. Most research has focused upon the use of caffeine prior to or during endurance work.

In 1978, Costill et al investigated the effects of caffeine ingestion on performance.[25] It had already been found that caffeine enhanced the release of free fatty acids (FFAs) into the bloodstream, and the subsequent increase in utilization of FFA metabolism. Two female and seven male cyclists were tested to exhaustion using 80% of their maximal aerobic capacity several times. For each trial the subject drank one of two mixtures, picked at random, 60 minutes prior to exercise. The authors found that caffeine ingestion prior to endurance work significantly ($p < 0.05$) improved total time to exhaustion. Interestingly, oxygen consumption and heart rate did not vary significantly, and the perception of effort was lower for the caffeine performance. These findings were corroborated in part by Ivy et al, although the latter authors found a significantly greater oxygen consumption associated with the increased endurance work following caffeine ingestion.[26] Sasaki et al examined the effect of combined feedings of caffeine

and sucrose on endurance performance.[27] They found that the best performances seemed to come from a combination of the two substances, but this was not statistically significantly different from either sucrose or caffeine ingestion alone, both of which resulted in improved endurance performance. McNaughton investigated the difference between two levels of caffeine and found that both resulted in improvements in performance, but did not differ significantly from each other.[28] Table 6–3 lists some of the caffeine levels for common beverages. The levels that have been used to produce a stimulant effect vary from 150 to 250 mg.

The negative aspect of caffeine ingestion stems from the same stimulant effect that resulted in a release of FFAs. Caffeine ingestion can cause an increase in the secretion of stomach acid, an increased incidence of ECG abnormalities, a decreased uptake of required nutrients from the gastrointestinal (GI) tract, and the irritability which is a side effect of central nervous system (CNS) stimulation.[29,30] Most of these effects are limited when the amount of caffeine is kept at a reasonable level; however, recreational athletes must be educated, as many have the idea that if a little is beneficial, a lot will be even better. Such potential overdose problems may be noticed at an even earlier stage with those already prone to problems with the GI tract or with their heart.

Depressants and Beta-Blockers

Barbiturate use is not something that enters most therapists' heads when considering ergogenic aids; however, its use must be considered when working with those in sports where fine control is required. The misuse of depressants has become increasingly common, not only among those seeking to "relax" after a hard competition, but also among those who believe that the depressant effect on the CNS will benefit their performance. Depressants have been utilized specifically in shooting and archery events. Within the past few years, athletes in these events, have moved away from the use of depressants towards the use of beta-blockers, having found that depressants not only relaxed muscles, but

TABLE 6-3. CAFFEINE CONTENT OF SELECTED BEVERAGES

Beverage	Caffeine (mg/serving)
Coca-Cola	65
Diet	45
Pepsi	43
Diet	36
Dr. Pepper	61
Coffee (5 oz brewed)	146
Coffee (5 oz instant)	53
Tea	20–50

also diminished performance. Beta-adrenergic blockers have been utilized, and they do result in the reduced heart rate which the athletes desire. Although the beta-blockers do have the necessary calming effect, their adverse effects can be severe. Even therapeutic doses may cause bronchospasm, hypotension, congestive heart failure, and bradycardia.[31] Thus, as with other pharmacological aids, the use of beta-adrenergic blockers should be discouraged.

Diuretics

Diuretics have been used occasionally to enhance performance indirectly in those sports where weight is a factor, such as wrestling. Many athletes using steroids also use diuretics in an attempt to flush the by-products of steroids from the body. Researchers do not believe that the by-products of steroids can actually be flushed from the body, as these by-products are produced during metabolism and thus are constantly being produced so that any "flushing" is temporary. Chronic use of diuretics can result in depletion of potassium, magnesium, calcium, and phosphorous levels due to the constant flushing of these minerals through the renal system.

NUTRITIONAL AIDS

Ever since competition began humans have been searching for some factor that would improve their performance beyond that of their competitors. Diet has played a major role in improving performance, although the scientific basis has not always been firmly established. In this section, the most common dietary supplements or beliefs are addressed as well as the problems some may cause when used incorrectly. For a more detailed examination of dietary needs, refer to chapter 8.

Vitamins

The Federal Drug Administration (FDA) has estimated that 40% or more Americans take vitamin supplements, and some researchers have found that approximately 85% of athletes use some vitamin supplement.[32] Unfortunately, although many claims have been made and continue to be made regarding the performance-enhancing effects of each of the vitamins, research has only proved effectiveness of supplementation if there was a preexisting deficiency for most vitamins. The focus here is on those vitamins that are most dominant in claims for ergogenic effects.

Vitamins may be divided into fat soluble, which are known to be stored in the body, and water soluble, which are normally flushed through the body's system and excesses excreted in the urine. The water-soluble vitamins include vitamin C and the various B vitamins.

The fat-soluble vitamins include vitamins A, E, K, and D, with the most claims for performance enhancement among these being made regarding vitamin E. It has long been known that excesses of the fat-soluble vitamins can cause toxicity due to storage within the body; however, it has only been in the last decade or two that toxic effects were noted with megadoses of water-soluble vitamins. Thus, the most commonly misused vitamins are the water-soluble vitamins, again, probably due to the concept that any excess would be excreted by the body. Table 6–4 presents a brief summary of the metabolic related function of the B vitamins, with associated performance enhancement claims and side effects caused by megadoses, and Table 6–5 presents the same information for the remainder of the water-soluble vitamins and the fat-soluble vitamins.[33]

Vitamin C has been associated with many ergogenic, as well as healing, properties. Due to its role in synthesis of catecholamines and cortisol, the need for vitamin C theoretically increases with an increased level of activity. Although some research has identified an increased need for ascorbic acid, the only performance benefits many of these studies were able to show was a reduced heart rate during work and recovery.[34] Well-designed research concerning the performance-enhancing effects of vitamin C has not found any improvements in oxygen consumption, anaerobic capacity, endurance performance, or strength.[32,34–36]. Keren and Epstein noted that most of the studies did not determine the dietary intake of ascorbic acid for their subjects, and that variation of intake could interact with the supplementation to affect the final performance findings of many of these studies.[37]

The B vitamins include individual vitamins such as thiamine, riboflavin, niacin, and pyridoxine, and what is normally called B complex. The B vitamins are involved as coenzymes or enzymes in the metabolic energy cycles or in the production of erythrocytes. In a review of some of the prominent literature, Keren and Epstein reported that much of the early research focused upon detriment to performance in the presence of a deficiency,[38–40] but that performance improved when the specific B vitamin was returned to normal levels.[40,41] Most of the well-designed studies, however, have not found beneficial effects ascribable to vitamin B supplementation in the absence of a preexisting deficiency.[41–43] In fact, supplementation of niacin or pyridoxine (B_6) might be contraindicated.[44] Manore and Leklem studied the effects of both carbohydrate or vitamin B_6 supplementation upon the plasma levels of FFAs

TABLE 6-4. THE B-VITAMINS: USE AND ABUSE

Compound	Exercise-Related Functions	Advertising Claims for Athletes	Side Effects and Toxicities
Vitamin B complex		Increases energy and endurance, enhances performance, delays fatigue	
Thiamine	Carbohydrate metabolism nervous system function		Interferes with absorption of other B vitamins
Riboflavin	Cellular energy release and respiration		Relatively nontoxic
Niacin	Cellular energy processes and respiration, carbohydrate metabolism and fat synthesis		Flushing, itchy skin, headache, nausea, low blood pressure, fainting, irregular heartbeat, liver damage
Pyridoxine (B_6)	Amino acid and protein metabolism, RBC formation		Liver damage, nerve damage (sensory ataxia), limb impairment of vibration sense
Folacin	Regulation of tissue processes, RBC formation		Gastric upset; sleep disturbances; malaise; irritability; masks certain anemias
Biotin	Synthesis of glycogen and fat, amino acid metabolism		Depresses secretion of gastric hydrochloric acid
Panthothenic	Energy and tissue metabolism		Diarrhea, water retention
B_{12}	Maintenance of nerve tissue, RBC formation		Liver damage, some allergic reactions

From Aronson V. Vitamins and minerals as ergogenic aids. Physician Sportsmed. *1986; 14(3): 209–212, with permission.*

TABLE 6-5. WATER- AND FAT-SOLUBLE VITAMINS: USE AND ABUSE

Compound	Exercise-Related Functions	Advertising Claims for Athletes	Side Effects and Toxicities
Vitamin C	Tissue maintenance and repair, resistance to infection	Protects against illness and infection, aids in rapid recovery from injury	GI upset, increases need for vitamin E, interferes with copper and iron status, may cause kidney stones and gout, interferes with pregnancy
Vitamin E	Maintenance of cell integrity, muscle metabolism	Improves performance, increases endurance	Depression, fatigue; flu-like symptoms; interferes with vitamins A and K; hypertension, phlebitis, clots; gynecomastia
Vitamin A	Maintenance of proper vision, resistance to infection	Improves vision and immunity to infection	Anorexia, hair loss, increases cranial pressure, hypercalcemia, bone and kidney damage, liver damage, birth defects
Vitamin D	Normal bone growth and development	Builds stronger bones	Anorexia; weakness; hypercalcemia; deposits in soft tissue; irreversible kidney damage, damage to heart, lungs, and tissues surrounding joints
Vitamin K	Normal blood clotting	Aids in recovery from injury	Interferes with normal clotting; liver damage

From Aronson V. Vitamins and minerals as ergogenic aids. Physician Sportsmed. *1986; 14(3): 209–212, with permission.*

and subsequent metabolic cycle.[45] They found that supplementation of vitamin B_6 decreased the level of plasma FFAs, thus increasing the utilization of glucose and glycogen stores. This type of effect is obviously detrimental to endurance performance (leading to earlier fatigue), and thus the authors conclude that the supplementation of B_6 above recommended levels is contraindicated for optimal performance. It should be pointed out, however, that Bergstom et al found no decrease in performance even though they did find the decreased muscle glycogen and high blood lactate levels associated with niacin supplementation.[46] The only research that supported supplementation was that of Early and Carlson, who found that B-complex supplementation could decrease the amount of fatigue for those who may have lost excessive amount of body water through sweating, such as in a hot environment.[47]

Of the fat-soluble vitamins, performance enhancement has most often been attributed to vitamin E. Sharman et al found no improvements in measures of VO_{2max} or endurance performance in swimmers when their diet was supplemented with vitamin E.[48] These findings were substantiated by Lawrence et al, who studied the effects of vitamin E and vitamin B_6 supplementation.[49] Williams suggests that early studies that found improved performances were poorly designed and conducted.[32] Importantly, Kobayashi has found that vitamin E may become an important factor at high altitude, where performance might be decreased due to reduced oxygen pressure.[50]

Amino Acids

Dietary protein provides a source for amino acids, of which there are approximately 20. The amino acids may be categorized as either essential or nonessential, either not synthesized within the body, or being synthesized, respectively. The amino acids participate in almost every conceivable manner within the body, and in special instances they provide energy. Due especially to their role in maintenance and growth of muscle tissue, it has been theorized that protein and its components may be required in greater amounts during participation in strenuous exercise.[38]

Support for an increased need for protein comes from research by Dohm, who found significant decreases in soluble and myofibrillar proteins following exercise to exhaustion in trained rats.[51] These findings have not been replicated with human subjects, however.[52] Increased need might not only occur when there has been protein degradation, but also if amino acids were being oxidized for energy.

Regardless of the theorized role of protein use during exercise, the majority of research found no improvements in performance to result from protein or amino acid supplementation. In fact, Laritcheva et al found that rats fed an excess of protein had a higher excretion rate with no changes in performance.[53] Haymes summarizes that although there is definite proof of increased excretion of nitrogen and other protein degradents, few studies have provided support for supplementation above the daily recommended allow-

ances.[38] An avenue of use for protein supplementation that has recently been introduced for potential performance benefits is that of the endorphin effects produced by L-tryptophan.

Segura and Ventura noted that L-trytophan had been shown to effect changes in the enkephalin-endorphin system, resulting in changes in the perception of pain.[54] They hypothesized that this effect might be used to enhance performance by delaying the perception of fatigue. In a study of 12 athletes, they found that time to exhaustion was significantly ($p < 0.05$) longer during the trial with L-tryptophan than with a placebo. There were no other differences between the placebo group and the L-tryptophan group, thus supporting the hypothesis that L-tryptophan might improve performance by means of delaying the perception of fatigue. This is interesting work that needs more corroborating evidence.

Two potential problems with amino acid supplementation are that of liver or kidney damage. The liver is the major site of amino acid degradation and as such may be stressed if required to degrade amounts greatly above normal for prolonged periods of time. As noted previously, supplementation is usually accompanied by an increased excretion rate.[52] Thus, the athlete must be cautious when supplementing for long periods of time, and must take in increased quantities of water to be used in the hepatic system.

Carbohydrate Loading

Carbohydrates are known to be the first and primary source of energy for high-intensity exercise and they are stored in both the liver and muscle as glycogen. Energy for muscular activity can only be derived from cellular stores or circulating blood glucose. As muscle stores and blood glucose become depleted, glycogen is released from the liver. It is believed that this is ultimately to prevent hypoglycemic effects on the central nervous system. Once the depletion patterns in exercising muscle had been identified by researchers, the question of altering available stores of carbohydrates was raised. Saltin and Hermansen conducted one of the first studies examining the effects of three different diets (percentages of carbohydrates) on work time.[55] Subjects were initially exercised to exhaustion, so as to deplete the available stores, and then were given one of three diets in random order. A significant increase in work time was found with a high carbohydrate diet and the muscle glycogen levels were also higher following exercise, thus indicating a sparing of some of the energy stores. These findings were similar to a later study by Karlsson and Saltin, who elaborated upon the research by looking at the muscle glycogen levels before and after the exercise bouts.[56] They were able to demonstrate that the increased work capacity was due to an increase in the amount of glycogen stored in the muscle following depletion and repletion through a high carbohydrate diet. These findings have been elaborated upon and corroborated several times since the original work.[57-59] Some of the later work made use of a low-carbohydrate diet to further deplete the muscle glycogen.[60] As a result of this research, supercompensation or carbohydrate loading was brought to the forefront as a method for improving endurance performance. The method that was derived from this research used a depletion of muscular stores of glycogen by first exercising subjects to exhaustion and then providing a high-fat, low-carbohydrate diet for a few days, finally repleting the muscle stores by means of a high-carbohydrate, low-fat diet for 2 to 3 days, with a concomitant reduction in work intensity.

One problem with the previously described regimen is that the athletes usually went through some form of carbohydrate phase, then repleted. As Costill noted, the depletion phase was psychologically difficult and physically draining.[61] He suggested that if the work intensity were reduced and dietary carbohydrates increased for a few days prior to the event, the muscles would still synthesize additional glycogen. Tremblay et al provided support for this hypothesis when they found that two trials—one with depletion and another with no depletion—did not differ significantly in total amount of glycogen stored.[62]

Nutritionists raised the question of possible deficiencies of necessary nutrients in a carbohydrate-loading diet and short- and long-term consequences. One study noted niacin and riboflavin levels markedly lower than the recommended daily allowances.[63] It should be noted, however, that the subjects were untrained and that the testing protocol was not similar to those previously used. Another potential disadvantage of carbohydrate loading is that for every gram of glycogen stored there are approximately 2.7 to 3.0 g of water stored with it. This could result in a weight gain of as much as 2 to 3 kg, dependent upon how much the athlete stored. Saltin points out that the extra water may aid in the prevention of dehydration and control of body temperature, thus ultimately benefiting performance in ways other than glycogen sparing.[64] For persons with potential heart problems, a more serious effect of carbohydrate loading is the edema in the heart muscle that may occur. Finally, it should be pointed out that muscle glycogen loading is really only advantageous for events that use a high percent of maximal oxygen uptake over a long duration (at least 1½ hours), and that the timing is critical, or an overshoot phenomenon may occur and the stores become depleted. Carbohydrate loading does not result in improved performance when the exercise involved is a short one or when its intensity is such that fat metabolism will be used (low).

Carbohydrate Feedings

Carbohydrate ingestion prior to or during competition has often been used in an attempt to delay or prevent

fatigue. Usually the carbohydrates are ingested in the form of a glucose solution or another similar sugar-based fluid. Carbohydrate feedings can be divided into two types: preexercise ingestion and ingestion during exercise (feedings have also been used following exercise to speed recovery).[65]

Carbohydrate feedings prior to exercise are based upon the concept that the additional carbohydrates will delay the use of glycogen stores within the muscle, thus delaying fatigue due to decreased stores and subsequently lowered blood glucose. Unfortunately, much of the early research found that glucose ingestion prior to performance was accompanied by a rapid rise in plasma insulin levels, which led to decreased blood glucose levels during the exercise bout without an increase in the FFA activity. Thus endurance performance was actually diminished rather than enhanced. Recent authors have postulated that perhaps the use of a sugar compound that was not as rapidly absorbed would ultimately provide the searched for enhancement to endurance. Okano et al addressed this hypothesis in a study of 12 trained males.[66] Using a double-blind crossover design, the authors tested each subject on two trials, one with a placebo and one with a fructose solution. They found that the subjects were able to exercise significantly ($p < 0.01$) longer following ingestion of a fructose solution. Furthermore, they found a significant difference ($p < 0.05$) between two levels of fructose solution, with subjects consuming 85 g fructose being able to pedal longer than those ingesting 60 g fructose. The authors noted that their findings were in direct contradiction to those of Hargreaves et al,[67] but felt that a portion of the difference could be attributed to methodology. In the study by Hargreaves, ten male subjects were given either a preexercise feeding that included 43 g sucrose, as well as fat and protein, or they were given an artificially sweetened drink solution of water.[67] Hargreaves et al found no differences between the exercise group and the control group for any of the oxygen consumption parameters measured during a 3-hour cycling period. Again, it should be noted that sucrose was used in the study by Hargreaves et al, whereas the study by Okano et al utilized a fructose solution, which has a slower absorption rate, thus theoretically avoiding the rapid shifts in blood sugar and FFAs.

Guezennec et al provided further evidence for enhanced performance potential using preexercise feedings of fructose as compared to the effects of glucose or corn starch ingestion.[68] Assigned by a randomized design, six males were tested on three separate occasions, prior to which they ingested either a solution of glucose, fructose, or corn starch. The authors noted that plasma insulin increased significantly for both glucose and corn starch trials, but not during the fructose trials. Computations based on CO_2 indicated that less of the fructose was oxidized over the exercise time period, thus indicating an increase in fat metabolism. There is still a need for more research in this area, but it appears that fructose may aid endurance performance. The major side effect from fructose ingestion prior to endurance exercise is nausea, GI distress, and diarrhea, which may result if the dose is too high.

Currently much of the focus upon carbohydrate feedings has been upon feeding during prolonged exercise, such as might be found during long bicycle races. As noted previously, blood glucose and muscle glycogen are among the first energy sources to be used during exercise, and may become depleted during endurance exercise.[55,56] In 1976, Ahlborg and Felig found that a carbohydrate feeding when the subject was near exhaustion would return the blood glucose levels toward normal.[69] Ivy et al examined the effect of glucose feedings on subsequent work production (subjects cycled at a set rate) as indicated by oxygen consumption parameters.[26] Subjects were given a glucose polymer every 15 minutes during 2-hour bicycle test. Although the glucose feeding did not appear to improve total performance, the authors noted an important increase in work production over the last 30 minutes.

Recently researchers have attempted to answer some of the questions that the previous work had raised concerning glucose feedings during endurance exercise. Ivy et al exercised ten male subjects to exhaustion using exercise bouts of 45% of maximum oxygen uptake during walking.[70] During the experimental session, the subjects were given a 20% solution of glucose totaling 120 g in four separate feedings. The authors found a significant ($p < 0.05$) improvement in the time to exhaustion for the group fed glucose as compared to the control group. Coyle et al have since corroborated these findings at work loads of 70% to 80% maximum, having found a delay in time to fatigue between 30 and 60 minutes.[71-73] In addition, it should be noted that the increased time to exhaustion in all of these studies was due to an increase in the percentage of blood glucose utilized. Further research in this area is needed to see if muscle glycogen is being spared, or if the shift to greater blood glucose utilization could have later detrimental effects. For further insight into the entire aspect of carbohydrates and their use in enhancing performance, Coyle recently presented a good overview of the topic that outlines the pertinent research and practical applications.[65]

Minerals and Electrolytes

For the purpose of simplicity, this section combines the substances defined as minerals, electrolytes, and trace elements. Many of these, like vitamins, have often been attributed to have performance-enhancing capabilities. Supplementation takes one of two forms: solid supplementation and fluid supplementation. The most common elements used for an ergogenic effect are sodium, potassium, calcium, magnesium, iron, and zinc. Table

TABLE 6-6. MINERALS: USES AND ABUSES

Compound	Exercise-Related Functions	Advertising Claims for Athletes	Side Effects and Toxicities
Sodium, potassium	Maintenance of normal fluid balance, regulation of body systems including heartbeat and hydration	Sweat loss necessitates	Salt tablets irritate the GI tract, cause dehydration and cramps
Zinc	Protein synthesis and tissue repair	Speeds wound healing; losses incurred with exercise necessitate supplementation	Anorexia; nausea; diarrhea; lethargy; dizziness; muscle pain; interferes with copper metabolism, calcium and iron absorption; may impair immune response, decrease blood levels of HDL, triggers bleeding ulcers
Iron	Oxygen transport to tissues for energy	Reduces fatigue, weakness; improves performance, endurance; supplementation required by all athletes	Overdoses have caused death in children; dangerous for adults with hemochromatosis

From Aronson V. Vitamins and minerals as ergogenic aids. Physician Sportsmed. *1986; 14(3):209–212, with permission.*

6-6 presents a synopsis of the exercise related function of some of these with their respective potential toxicities. For a more detailed examination of nutritional requirements, refer to chapter 8.

Calcium. The mineral calcium has received much attention, perhaps due to its function in muscle contraction, blood plasma and bone formation, and homeostasis. Two areas of concern with athletes that are commonly cited are the loss of calcium during strenuous exercise in the heat and the possible increased need for calcium for young competitive females.

Normal loss of calcium is variable, although plasma concentrations of calcium are kept within a fairly constant range. Calcium loss may be increased through profuse sweat losses, reaching up to 1 g/day.[74] Thus, most claims are based upon the need to replenish the blood plasma levels that have been diminished during strenuous exercise. These losses are readily replaced through a normal diet, however.[75] Johnson et al examined the effect of electrolyte supplementation during exercise in the heat, using a variety of solutions, as well as plain water.[76] They found that there were no significant differences in calcium loss between any of the solutions and noted that intake of any of the electrolytes above normal was paralleled by an increase in the excretion rate of that same electrolyte. Furthermore, the differences in performance were minimal and not attributable to any single electrolyte.

Calcium is a nutrient of concern with female athletes, especially those competing in endurance events. Previous research has identified a link between bone density and the normal hormonal cycle in women.[77] A problem that arises with some women in endurance events is that of amenorrhea. Unfortunately, the results in the young female (osteopenia) are similar to those of a woman following menopause.[78,79] Recent evidence highlights the increased incidence of stress fractures and injuries with females who have a lower bone density that may have resulted from amenorrhea.[80] In such cases, moderate supplementation may be of some help in retarding the loss of bone, but the underlying cause of the calcium loss must eventually be addressed. Although in many women, regular menstruation may be restored by a reduction in the intensity of training, yet some authors feel that the loss of bone density that was incurred during the cessation of menstruation is irreversible.[81]

Sodium and Potassium. Two minerals that are often misused are sodium and potassium. Although it has been known for many years that sodium tablets are not necessary for the athlete and may in fact cause more harm than good, this misconception is still around. Losses in the sweat may reach as much as 129 mEq for sodium and 13 mEq for potassium.[82] Gisolfi notes that sodium reabsorption is enhanced during increased sweat losses, and that the losses of potassium are not that great.[82] Johnson et al at first seem to refute this in their study of electrolytes and performance.[76] The authors found negative sodium and potassium balances following repeated bouts of exhaustive exercise in the heat; however, they noted that a well-balanced diet appeared to maintain normal levels of plasma electrolytes, as increased ingestion was equaled by increased excretion of the electrolytes. Thus the evidence support-

ing a need for supplementation above normal dietary intakes has not currently been validated.

Iron. Iron has received much attention due to its role in erythrocyte formation and transportation of oxygen. Iron may be lost via sweat, menstrual flow, increased breakdown due to increased activity, and a variety of other ways. In 1970, Andersen and Barkve noted that as many as 25% of the Swedish women of childbearing age were probably iron deficient due to losses during menstruation.[83] They examined the effects of iron deficiency anemia upon cardiorespiratory function of five women over a prolonged period of time. These women were tested while iron deficient and then following iron supplementation therapy, once normal hematologic values were reached. The authors found that the recovery from exercise was prolonged when the subject was anemic, and that the subjects tended to exercise more anaerobically than aerobically when iron deficient. They concluded that "iron deficiency anaemia impairs the working capacity of patients by placing an excessively increased load on the cardiorespiratory functions."[83] Haymes cited a similar incidence of iron deficiency among women in the United States, and after giving a brief review of the literature, concluded that iron deficiency anemia negatively affects aerobic performance.[38] As found in Andersen and Barkve's study, oxygen consumption parameters appeared to return toward normal values following supplementation therapy.

Edgerton et al examined the relation of iron deficiency anemia to exercise performance by using rats in several associated training studies.[84] Within each project the authors studied anemia from a different aspect, such as (1) the repletion of iron stores to normal, (2) the effects of training as related to iron status, and (3) the interaction of these variables with status of iron deficiency. Among the important findings of this extensive study were a significantly ($p < 0.01$) decreased exercise time when anemic, a change in heart and spleen weight due to anemia, and a decreased body weight during iron deficient status. Importantly, they also found that repletion of iron status was rapidly associated with improvements in aerobic capacity.

Does supplementation above normal levels lead to improved aerobic performance? Most of the literature suggests that if the subject's hemoglobin is within normal limits, supplementation does not increase the amount of serum iron and hemoglobin levels or result in improved aerobic performance.[38,85] There is some evidence to suggest the prolonged strenuous exercise in the heat may lead to increased iron losses via sweat, therefore leading to the hypothesis that athletes—especially women—exercising in hot climates should supplement their diet. Little evidence has substantiated this theory, however. Current recommendations are to

attempt to supply the recommended daily allowance (RDA) through a balanced diet, and, if a supplement is given, to keep the levels within those of the RDA guidelines.

PHYSIOLOGICAL AIDS

Physiological aids include many types of aids, some which are considered ethical, such as altitude training, and others, such as blood doping, that are controversial. This section discusses some of the currently popular aids, including blood doping, bicarbonate loading, use of oxygen, and altitude training. It is important to realize that many things may act as physiological aids, such as warmup, and are usually considered appropriate performance components. In general, those aids that improve performance by maximizing the body's normal reaction to training are considered acceptable, whereas performance improvements gained by the use of substances other than those already in the body are usually considered unacceptable.

Blood Doping

Blood doping is a topic that has received much attention, and, like anabolic steroids, raises questions of ethics. Proponents suggest that there is not an ethical problem, as the blood which is being injected is that of the athlete himself or herself; however, there are many who question the validity of this argument. The American College of Sports Medicine published a position stand regarding blood doping in 1987. The college stated that "the use of blood doping as an ergogenic aid for athletic competition is unethical and unjustifiable," thus supporting the International Olympic Committee (IOC) position regarding blood doping as an abnormal means of improving performance.[86]

The theoretical basis of blood doping is that if one can increase the amount of circulating hemoglobin, there should be a concomitant increase in the amount of oxygen delivered to the working tissues, and thus an increased aerobic work capacity. Increased aerobic capacity can be achieved through training at altitude, in which case the increase in hemoglobin is brought about by an increase in erythrocyte production at the bone marrow. With blood doping, an amount of blood is withdrawn from the subject, following which the body increases erythropoiesis to bring the circulating level of erythrocytes back to normal level. After a few weeks, the subject is reinfused with the previously withdrawn blood, thus substantially increasing the amount of circulating hemoglobin.

In 1972 Ekblom et al studied the effects of reinfusion of blood on the cardiorespiratory parameters of seven male subjects.[87] Reinfusion of blood resulted in a significant ($p < 0.05$) increase in maximal work time

and maximal oxygen consumption. Ekblom et al conducted a similar study in 1976, finding similar increases in maximal oxygen consumption and endurance when five trained athletes were reinfused with packed red blood cells (RBCs).[88] Williams et al examined the effects of reinfusion of blood upon maximal aerobic capacity as reflected in time to exhaustion and perceived exertion for 16 trained runners.[89] In contrast to the previous work, these researchers found no significant differences in total work capacity or perceived exertion. They suggest that the reinfusion of packed RBCs could lead to polycythemia, with an increase in blood viscosity, which could result in decreased cardiac output, blood flow velocity, and so on. Gledhill reviewed the issue of blood doping in 1982 and suggested that many of the studies that had found no improvements in maximal oxygen consumption or endurance had failed to use appropriate methodologies.[90]

As previously mentioned, blood doping is primarily an ethical question. Although the IOC has banned blood doping, detection of blood doping is not reliable and it is thus necessary to rely upon the integrity of the athlete. The only physical complication that accompanies reinfusion of blood is an increased risk of infection, but that risk is limited with the use of autologous blood. Many athletes do not feel that blood doping is unethical, and thus there have been numerous reports of athletes using this method, especially within the endurance cycling and running events. Techniques are improving for the detection of blood doping; however, this is still an area about which the sports physical therapist must be informed and where ethical questions are of great importance.

Sodium Bicarbonate

A variety of ergogenic aids have been associated with endurance performance, but the number of aids for anaerobic events is limited, often including only those aids that affect performance by increasing muscle mass. One physiological aid that theoretically would improve performance is that of bicarbonate loading. During intense, short-duration exercise, energy is produced through metabolic pathways that have a by-product of lactic acid. As metabolic acidosis limits the effectiveness of the contracting muscle, if one could delay the acidosis, one could theoretically improve performance. As early as 1931, Dennig et al showed that if metabolic alkalosis was produced prior to exercise, then anaerobic performance could be improved.[91] The question has been investigated throughout the years and is still an area of interest to physiologists.

More recently, Wilkes et al examined the effects of induced alkalosis upon 800-m race time for six competitive athletes and found a significant ($p < 0.05$) increase in postexercise pH, which indicated an increased buffering of the lactic acid produced during the

event.[92] In addition, the competitive times for the bicarbonate-loaded group were significantly ($p < 0.05$) faster than the times for either the control or placebo groups. The authors mentioned, however, that many of the athletes suffered "minor acute GI distress" following the experimental races.

Horswill et al attempted to determine the quantity of bicarbonate necessary to produce the needed increase in blood pH by studying the effects of various dosages upon anaerobic performance using a cycle ergometer.[93] They found no improvements in performance but did note that they may have used insufficiently high levels of bicarbonate to produce the necessary changes associated with improved performance. The greatest amount of bicarbonate in this study was 0.20 g·kg^{-1} and previous research that had found improvements in performance had utilized as much as 0.30 g·kg^{-1}.

As mentioned by Wilkes et al, there is currently no ban upon the use of bicarbonate loading as an ergogenic aid to performance.[92] It is important, however, to consider the ethics of its use for performance. It should also be noted that the side effects of bicarbonate loading, although usually not life threatening, can be significant. The GI distress noted in some of the studies takes the form of severe cramps and eventually diarrhea. If the dosage is too high or taken too early or if the race is delayed, the athlete may not be able to make it to the starting line due to the cramps or diarrhea. As the normal balance of the buffer system of the blood has been affected, other side effects might also include headaches and respiratory acidosis.

Oxygen

Oxygen is a popular ergogenic aid in many different sports, often being used to speed recovery. Wilmore separated the research into three categories: prior to exercise, during exercise, and following exercise.[94] Research findings concerning supplementation with oxygen prior to exercise were contradictory, although Wilmore suggested that the improved performances relied upon a short interval between oxygen inhalation and the event, as well as upon the length of the event itself. Oxygen inhalation during exercise generally increased the amount of work performed, with lower physiological costs to the individual. There did not seem to be any benefit associated with postexercise oxygen inhalation.

In 1983, Morris reviewed the literature and came to the same conclusions as Wilmore.[95] He noted that research findings varied according to methodology of oxygen supplementation, time of supplementation, parameters used to assess the effects of oxygen inhalation, and so forth. Upon review of the literature directly assessing performance or performance components, he concluded that oxygen inhalation prior to or following

exercise resulted in minimal changes. Furthermore, he noted that although improvements in performance had been recorded when oxygen was inhaled during exercise, the mechanism was still unknown.

Altitude Training

As mentioned in the section on blood doping, it has been theorized that if the amount of circulating hemoglobin could be increased, there would be an associated ability of the blood to carry and deliver increased amounts of oxygen to the working tissues. Decreased Po_2, such as found at high altitudes, stimulates erythropoiesis. Thus, it has been found that those training at high altitudes have higher hematocrits than those training at sea level, due to the erythropoiesis. Athletes who reside at sea level and subsequently go to high altitude to train for a period of time will also have higher hemoglobin levels; however, the hemoglobin levels will return toward normal with a few days of returning to sea level. Morris noted that many athletes were unable to train at the same intensity at high altitude, which resulted in a slight detraining effect.[95] Therefore, the potential advantage of the increased hemoglobin level might be balanced by the disadvantage of detraining.

SUMMARY

Several ergogenic aids have been discussed within this chapter: pharmacological aids such as anabolic steroids, stimulants, depressants, and diuretics; nutritional aids such as vitamins, amino acids, and carbohydrates; and physiological aids such as blood doping, bicarbonate loading, and human growth hormone; however, volumes have been written concerning these aids. If more information is desired regarding a specific aid, refer to one of the many texts or to one of the excellent review articles listed in the references. Education is probably one of the most important roles the sports physical therapist will play regarding ergogenic aids. This education should address not only the physical aspects of the use of ergogenic aids, but also the ethical and legal questions. Ignoring the use and misuse of ergogenic aids is acting like the ostrich who sticks its head in the sand and thinks the problem no longer exists.

REFERENCES

1. Burkett LN, Falduto MT. Steroid use by athletes in a metropolitan area. *Physician Sportsmed.* 1984; 12(8):69–74.
2. Taylor WN, Black AB. Pervasive anabolic steroid use among health club athletes. *Ann Sports Med.* 1987; 3(3):155–159.
3. Sweeney GD. Drugs—Some basic concepts. *Med Sci Sports Ex.* 1981; 13(4):247–251.
4. Lamb DR. Anabolic steroids. In: Williams, MH, ed. *Ergogenic Aids in Sport*. Champaign, Ill: Human Kinetics Publishers Inc; 1983; 164–182.
5. Bauman DH, Richerson JT, Britt AL. A comparison of body and organ weights, physiologic parameters, and pathologic changes in target organs of rats given combinations of exercise, anabolic hormone, and protein supplementation. *Am J Sportsmed.* 1988; 16(4):397–402.
6. Percy EC. Ergogenic aids in athletics. *Med Sci Sports.* 1978; 10(4):298–303.
7. Freed DLJ, Banks AJ, Longson D, et al. Anabolic steroids in athletics: Crossover double blind trial on weight lifters. *Br Med J.* 1975; 2:471–473.
8. Era P, Alen M, Rahkila P. Psychomotor and motor speed in power athletes self-administering testosterone and anabolic steroids. *Res Q Ex Sport.* 1988; 59(1):50–56.
9. Kiraly CL. Androgenic–anabolic steroid effects on serum and skin surface lipids, on red cells, and on liver enzymes. *Int J Sports Med.* 1988; 9:249–252.
10. Creagh TM, Rubin A, Evans EJ. Hepatic tumours induced by anabolic steroids in an athlete. *J Clin Pathol.* 1988; 41:441–443.
11. Hurley BF, Seals DR, Hagberg JM, et al. High-density-lipoprotein cholesterol in bodybuilders v powerlifters. *JAMA.* 1984; 252:507–513.
12. Kantor MA, Bianchini A, Bernier D, et al. Androgens reduce HDL2-cholesterol and increase hepatic triglyceride lipase activity. *Med Sci Sports Ex.* 1985; 17:462–465.
13. McNutt RA, Ferenchick GS, Kirlin PC, et al. Acute myocardial infarction in a 22-year-old world class weight lifter using anabolic steroids. *Am J Cardiol.* 1988; 62:164.
14. Mochizuki RM, Richter KJ. Cardiomyopathy and cerebrovascular accident associated with anabolic-androgenic steroid use. *Physician Sportsmed.* 1988; 16(11):109–114.
15. Pearson AC, Schiff M, Mirosek D, et al. Left ventricular diastolic function in weight lifters. *Am J Cardiol.* 1975; 58:1254–1259.
16. Behrendt H, Boffin H. Myocardial cell lesions caused by anabolic hormone. *Cell Tissue Res.* 1977; 181:423–426.
17. Salke RC, Rowland TW, Burke EJ. Left ventricular size and function in body builders using anabolic steroids. *Med Sci Sports Ex.* 1985; 17:701–704.
18. Wood TO, Cooke PH, Goodship AE. The effect of exercise and anabolic steroids on the mechanical properties and crimp morphology of the rat tendon. *Am J Sportsmed.* 1988; 16:153–158.
19. Pope HG, Katz DL. Affective and psychotic symptoms associated with anabolic steroid use. *Am J Psychiatry.* 1988; 145:487–490.
20. Pope HG, Katz DL. Bodybuilders psychosis. *Lancet.* 1987; 1:865.
21. Tennant F, Black DL, Voy RO. Anabolic steroid dependence with opioid-type features. *New Engl J Med.* 1988; 319:578.
22. The Use of Anabolic-Androgenic Steroids in Sports. American College of Sports Medicine Position Stand. *Med Sci Sports Ex.* 1987; 19:534–539.
23. Ivy JL. Amphetamines. In: Williams MH, ed. *Ergogenic Aids in Sport*. Champaign, Ill; Human Kinetics Publishers Inc; 1983: 101–127.

24. Chandler JV. The effects of amphetamines on selected physiological components related to athletic success. *Med Sci Sports.* 1978; 10(1):38. Abstract.

25. Costill DL, Dalsky GP, Fink WJ. Effects of caffeine ingestion on metabolism and exercise performance. *Med Sci Sports.* 1978; 10(3):155–158.

26. Ivy JL, Costill DL, Fink WJ, et al. Influence of caffeine and carbohydrate feedings on endurance performance. *Med Sci Sports.* 1979; 11(1):6–11.

27. Sasaki H, Maeda J, Usui S, et al. Effect of sucrose and caffeine ingestion on performance of prolonged strenuous running. *Int J Sports Med.* 1987; 8(4):261–265.

28. McNaughton L. Two levels of caffeine ingestion on blood lactate and free fatty acid responses during incremental exercise. *Res Exerc Sport.* 1987; 58(3):255–259.

29. van der Merwe PJ, Muller FR, Muller FO. Caffeine in sport: Urinary excretion of caffeine in healthy volunteers after intake of common caffeine-containing beverages. *S Afr Med J.* 1988; 74(4):163–164.

30. Van Handel P. Caffeine. In: Williams MH, ed. *Ergogenic Aids in Sport.* Champaign, Ill: Human Kinetic Publishers Inc, 1983; 128–163.

31. Lombardo JA. Stimulants. In: Strauss RH, ed, *Drugs and Performance in Sports.* Philadelphia, Pa: W B Saunders; 1987; 87–102.

32. Williams M. Vitamin supplementation and physical performance. In: Fox EL, ed. *Nutrient Utilization During Exercise, Ross Symposium.* Columbus, Ohio: Ross Laboratories; 1983; 26–30.

33. Aronson V. Vitamins and minerals as ergogenic aids. *Physician Sportsmed.* 1986; 14(3):209-212.

34. Van Huss WD. What made the Russians run? *Nutr Today.* 1966; 1:20–23.

35. Bailey DA, Carron AV, Teece KG, et al. Effect of vitamin C supplementation upon the physiological response to exercise in trained and untrained subjects. *Int J Vitamin Res.* 1970; 40:435–440.

36. Gey G, Cooper K, Bottenberg R. Effects of ascorbic acid on endurance performance and athletic injury. *JAMA.* 1970; 211:105.

37. Keren G, Epstein Y. The effect of high dosage vitamin C intake on aerobic and anaerobic capacity. *J Sports Med Phys Fitness.* 1980; 20:145–148.

38. Haymes EM. Protein, vitamins, and Iron. In: Williams MH, ed. *Ergogenic Aids in Sport.* Champaign, Ill: Human Kinetics Publishers Inc; 1983; 27–55.

39. Johnson RE, Darling RC, Forbes WH, et al. The effects of a diet deficient in part of the vitamin B complex upon men doing manual labor. *J Nutr.* 1942; 24:585–596.

40. Archdeacon J, Murlin J. The effect of thiamine depletion and restoration on muscular efficiency and endurance. *J Nutr.* 1944; 28:241–254.

41. Berryman GH, Henderson CR, Wheeler NC, et al. Effects in young men consuming restricted quantities of B-complex vitamins and protein, and changes associated with supplementation. *Am J Physiol.* 1947; 148:618–647.

42. Tin-May-Than, Ma-Win-May, Khin-Sann-Aung, et al. The effect of vitamin B12 on physical performance capacity. *Br J Nutr.* 1978; 40:269.

43. DeVos A, Leklem J, Campbell D. Carbohydrate loading, vitamin B6 supplementation, and fuel metabolism during exercise in man. *Med Sci Sports Ex.* 1982; 14:137.

44. Coleman EC. Vitamin/mineral supplements—Use and abuse. *Sports Med Dig.* 1988; 10(8):5.

45. Manore MM, Leklem JE. Effects of carbohydrate and vitamin B6 on fuel substrates during exercise in women. *Med Sci Sports Ex.* 1988; 20:233–241.

46. Bergstrom J, Hultman E, Jorfeldt L, et al. Effect of nicotinic acid on physical working capacity and metabolism of muscle. *J Appl Physiol.* 1969; 26:170–176.

47. Early R, Carlson B. Water soluble vitamin therapy on the delay of fatigue from physical activity in hot climate. *Int Z Agnew Physiol.* 1969; 27:43.

48. Sharman IM, Down MG, Sen RN. The effect of vitamin E on physiological function and athletic performance on trained swimmers. *J Sports Med Phys Fitness.* 1976; 16:215.

49. Lawrence J, Smith J, Bower R, et al. The effect of alpha-tocopherol (vitamin E) and pyridoxine HCL (vitamin B6) on the swimming endurance of trained swimmers. *J Am Coll Health Assoc.* 1975; 23:219–222.

50. Kobayashi Y. *Effect of Vitamin E on Aerobic Work Performance in Men During Acute Exposure to Hypoxic Hypoxia.* Albuquerque, NM: University of New Mexico; 1974.

51. Dohm GL. Protein metabolism in exercise. In: Fox EL, ed. *Nutrient Utilization During Exercise, Ross Symposium.* Columbus, Ohio: Ross Laboratories; 1983; 8–13.

52. Lemon PWR, Nagle FJ. Effects of exercise on protein and amino acid metabolism. *Med Sci Sports Ex.* 1981; 13(3):141–149.

53. Laritcheva KA, Yalovaya NI, Shubin VI, et al. Study of energy expenditure and protein needs of top weight lifters. In: Parizkova J, Rogozkin VA, eds. *Nutrition, Physical Fitness, and Health.* Baltimore, Md: University Park Press; 1978.

54. Segura R, Ventura JL. Effect of L-tryptophan supplementation on exercise performance. *Int J Sports Med.* 1988; 9:305–310.

55. Saltin B, Hermansen L. *Glycogen Stores and Prolonged Severe Exercise.* Symposia of the Swedish Nutrition Foundation, Nutrition and Physical Activity; 1967; 32–46.

56. Karlsson J, Saltin B. Diet, muscle glycogen and endurance performance. *J Appl Physiol.* 1971; 31(2):203–206.

57. Jette M, Pelletier O, Parker L, et al. The nutritional and metabolic effects of a carbohydrate-rich diet in glycogen supercompensation training regimen. *Am J Clin Nutr* 1978; 31:2140–2148.

58. Essen B. Intramuscular substrate utilization during prolonged exercise. *Ann NY Acad Sci* 1977; 301:30–43.

59. Maughan RJ, Williams C, Campbell DM, et al. Fat and carbohydrate metabolism during low intensity exercise: Effects of the availability of muscle glycogen. *Eur J Appl Physiol.* 1978; 39:7–16.

60. Kochan RG, Lamb DR, Lutz SA, et al. Glycogen synthase activation in human skeletal muscle: effects of diet and exercise. *Am J Physiol.* 1979; 236(6):E660-E666.

61. Costill DL. A scientific approach to distance running. *Track Field News.* 1979; 120–122.

62. Tremblay A, Sevigny J, Allard C, et al. Diet and muscle glycogen in runners. *Track Field Q Rev.* 1977; 77(4):63. Abstract.

63. Sherman WM. Carbohydrates, muscle glycogen, and muscle glycogen supercompensation. In: Williams MH, ed. *Ergogenic Aids in Sports.* Champaign, Ill: Human Kinetics Publishers Inc; 1983; 3–26.

64. Saltin B. Fluid, electrolyte, and energy losses and their replenishment in prolonged exercise. In: Parizkova J, Rogozkin VA, eds. *International Series on Sport Sciences: Nutrition, Physical Fitness, and Health*, Baltimore, Md: University Park Press; 1978; 7:76–97.

65. Coyle EF. Carbohydrates and athletic performance. *Sports Sci Exchange.* 1988; 1(7).

66. Okano G, Hidekatsu T, Morita I, et al. Effect of preexercise fructose ingestion on endurance performance in fed men. *Med Sci Sports Ex.* 1988; 20(2):105–109.

67. Hargreaves M, Costill DL, Coggan A, et al. Effect of carbohydrate feedings on muscle glycogen utilization and exercise performance. *Med Sci Sports Ex.* 1984; 16(2):219–222.

68. Guezennec CY, Satabin P, Duforez F, et al. Oxidation of corn starch, glucose, and fructose ingested before exercise. *Med Sci Sports Ex.* 1989; 21(1):45–50.

69. Ahlberg G, Felig P. Influence of glucose ingestion on fuel-hormone response during prolonged exercise. *J Appl Physiol.* 1976; 41:683–688.

70. Ivy JL, Miller W, Dover V, et al. Endurance improved by ingestion of a glucose polymer supplement. *Med Sci Sports Ex.* 1983; 15(6):466–471.

71. Miller JM, Coyle EF, Sherman WM, et al. Effect of glycerol feeding on endurance and metabolism during prolonged exercise in man. *Med Sci Sport Ex.* 1983; 15(3):237–242.

72. Coyle EF, Hagberg JM, Hurley BF, et al. Carbohydrate feeding during prolonged strenuous exercise can delay fatigue. *J Appl Physiol.* 1983; 55:230–235.

73. Coyle EF, Coggan AR, Hemmert MK, et al. Muscle glycogen utilization during prolonged strenuous exercise when fed carbohydrate. *J Appl Physiol.* 1986; 61:165–172.

74. Avioli LV. Major minerals: Calcium and phosphorous. In: Goodhart RS, Shils ME, eds. *Modern Nutrition in Health and Disease.* Philadelphia, Pa: Lea and Febiger; 1978; 294–309.

75. Bohmer D. Loss of electrolytes by sweat in sports. In: Katch FI, ed. *The 1984 Olympic Scientific Congress Proceedings; Sport Health, and Nutrition.* Champaign, Ill: Human Kinetics Publishers Inc; 1984; 2:67–74.

76. Johnson HL, Nelson RA, Consolazio CF. Effects of electrolyte and nutrient solutions on performance and metabolic balance. *Med Sci Sports Ex.* 1988; 20(1):26–33.

77. Riggs BL, Wahner HW, Dunn WL, et al. Differential changes in bone mineral density of the appendicular and axial skeleton with aging. *J Clin Invest.* 1981; 67:328–335.

78. Drinkwater BL, Nilson K, Chesnut CH, et al. Bone mineral content of amenorrheic and eumenorrheic athletes. *N Engl J Med.* 1984; 311:277–281.

79. Cann CE, Martin MC, Genant HK, et al. Decreased spinal mineral content in amenorrheic women. *JAMA.* 1984; 251:626–629.

80. Lloyd T, Triantafyllou SJ, Baker ER, et al. Women athletes with menstrual irregularity have increased musculoskeletal injuries. *Med Sci Sports Ex.* 1986; 18(4):374–379.

81. Cann CE, Cavenaugh DJ, Schnurpfiel K, et al. Menstrual history is the primary determinant of trabecular bone density in women runners. *Med Sci Sports Ex.* 1988; 20(2S):S59. Abstract.

82. Gisolfi CV. Water and electrolyte metabolism in exercise. In: Fox EL, ed. *Nutrition Utilization During Exercise. Ross Symposium.* Columbus, Ohio: Ross Laboratories, 1983; 21–25.

83. Anderson HT, Barkve H. Iron deficiency and muscular work performance. *Scand J Clin Lab Invest.* (Suppl) 1970; 114:8–39.

84. Edgerton VR, Bryant SL, Gillespie CA, et al. Iron deficiency anemia and physical performance and activity of rats. *J Nutr.* 1972; 102:381–400.

85. Cooter GR, Mowberry KW. Effects of iron supplementation on serum iron depletion and hemoglobin levels in female athletes. *Res Q.* 1978; 114–118.

86. Blood Doping as an Ergogenic Aid. American College of Sports Medicine Position Stand. *Med Sci Sports Ex.* 1987; 19(5):540–543.

87. Ekblom B, Goldbarg AN, Gullbring B. Response to exercise after blood loss and reinfusion. *J Appl Physiol.* 1972; 33(2):175–180.

88. Ekblom BG, Wilson G, Astrand PO. Central circulation during exercise after venesection and reinfusion of red blood cells. *J Appl Physiol.* 1976; 40:379–383.

89. Williams MH, Lindhjem M, Schuster R. The effect of blood infusion upon endurance capacity and ratings of perceived exertion. *Med Sci Sports.* 1978; 10(2):113–118.

90. Gledhill N. Blood doping and related issues: A brief review. *Med Sci Sports Ex.* 1982; 14(3):183–189.

91. Dennig H, Talbot JH, Edwards HT, et al. Effects of acidosis and alkalosis upon the capacity for work. *J Clin Invest.* 1931; 9:601–613.

92. Wilkes D, Gledhill N, Smyth R. Effect of acute induced metabolic alkalosis on 800-m racing time. *Med Sci Sports Ex.* 1983; 15(4):277–280.

93. Horswill CA, Costill DL, Fink WJ, et al. Influence of sodium bicarbonate on sprint performance: Relationship to dosage. *Med Sci Sports Ex.* 1985; 20(6):566–569.

94. Wilmore JH. Oxygen. In: Morgan WP, ed. *Ergogenic Aids and Muscular Performance.* New York, NY: Academic Press; 1972; 321–342.

95. Morris AE. Oxygen. In: Williams MH, ed. *Ergogenic Aids in Sport.* Champaign, Ill: Human Kinetic Publishers Inc; 1983; 185–201.

7

Drugs, Athletes, and Drug Testing

Gary Alan Green

INTRODUCTION

"Cocaine has probably joined rotator-cuff injuries, torn ligaments, and broken bones as a potential occupational hazard for athletes."[1]

"New Drug Epidemic: Steroids. As many as one million athletes in this country may be using steroids."[2]

These headlines in *The New York Times* announced that drug abuse among athletes has become a problem of increasing concern. A daily sports page that is devoid of a story about an athlete and drugs is almost as rare today as a perfect game in baseball. Whether it is an Olympic competitor failing a drug test or a collegiate athlete being arrested for driving while intoxicated, there appears to be a national fascination with the use of substances by athletes. It has become necessary for those professionals who deal with the medical needs of athletes to become knowledgeable about the possible drugs of abuse. This chapter presents a historical perspective of drugs in sport and an overview of the current problem. From there, some of the more popular drugs that are used and abused by athletes are discussed, with an emphasis on recognition, reasons for use, adverse reactions, and avenues for deterrence. Finally, this chapter evaluates various types of drug testing and discusses current regulations by some of the major governing bodies of sports.

HISTORY OF DRUG USE IN SPORTS

Searching for a competitive edge in athletics through the use of foreign substances is an ancient theme. The first recorded reference was by the Greek author Homer, writing in the eighth century BC, who described the ingestion of mushrooms by Greek athletes to enhance performance.[3] Other cultures believed in the value of various substances to improve athletic performance. The stimulant properties of the coca leaf were first discovered by the Incas of South America.

Incan rulers used the coca leaf as a reward for runners carrying fresh foods long distances and coca itself helped the runner endure.[4] The word "doping," which has become a synonym for drug use, was derived from the Kaffir tribe of Southeast Africa who used a local liquor called "dop" as a stimulant.[3] The drive to increase performance led European athletes of the nineteenth century to reportedly use caffeine, alcohol, nitroglycerine, ethyl ether, and opium to gain a competitive advantage.[3] It therefore appears that the impetus to discover a substance that can increase athletic performance is a cross-cultural phenomenon that predates efforts to control such drugs.

PATTERNS OF USE AMONG ATHLETES

Given the massive amount of media attention, the assumption follows that drug use is endemic among athletes at all levels of competition. Several studies have attempted to evaluate the differences between athletes and nonathletes with respect to patterns of drug use. The validity of such studies is difficult to determine because of their reliance on self-reporting and variable response rates. A conference was organized by the American Medical Association's House of Delegates in 1985 in which representatives from 16 sports and medical organizations were invited to discuss the existing data. They reviewed three major studies of athletes since 1978 that employed self-reporting surveys. All three of the studies were conducted among college athletes at a variety of schools in order to provide the greatest diversity.

The first study was performed by Toohey in 1978 who assessed nonmedical drug use among intercollegiate athletes at six colleges.[5] He compared the patterns of use of marijuana, alcohol, barbiturates, LSD, cocaine, and amphetamines among athletes and nonathletes. The study reported that, with the exception of amphetamines, there was no difference in drug use be-

tween the two groups. Emphasizing that athletes are subject to the same social processes as the rest of the population, the report concluded that: "Athletes do not represent a special subpopulation within our society with respect to drug use and the athlete is as much a part of the culturization that has taken place with respect to drug use as any other individual in the university population."[5]

The National Collegiate Athletic Association (NCAA), which is the governing body for intercollegiate athletics, commissioned their first survey on drug use in 1981. Responses were solicited from athletes, coaches, athletic trainers, and team physicians from colleges in the Big Ten athletic conference. A total of 1140 male athletes competing in four sports were surveyed at the ten schools. The data were significant for the numbers and patterns of use of alcohol, marijuana, cocaine, amphetamines, and hypnotics during their competitive season and during the off-season. The results are summarized in Table 7–1. Alcohol was the most abused drug throughout the year and the other drugs were rarely taken.[5]

Armed with that initial information, the NCAA embarked on a more comprehensive evaluation in 1983, which was conducted by investigators at Michigan State University. A total of 2048 student athletes completed questionnaires, which represented a 72% response rate. These athletes were drawn from five men's and five women's sports who were enrolled at 11 colleges. The schools were divided among Division I, II, and III (large, medium, and small colleges, respectively) and the patterns of drug use of 14 substances were evaluated.[6] The results are listed in Table 7–2 and reveal the percentages of athletes that had used seven drugs in the preceding 12 months.

Having established the relative frequency of drug use among collegiate athletes, it is useful to compare a cohort group of college students. Anderson recently reviewed data from surveys of drug use by both athletes and nonathletes at the college level.[2] The results are summarized in Table 7–3 and indicate that for most substances, athletes have comparable or lower usage rates than their nonathlete peers. The only exception to

TABLE 7-2. 1983 SURVEY OF DRUG USE BY INTERCOLLEGIATE ATHLETES

Drug	Percentage of Athletes
Alcohol	88%
Amphetamines	8%
Anabolic Steroids	6.5%
Anti-inflammatories	31%
Caffeine	68%
Cocaine	17%
Marijuana	36%

From Anderson WA, McKeag DB. The Substance Use and Abuse Habits of College Student Athletes. *National Collegiate Athletic Association; June 1985.*

this is anabolic steroids, which was not surveyed among the nonathletes.

These studies support the relatively low rates of drug use among athletes as compared to nonathletes. This is reflective of the fact that, prior to college, athletes in our society are not segregated from the general population. According to the 1983 NCAA study, most patterns of drug use are established in junior high and high school.[6] These data are summarized in Table 7–4, which lists the age at which athletes first tried eight recreational drugs. These studies all support the conclusion that athletes differ very little from their nonathlete colleagues with respect to recreational drug use. It appears that an effective drug education program would ideally focus on junior high and high school students, regardless of athletic status. If athletics do confer a greater risk for drug use, then it is only with respect to ergogenic aids.

CLASSIFICATION OF DRUG USE

It is impossible to examine the category "drugs" as a whole; the reasons for use vary depending on the effect of the drug and the athlete's intent. The International

TABLE 7-1. 1981 NCAA SURVEY OF DRUG USE AMONG ATHLETES

Drug	Percentage Using Regularly	Percentage Using Intermittently
Alcohol	36%	26%
Marijuana	11%	9%
Cocaine	5%	2%
Amphetamines	5%	1%
Hypnotics	2%	1%

From Bell JA, and Doege TC, Athlete's use and abuse of drugs. Phys Sports Med *1987; 15(3):99–108.*

TABLE 7-3. DRUG USE AMONG COLLEGE STUDENTS AND ATHLETES

Drug	Students	Athletes
Alcohol	92%	88%
Amphetamines	12%	8%
Anabolic steroids	N/A	5%
Barbiturates/tranquilizers	6%	2%
Cigarettes	23%	5%
Cocaine	17%	17%
Marijuana	42%	36%
Smokeless tobacco	19%	20%

From McKeag D. Drug use and abuse in athletics: Clinical workshop. American College of Sports Medicine Annual Meeting, Baltimore, 1989.

TABLE 7-4. FIRST USE OF RECREATIONAL DRUGS

Drug	Junior High or Before (%)	High School (%)	First-Year College (%)	After First Year (%)
Cigarettes[a]	41	34	14	12
Smokeless tobacco	16	53	24	7
Alcohol	24	65	8	3
Marijuana/hashish[a]	25	58	10	6
Cocaine	4	42	24	30
Psychedelics[a]	13	44	21	20
Barbiturates/tranquilizers[a]	31	31	17	17
Amphetamines[a]	8	58	21	14

[a]Percentages do not total 100% because of rounding.
From Duda M. NCAA: Only 4% of athletes used steroids. Physician Sports Med. 1985; 13(8):30.

Olympic Committee (IOC) and the NCAA have developed classification schemes for drug use that are summarized in Tables 7–5 and 7–6. Discussed in more detail later in this chapter, these classification systems are primarily devoted to the athlete who attempts to gain a competitive edge by the use of foreign substances. Although this may certainly be useful at the elite level, it is insufficient for athletes at lower levels of competition.

For the purposes of this chapter, drugs are divided into ergogenic, recreational, and therapeutic substances. Table 7–7 combines the IOC and NCAA systems into this classification scheme. Under this method, drugs are classified according to their reasons for use and desired effect. This becomes significant in understanding the athlete and potential avenues for treatment and deterence. Table 7–7 provides examples of each type of drug and an outline for discussion in this chapter; it does not represent all drugs of abuse by athletes. Patterns of drug use are changing rapidly and the examples in this chapter provide a method for evaluating substances as they emerge.

ERGOGENIC DRUGS

Ergogenic, or performance-enhancing, drugs are used by athletes in order to gain a competitive advantage. In 1964, the IOC adopted the following definition of "doping": The administration to, or the use by, a competing athlete of any substance foreign to the body or any physiological substance taken in abnormal quantity or by an abnormal route of entry into the body, with the sole intention of increasing, in an artificial and unfair manner, an athlete's performance in competi-

TABLE 7-5. IOC CLASSIFICATION OF BANNED DRUGS

I. Doping classes
　A. Stimulants
　　1. Psychomotor stimulants
　　2. Sympathomimetic amines
　　3. Miscellaneous central nervous system stimulants (including caffeine)
　B. Narcotics
　C. Anabolic steroids
　D. β-blockers
　E. Diuretics
II. Doping methods
　A. Blood doping
　B. Pharmacological, chemical, and physical manipulation of the urine
III. Classes of drugs subject to certain restrictions
　A. Alcohol[a]
　B. Local anesthetics[b]
　C. Corticosteroids[c]
　D. β₂ agonists[d]

[a]Not prohibited but levels (breath or blood) may be requested by an internal federation.
[b]Permitted when medically indicated and documented in writing to IOC Medical Commission.
[c]Banned, except when used topically, via inhalation, locally, or intra-articularly and documented in writing to IOC medical Commission (oral, intravenous, and intramuscular use banned).
[d]Permitted in the aerosol or inhalant form for the treatment of asthma and accompanied by physician note to the IOC Medical Commission prior to competition.

TABLE 7-6. NCAA CLASSIFICATION OF BANNED DRUGS

I. Psychomotor and central nervous system stimulants
II. Sympathomimetic amines
III. Anabolic steroids
IV. Substances banned for specific sports
　A. Rifle shooting
　　1. Alcohol
　　2. β-blockers
V. Diuretics
VI. Street drugs
　A. Amphetamine/methamphetamine
　B. Cocaine
　C. Heroin
　D. Marijuana/THC
　E. Others

TABLE 7-7. DRUG CLASSIFICATION

Ergogenic Aids	Recreational Drugs	Therapeutic Drugs
Anabolic steroids	Alcohol	NSAIDS
Human growth hormone	Cocaine	Analgesics
Stimulants	Marijuana	β_2 aerosols
Amphetamines	Tobacco	
Sympathomimetic amines		
Caffeine		
Blood doping		
Diuretics		

tion.[7] This covers a broad range of substances and practices that are summarized in Table 7–5. When it comes to segregating athletes with regard to drug use, the use of ergogenic aids is where athletes differ most from nonathletes.

Anabolic Steroids

Anabolic steroids have attracted the most publicity and their use appears to be increasing. There has been a great deal of confusion as to their definition, mechanism of action, and properties. Anabolic steroids are testosterone or testosterone-like synthetic drugs that have both anabolic and androgenic effects. These substances are used by athletes for their ability to increase protein synthesis (anabolic effects). Unfortunately, anabolic steroids also enhance the development of male secondary sexual characteristics (androgenic effects) and have numerous adverse side effects.

Although the history of anabolic steroids is unclear, they were probably developed in the 1930s and first used medically in World War II to help restore positive nitrogen balance to starvation victims.[8] There are also anecdotal reports of their use by German troops in order to increase aggressiveness during the same period.[9] Today, anabolic steroids are used medically in the treatment of certain refractory anemias, as replacement therapy in hypogonadal males and in the management of burn victims. Despite conflicting claims from the Soviet Union and the United States, it seems likely that these drugs were "discovered" by international, elite athletes sometime during the 1950s.[10] Since that time, their use has continually escalated.

Although it is difficult to evaluate, several recent studies have attempted to determine the prevalence of anabolic steroid usage. Buckley et al conducted an extensive study among 3403 12th-grade male students attending 46 high schools in 24 states.[11] Overall, 6.6% of the respondents had used anabolic steroids and 47% took the drug to improve athletic performance. Among the unexpected data from this study were the facts that 35% of the anabolic steroid users were not connected with any school-sponsored athletic activity and 27% used anabolics in order to improve appearance. This suggests that steroids are being used not only by athletes but by nonathletes as well. There are estimated to be one million anabolic steroid users in the United States and a $100 million black market industry.[12]

At the cellular level, it appears that anabolic steroids increase protein synthesis after binding to cytoplasmic proteins and being transported to the nucleus of the cell. From there, a DNA-dependent RNA polymerase is activated, resulting in the production of messenger RNA (mRNA) encoded for protein synthesis.[13] Although this mechanism has been known for some time, there has been a great deal of controversy regarding the effects of anabolic steroids in human subjects. Several studies have demonstrated no gains in strength when anabolic steroids were given to men.[14–17] These studies were limited, either by using nonathletes as subjects or administering steroids in far smaller doses than athletes commonly employ. Once these errors were corrected, clinical trials demonstrated that anabolic steroids could contribute to increases in strength.[18–20]

The reluctance of health care professionals to acknowledge that anabolic steroids could increase strength damaged some physicians' credibility among athletes. Athletes could see the effects of steroids in the gym and felt that they increased strength, and yet the health care community seemed unwilling to recognize that anabolic steroids "worked." To address these concerns, the American College of Sports Medicine reviewed all of the previous studies and concluded the following[21]:

1. In the presence of an adequate diet, anabolic steroids can contribute to increases in body weight and lean mass.
2. The gains in muscular strength achieved through high-intensity exercise and proper diet can occur by increased use of anabolic steroids in some individuals.
3. Anabolic steroids do not increase aerobic power.

In order to effectively educate athletes about anabolic steroids, accurate and reliable information must be dispensed.

One of the limitations of studying the effects of anabolic steroids in the laboratory is that athletes commonly use these drugs at dosages that far exceed therapeutic recommendations and in multiple combinations. The practice of combining oral and injectable steroids is called "stacking" and involves cycles of use in a pyramidal fashion to achieve the maximal effect. Table 7–8 details the use of anabolic steroids by a weightlifter and a comparison with the recommended therapeutic dosages. In addition to drugs approved for human use, athletes often obtain veterinary steroids of unknown

TABLE 7-8. ANABOLIC STEROID USE BY A WEIGHTLIFTER

Drug	Dose	Therapeutic Dose
Testosterone cypionate (Depo-Testosterone)	200 mg intramuscularly every 3 days	200 mg every 3 weeks
Nandrolone decanoate (Deca-Durabolin)	100 mg intramuscularly every 3 days	100 mg every week
Oxandrolone (Anavar)	25 mg orally daily	2.5–10 mg daily
Methandrostenolone (Dianabol)	40 mg orally daily	5 mg daily
Bolasterone (Finaject)	30–40 mg subcutaneously every 2–3 days	

From Brower KJ, et al. Anabolic–androgenic steroid dependence. J Clinical Psychiatry. 1989; 50:31–33.

potency on the black market. Table 7–9 lists some of the anabolic steroids commonly used by athletes.

The gains that are possible through the use of anabolic steroids are offset by the potential adverse reactions. The most significant risks are the negative effects on the cardiovascular system. Anabolic steroids cause an increase in total cholesterol and low-density-lipoprotein (LDL) cholesterol, and a decrease in high-density-lipoprotein (HDL) cholesterol.[21] Salt and water retention also occurs, resulting in the development of hypertension; combined with the adverse effects on lipids, anabolic steroids greatly increase the risk of coronary artery disease. As an example, anabolic steroids were recently implicated as the cause of an acute myocardial infarction in a 22-year-old world class weightlifter.[22] It is not yet clear whether these adverse effects are reversible after cessation of anabolic steroids.

The gastrointestinal system can also be affected by anabolic steroids. The most serious consequences seem to be in the liver, where hepatomas and peliosis hepatis—the formation of blood-filled cysts—have been reported.[23,24] The hepatic consequences appear to be increased with the use of the 17 α-alkylated oral

TABLE 7-9. COMMON ANABOLIC STEROIDS

Generic Name	Trade Name
Oral	
Fluoxymesterone	Android-F, Halotestin
Methyltestosterone	Android-5, Testred, Virilon
Oxandrolone	Anavar
Oxymetholone	Anadrol-50
Stanazolol	Winstrol
Ethylestrenol	
Mesterolone	
Injectable	
Nandrolone decanoate	Deca-Durabolin, Kabolin
Nandrolone phenpropionate	Durabolin
Testosterone cypionate	Depo-Testosterone, Virilon IM
Testosterone enanthate	Testaval 90/4
Testosterone propionate	

preparations due to their first pass effect through the liver. By virtue of their shorter half-lives, oral preparations are being used by athletes in order to avoid detection by drug testing. As a result, there may be an increasing incidence of liver complications in the future.

Evidence has been mounting about the psychological effects of anabolic steroids, including mood swings, aggressive behavior, and changes in libido among chronic users.[21] Two recent articles describe a dependence pattern involving an opioid-type withdrawal state following the cessation of anabolics.[25,26] In addition, Pope and Katz interviewed chronic steroid users and found that 22% demonstrated a full affective syndrome and 12% displayed psychotic symptoms while using anabolic steroids.[27] The studies emphasize the powerful effects that these drugs can have on behavior.

The effects of excess androgens on the male reproductive system are secondary to the suppression of gonadotropins. Anabolic steroids act as weak androgens and may lead to a decreased sperm count and decreased testicular size. There has also been a case of adenocarcinoma of the prostate in a 40-year-old body builder who abused anabolic steroids.[28] In addition, the conversion of excess androgens to estrogenic compounds may result in gynecomastia.[21] Although many of these responses are reversible, they may serve as clinical signs of current anabolic steroid usage.

The side effects experienced by women are based on the relatively small amount of daily testosterone secretion as compared to men (0.25 mg versus 5 to 6 mg for men).[29] Women may suffer from the virilizing actions of the drugs, including male-pattern alopecia, acne, and breast reduction. These are all probably reversible after the cessation of anabolic steroids, but hirsutism, clitoromegaly, and deepening of the voice are probably irreversible.[21] In addition, women using anabolic steroids generally have reduced luteinizing hormone (LH), follicle-stimulating hormone (FSH), estrogen, and progesterone, resulting in menstrual irregularities.

A special note of caution needs to be included re-

garding the use of anabolic steroids in children who are still growing. Buckley et al found that 38% of anabolic steroid users began using the drug before the age of 15.[11] In growing children, anabolic steroids will cause a premature, irreversible closure of the epiphyses, leading to a loss of full, adult stature.[30] Given the increasing availability of anabolic steroids at the junior high and high school levels, this point must be emphasized in the education of young people and their parents.

Miscellaneous side effects that have been reported include weakening of the tendons and spontaneous ruptures of the musculotendon unit.[31,32] There has been ample documentation of the effects on the skin, leading to an increase in sebaceous glands and resultant acne.[33] In addition, potentially lethal consequences may develop from the use of injectable anabolic steroids and shared needles, including AIDS, hepatitis, and endocarditis. Despite the many possible complications, the prevalence of such effects is difficult to determine because there have been no long-term studies of anabolic steroid use.

Athletes are often willing to assume or ignore the potential adverse reactions in order to improve their performance. The use of anabolic steroids is opposed by the American College of Sports Medicine, the NCAA, the IOC, and the United States Olympic Committees. The penalty for detection varies, depending on the sport and organization involved. The Canadian Olympian Ben Johnson received a lifetime ban and was estimated to have lost $10 to $15 million in endorsements following his positive test for the anabolic steroid stanazolol in 1988. Contrast this with Brian Bosworth, a football player for the University of Oklahoma who tested positive in 1986 for an anabolic steroid, nandrolone. Although he was banned from the Orange Bowl, he later signed a multimillion dollar professional football contract and received offers to endorse several products. As anabolic steroids become more popular, they are no longer confined to the traditional "power" sports such as football and weight lifting. Health care professionals need to consider the use of anabolic steroids among all athletes.

Human Growth Hormone

The increased awareness of anabolic steroids, coupled with the improved sensitivity of drug testing has led athletes to seek alternatives. One of the more popular substances is human growth hormone (hGH) because it is not currently detectable by drug testing. Human growth hormone is a polypeptide consisting of 191 amino acids and with a molecular weight of 21,500. In the normal adult, 5 to 10 mg are stored in the anterior pituitary gland and mature males have a daily production rate of 0.4 to 1.0 mg.[34] The effects of hGH were first realized by animal breeders in the 1930s who found that animals given an extract of specific pituitary

glands developed increased muscle mass, decreased body fat, and an accelerated growth rate. In the 1950s, it was discovered that hGH contributed to the production of somatomedins, which in turn increased growth. With the advent of radioimmunoassay in 1961, it became possible to measure hGH levels in the plasma. Human growth hormone was isolated and purified from cadaveric pituitary glands for medical use until 1985 when synthetic hGH was licensed.

Most of the medical research on the effects of hGH have been conducted on children with hypopituitarism who have been given replacement hormone. There have been no documented scientific reports on excess growth hormone in athletes with normally functioning pituitary glands. When hGH is given to deficient children, a positive nitrogen balance develops and skeletal and soft tissue growth accelerates.[34] The effects on muscle have been difficult to determine and several experiments have led to conflicting data on improvements in strength.[35-37] Much of the research has been accomplished with animal studies and it is difficult to determine the capacity of hGH to increase muscular force of contraction or to improve performance in humans.

The metabolic effects of hGH have been studied using hypophysectomized animals. It has been found that hGH stimulates lipid mobilization from the adipose tissue, and increased rates of protein synthesis have been observed.[34] Human growth hormone exhibits an anti-insulin effect at the cellular level by inhibiting the uptake of glucose. Overall, hGH acts as a counterregulatory hormone to increase the serum concentration of glucose.

The medical use of hGH is limited to the treatment of hGH-deficient children. It has been well documented to be effective in increasing the stature of these patients[38] as well as some short-statured children who are not hGH deficient.[39] It is estimated that in the United States there are approximately 9000 patients who fit these criteria in which hGH would be medically indicated. The Food and Drug Administration (FDA), however, has become increasingly alarmed by the number of complaints from endocrinologists and team physicians about requests for hGH.[40] In 1983, it was reported that evidence of hGH was found in several urine specimens at the World Track and Field Championships in Helsinki and it is thought to be widely used by bodybuilders and power athletes.[34] A recent study among high school football players found a 2% use of growth hormone.[41]

The rising use of hGH has triggered concern about side effects, many of which are irreversible. Acromegaly is a potentially serious consequence in athletes using megadoses of hGH. The therapeutic dose of hGH in deficiency states is approximately 1 mg/day for a 50-kg individual; there have been reports of athletes consuming up to 20 times this dosage.[40] It is estimated that

a patient with acromegaly will produce 1.5 to 9 mg/day of hGH,[42] which may be as little as a twofold increase over the normal rate of production. Thus, hGH has a relatively narrow therapeutic index. With athletes consuming megadoses of hGH, the risk of acromegaly is high. The complications of acromegaly include diabetes, arthritis, myopathies, and the characteristic coarsening of the bones of the hands, feet, and face.[34]

An additional concern is infection with a slow virus that is the etiologic agent of Creutzfeldt–Jakob disease. The development of this lethal disease has been documented following the use of hGH derived from cadaveric pituitary glands.[43] Although the risk is obviously diminished in patients who obtain legitimate prescriptions for biosynthetic hGH, athletes often obtain illegal substances from the black market, thereby placing themselves at risk for this catastrophic neurological disease. Although hGH is banned by the IOC, there currently exists no reliable testing method to detect its use. Clinical suspicion based on the adverse effects should be the guide for those health care professionals involved in the care of athletes.

Amphetamines and Sympathomimetic Amines

Athletes have long experimented with amphetamines in order to avoid fatigue and increase concentration. The role of amphetamines in sport has been well known since the 1960 Summer Olympics when the Danish cyclist Kurt Enemar Jensen died from an overdose of amphetamines and Roniacol. The use of amphetamines became widespread in the National Football League during the 1970s, and the term "Sunday Syndrome" was coined to describe a pattern of use among those athletes.[44] Amphetamines and weaker sympathomimetic amines such as phenylpropanolamine, phenylephrine, ephedrine, and pseudoephedrine are synthetic congeners of naturally occurring catecholamines[45] that were manufactured following the isolation of epinephrine in 1899.[46] Amphetamines were first used medically in the 1930s for the treatment of nasal congestion, narcolepsy, and obesity.[45]

There have been several theories proposed to explain amphetamines' effects on the nervous system. Potential mechanisms include increased output of endogenous catecholamines, release of bound catecholamines, inhibition of monoamine oxidase, a decrease in catecholamine reuptake, and acting as a false neurotransmitter.[45] It is likely that all of these contribute in some way to the observed physiological responses to amphetamine ingestion. These include increased heart rate and blood pressure, bronchodilation, an increased metabolic rate, and increased free fatty acid mobilization.

The effects of the other sympathomimetic amines depend on the relative selectivity of each individual drug toward the neurological receptors α, β_1, and β_2. Drugs that are primarily α selective tend to cause smooth muscle contraction that results in vasoconstriction. Agents that stimulate β_1 sites increase intracellular cyclic adenosine monophosphate (cAMP) and this increases heart rate and the force of contraction. β_2 stimulation relaxes smooth muscle and leads to bronchodilation and stimulation of skeletal smooth muscle.[47] Although the sympathomimetic amines are classified according to their primary receptor site of action, each individual drug possesses some degree of reactivity for the other receptors. The most famous case of an athlete using these drugs was the American swimmer Rick DeMont, who was disqualified from the 1972 Olympics for using ephedrine.

Numerous studies have been conducted to determine if amphetamines and sympathomimetic amines can improve athletic performance and the data has been conflicting. Although Smith and Beecher reported that 75% of their subjects improved their performance with amphetamines,[48] Chandler and Blair were unable to reproduce this effect.[49] The basis for this discrepancy may lie in the nature of the tasks. Amphetamines seem to improve simple, repetitive tasks, but not more complicated maneuvers. The sympathomimetic amines were touted as ergogenic aids, but two recent studies demonstrated no such effect on performance.[50,51]

There are many adverse reactions associated with these stimulants, as well as a high potential for amphetamine addiction. The central nervous system (CNS) is affected and the athlete may experience restlessness, insomnia, tremors, frank psychosis, anxiety, and cerebral hemorrhage. Amphetamine affects the cardiovascular system by lowering the threshold for cardiac arrhythmias and may induce angina. Of particular concern to athletes is that these drugs can disrupt thermoregulation and predispose an athlete exercising in warm weather to heat illness. The sympathomimetic amines can provoke similar symptoms, although to a much lesser degree. All of the drugs in this category, with the exception of some aerosolized β_2 agonists used in the treatment of asthma, are banned by the IOC. In August of 1989, the NCAA removed sympathomimetic amines from their list of banned substances, but amphetamines are not allowed.

Caffeine

The knowledge that caffeine-containing plants could be brewed into a beverage has probably been common since the paleolithic age. Caffeine is a CNS stimulant that is a naturally occurring alkaloid derived from aqueous extracts of *Coffea arabica* and *Cola acuminata*.[46] Caffeine is classified as a xanthine and is related chemically to theobromine and theophylline; it is commonly found in coffee, tea, colas, and over-the-counter stimulants. It is estimated that coffee is consumed in

98% of American homes with an annual per capita consumption of 16 lb.[46]

Athletes have been attracted to caffeine both for its stimulant properties and the potential to increase power and work. During the 1976 Summer Olympic Games, a significant number of athletes were found to have large quantities of caffeine in their urine.[52] Although Anderson and McKeag found that 68% of the intercollegiate athletes surveyed used caffeine, 82% consumed it less than three times per day.[53] This suggests that athletes are using caffeine recreationally, rather than for ergogenic effects.

There has been a great deal of investigation concerning caffeine's ability to enhance performance. Evidence suggests that caffeine may enhance the mobilization of free fatty acids (FFAs), thus increasing the rate of lipid metabolism.[54] At the cellular level, the observation of improved muscular contraction is likely secondary to an increased permeability of calcium in the sarcoplasmic reticulum.[55] These effects have been difficult to corroborate in human studies and doubts have been raised about caffeine's effectiveness.[56,57] To summarize the literature, it seems likely that if there is any benefit, it is limited to an improvement in endurance capacity.[45]

At higher doses, caffeine can produce adverse reactions similar to the amphetamines. Anxiety, insomnia, headache, tremors, hypochondriasis, and addiction with a withdrawal state are all symptoms of CNS involvement. Tachycardia and tachyarrhythmias, especially paroxysmal atrial tachycardia, can result from caffeine use. In addition, caffeine has a diuretic effect that can lead to dehydration in the athlete exercising in hot weather.[45] Caffeine also causes an increase in gastric acid secretion that can produce ulcer disease and gastritis.

The potential for abuse as an ergogenic aid has led the IOC and the NCAA to ban caffeine and check urinary concentrations. The IOC has determined a maximum urinary concentration of 12 μg/mL, whereas the NCAA allows 15 μg/mL. There has been concern on the part of athletes undergoing drug testing as to how much caffeine can be consumed before a positive test results. A recent study attempted to examine that issue and found that an individual had to consume almost 1000 mg of caffeine within 3 hours to exceed 12 μg/mL.[58] The average cup of brewed coffee contains between 55 and 85 mg/mL of caffeine and it can therefore be assumed that if an athlete has a level above 12 μg/mL it is not merely the result of casual imbibing. Table 7–10 lists the caffeine content of various beverages and over-the-counter caffeine-containing drugs.

Blood Doping

Blood doping is the practice whereby blood is removed from an athlete and stored in a frozen state to be reinfused at a later date. The result is an increased red

TABLE 7-10. CAFFEINE CONTENT OF COMMONLY USED SUBSTANCES

Substance	Caffeine Concentration (mg/mL)	Caffeine Level[a] (μg/mL)
Coffee	55–85	1.5–3 (1 cu)
Tea	55–85	1.5–3 (1 cu)
Cola	10–15	0.75–1.5 (1 cu)
Medications	(mg/tab)	
Cafergot	100	3–6
NoDoz	100	3–6
Anacin	32	2–3
Midol	32	2–3

[a]Level dependent on size of athlete and rate of metabolism. These figures represent general estimates based on average size and rate of metabolism.

blood cell (RBC) mass and an improvement in oxygen-carrying capacity. This practice, also known as blood boosting or blood packing, received a great deal of publicity when it became known that seven United States cyclists had engaged in blood doping at the 1984 Summer Olympics. The first medical experiments using this technique were in 1947 when armed forces personnel received 2000 mL of freshly donated blood from matched donors.[59] Those investigators reported a 34% increase in endurance compared to controls, and this was reproduced when blood was frozen at $-80°$C.

Previous studies have demonstrated that maximal VO_2 correlates with red cell mass through an increased delivery of oxygen to active muscle.[60] Researchers have sought to determine the effects of an increased red cell mass on performance. Buick et al studied elite runners following blood doping and found an increased hemoglobin concentration and a general improvement in maximal oxygen consumption.[61] In addition, the total exercise time was significantly increased.[61] Although blood doping is currently unable to be detected, rumors of this practice have been widespread for the past 20 years.

Blood doping is not a benign practice. The use of improperly matched donor blood carries the risk of potentially fatal transfusion reactions. Immunologic complications occur in approximately 3% of all transfusions.[61] In addition, infectious problems such as hepatitis and AIDS are possible risks in all heterologous transfusions. Although the use of autologous blood reduces the possibility of infection and immune reactions, however, improperly stored blood can lead to serious complications. Experimental protocols are being developed to detect blood doping, but there is no current method available at this time. Despite this, the IOC and NCAA ban the practice of blood doping. Blood doping violates the spirit of the IOC rules because it is a "physiologic substance taken in abnormal quantity and by an abnormal route . . . with the sole intention

of increasing in an unfair and artificial manner . . . performance."

As the risks of blood doping become more publicized and testing methods are developed, it is expected that athletes will begin using the hormone erythropoietin to achieve increased red cell mass. Erythropoietin can now be synthesized by a recombinant process and is available for kidney failure patients who suffer from anemia. There is the possibility that this will become increasingly popular with athletes.

RECREATIONAL DRUGS

Most surveys have demonstrated that use and abuse of recreational drugs is no greater among athletes than it is in the general population. For the purposes of this chapter, social or recreational substances are considered to be the legal drugs alcohol and tobacco, as well as the street drugs cocaine, marijuana, LSD, PCP, barbiturates, and heroin. All these drugs are readily available and athletes are exposed to the same temptations and pressures as the rest of the population. Accordingly, an athlete's reasons for using recreational drugs are similar to those of the nonathlete. A significant aspect of McKeag's study of intercollegiate athletes was that those who took recreational drugs tended to use them with their nonathlete peers. In addition, they usually obtained the substances outside of the athletic program.[53] This chapter reviews some of the more frequently used drugs and focuses on side effects as they relate to performance.

Alcohol

Several studies have concluded that alcohol is the most widely used drug by students and athletes at the high school and college level.[62] The fermenting of alcoholic beverages has been known since ancient times and was considered to be the elixir of life in the Middle Ages.[46] The current per capita consumption of alcohol is estimated to be 2.7 gal/yr and alcohol is consumed by 70% of the population.[63] Surveys indicate that 10% of males and 3% to 5% of women will develop alcoholism—15 to 20 million people—leading to 1 to 1.5 million cases of cirrhosis.[29] It has been suggested that alcoholics have a tenfold higher rate of carcinoma than the general population and that moderate alcohol consumption among women is associated with a 50% to 100% increase in the rate of breast cancer.[64] Finally, alcohol is directly responsible for at least 200,000 deaths per year.[63]

Numerous publications are devoted to the general health effects of chronic alcohol consumption; alcohol can affect nearly every organ in the body. This chapter is limited to the effects of alcohol on athletic performance. In sports requiring precise hand–eye coordina-

tion, small to moderate amount of alcohol will impair reaction time and lead to a deterioration in psychomotor performance.[65] It also appears that the acute ingestion of alcohol does not significantly alter basic metabolic functions that are necessary for an exercising individual. Thus, alcohol offers no physiological benefit to an active individual.[65] The American College of Sports Medicine concluded that alcohol ingestion will not improve muscular work capacity and may in fact lead to decreased performance levels.[65] There has also been evidence to suggest that alcohol may adversely affect thermoregulation while exercising in a cold environment.[66] Alcohol has direct effects on muscle and a long-term study revealed that alcohol is toxic to striated muscle in a dose-dependent fashion.[67]

Alcohol abuse is the leading drug problem among athletes and needs to be addressed through education by those health care professionals concerned with athletes. Although the percentage of athletes who consume alcohol is similar to nonathletes, there may be important distinctions in patterns of use. A recent survey revealed that intercollegiate athletes drank more alcohol at a sitting and were more likely to drive or ride with someone under the influence of alcohol than were their nonathlete peers.[68] The American Medical Association defines alcoholism as "an illness characterized by significant impairment that is directly associated with persistent and excessive use of alcohol. Impairment may involve physiological, psychological or social dysfunction."[63] It is important to note that under this definition, the actual amount of alcohol consumed is not a criteria for alcoholism. An effective educational program for athletes should include discussion of the negative effects of alcohol on performance.

Cocaine

The increasing availability of cocaine and "crack" has generated a tremendous amount of concern among health officials. Although it is estimated that 30 million Americans have tried cocaine and that there are at least 5 million regular users,[69] it was the tragic cocaine-related deaths of sports figures Len Bias and Don Rogers in 1986 that focused national attention on the problem. Cocaine is a naturally occurring alkaloid that is derived from the leaves of the *Erythroxylon coca* plant.[70] Since its discovery by the European scientific community in the late 19th century, it has enjoyed cyclical peaks of popularity.

Cocaine has actions both as a topical anesthetic and a stimulant of the cardiorespiratory and central nervous systems. The mechanism responsible for these effects is the inhibition of presynaptic reuptake of norepinephrine and dopamine. This produces an excess of neurotransmitter at the postsynaptic receptor sites leading to an increased sympathetic response. The results are vasoconstriction, an increase in blood pressure and

heart rate, and a lowered threshold for ventricular arrhythmias and seizures. The increased availability of neurotransmitters is also responsible for a feeling of euphoria and increased peripheral reflex speed. In addition, cocaine use may cause hyperglycemia, mydriasis, and hyperthermia.[71] At the local level, cocaine acts as an anesthetic by stabilizing neuronal axons and blocking nerve impulse initiation and conduction. Combined with its vasoconstrictive properties, cocaine is an excellent local anesthetic and is used in ophthalmological surgery.[72]

Cocaine is readily absorbed by a number of methods. Common routes include sniffing or snorting through the nose, smoking the freebase form, intravenous injection, and smoking the newest form, "crack" cocaine. Crack is a relatively inexpensive ready-to-smoke form of freebase cocaine that has reached epidemic proportions in urban areas. When it is smoked in a pipe or mixed with tobacco in a cigarette, it produces a popping sound: hence the nickname "crack." The danger of crack use is that it produces an effect comparable to intravenous injection with a rapid onset of action lasting only 5 to 10 minutes. It is estimated that a recreational user of intranasal cocaine consumes 1 to 3 g/wk.[71]

Although cocaine does not discriminate in its effects on athletes, performance may be impaired in a number of ways. Symptoms of cocaine use include tremulousness, agitation, restlessness, insomnia, anxiety, and a powerful addiction.[73] Judgment can be significantly impaired while one is under the influence of cocaine, endangering the athlete and other competitors. Exercise may also accentuate the cardiovascular response to cocaine use. Another concern for the athlete is cocaine-induced hyperpyrexia, which is caused by a combination of excess heat production from increased muscular activity and vasoconstriction that inhibits heat loss.[74] In addition, cocaine probably has a direct effect on the thermoregulatory center of the brain.[72] An athlete exercising in a warm environment would be more susceptible to hyperthermia while using cocaine. It has been proposed that elite sprint-trained athletes may be at greater risk for severe lactic acidosis and cocaine-induced seizures due to a higher percentage of glycolytic muscle fibers.[75]

The treatment of an athlete who is abusing cocaine highlights the difficulty of any recreational drug abuse problem. Frequently, the most challenging aspect is to identify the athlete with a significant problem because denial is a key ingredient to the addiction. The repeated treatment failures of several prominent professional players, despite the loss of lucrative salaries, is testimony to the addictive power of cocaine. Coaches, trainers, therapists, teammates, and team physicians should be aware of behavioral changes that may be sec-

ondary to cocaine usage. A player's performance is often a poor indicator of drug use; many athletes have been able to maintain a high level of play while their personal lives were deteriorating. The signs of drug abuse in an athlete are often ignored as long as performance is maintained at an acceptable standard. One final conclusion offered by McKeag was that no consistent profile of the athlete who used recreational drugs could be found.[76]

Marijuana

Marijuana is a naturally occurring cannabinoid that contains the psychoactive ingredient delta-9-tetrahydrocannabinol (THC) that is responsible for its properties as a euphoriant. Current estimates are that 43 million Americans have experimented with marijuana and there are at least 17 million regular users.[77] Anderson and McKeag's survey of intercollegiate athletes revealed that 36% had used marijuana and that 83% of that group had first tried the drug in junior high or high school.[53] These patterns of use are consistent with those found in the general population and serve to emphasize the fact that athletes are influenced by the same societal pressures as nonathletes.

THC can be readily absorbed from either the lungs or the gastrointestinal tract and exerts its effects on several areas of the body. The effects are dependent on the route of administration, dosage, setting, and prior experiences of the individual with the drug. The CNS is primarily affected by impaired motor skills, decreased short-term memory, difficulty concentrating, and a decline in work performance.[3] Tachycardia is the most prominent reaction, involving the cardiovascular system, and this can be ablated by the use of a β-blocker. In addition, acute ingestion of marijuana results in an increased systolic blood pressure while supine and a decreased upright blood pressure.[46] Marijuana can inhibit sweating, which increases core body temperature.[46] Long-term marijuana use can also cause problems of the male reproductive system, including decreased plasma testosterone, gynecomastia, and oligospermia.[78]

The acute effects of marijuana use on performance have been studied by Renaud and Cormier.[79] Subjects were studied on a cycle ergometer by pedaling to exhaustion and measuring several parameters of exercise in the nonsmoking state and 10 minutes after smoking marijuana. Renaud and Cormier found that although marijuana did induce a bronchodilation, there was no effect on pulmonary tidal volume, arterial blood pressure, and carboxyhemoglobin as compared to controls. The key feature of the study was that marijuana use did result in a reduction of maximal exercise performance with a premature achievement of maximal oxygen uptake.[79] Athletes tend to be highly concerned about

their level of play and the information about marijuana's negative effects on performance may be part of a successful educational program.

The IOC is primarily concerned with ergogenic drugs and thus does not specifically ban marijuana. The NCAA considers marijuana a street drug and tests for urine levels above 25 ng/mL. Owing to its high lipid solubility, THC has a long half-life and can be detected in the urine for 2 to 4 weeks by drug testing. Depending on an individual's percentage of body fat, the concentration sensitivity of the test, and the length of time between exposure and testing, passive inhalation of secondary marijuana smoke can result in a positive drug test. Athletes who are eligible to be drug tested should be advised to avoid these situations.

Tobacco

Tobacco is a major health hazard that is responsible for approximately 90,000 deaths from lung cancer and contributes significantly to 125,000 deaths from coronary artery disease each year. The costs attributable to smoking-related medical care and lost productivity in the United States are estimated to be $55 billion annually.[29] Athletes' awareness of the adverse effects of cigarette smoking is reflected in their low rate of this practice. Anderson and McKeag found that 5% of intercollegiate athletes had smoked cigarettes in the previous year and only half of that group had continued to smoke.[53] In addition, 88% of the smokers consumed less than one-half pack per day.[53] Cigarette smoking appears to be a minimal problem among athletes.

Of much greater concern is the increasing use of smokeless tobacco among the athletic population. During one game of the 1986 World Series, there was almost 24 minutes of television air time devoted to players and coaches chewing and dipping smokeless tobacco.[80] Advertisers have utilized famous sports personalities to convey the notion that the use of smokeless tobacco is a "safe" practice, and this has resulted in its use by young children. The results of a survey of more than 2000 Oklahoma children is summarized in Table 7–11.[81] This is consistent with similar rates of use among adolescents across the country, which estimate that approximately 8% to 10% of males aged 5 to 19 regularly use smokeless tobacco.[81] Anderson and McKeag's study of intercollegiate athletes revealed that 20% had used smokeless tobacco in the previous year, with 18% being regular users.[53] Other surveys of athletes have found a 34% rate of regular use among professional baseball players and a 30% usage rate in Alabama high school football players.[82] Clearly, this is a problem that is of increasing concern.

Advertising claims to the contrary, the use of smokeless tobacco has many negative health conse-

TABLE 7-11. REGULAR USE OF SMOKELESS TOBACCO BY SCHOOL CHILDREN

Grade in School	Percentage Using Smokeless Tobacco Regularly	
	Boys	Girls
Third grade	13%	2%
Fifth grade	21%	5%
Seventh grade	22%	7%
Ninth grade	33%	2%
Eleventh grade	39%	1%

From Glover ED, et al. Implication of smokeless tobacco use among athletes. Physician Sports Med. *1988; 14(12):95–105.*

quences. Significant consequences include a 50-fold increase in oral carcinomas among long-term snuff users, a 2.4-fold increase in the incidence of dental caries over control group subjects, and increases in gingival disease and precancerous leukoplakia lesions.[81] Smokeless tobacco has a high nicotine content that leads to an addiction similar to that of cigarette smoking. A user who consumes 8 to 10 dips or chews per day receives a nicotine dose equivalent to 30 to 40 cigarettes daily.[83] A study of college athletes who used smokeless tobacco revealed that 23% used it six or more times per day.[53] The American Academy of Oral Medicine concluded that "smokeless tobacco is not an innocuous substitute for cigarette smoking [and] its use should be recognized as potentially hazardous and therefore discouraged by all health professionals."[84]

Athletes have long touted smokeless tobacco for its properties as a stimulant that would increase concentration and improve reaction time. In order to investigate these claims, a study was conducted to test neuromuscular reactivity and heart rate among athletes and nonathletes. The study concluded that although smokeless tobacco did increase heart rate, no significant increases were noted in reaction time, movement time, or total response time among either athletes or nonathletes.[85] Interestingly, a survey of major league baseball players who were long-time users of smokeless tobacco revealed that only 10% felt that smokeless tobacco improved concentration and none felt that it sharpened reflexes.[83]

The addictive natures of tobacco and alcohol make it imperative that education is begun at a young age. Compare the annual mortality from tobacco and alcohol with the total of 643 cocaine-related deaths that were reported in all of 1985.[86] With all of the media attention given to anabolic steroids, cocaine, and other drugs, it is important to remember that tobacco and alcohol are still the most abused drugs and are responsible for the vast majority of morbidity and mortality caused by drug use. Comparing two legends of baseball

provides an example as to why interventions are needed by health care professionals. Babe Ruth was one of the great stars of baseball and died at age 52 following a career that was marked by the heavy use of tobacco and alcohol. Contrast this with another early star, Honus Wagner who was a teetotaler and an outspoken critic of tobacco. Wagner retired from baseball 3 years after Ruth first signed a professional contract and he went on to outlive Ruth by 7 years, dying at the age of 59 in 1955.[83]

THERAPEUTIC DRUGS

The final category of drugs are those that are supplied by a physician to treat an illness, injury, or underlying condition. The distinction between these substances and ergogenic aids is that therapeutic drugs allow an athlete to compete while overcoming a medical condition. The drugs in this category would not give a competitor an advantage over an otherwise healthy opponent. An example of this would be the use of an albuterol inhaler to prevent wheezing and dyspnea in an athlete with exercise-induced asthma. Drugs that are allowed by the IOC and NCAA are those substances that have been shown to be safe and do not provide the athlete with an unfair competitive advantage. Therapeutic drugs do not generally produce problems unless the drugs cause an athlete to compete unsafely. The injudicious use of an analgesic that results in the masking of further injury would be an example of the misuse of a therapeutic drug. Great care is required in prescribing drugs to competitive athletes.

Nonsteroidal Anti-Inflammatory Drugs

Nonsteroidal anti-inflammatory drugs (NSAIDs) have become the mainstay of treatment for the sprains and strains of athletic injuries and are the most commonly used class of therapeutic drugs among athletes. Nonsteroidal anti-inflammatory drugs have changed the traditional RICE therapy (rest, ice, compression, elevation) for athletic trauma to RICEM, with the "M" standing for medication. Anderson and McKeag found that 31% of the intercollegiate athletes in their study had used NSAIDs during the previous year.[53] Including aspirin and over-the-counter ibuprofen, over 26 billion tablets of NSAIDs were consumed in the United States in 1984.[87]

Nonsteroidal anti-inflammatory drugs are a class of drugs that have both analgesic and anti-inflammatory properties by virtue of their inhibition of prostaglandin synthesis, nonsteroidal anti-inflammatory drugs owe their development to the salicylates, which were first isolated from the willow bark in 1829 and used primarily as analgesics and antipyretics.[88] In 1960, indomethacin became the first synthetic derivative of salicylic acid to be marketed for its anti-inflammatory properties. The NSAIDs have proved to be very popular drugs and there are at least ten different compounds with varying half-lives, potencies, and absorption. In addition to their use in soft-tissue injuries, nonsteroidal anti-inflammatory drugs are effective in the treatment of rheumatoid arthritis, other rheumatological conditions, degenerative joint disease, pain management, and dysmenorrhea.

Although the exact mechanism by which the NSAIDs act to reduce inflammation is unclear, there have been several observations regarding the effect of prostaglandin synthesis inhibition.[88] Superoxides are known to be degradative substances that are present in inflammatory states and superoxide generation is diminished by NSAIDs. Nonsteroidal anti-inflammatory drugs have also been shown to inhibit both the migration of leukocytes and the release of lysosomal enzymes from leukocytes, thereby decreasing the inflammatory response. Nonsteroidal anti-inflammatory drugs have additional effects on the adenylate cyclase system and compete with prostaglandins for binding at receptor sites. The net result is to decrease the mediators of pain and inflammation. A recent animal study has shown that NSAIDs may also promote healing in damaged ligaments.[89]

Although the NSAIDs have proved to be effective and well-tolerated, significant adverse reactions do occur. The most prominent are the gastrointestinal manifestations, which can include nausea, dyspepsia, gastritis, ulceration, and bleeding. It has been reported that 2% to 10% of patients with rheumatoid arthritis have had to discontinue NSAIDs due to some form of gastrointestinal toxicity.[90] Hepatic toxicity has also been reported with some NSAIDs, and benoxaprofen was withdrawn from the market following several cases of hepatic failure.

The kidneys can be affected through sodium and water retention, hyperkalemia, papillary necrosis, interstitial nephritis, proteinuria, and eventual renal failure. Suprofen was shown to cause a syndrome of flank pain and a reversible form of acute renal failure; it was later withdrawn by the manufacturer.[91] Although renal complications are uncommon, it has been found that renal pathology occurs more frequently in hypovolemic patients taking NSAIDs. Other adverse reactions include bone marrow suppression, reversible inhibition of platelet aggregation, and possibly decreased coagulation. Headache, tinnitus, dizziness, and sedation are possible CNS symptoms following the use of NSAIDs.

Nonsteroidal anti-inflammatory drugs have been shown to uncouple oxidative phosphorylation, and this may have negative effects in athletes. Inhibition of this enzymatic process alters oxygen consumption and directly stimulates ventilation and sweating. All of this can lead to dehydration and make an athlete suscepti-

ble to heat illness while exercising in warm weather.[92] As NSAIDs become "standard practice" in the treatment of athletic injuries, it is important to keep in mind that there are significant side effects that should be anticipated. This serves to emphasize that NSAIDs, and all therapeutic medications, should be used judiciously and only where indicated.

DRUG TESTING

The increasing concern over substance abuse in athletics has led to various attempts to control such behavior through the use of drug testing. The first "athletes" to undergo drug testing were thoroughbred race horses and the first athlete to fail a drug test and endure public humiliation was Dancer's Image in the 1968 Kentucky Derby. Testing for human athletes was first begun on a nonpunitive basis at the 1964 Summer Olympics in Tokyo and formal testing began with the 1968 Olympic Games.[3] In 1986, the NCAA promulgated legislation that authorized drug testing at all NCAA-sanctioned championships and postseason bowl games after August 1986. A great deal of controversy has been generated over the ethical right to test an athlete's urine. Because discussion of this issue is beyond the scope of this chapter, this section concentrates on the methods of drug detection and the manner in which it is employed by sports organizations.

Two of the major considerations in drug testing are reliability and cost. The former concerns the accuracy of the results. A lack of specificity can lead to false positives and jeopardize an athlete's career. If a test is not sufficiently sensitive, there will be a number of false negatives and the deterrence potential will be lost. A 1985 study by the Centers for Disease Control (CDC) found no national standards for drug testing laboratories and concluded, "Laboratories are often unable to detect drugs at concentrations called for by their contracts."[93] The first step in an effective drug testing program is a reliable laboratory using the highest-quality equipment and technicians available.

Another issue involving drug testing is the cost of starting and maintaining a program. The cost of equipping the Montreal drug testing laboratory for the 1976 Olympics was estimated to be $3 million and the UCLA Olympic Analytic Laboratory required $1.8 million for the 1984 Games. The NCAA currently budgets $1 million annually for its drug testing program.[94] With a cost of approximately $125 for each urine test for anabolic steroids, strong consideration must be given before allocating resources for drug testing. If funding is insufficient to provide highly reliable testing, then the program cannot be effective.

There are several methods of urine drug testing that are currently available. Thin layer chromatogra-

phy (TLC) is the least expensive test, but it has poor specificity and cannot provide a positive substance identification. It must be coupled with another testing method in order to be effective. Radioimmunoassay (RIA) and the enzyme-multiplied immunoassay test (EMIT) are the most commonly employed screening tests. The former was used as a screening tool for amphetamines, morphine, and benzoylecgonine during the 1984 Olympic Games.[95] Although the manufacturers maintain that the test has a 97% to 99% accuracy rate, this is not always the case.[94] The seriousness of a drug test and the impact a positive test has on an athlete's career requires that a second, confirmatory test be performed. The gas chromatography–mass spectroscopy (GC/MS) test is the "gold standard" of testing and provides a "fingerprint" for each substance positively identified. This is the only drug test that can be used as legally admissible evidence in court. For these reasons, all state-of-the-art drug testing laboratories use GC/MS as the confirmatory test. Unfortunately, the high cost of the equipment and procedures make this test prohibitive for all but the most sophisticated laboratories. A 1986 survey of NCAA schools that were conducting drug testing found that several methods were employed (percentage of schools using each test in parenthesis): GC/MS (72%), RIA (56%), TLC (30%), and GC alone (25%).[96] Prime targets for any legal challenge to drug testing would be the reliability of the laboratory and the testing procedure.

The challenge of testing for anabolic steroids is an example of the cat and mouse games that are played by athletes and sports organizations. The increasing sophistication of testing for anabolic steroids caused athletes to turn to testosterone, which could not be detected. In order to combat this practice, the ratio of testosterone to epitestosterone is now performed with drug testing. The usual ratio of testosterone to its isomer epitestosterone is 1:2, but the use of exogenous testosterone elevates the serum level of testosterone out of proportion to epitestosterone. A ratio of greater than 6:1 is considered to be evidence of exogenous testosterone use. One caveat that has recently developed from a Swedish study is that ethanol ingestion may increase the testosterone–epitestosterone ratio.[97] Athletes have also begun using diuretics and probenecid as "masking" agents for anabolic steroids. This led the IOC, and other organizations, to ban the use of these substances.

There are several problems associated with drug testing, and a negative test result needs to be interpreted with caution. There are a number of ways that drug testing can be circumvented by athletes. The first involves the previously mentioned practice of masking agents to prevent detection. A simpler method involves the determination of drug half-life and elimination time from the urine. An athlete can then discontinue the drug at a safe interval before the test. The Olympics

TABLE 7-12. DRUG CLEARANCE TIMES

Drug	Elimination Time
Stimulants, i.e., amphetamines	1–7 days
Cocaine	
Occasional use	6–12 hours
Repeated use	3–5 days
Codeine and narcotics in cough medicine	24–48 hours
Tranquilizers	4–8 days
Marijuana	3–5 weeks
Anabolic steroids	
Fat soluble, injectable	6–8 months
Water soluble, oral	3–6 weeks
Over-the-counter cold preparations containing ephedrine, etc.	48–72 hours

and NCAA championships conduct drug testing in an announced fashion either before or after an event. Table 7–12 lists the detection and elimination times for several substances. Random, unannounced testing is the only reliable method to overcome this problem. In addition, athletes have invented several unique methods of providing a "clean" urine sample, including self-catheterization. This problem can be addressed through constant supervision of the entire collection and drug testing procedure.

It is difficult to judge the overall effectiveness of drug testing as a deterrent to drug use by athletes. Of 407 football players at Division I schools surveyed by the NCAA in 1987, 63% felt that drug testing was a deterrent to drug use.[98] Frequent studies point to the low rates of positive drug tests as proof of the effectiveness of drug testing. It is difficult, however, to reconcile the disparity between positive drug tests (0.72% at the 1984 Olympics and 2.5% by the NCAA) and the prevalence of drug use by athletes that has been demonstrated in numerous studies. It is clear that for a testing program to be effective it must be conducted in a random, unannounced fashion and must test for the correct substances.

There has been a great deal of controversy regarding the legal issues surrounding drug testing. Most of the legal challenges have centered on an athlete's right to privacy and laws against illegal search and seizure. There have been numerous court cases but no clear determination as to an organization's right to test athletes. The ambiguity of the courts has led some programs, such as University of California at Berkeley, to discontinue drug testing in order to avoid a suit by the American Civil Liberties Union. Due to the unresolved controversy, it is essential to involve legal counsel in the early stages of organizing a drug testing program. As a general rule, a program that tests only for "probable cause" is more defensible in court than one that tests in a random fashion.

Drug testing is conducted by several organizations at the local, national, and international level. At the Olympic level, drug testing is conducted by the IOC and USOC at all sanctioned events such as the Olympics, Olympic Trials, and Olympic Festivals. All of these tests are conducted on an announced basis. In order to combat the use of drugs at other times, The Athletic Congress (TAC) has recently formulated a plan to test top athletes throughout the year on a random basis beginning October 1, 1989. This reflects the growing realization of the ineffectiveness of announced testing at championships.

Collegiate athletes were introduced to drug testing in 1986 when the NCAA began testing at postseason football games and championship events at the Division I, II, and III levels. This led to an explosion of testing among NCAA member schools. A 1986 survey of 257 NCAA affiliated schools found that 28% had some type of drug testing program in place and 52% of the remaining schools were considering implementation.[96] According to that study, the drugs that schools were screening for most commonly were cocaine (99%), amphetamines (97%), cannabinoids (96%), and anabolic steroids (60%).[96]

The professional associations have also become involved with drug testing.[99] Major league baseball currently conducts random tests for cocaine, marijuana, heroin, and morphine only among those players with specified drug testing clauses in their contracts. In addition, managers, executives, owners, and umpires can be tested at random. The National Basketball Association has perhaps the most comprehensive and enlightened educational and drug testing program. Individual players can be tested with "reasonable cause" for cocaine and heroin without prior notice, but a player who voluntarily admits to a problem can undergo treatment without penalty. Due to the National Football League's collective bargaining agreement with the players, random testing cannot be conducted. Currently, drug testing is only done in preseason camps and scouting sessions in an announced fashion for "street drugs," anabolic steroids, and amphetamines. It is interesting to note that of all the money spent on drug testing, none of the tests are for alcohol, the most abused drug among athletes.

DRUG EDUCATION

The publicity surrounding drug testing has obscured the function of education in preventing drug abuse. Although drug testing plays an important role, it can be considered as a "final exam." An educational program must be initiated at a young age in order to be effective; the collegiate level is probably too late. Anderson and McKeag demonstrated that most patterns of drug use are established in junior high and high school

(Table 7–4).[53] Educational intervention can be most successful in deterring recreational drug use because these substances usually have a negative impact on performance. An athlete's performance is integral to self-esteem and an educational program can focus on the effects of recreational drugs on performance. A recent survey of college football players found that 34% felt that special seminars and courses would discourage drug use.[98] Education views drug use as a symptom and seeks not only to educate about the hazards of drug use, but also to deal with underlying issues of self-esteem, peer pressure, and feelings of inadequacy. These can all contribute to a variety of adjustment problems, of which drug abuse is only one. Although education may be useful in alerting athletes to the risks involved with ergogenic aids, the positive reinforcement of improved performance makes drug testing a necessary component of deterrence.

CONCLUSIONS

The problem of drugs and athletes is one that will increasingly challenge the health care system and require innovations in scientific research, drug testing, and education. Basic research is required to accurately assess drugs for their positive and negative effects on performance and consequences. For many substances, such as anabolic steroids, the long-term effects are unknown, and this leads to confusion on the part of athletes and physicians. In addition, research is needed to carefully evaluate new drugs and practices as they appear so that athletes can be advised with facts, rather than stories told at the local gym.

In order for drug testing to become an effective deterrent, it must keep up with the popular trends of abuse. Athletes are currently able to exploit the limitations of testing by using hGH and engaging in blood doping. Drug testing must be able to accurately detect the drugs of abuse and be given at random intervals throughout the year, while maintaining the highest standards of reliability.

New directions are needed in education as well. In the past, education has focused on recognizing the symptoms of drug abuse, which is often too late. It is necessary to evaluate the atmosphere in which drug abuse occurs and individual vulnerabilities. In this way, changes can be made to help decrease the outside pressures to abuse drugs and provide the athlete with the coping skills to resist drug use. Some of the more innovative programs train athletes in decision-making skills and teach individuals how to approach potentially difficult situations.

The patterns of drug abuse are changing rapidly, and health care professionals need to follow the current trends. New ergogenic aids appear in local gyms and "muscle" magazines almost daily and it is difficult for the scientific community to keep pace. The drugs discussed in this chapter are some of the commonly abused substances, but athletes engage in many other practices. This chapter is meant to serve as a guide and provide a method of evaluating new drugs as they become popular. If one understands the demands of the sport and the mechanism of action of each drug, the patterns of abuse and side effects can be predicted. Medical professionals need to be aware of "sport-specific" drugs of abuse and be able to recognize, counsel, and treat athletes with drug problems.

REFERENCES

1. Goodwin M. In sport, cocaine's here to stay. *New York Times.* May 1, 1987.
2. Anderson D. New drug epidemic: Steroids. *New York Times.* July 10, 1988.
3. Puffer JC. The use of drugs in swimming. *Clin Sports Med* 1986; 5:77–88.
4. Kunkel DB. Cocaine then and now. Part 1. *Emerg Med.* June 15, 1986; 125–138.
5. Bell JA, Doege TC. Athlete's use and abuse of drugs. *Phys Sports Med.* 1987; 15(3):99–108.
6. Duda M. NCAA: Only 4% of athletes used steroids. *Phys Sports Med.* 1985; 13(8):30.
7. Memorandum of Agreement between the United States Olympic Committee and the National Governing Boards. 1985. 1.
8. Loughton SV, Ruhline RO. Human strength and endurance responses to anabolic steroids and training. *J Sports Med Phy Fit.* 1977; 17:285–296.
9. Cowart V. Steroids in sports: After four decades, time to return these genies to the bottle? *JAMA.* 1987; 257(4):421–427.
10. Wilson JD. Androgen abuse by athletes. *Endocrine Rev* 1988; 9(2):181–199.
11. Buckley WE, et al. Estimated prevalence of anabolic steroid use among male high school seniors. *JAMA.* 1988; 260:3441–3445.
12. Marshall E. The drug of champions. *Science.* 1988; 242:183–184.
13. Windsor RE, Dumitru D. Anabolic steroid use by athletes. *Postgrad Med.* 1988; 84(4):37–49.
14. Hervey GR. Are athletes wrong about anabolic steroids? *Br J Sports Med.* 1975; 9:74–77.
15. Johnson LD, et al. Effects of anabolic steroid treatment on endurance. *Med Sci Sports Exerc.* 1975; 7:287–289.
16. Loughton SV, Ruhline RO. Human strength and endurance responses to anabolic steroids and training. *J Sports Med Phys Fit* 1977; 17:285–296.
17. Stromme SB, Meen HD, Aakvaag A. Effects of an androgenic–anabolic steroid on strength development and plasma testosterone levels in normal males. *Med Sci Sports Exerc.* 1974; 6:203–208.
18. Ariel G. The effect of anabolic steroid upon skeletal muscle contractile force. *J Sports Med Phys Fit.* 1973; 13:187–190.

19. Hervey GR, et al. Effects of methandienone on the performance and body composition of men undergoing athletic training. *Clin Sci*. 1981; 60:457–461.

20. Stamford BA, Moffatt R. Anabolic steroid effectiveness as an ergogenic aid to experienced weight trainers. *J Sports Med Phys Fit*. 1974; 14:191–197.

21. American College of Sports Medicine. Stand on the use of anabolic–androgenic steroids in sports. *American College of Sports Medicine*. 1984.

22. McNutt RA, et al. Acute myocardial infarction in a 22-year-old world class weight lifter using anabolic steroids. *Am J Cardiol*. 1988; 62:164.

23. Farrell G, et al. Androgen-induced hepatoma. *Lancet*. 1975; ii:430–433.

24. Bagheri S, et al. Peliosis hepatis. *Ann Intern Med*. 1974; 81:610–618.

25. Tennant F, Black DL, Voy RO. Anabolic steroid dependence with opioid-type features. *N Engl J Med*. 1988; 319:578.

26. Brower KJ, et al. Anabolic–androgenic steroid dependence. *J Clinical Psychiatry*, 1989; 50:31–33.

27. Pope HG, Katz DL. Affective and psychotic symptoms associated with anabolic steroid use. *AM J Psychiatry*. 1988; 145:487–490.

28. Roberts JT, Essenhigh DM. Adenocarcinoma of prostate in a 40 year old body-builder. *Lancet*. 1986; 2:742.

29. Braunwald E, et al, eds. *Harrison's Principles of Internal Medicine*. 11th ed. New York, NY: McGraw-Hill; 1987.

30. Lamb D. Anabolic steroid in athletics. *Am J Sports Med*. 1984; 12:31–37.

31. Kramhoft M, Solgaard S. Spontaneous rupture of the extensor pollicis longus tendon after anabolic steroids. *J Hand Surg*. 1986; 11(1):87.

32. Back BR, et al. Triceps rupture: A case report and literature review. *Am J Sports Med*. 1987; 15:285–289.

33. Kiraly CL, et al. Effect of testosterone and anabolic steroids on the size of sebaceous glands in power athletes. *Am J Dermatopathol*. 1987; 96:515–519.

34. Macintyre JG. Growth hormone and athletes. *Sports Med* 1987; 4:129–142.

35. Ahren K, et al. Cellular mechanisms of the acute stimulatory effect of growth hormone. In: Pecile, Muller, eds. *Growth Hormone and Related Polypeptides. Proceedings of the 3rd International Symposium, Milan*. September 17–20, 1975. Amsterdam; Excerpta Medica; 1975.

36. Goldberg AL. Relationship between growth hormone and muscle work in determining muscle size. *J Physiol*. 1969; 216:655–666.

37. Kostyo JL, Reagan CR. The biology of growth hormone. *Pharmacol Therapeut*. 1976; 2:591–604.

38. Underwood LE. Report of the conference on uses and possible abuses of biosynthetic human growth hormone. *N Engl J Med*. 1984; 311:606–608.

39. VanVilet G, et al. Growth hormone treatment for short stature. *N Engl J Med*. 1983; 309:1016–1022.

40. Cowart V. Human growth hormone: The latest ergogenic aid? *Physician Sports Med*. 1988; 16(3):175–185.

41. Trevisan L, et al. A sequential study of anabolic steroid use and availability among high school football players. *Med Sci Sports Exerc*. 1989; 21(2)(suppl):525.

42. Adhoc Committee on Growth Hormone Usage, the Lawson Wildins Pediatric Endocrine Society, and the Committee on Drugs. Growth hormone in the treatment of children with short stature. *Pediatrics*. 1983; 72:891–894.

43. Koch TK, et al. Creutzfeldt–Jakob Disease in a young adult with idiopathic hypopituitarism: Possible relation to the administration of cadaveric human growth hormone. *N Engl J Med*. 1985; 313:713–733.

44. Mandell AJ. The Sunday Syndrome: A unique pattern of amphetamine use indigenous to american professional football. *Clin Toxicol*. 1979; 15:225–232.

45. Lombardo JA. Stimulants and athletic performance: Amphetamines and caffeine. *Phys Sports Med*. 1986; 14(11):128–139.

46. Gilman Ag, Goodman LS, Rall TW, Murad F, eds. *Goodman and Gilman's The Pharmacologic Basis of Therapeutics*. 7th ed. New York: Macmillan Publishing Co; 1985.

47. De Meersman R, et al. The effects of a sympathomimetic drug on maximal aerobic activity. *J Sports Med* 1986; 26:251–257.

48. Smith GM, Beecher HK. Amphetamine sulfate and athletic performance. *JAMA*. 1959; 170:542–557.

49. Chandler JV, Blair SN. The effects of amphetamines on selected physiological components related to athletic success. *Med Sci Sports Exerc*. 1980; 12:65–69.

50. Sidney KH, Lefoe NM. The effects of Tedral upon athletic performance: A double blind cross-over study. Quebec City International Congress of Physical Activity Sciences; 1976.

51. DeMeersman R, Getty D, Schaefer DC. Sympathomimetics and exercise enhancement: All in the mind? *Pharmacol Biochem Behav*. 1987; 28:361–365.

52. Laurin CA, Letorneau G: Medical report on the Montreal Olympic Games. *Am J Sports Med*. 1978; 6:54–61.

53. Anderson WA, McKeag DB. The substance use and abuse habits of college student athletes. National Collegiate Athletic Association. June 1985.

54. Ivy JL, et al. Role of caffeine and glucose ingestion on metabolism during exercise. *Med Sci Sports Exerc*. 1978; 10:66.

55. Welch JM, et al. Effect of caffeine on skeletal muscle function before and after fatigue. *J Appl Physiol*. 1983; 54:1303–1305.

56. Butts NK, Crowell D. Effects of caffeine ingestion on cardiorespiratory endurance in men and women. *Res Q Exerc Sport*. 1985; 56:301–305.

57. Casal DC, Leon AS. Failure of caffeine to affect substrate utilization during prolonged running. *Med Sci Sports Exerc*. 1985; 17:174–179.

58. Van Der Merwe PJ, et al. Caffeine in sport: Urinary excretion of caffeine in healthy volunteers after intake of common caffeine-containing beverages. *S Afr Med J*. 1988; 74:163–164.

59. Pace N, et al. The increase in hypoxia tolerance of normal men accompanying the polycythemia induced by transfusion of erythrocytes. *Am J Physiol*. 1947; 148:152–163.

60. Klein HG. Sounding Board: Blood transfusion and athletics. *N Engl J Med*. 1985; 312:854–856.

61. Buick FJ, et al. Effect of induced erythrocythemia on

aerobic work capacity. *J Appl Physiol.* 1980; 48:636–642.

62. McKeag D. Drug use and abuse in athletics: Clinical workshop. American College of Sports Medicine Annual Meeting, Baltimore, 1989.

63. Millhorn HT. The diagnosis of alcoholism. *Am Fam Physician.* 1988; 37:175–183.

64. Schatzkin A, et al. Alcohol consumption and breast cancer. *N Engl J Med.* 1987; 316:1169–1185.

65. American College of Sports Medicine. Position statement on the use of alcohol in sports. *Med Sci Sports Exerc.* 1982; 14:ix–x.

66. Graham T, Dalton J. Effect of alcohol on man's response to mild physical activity in a cold environment. *Aviat Space Environ Med.* 1980; 51:793–796.

67. Urbano–Marquez A, et al. The effects of alcoholism on skeletal and cardiac muscle. *N Engl J Med.* 1989; 320:409–415.

68. Nattiv A. Lifestyle and health risk behaviors of intercollegiate athletes. 1989, in press.

69. Roth D, et al. Acute rhabdomyolysis associated with cocaine intoxication. *N Engl J Med.* 1988; 319:673–677.

70. Cantwell JD, Rose FD. Cocaine and cardiovascular events. *Phys Sports Med.* 1986; 14(11):77–82.

71. Cregler L, Mark H. Special report: Medical complications of cocaine abuse. *N Engl J Med.* 1986; 315:1495–1500.

72. Kunkel DB. Cocaine then and now: Part II. *Emerg Med.* July 15, 1986; 168–173.

73. Lombardo J. Stimulants and athletic performance. *Phys Sports Med.* 1986; 14:85–90.

74. Green G. Drugs and the athlete. *Del Med J.* 1987; 59:565–576.

75. Giammarco RA. The athlete, cocaine, and lactic acidosis: A hypothesis. *Am J Med Sci.* 1987; 294:412–414.

76. McKeag D. Personal communication. February 1987.

77. Powell DR. Does marijuana smoke cause lung cancer? *Primary Care Cancer.* Oct 1987:15.

78. Biron S, Wells J. Marijuana and its effects on the athlete. *Athlet Train.* 1983; 18:295–303.

79. Renaud AM, Cormier Y. Acute effects of marihuana smoking on maximal exercise performance. *Med Sci Sports Exerc.* 1986; 18:685–689.

80. Jones R. Use of smokeless tobacco in the 1986 World Series. *N Engl J Med.* 1987; 316:952.

81. Glover ED, et al. Implications of smokeless tobacco use among athletes. *Physician Sports Med.* 1988; 14(12):95–105.

82. Bergert N: The dangers of smokeless tobacco. *Sports Med Dig.* 1989; 11(6):1–8.

83. Connolly GN, Orleans CT, Kogan M. Use of smokeless tobacco in major-league baseball. *N Engl J Med.* 1988; 318:1281–1284.

84. Eskow RN. Hazards of smokeless tobacco. *N Engl J Med.* 1987; 317:1229.

85. Edwards SW, Glover ED, Schroeder KL. The effects of smokeless tobacco on heart rate and neuromuscular reactivity in athletes and nonathletes. *Phys Sports Med* 1987; 15(7):141–146.

86. Drug Abuse Warning Network. Bethesda, Maryland. 1985 statistics.

87. Sedor JR, Davidson EW, Dunn MJ. Effects of nonsteroidal anti-inflammatory drugs in healthy subjects. *Am J Med.* 1986; 81(suppl 2B):58–83.

88. Amadio P, Cummings DM. Nonsteroidal anti-inflammatory agents: An update. *Am Fam Physician.* 1986; 34(4):147–154.

89. Dahners LE, Gilbert JA, Lester GE, et al. The effect of a nonsteroidal antiinflammatory drug on the healing of ligaments. *Am J Sports Med.* 1988; 16(6):641–646.

90. Butt JH, Barthel JS, Moore RA. Clinical spectrum of upper gastrointestinal effects of nonsteroidal anti-inflammatory drugs. *Am J Med.* 1988; 84(suppl 2A):5–14.

91. Hart D, Ward M, Lifschitz MD: Suprofen-related nephrotoxicity: A distinct clinical syndrome. *Ann Intern Med.* 1987; 106:235–238.

92. Day RO. Effects of exercise performance on drugs used in musculoskeletal disorders. *Med Sci Sports Exerc.* 1981; 13:272–275.

93. Hansen H, et al. Crisis in drug testing. *JAMA.* 1985; 253:2382–2387.

94. Puffer JC. Drugs and doping in athletics. In: Million MB, ed. *Office Management of Athletic Injuries.* Philadelphia, Pa: Hanley and Belfus, Inc; 1987: 37–48.

95. Catlin DH, Kammerer RC, Hatton CK, et al. Analytic chemistry at the games of the XXIIIrd olympiad in Los Angeles, 1984. *Clin Chem.* 1987; 33:319–327.

96. Summary Report of Drug Screening Questionnaire; December 1986.

97. Falk O, et al. Effect of ethanol on the ratio between testosterone and epitestosterone in urine. *Clin Chem.* 1988; 34:1482–1484.

98. Abdenour TE, Miner MJ, Weir N. Attitudes of intercollegiate football players toward drug testing. *Athlet Train.* 1987; 22:199–201.

99. Wagner JC. Substance-abuse policies and guidelines in amateur and professional athletics. *Am J Hosp Pharm* 1987; 44:305–310.

8

Nutritional Considerations

Millicent Owens

INTRODUCTION

Eat this food, take this vitamin pill, drink this beverage, and your performance will improve! Promises about the magical properties of nutrition are common in athletics. To sort through the claims and decide which are true and which are false requires at least a basic understanding of nutrition and frequently a very careful examination of the nutritional claims. The goal of this chapter is to provide an overview of nutrition, especially as it relates to athletic performance.

OVERVIEW OF THE DIGESTIVE PROCESS

The processing of food by the digestive system involves five activities—ingestion, movement, digestion (mechanical and chemical), absorption, and defecation. Ingestion occurs when food is placed in the mouth. Some mechanical digestion occurs as the food is chewed. After leaving the mouth, food moves down the esophagus to the stomach, where both mechanical and chemical digestion occurs. Absorption of alcohol, water, and some electrolytes can occur in the stomach, but no other food products are absorbed there. With the aid of several enzymes and other secretions most food is digested to a thin liquid substance called chyme. Chyme exits the stomach by squirting through the pyloric sphincter into the small intestine. The small intestine can be divided into three parts—the duodenum, the jejunum, and the ileum. Chemical digestion continues but the major activity occurring in the small intestine is absorption. Food products not absorbed in the small intestine pass into the large intestine. A small amount (though for some nutrients a significant amount) of absorption occurs in the large intestine. The liquid chyme is formed into solid or semisolid matter (feces), a high percentage of which is bacteria, in preparation for elimination from the body.

PROTEINS

The majority of protein digestion occurs in the stomach and upper portion of the small intestine. A variety of enzymes are necessary to break proteins into their component amino acids. Amino acids are then absorbed by carrier systems through the small intestine wall into the portal blood system. Amino acids circulate in the blood until they are absorbed by an organ or cell that needs them. When the appropriate number and type of amino acids to make a specific protein are present, the cell reassembles them into a protein. This reassembly process is called anabolism.

Proteins are widely distributed throughout the body and serve in a wide variety of functions. These functions can be placed in three general categories—(1) maintenance and growth, (2) regulation of body processes, and (3) energy. Proteins for maintenance and growth include the chief solid matter of endocrine glands, organs, and muscles. Proteins are also major constituents of the matrix of bones, skin, nails, hair, and blood cells. In the normal healthy human, protein is found in all body fluids except bile and urine. Proteins involved in regulatory processes of the body have highly specialized functions. Examples of regulatory proteins include nucleoproteins (RNA and DNA), contractile proteins (myosin and actin), hormonal proteins, immune system proteins, and transport proteins. Proteins are also a potential energy source for the body. Each gram of protein yields approximately 4 kcal of energy. In a healthy individual protein is only used as the primary energy source when carbohydrate and fat are unable to provide sufficient calories. Under normal exercise conditions, however, protein contributes 5% to 18% of the energy used.[1,2]

When protein ingestion increases above body requirements, digestion and absorption still occur; however, the excess amino acids are deaminized and used for energy or stored as fat. As a result, the amount of

urinary nitrogen increases, which may stress the kidneys. Excessive amounts of protein may also lead to dehydration. When protein intake is inadequate, amino acids are lost from body tissues faster than they can be replaced.

Protein can be found in foods of plant or animal origin. Protein from animal sources, such as eggs, meat, fish, poultry, and dairy products, is referred to as complete protein. In general, proteins from plant sources are referred to as incomplete proteins, the exception being quinoa, a grain that appears to be a complete protein. A complete protein contains enough of the essential amino acids to maintain the normal body processes in which protein is involved.

Essential amino acids are those that the human body cannot synthesize at a sufficiently rapid rate to meet body needs. The essential amino acids are threonine, valine, leucine, isoleucine, methionine, lysine, phenylalanine, tryptophan, and histidine.

Nonessential amino acids are those that the body can produce from excess essential amino acids or from the chemical combination of a nitrogen source and a carbon skeleton, both of which are available in the body. Diet must supply the essential amino acids and sufficient nitrogen for synthesis of the nonessential amino acids.

A person following a vegetarian diet, even a strict vegetarian (or vegan), can obtain adequate protein from their diet. Plant foods can provide more than enough of all the essential and nonessential amino acids. It is necessary to conscientiously eat a variety of plant foods to meet protein needs. Until recently it was generally believed that it was necessary to follow a strategy of mutual supplementation in order for a strict vegetarian to meet his or her protein needs. Mutual supplementation is the practice of combining plant proteins so that one food that is low in an essential amino acid is complemented with another food high in this essential amino acid. For example, beans, which are deficient in tryptophan and methionine, would be consumed with rice, which has a high tryptophan and methionine content. It now appears possible to consume adequate amounts of essential amino acids without strict adherence to mutual supplementation principles.[3] Other nutrients, such as vitamin B_{12}, iron, calcium, and zinc, may be difficult for vegetarians to obtain in sufficient quantities from their diet. Infants, children, and pregnant women need to be particularly conscious of the protein and nutrient content of the foods they consume if they are following a vegetarian diet.

For a healthy adult, the recommended dietary allowance (RDA) for protein is 0.8 g/kg of body weight (Table 8–1).[4] The allowance is greater in infants, children, and pregnant women to allow for growth and development. Protein requirements for athletes are probably greater. Brotherhood has estimated the protein requirement for endurance athletes to be 1.0 to 1.2 g/kg body weight and the requirement for the power athlete to be 1.3 to 1.6 g/kg body weight.[5] Lemon et al suggest 1.8 g/kg body weight for exercising adults and 2.0 g/kg body weight for exercising adults who may "belong to any group with elevated protein needs."[6] At least two other studies[7,8] have suggested protein levels of 2.0 g/kg body weight or higher for power athletes; however, inadequate research controls or methods or both cause these studies to be questionable.[9] A carefully controlled metabolic study including power athletes suggests a protein intake of 1.2 g/kg of body weight may be adequate.[9] Protein requirements can be easily met through diet without protein supplements or special high-protein foods.

CARBOHYDRATES

Carbohydrates are monosaccharides, disaccharides, or polysaccharides. Examples of monosaccharides with dietary importance are glucose (also known as dextrose), galactose, and fructose. Disaccharides, or double sugars, include sucrose (table sugar), lactose (milk sugar), and maltose (the sugar resulting from the malting and fermentation of grain products). Polysaccharides include starch, dextrin, glycogen, and a variety of indigestible polysaccharides generally called fiber.

Carbohydrate digestion occurs primarily in the small intestine where disaccharides and polysaccharides (except fiber) are broken into their component monosaccharides by specific enzymes. For example:

$$\text{starch} \xrightarrow{\quad\text{amylase}\quad} \text{glucose}$$

$$\text{sucrose} \xrightarrow{\quad\text{sucrase}\quad} \text{glucose} + \text{fructose}$$

$$\text{maltose} \xrightarrow{\quad\text{maltase}\quad} \text{glucose} + \text{glucose}$$

$$\text{lactose} \xrightarrow{\quad\text{lactase}\quad} \text{glucose} + \text{galactose}$$

Generally, only monosaccharides are absorbed. Absorption occurs in the small intestine, mostly in the jejunum. The process by which they are absorbed through the intestinal wall into the portal blood system is complex. It involves a form of active transport utilizing a selective carrier system. The absorption of fructose is slightly different than that of other monosaccharides. Once absorbed into the portal vein, monosaccharides go to the liver. In the liver, all monosaccharides are converted to glycogen (glycogenesis). The liver reconverts this glycogen to glucose (glycogenolysis) according to body needs. Current research indi-

TABLE 8-1. FOOD AND NUTRITION BOARD, NATIONAL ACADEMY OF SCIENCES-NATIONAL RESEARCH COUNCIL RECOMMENDED DAILY DIETARY ALLOWANCES[a]—REVISED, 1980.

	Age (yr)	Weight kg	Weight lb	Height cm	Height in.	Protein (g)	Vitamin A (μg RE)[b]	Vitamin D (μg)[c]	Vitamin E (mg α-TE)[d]	Vitamin C (mg)	Thiamin (mg)	Riboflavin (mg)	Niacin (mg NE)[e]	Vitamin B6 (mg)	Folacin (μg)[f]	Vitamin B12 (μg)	Calcium (mg)	Phosphorus (mg)	Magnesium (mg)	Iron (mg)	Zinc (mg)	Iodine (μg)
Infants	0.0-0.5	6	13	60	24	kg × 2.2	420	10	3	35	0.3	0.4	6	0.3	30	0.5[g]	360	240	50	10	3	40
	0.5-1.0	9	20	71	28	kg × 2.0	400	10	4	35	0.5	0.6	8	0.6	45	1.5	540	360	70	15	5	50
Children	1-3	13	29	90	35	23	400	10	5	45	0.7	0.8	9	0.9	100	2.0	800	800	150	15	10	70
	4-6	20	44	112	44	30	500	10	6	45	0.9	1.0	11	1.3	200	2.5	800	800	200	10	10	90
	7-10	28	62	132	52	34	700	10	7	45	1.2	1.4	16	1.6	300	3.0	800	800	250	10	10	120
Males	11-14	45	99	157	62	45	1000	10	8	50	1.4	1.6	18	1.8	400	3.0	1200	1200	350	18	15	150
	15-18	66	145	176	69	56	1000	10	10	60	1.4	1.7	18	2.0	400	3.0	1200	1200	400	18	15	150
	19-22	70	154	177	70	56	1000	7.5	10	60	1.5	1.7	19	2.2	400	3.0	800	800	350	10	15	150
	23-50	70	154	178	70	56	1000	5	10	60	1.4	1.6	18	2.2	400	3.0	800	800	350	10	15	150
	51+	70	154	178	70	56	1000	5	10	60	1.2	1.4	16	2.2	400	3.0	800	800	350	10	15	150
Females	11-14	46	101	157	62	46	800	10	8	50	1.1	1.3	15	1.8	400	3.0	1200	1200	300	18	15	150
	15-18	55	120	163	64	46	800	10	8	60	1.1	1.3	14	2.0	400	3.0	1200	1200	300	18	15	150
	19-22	55	120	163	64	44	800	7.5	8	60	1.1	1.3	14	2.0	400	3.0	800	800	300	18	15	150
	23-50	55	120	163	64	44	800	5	8	60	1.0	1.2	13	2.0	400	3.0	800	800	300	18	15	150
	51+	55	120	163	64	44	800	5	8	60	1.0	1.2	13	2.0	400	3.0	800	800	300	10	15	150
Pregnant						+30	+200	+5	+2	+20	+0.4	+0.3	+2	+0.6	+400	+1.0	+400	+400	+150	h	+5	+25
Lactating						+20	+400	+5	+3	+40	+0.5	+0.5	+5	+0.5	+100	+1.0	+400	+400	+150	h	+10	+50

[a]The allowances are intended to provide for individual variations among most normal persons as they live in the United States under usual environmental stresses. Diets should be based on a variety of common foods in order to provide other nutrients for which human requirements have been less well defined. See text for detailed discussion of allowances and of nutrients not tabulated.

[b]Retinol equivalents. 1 retinol equivalent = 1 μg retinol or 6 μg β carotene.

[c]As cholecalciferol. 10 μg cholecalciferol = 400 IU of vitamin D.

[d]α-tocopherol equivalents. 1 mg δ-α tocopherol = α-TE.

[e]1 NE (niacin equivalent) is equal to 1 mg of niacin or 60 mg of dietary tryptophan.

[f]The folacin allowances refer to dietary sources as determined by Lactobacillus casei assay after treatment with enzymes (conjugases) to make polyglutamyl forms of the vitamin available to the test organism.

[g]The recommended dietary allowance for vitamin B₁₂ in infants is based on average concentration of the vitamin in human milk. The allowances after weaning are based on energy intake (as recommended by the American Academy of Pediatrics) and consideration of other factors, such as intestinal absorption.

[h]The increased requirement during pregnancy cannot be met by the iron content of habitual American diets nor by the existing iron stores of many women; therefore the use of 30–60 mg of supplemental iron is recommended. Iron needs during lactation are not substantially different from those of nonpregnant women, but continued supplementation of the mother for 2 to 3 months after parturition is advisable in order to replenish stores depleted by pregnancy.

From Committee on Dietary Allowances, Food and Nutrition Board, National Research Council. Recommended Dietary Allowances. 9th ed. Washington, D.C.: National Academy of Sciences; 1980, with permission.

cates that it may not be necessary for glucose to go to the liver and through glycogenesis before being utilized. This theory, referred to as "the glucose paradox," is still under investigation.[10] The liver is also the site of lipogenesis (by which excess glucose is converted to fat), and stored glycerol resulting from lipid breakdown is converted to glucose when the body requires it.[11] Fatty acids cannot be converted to glucose in humans.[11]

Lactic acid is a normal by-product of carbohydrate metabolism. In order to understand how lactic acid is produced, some of the basic biochemical pathways describing the cellular metabolism of glucose must be examined. The pathway for glycolysis (Embden–Meyerhof pathway) and the citric acid cycle

(Krebs cycle) are shown in Fig 8–1. One end product of glycolysis, which is an anaerobic process, is pyruvic acid.

Under aerobic conditions most pyruvic acid enters the citric acid cycle. Glycolysis has a net yield of 2 adenosine triphosphate (ATP) per molecule of glucose whereas the citric acid cycle has a net yield of 36 to 38 ATP. The largest amount of ATP, and thus energy, results when aerobic conditions are present and the citric acid cycle is functioning. Under normal aerobic conditions, a small amount of pyruvic acid is converted to lactic acid. This lactic acid is reconverted to glucose via the Cori cycle (Fig 8–2). When anaerobic conditions exist, however, pyruvic acid is unable to enter the aero-

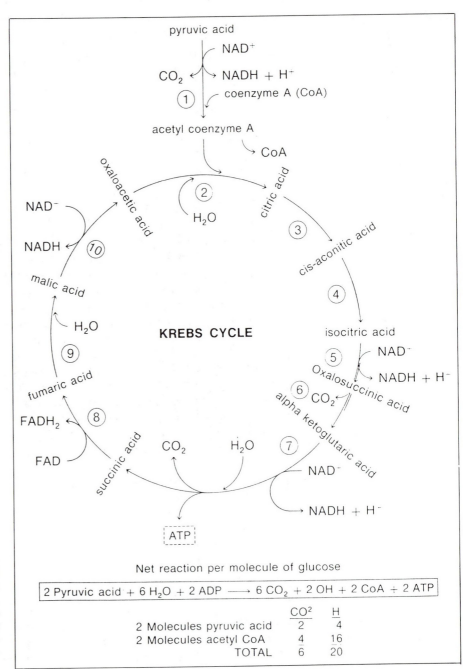

Figure 8–1. Glycolysis (Embden–Meyerhof pathway) and the citric acid cycle (Krebs cycle). *(From Robinson CH, Lawler MR. Normal and Therapeutic Nutrition. 16th ed. New York, NY: Macmillan Publishing Co; 1982; 166, with permission.)*

Net reaction per molecule of glucose

$$2 \text{ Pyruvic acid} + 6\ H_2O + 2\ ADP \longrightarrow 6\ CO_2 + 2\ OH + 2\ CoA + 2\ ATP$$

	CO^2	H
2 Molecules pyruvic acid	2	4
2 Molecules acetyl CoA	4	16
TOTAL	6	20

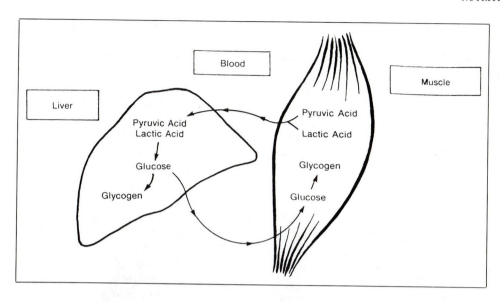

Figure 8-2. Cori cycle. *(From McArdle WD, Katch FI, Katch VL. Exercise Physiology: Energy, Nutrition and Human Performance. 2nd ed. Philadelphia, Pa: Lea & Febiger; 1986; 62, with permission.)*

bic citric acid cycle and more lactic acid is produced than the Cori cycle can process. Therefore, lactic acid builds up in the muscle. When aerobic conditions return, the lactic acid is reconverted to pyruvic acid and enters the citric acid cycle.

The primary function of carbohydrate is to provide energy. Each gram of carbohydrate yields approximately 4 kcal of energy. Glycogen can be stored in the liver or in muscle and is the principal storage form of carbohydrate. Glycogen is converted to glucose on the basis of need. Glucose is essential to every cell in the body, especially to the cells of the brain and nervous system. Blood glucose (sometimes called blood sugar) is normally maintained within a standard range. Blood glucose levels below (hypoglycemia) or above (hyperglycemia) this range result in conditions that are less than optimum. Liver glycogen is used to help maintain the blood sugar level, but muscle glycogen cannot directly help to maintain the blood sugar level. It does so indirectly when lactic acid resulting from anaerobic glycolysis of muscle glycogen is processed through the Cori cycle. Muscle glycogen provides energy only for cells of the muscle in which it is stored. When inadequate carbohydrate is ingested, the liver converts stored fat to glucose in order to maintain normal blood glucose levels.

Foods that provide carbohydrate can be divided into three general categories—simple carbohydrates, complex carbohydrates, and fiber. There are no strict biochemical definitions of these categories. In general, foods referred to as simple carbohydrates have a high percentage of monosaccharides or disaccharides, are easily digested and quickly absorbed. Foods such as sugar, honey, frosting, fruit juices, and some candy are frequently referred to as sources of simple carbohydrates.

Complex carbohydrates have a high percentage of polysaccharides, and take longer to digest and absorb.

Foods such as whole-grain breads, pasta, waffles, and pancakes are examples of foods containing complex carbohydrate. There are many carbohydrate foods that are difficult to classify as either complex or simple. For example, fresh fruits contain predominantly monosaccharides and disaccharides; however, because of their relatively high fiber content they are not easily digested. The presence of fat or fiber increases the time necessary to digest carbohydrates.

Fiber refers to the indigestible polysaccharides including cellulose, hemicellulose, pectin, gums, and mucilages. Current analytical methods measure the total fiber content of a food. Older methods of analysis resulted in a value for crude fiber content. Crude fiber is the residue that remains after a food sample has been treated with acid followed by alkali under standard conditions. Because many dietary fibers are destroyed by this method, crude fiber measurements do not accurately reflect total fiber content. Fiber can be categorized as water soluble or water insoluble. Water-insoluble fibers include cellulose, many hemicelluloses, and lignin. Examples of foods containing insoluble fiber include wheat bran, whole grains, and whole-wheat bread. Water-insoluble fibers produce bulkier bowel movements (assuming adequate water is consumed), help food pass more rapidly through the intestinal tract, and aid in the relief of constipation. Water-soluble fibers include gums, mucilages, and pectin. They are found mainly in oats, including oat bran, fresh fruits, and dried peas and beans. These fibers appear to aid in the reduction of blood cholesterol and aid diabetics in their control of blood sugar.

The dietary goals for the United States suggest that approximately 58% of the calories in a diet should be derived from carbohydrate.[12] Athletes would probably benefit from a higher percentage of calories being derived from carbohydrate.[13] One study suggests athletes should obtain 70% of calories from carbohydrate.[14]

In an effort to increase muscle glycogen stores, many athletes "carbohydrate load" (also known as glycogen loading or glycogen supercompensation). Muscle glycogen depletion occurs after about $1\frac{1}{2}$ to 2 hours of exercise at 75% of aerobic capacity if the average American diet is consumed (46% carbohydrate). The length of time until glycogen depletion occurs can be increased to 3 hours or more, however, at the same intensity of exercise when a carbohydrate loading regimen (Fig 8–3) is followed.[15] Normal glycogen stores can sustain exercise for 80 to 90 minutes. Therefore, carbohydrate loading is useful only for events lasting longer than 80 to 90 minutes.[13,15]

Carbohydrate loading does not increase the athlete's pace at the beginning of a race; however, it allows an athlete to maintain intensity longer.[13,15] The carbohydrate loading regimen is a weeklong process with the seventh day being the day of the event. Older methods of carbohydrate loading required a low carbohydrate diet and intense exercise on the first 3 days, followed by 3 days of a high carbohydrate diet and no exercise.[16] The low-carbohydrate phase of the regimen was very difficult to endure; hypoglycemia, nausea, and irritability were common side effects. The current method of carbohydrate loading is shown in Figure 8–3. It is as effective as older methods in storing muscle glycogen.

Glycogen loading is muscle specific. In other words, muscle that is exercised will increase glycogen stores to a greater extent than muscle that is not exercised.[17] In order to be effective, the same muscles used during the event need to be used during the exercise portion of carbohydrate loading. For elite athletes who normally eat a high-carbohydrate diet, carbohydrate loading may not be effective as they already have high muscle glycogen stores. There are drawbacks associated with carbohydrate loading. Weight gain caused from water retention results in an uncomfortable bloated feeling in some athletes. Water is stored with glycogen in the liver and the muscle. The motility in the intestinal tract is sometimes affected, causing a change in bowel habits. If the need to defecate occurs during an inconvenient time, it can be quite disconcerting to the athlete.

It has been assumed that the ingestion of simple carbohydrate within 1 hour of exercise impairs performance due to increased insulin levels and resulting lowered blood glucose levels. This assumption is not supported by current research, which indicates that preexercise carbohydrate feedings may actually provide ergogenic benefits.[17–20]

At times an athlete is unable (or unwilling) to increase dietary carbohydrate intake enough to consume a large percentage of calories from carbohydrate. In these instances, a liquid carbohydrate supplement may be useful.

LIPIDS

Lipids are fats, oils, and fatlike substances that have a greasy feel and are insoluble in water. They include fatty acids, glycerol, monoglycerides, diglycerides, triglycerides, cholesterol, and phospholipids. Most lipid digestion occurs in the small intestine, although a small amount occurs in the stomach. Once the dietary fat has been digested to monoglycerides, diglycerides, fatty acids, and glycerol it combines with bile to form micelles. The micelles are then absorbed through the intestinal wall and enter the lymph circulation.

Because lipids are insoluble in water they cannot circulate through the blood in their free state. To allow for the circulation of lipids in the blood, proteins combine with lipid and form lipoproteins. There are three lipoproteins—high-density lipoproteins (HDLs), low-density lipoproteins (LDLs), and very low-density lipoproteins (VLDLs). LDLs and VLDLs transport lipids, including cholesterol, from the liver to the cells. HDLs carry lipids from the cells back to the liver.

The chemical structure describes the differences between types of lipids. The main constituents of lipids are fatty acids. Fatty acids, which vary in length and degree of saturation, are attached to a glycerol backbone. Some examples are shown in Fig 8–4. Depending on the number of fatty acids attached to the glycerol, a monoglyceride, diglyceride, or triglyceride is formed. The degree of saturation of the fatty acids in a food can be determined by examining the food. Usually, foods containing a high percentage of saturated fatty acids retain their shape at room temperature (e.g., margarine), whereas foods containing a high percentage of

Figure 8–3. Carbohydrate loading regimen. *(From Coleman E. Eating for Endurance. Palo Alto, Calif: Bull Publishing Co; 1988; 40–49, with permission.)*

	Day 1	Day 2	Day 3	Day 4	Day 5	Day 6	Day 7
TRAINING	90 Min. 70–75% VO$_2$max	40 Min. 70–75% VO$_2$max	40 Min. 70–75% VO$_2$max	20 Min. 70–75% VO$_2$max	20 Min. 70–75% VO$_2$max	Rest	EVENT
EATING	50% Carbohydrate	50% Carbohydrate	50% Carbohydrate	70% Carbohydrate	70% Carbohydrate	70% Carbohydrate	EVENT

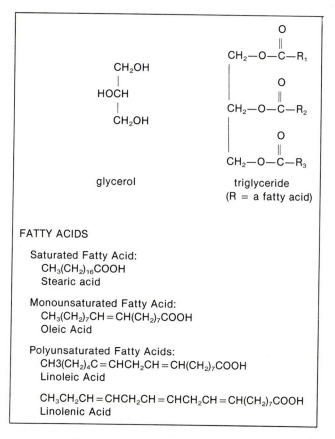

FATTY ACIDS

Saturated Fatty Acid:
$CH_3(CH_2)_{16}COOH$
Stearic acid

Monounsaturated Fatty Acid:
$CH_3(CH_2)_7CH=CH(CH_2)_7COOH$
Oleic Acid

Polyunsaturated Fatty Acids:
$CH3(CH_2)_4C=CHCH_2CH=CH(CH_2)_7COOH$
Linoleic Acid

$CH_3CH_2CH=CHCH_2CH=CHCH_2CH=CH(CH_2)_7COOH$
Linolenic Acid

Figure 8-4. Examples of fatty acids.

polyunsaturated fatty acids (PUFAs) are liquid at room temperature (e.g., oil). Two notable exceptions to this general rule are coconut oil and palm oil. Although liquid at room temperature, they are considered to be saturated fats.

Cholesterol is one of several lipids called sterols. It can be manufactured by the liver from protein, lipid, or carbohydrate and has essential functions. Cholesterol is a precursor for bile salts and steroid hormones. It is also a key regulator of cell membrane fluidity. The body conserves cholesterol by recycling it from the liver to the gallbladder to the small intestine and back to the gallbladder again. Only small amounts of cholesterol are excreted from the body in the feces. Cholesterol in the diet is found only in foods of animal origin. Examples include meat, poultry, butter, eggs, and dairy products.

The primary function of lipid is to provide energy. The high energy density and low solubility of fats make them an ideal form in which to store potential energy. Each gram of fat provides approximately 9 kcal of energy. Any excess fat is stored as adipose tissue. Adipose tissue, especially the subcutaneous layer, provides insulation and protection against cold weather by preventing excess loss of body heat. Adipose tissue also provides physical protection for several vital organs, including the kidneys.

Lipids function as fat-soluble vitamin carriers and provide essential fatty acids. Essential fatty acids include linoleic acid, arachidonic acid, and linolenic acid. Fats reduce gastric motility and remain in the stomach longer than carbohydrate or protein. This may delay feelings of hunger in some people.

Increased risk for cardiovascular disease is associated with some lipids. A high intake of saturated fats is related to increased risk for cardiovascular disease. Conversely, a high intake of PUFAs and monounsaturated fatty acids is felt to be beneficial in relationship to cardiovascular disease.[21] A relationship between a high intake of PUFAs and an increased risk for some types of cancer may be possible. If this relationship exists, however, it is complex and further research is necessary to explain it.[22-24] Although an elevated serum cholesterol is an unfavorable factor in cardiovascular disease, the HDL–LDL ratio is at least as important. The higher the HDL and the lower the LDL the better. It is felt that the intake of saturated fat increases the LDL levels, as well as serum cholesterol levels. Exercise assists in raising HDL levels.[25] In some people, a high dietary cholesterol intake appears to increase serum cholesterol levels. In others, dietary cholesterol intake appears to have a minimal effect on serum cholesterol. Diet is only one risk factor for cardiovascular disease. Other factors include heredity, obesity, smoking, stress, blood pressure, and exercise. Elevated serum cholesterol frequently results when anabolic–androgenic steroids are being taken. This hypercholesterolemia appears to be largely due to an increase in LDL levels.[26,27]

ENERGY BALANCE

Determining the appropriate body weight for an athlete can be difficult. Optimally, one first needs to know an athlete's body composition, especially percentage of body fat, and the desirable body composition for the event in which the athlete participates. If body composition were ignored and only body weight was used, it would be easy for a football player to appear overweight or a ballet dancer to appear underweight. To accurately determine if either of these athletes needed to lose or gain weight, body fat percentages and some general background would need to be obtained. A 6-ft, 230-lb football player with 8% body fat would not have excess fat on his body and would not be considered an overly fat athlete. If this same football player had 30% body fat, however, he would be considered overly fat and a dietary modification in conjunction with exercise would be appropriate.

Body fat can be most accurately estimated using either water displacement or underwater weighing. To achieve accurate results both of these techniques should be performed with well-maintained and calibrated

equipment under the supervision of trained personnel. Another method of estimating body fat uses skinfold calipers to obtain skinfold measurements. These measurements are then used to obtain body fat percentage. This method is less expensive since it can be used when water equipment is not available. Although accuracy is improved when skinfold measurements are taken by experienced personnel and by using multiple skinfolds, this method is less accurate than the water techniques. Recently, equipment based on an electrical impedance technique has been introduced. Although this method still needs further examination under scientific conditions before accuracy can be determined, it does appear promising.

Although it is best to determine body fat percentage before recommending that an athlete lose or gain weight, standard weight/height tables or a "rule of thumb" are still used by many to determine the need for body weight adjustment. The American Dietetic Association's rule of thumb is:[28]

- Men: for the first 5 ft allow 106 lb; for every inch over 5 ft add 6 lb
- Women: for the first 5 ft allow 100 lb; for every inch over 5 ft add 5 lb

Although not the very best methods, these provide a measure of general body weight with acceptable accuracy, especially for the nonathletic population. Also, in some situations they provide the only method of assessing body weight when equipment or trained personnel are not available. Once the need for weight loss or weight gain has been established, an appropriate program, usually combining dietary modification and exercise, is designed. Often the first step in dietary modification is estimating caloric needs. A number of different formulas exist to estimate caloric needs. Probably the most popular is the Harris–Benedict equation for basal energy expenditure:

- Men:

$66 + (6.2 \times$ weight [lb]$) + (12.7 \times$ height [in]$) - (6.8 \times$ age [yr]$) =$ basal energy expenditure (kcal)

- Women:

$655 + (4.4 \times$ weight [lb]$) + (4.3 \times$ height [in]$) - (4.7 \times$ age [yr]$) =$ basal energy expenditure (kcal)

To estimate total caloric needs, basal energy expenditure is multiplied by an activity factor ranging from 1.3 to 1.35 for sedentary individuals to 1.7 to 2.0 for strenuous activity. The following guidelines offer another method for estimating total calorie needs:

- 13 kcal/lb for sedentary activity
- 15 kcal/lb for moderate activity
- 20 kcal/lb for strenuous activity

Several types of dietary modification exist to achieve the desired caloric level and the resulting weight loss or gain. The effectiveness of a method depends on a variety of factors, including the effectiveness of the diet counselor (registered dietitian, coach, trainer, etc.), the "livability" of the diet (how realistic is the diet), motivational factors on the part of the athlete and the counselor, and the nutritional safety of the diet. Some weight loss regimens are dangerous.

To achieve weight loss the calories (energy) expended must be greater than the calories ingested. The most effective weight loss techniques involve a reduction in fat intake, because fat is the most calorically dense food nutrient, combined with a moderate increase in aerobic exercise. Suggestions for weight loss are presented in Fig 8–5.

For individuals who have been obese for a long period of time or have a family history of obesity, or both, weight loss may be particularly difficult. Achieving or maintaining weight loss also may be difficult for persons who have dieted in the past, especially those who have followed low-calorie diets to achieve weight loss.

Gaining weight can be as difficult as losing weight. To gain weight the energy expenditure must be less than the energy intake, meaning caloric intake must be increased, exercise decreased, or both. Although fat is the most calorically dense nutrient, it is not recommended that its intake be raised above 30% of total caloric intake because of the increased risk of cardiovascular disease. Suggestions for weight gain are shown in Fig 8–6.

EATING DISORDERS

Eating disorders such as anorexia nervosa and bulimia are becoming more common in the athletic population.[29] Several criteria must be met before anorexia nervosa or bulimia can be diagnosed.[30] In general, anorexia is the prolonged refusal to consume an adequate amount of calories and is accompanied by a distortion in the patient's body image and an intense fear of obesity. Bulimia is characterized by periods of binge eating followed by episodes of purging. Both disorders are seen most frequently in the female population, although males have also been diagnosed with the disease. Both anorexia and bulimia are considered to be primarily psychological disorders. They can be extreme or mild in their manifestations.[30] After the problem has been identified, effective treatment usually requires the skills of a psychology professional supported by a nutrition professional. In advanced cases, hospitalization may be necessary.

1. *Decrease dietary fat*
   a. Decrease or eliminate fat:
      Fats: margarine, butter, shortening, oil, salad dressing, mayonnaise, cream cheese
      High fat foods: olives, avocados, cheese, pastry, cream, gravy
      Foods cooked in fat: fried chicken, doughnuts, potato chips, corn or tortilla chips, cream soups
   b. Substitute low fat products for high fat products:
      whole milk _____ low-fat (2%–1 1/2% fat) or nonfat (1/2%–0% fat) milk
      mayonnaise _____ reduced calorie mayonnaise
      doughnuts _____ bagels
      sour cream _____ yogurt
      ice cream _____ ice milk
2. *Increase complex carbohydrates:*
   These foods are relatively low calorie and have "bulk" thus may increase feelings of fullness. (Be careful of high-calorie toppings though)
   Examples of complex carbohydrates are: pasta, whole grain breads, fresh fruits, beans, split peas, and rice.
3. *Decrease simple sugars:*
   These foods are considered to provide "empty calories" because they contain predominantly sucrose with relatively few nutrients.
   Examples of foods that contain large amounts of simple sugars are: regular soda, candy, pie, jelly, and syrup.
4. *Have smaller portions and eat these slowly:*
   This helps by aiding a person to feel full before overeating.

Figure 8-5. Dietary suggestions for weight loss.

VITAMINS

Originally vitamins were classified as water soluble or fat soluble, based on what appeared to be their properties at that time. Although continued research has shown that the terms no longer describe unique properties of each group, the classification has continued to be used. Within each of the classes the vitamins differ widely in their properties, functions, and distribution. Vitamins function by facilitating metabolism of fats, carbohydrates, and proteins. Although vitamins are absolutely essential for proper functioning of the body, excess amounts are not necessary. Any substance taken in excessive amounts can be toxic.

Although it is commonly believed that vitamin and mineral supplements will enhance athletic performance, there is no research to support this belief. A 3-month, double-blind, crossover, placebo-controlled study of 30 male competitive runners showed that vitamin-mineral supplementation had no effect on several measures of athletic performance.[31]

Food sources, functions and the US RDAs for the major vitamins are shown in Table 8–2.

Water-Soluble Vitamins

There are two divisions of water-soluble vitamins—ascorbic acid (vitamin C) and the B vitamins.

Vitamin C. Vitamin C is found in a wide variety of fruits and vegetables. One of the principal functions of vitamin C involves the synthesis of collagen. Vitamin C is required to hydroxylate proline and lysine, which

1. Eat more frequently.
   In addition to breakfast, lunch, and dinner, snacks such as cheese and crackers, yogurt, and bagels are useful.
2. Remember to eat.
   Often people who are busy forget to eat. For some reason hunger does not affect them until it is extreme.
3. Trade lower calorie foods for ones with more calories.
   orange juice _____ grape juice
   flaked cold cereal _____ granola cold cereal
   bagel_____ doughnut
   saltine crackers _____ graham crackers
4. As a last resort consider a supplement.
   This should be a well-balanced (carbohydrate, protein and fat) supplement which is calorically dense. Often a liquid supplement is effective.

Figure 8-6. Dietary suggestions for weight gain.

TABLE 8-2. VITAMINS

Vitamin	Sources	Functions	US RDA
Vitamin C	Broccoli, brussel sprouts, green and sweet peppers, cantaloupe, grapefruit, oranges, strawberries	Formation of collagen, resistance to infection, aids in use of iron	60 mg
Thiamin	Pork, liver, enriched or whole-wheat cereals and breads, wheat germ	Involved in DNA and RNA formation and nerve function	20 mg
Riboflavin	Milk, yogurt, cottage cheese, meats	Involved, as FAD and FMN, in energy metabolism	1.7 mg
Niacin	Liver, fish, poultry, eggs, whole grain cereals	Involved, as NAD and NADP, in energy metabolism	20 mg
Folacin	Green leafy vegetables, oranges, liver, legumes	Involved in synthesis of DNA, red blood cells and protein	0.4 mg
Vitamin B_6	Liver, spinach, cabbage, fish, poultry, whole grains, legumes	Protein synthesis, fatty acid metabolism, and red blood cell formation	2.0 mg
Vitamin B_{12}	Meat, fish, poultry, eggs, milk and dairy products	Part of a key enzyme	6.0 μg
Biotin	Milk, dairy products, egg yolk, vegetables	Carbohydrate, fat, and protein metabolism	0.3 mg
Pantothenic acid	Whole grains, meats, milk, eggs, legumes	Coenzyme A is important in fat and carbohydrate metabolism	10 mg
Vitamin A	Broccoli, carrots, sweet potato, winter squash, apricots, cantaloupe, persimmon	Assists in formation and maintenance of skin and mucous membranes, involved in vision	5000 IU
Vitamin D	Vitamin D–fortified milk and margarine, egg yolk, cod liver oil	Involved with maintaining calcium in bone and serum, aids in calcium absorption	400 IU
Vitamin E	Wheat germ, safflower oil, cottonseed oil	Functions as an antioxidant, protecting vitamins A and C as well as PUFAs	30 IU

are constituents of collagen. This role in collagen synthesis is a major reason for vitamin C's importance in wound healing. Vitamin C functions as an antioxidant, preventing excessive oxidation of vitamin A, vitamin E, and PUFAs. It also enhances iron absorption by reducing ferric iron to ferrous iron, which is absorbed more efficiently. It is also involved in other areas of iron metabolism.

B Vitamins. The B vitamins refer to a large group of vitamins and include thiamin (vitamin B_1), riboflavin (vitamin B_2), niacin, vitamin B_6, pantothenic acid, biotin, vitamin B_{12}, and folacin.

Thiamin was first identified in the prevention of beriberi, a disease characterized by polyneuritis, cardiac abnormalities, and edema. Beriberi was common in cultures where polished rice was the primary food consumed. It was found that the disease could be prevented if the rice polishings (the outer kernel of the rice) were added to the diet. The factor responsible for the preventive effects of the rice polishings was found to be thiamin.

Thiamin is widely distributed among foods, but, other than in brewer's yeast and wheat germ, is not found in especially high concentrations in any food. Thiamin is found in whole-grain or enriched breads and cereals, as well as in pork, liver, legumes, and egg yolk. Thiamin is extremely important in carbohydrate metabolism, being necessary in the conversion of pyruvic acid to acetyl coenzyme A, and in the Krebs cycle for the conversion of α-keto glutaric acid to succinic acid. Thiamin is also involved in nerve functioning and is a necessary cofactor in the pentose shunt (formation of ribose).

Riboflavin is another B vitamin widely distributed in foods. Good sources of riboflavin include liver, milk, yogurt, meat, and enriched grain products. The primary function of riboflavin is as a constituent of flavin mononucleotide (FMN) and flavin adenine dinucleotide (FAD). Flavin mononucleotide and flavin adenine dinucleotide are coenzymes required in many processes that produce ATP. Sustained riboflavin deficiency results in cheilosis, which is cracking and dry scaling of the lips and angles of the mouth.

Niacin has two biologically active forms, nicotinic acid and nicotinamide. It is found in a wide variety of foods, including fish, liver, and mushrooms. Niacin is a constituent of two coenzymes that function as hydrogen

acceptors—nicotinamide adenine dinucleotide (NAD) and nicotinamide adenine dinucleotide phosphate (NADP). Nicotinamide adenine dinucleotide and nicotinamide adenine dinucleotide phosphate are involved in many energy-producing pathways, especially those associated with carbohydrate metabolism. Deficiency initially manifests itself as general weakness, irritability, headache, and abdominal pain. If the deficiency continues, pellagra may develop, the final stages of which are characterized by dermatitis, diarrhea, dementia, and death.

Vitamin B_6 can be found as pyridoxine, pyridoxal, or pyridoxamine, any one of which can form the active form of vitamin B_6, pyridoxal phosphate. The principal food sources of vitamin B_6 are meat, fish, and poultry. Milk, sweet potatoes, potatoes, and other vegetables are also sources of vitamin B_6. Vitamin B_6 is a constituent of a large number of coenzymes, most of which are involved in protein metabolism. Excessive intake of vitamin B_6 can result in neurological dysfunction.[32]

The active form of pantothenic acid is coenzyme A. Coenzyme A functions in the metabolism of carbohydrates and fats. Pantothenic acid is distributed throughout the food supply. Meats, egg yolks, and legumes are all excellent sources of pantothenic acid, and milk, fruits, and vegetables are good sources. No clear deficiency symptoms have been described, perhaps because pantothenic acid is so widely distributed.

Biotin is another B vitamin involved as a coenzyme in carbohydrate and fat metabolism. It is found in egg yolk, legumes, organ meats, and nuts. Biotin deficiency in humans has been described only when large amounts of raw egg whites, which bind biotin, were consumed on a daily basis. All deficiency symptoms were reversed by the administration of biotin.

Folacin is a generic term for folic acid, pteroylglutamic acid, and other similar compounds. Good sources of folacin include brewer's yeast, spinach, asparagus, and turnip greens. Folacin forms coenzymes called tetrahydrofolates (THFs), which link with carbon containing groups. These groups are further processed in a number of pathways. Folacin is essential in DNA synthesis, protein synthesis, and formation of normal red blood cells (RBCs).

Vitamin B_{12} functions as an enzyme that activates THF. Tetrahydrofolate is involved in RNA, DNA, and protein synthesis. Vitamin B_{12} also works as an enzyme in the conversion of homocysteine to methionine. Vitamin B_{12} is found only in foods of animal origin—meat, fish, poultry, eggs, milk, and dairy products. As a result, a deficiency is possible in persons who follow a strict vegetarian diet. For those who do not follow a strict vegetarian diet, vitamin B_{12} deficiency is usually due to a defect in absorption. Two disorders resulting from an absorption defect are pernicious anemia and megaloblastic anemia.

Fat-Soluble Vitamins

There are four vitamins that are classified as fat soluble—vitamin A, vitamin D, vitamin E, and vitamin K.

Vitamin A. The most widely recognized function of vitamin A is its relationship with vision. Vitamin A is necessary for maintaining normal vision in dim light. Vitamin A is also necessary for the synthesis of healthy skin and mucous membranes and for normal skeletal and tooth development. Only animal foods such as fish–liver oil, milk, butter, liver, and egg yolk contain preformed vitamin A (retinol). Preformed vitamin A is also added to some foods in processing, such as fortified margarine. Another form of dietary vitamin A is carotenoids, such as β-carotene. Carotenes are converted to vitamin A in the body. Carotenes are found in plant foods that have dark green or orange–yellow color. There is a direct correlation between the darkness of the color and the amount of carotene. Examples of food sources of β-carotene include carrots, pumpkin, sweet potatoes, apricots, spinach, beet greens, asparagus, and broccoli. Because vitamin A can be ingested in three different forms (retinol, β-carotene, and other carotenoids) a uniform method of measuring absorption and conversion was required. There are two methods of measuring vitamin A. One uses international units (IUs) and the other uses retinol equivalents (REs). The RE system offers a more precise method of measure. The relationship among REs, IUs, and vitamin A forms is as follows:

$$1 \text{ RE} = 1 \text{ } \mu g \text{ retinol} = 3.33 \text{ IU,}$$
$$1 \text{ RE} = 6 \text{ } \mu g \text{ beta-carotene} = 10 \text{ IU,}$$
$$1 \text{ RE} = 12 \text{ } \mu g \text{ other carotenoids} = 10 \text{ IU.}$$

Vitamin A deficiency can cause night blindness (nyctalopia), epithelial changes such as keratinization of the eye, nasal membranes, middle ear, lungs, and other organs, and xerophthalmia. Deficiency symptoms can advance to the point of being irreversible. Although deficiency of vitamin A should always be avoided, so should excessive intake, as this may be toxic to adults and children. Mild symptoms of hypervitaminosis A include nausea, irritability, anorexia, and drying of the skin. More serious symptoms include bone and joint pain, bone fragility and enlargement of the liver and spleen.

Vitamin D. The most common means of obtaining vitamin D is through exposure to sunlight. When ultraviolet rays from sunlight reach the skin, they convert the vitamin D precursor, 7-dehydrocholesterol, into vitamin D. Vitamin D is not found in large amounts in any food except fortified foods (vitamin D–fortified milk) and fish liver oils (e.g., cod liver oil). An active form of vitamin D, 1,25 dihydroxycholecalciferol (1,25 $(OH)_2$ D_3), is necessary for calcium absorption in the

intestine. 1,25 $(OH)_2$ D_3 also promotes phosphorus absorption. The involvement of 1,25 $(OH)_2$ D_3 with calcium and phosphorus permits bone to mineralize normally and maintains the correct concentration of calcium in the extracellular fluids for muscle contraction and nerve irritability. Vitamin D deficiency affects bone and teeth development and may result in rickets, tetany, and osteomalacia. Overconsumption of vitamin D can result in damage to the kidney characterized by weakness, lethargy, anorexia, and constipation. Hypercalcemia is also seen with excess vitamin D intake.[33]

Vitamin E. Vitamin E (tocopherol) appears to function primarily as an antioxidant. It protects vitamin A and vitamin C from oxidation. It also helps prevent membrane damage by preventing the oxidation of PUFAs and phospholipids. Vitamin E is widely distributed in foods, especially vegetable oils. In adults, symptoms of vitamin E deficiency are rarely seen except in starvation or in individuals with fat malabsorption disorders. Deficiency symptoms have been observed in premature and low-birth-weight infants, and in children with cystic fibrosis.

Vitamin K. Vitamin K is essential for the formation of prothrombin and other clotting proteins. It is synthesized by bacteria in the large intestine. It is also found in some vegetables, such as spinach, cauliflower, and cabbage, and in pork liver. A dietary deficiency is usually not the cause of vitamin K deficiency. Premature infants and hypoxic infants are the most susceptible to vitamin K deficiency. In adults, a deficiency is usually caused by an interference of intestinal synthesis, or a failure in absorption.

MINERALS

Sodium

Sodium and potassium are the two principal electrolytes found in the body. Sodium is found in extracellular fluid, where it helps maintain normal osmotic pressure and water balance. It is also involved in the maintenance of normal nerve function, contraction of muscles (including the heart), and permeability of cell membranes. Sodium is so essential that when intake is extremely restricted mechanisms exist to conserve existing body supplies. Humans who have restricted their sodium intake to 500 mg/day or less have been able to maintain a sodium balance.[34] Under normal conditions, lack of sodium is not a problem. The main source of sodium is sodium chloride (salt) used at the table, in cooking, and in food processing. One teaspoon of salt contains appropriately 2000 mg of sodium. Sodium occurs naturally in foods such as milk, egg whites, meat, spinach, beets, and celery. Although most drinking water is low in sodium, a few locations have significant levels of naturally occurring sodium. The sodium level of water is also increased by most home water-softening equipment.

Salt tablets should be avoided. They significantly increase water requirements and can have dangerous side effects.[35] If increased sodium intake is desired, liberal use of salt on food or the use of a sports drink containing electrolytes should be more than adequate to meet needs.

Potassium

Potassium is the major intracellular electrolyte and helps maintain osmotic pressure and fluid balance inside the cell. Some potassium is bound to phosphate and is required in the conversion of glucose to glycogen. Along with other substances, potassium is required for transmission of nerve impulses and contraction of muscle fiber. Potassium is widely distributed in foods and is found in meat, fruits (especially cantaloupes, dried prunes, apricots, and bananas), and vegetables (especially potatoes, spinach, squash, and asparagus).

Potassium deficiency can occur in severe malnutrition, anorexia nervosa, chronic alcoholism, or an illness causing extensive diarrhea or vomiting. Burns, treatment of diabetic acidosis, and therapeutic drug use can also cause potassium deficiency. Potassium deficiency causes hypokalemia (low plasma levels of potassium), the symptoms of which include nausea, vomiting, muscle weakness, hypotension, tachycardia, arrhythmia, and possibly cardiac arrest.

For athletes, hyperkalemia (elevated plasma levels of potassium) resulting from dehydration may be a problem. There are also some medical situations (e.g., renal failure, adrenal insufficiency) that can cause hyperkalemia. Characteristic symptoms of hyperkalemia include abnormal sensations in the face, tongue, and extremities, muscle weakness, difficult respiration, cardiac arrhythmias, and possibly cardiac arrest.

Iron

Iron is an essential component of hemoglobin, which carries oxygen from the lungs to the tissues. Iron is also an important constituent of catalases and cytochromes and is a required cofactor for other enzymes. For menstruating or pregnant women, it is difficult, but not impossible to obtain adequate iron from the diet. Athletes may also have increased iron needs due to poor absorption and increased iron losses in sweat.[36] Dietary iron is found in two forms, heme iron and nonheme iron. Heme iron can only be found in meat, fish, and poultry. These foods contain about 40% of their iron as heme iron and the remainder as non-heme iron.[37] Other sources of nonheme iron include legumes and enriched cereals. Heme iron is better absorbed than nonheme iron. Consuming a good source of vitamin C during the

same meal as an iron source can increase the amount of iron absorbed.

The result of inadequate iron consumption is iron-deficiency anemia. Typically, a hemoglobin value below normal ranges indicates anemia. In athletes, the diagnosis of iron-deficiency anemia requires additional consideration. Athletes, especially elite endurance athletes, normally have lower hemoglobin values than the general population (Table 8–3). Once iron-deficiency anemia has been diagnosed in an athlete, the cause should be determined. Usually, there is an inadequate consumption of dietary iron; however, footstrike hemolysis also may play a role.[38] With supplementation, iron overload may occur if excessive quantities of iron are taken. This may cause deficiencies of some trace minerals such as zinc and copper.[36]

Calcium

Approximately 99% of the body's calcium is found in bone and teeth. Bone not only serves as a skeleton but also provides calcium reserves, so the plasma calcium concentration can remain stable. The remaining 1% of the calcium has a variety of important functions. Calcium activates several enzymes, aids in absorption by increasing cell membrane permeability, and is required for the synthesis of acetylcholine, which is necessary for nerve impulse transmission. Calcium regulates contraction and relaxation of muscles and is necessary for blood clotting. The primary sources of calcium are milk and dairy products, although calcium can also be found in spinach, rhubarb, and canned sardines with bones. Unfortunately, the phytic acid in spinach, rhubarb, and other vegetables binds calcium, making it less available. Vitamin D aids in calcium absorption by assisting in the formation of calcium-binding protein.

Lack of dietary calcium is usually not exhibited by a low serum calcium. Bone serves as a calcium reservoir and maintains a stable serum calcium. A long-term calcium deficiency, even of mild proportions, can cause the reduction of total bone mass, resulting in osteoporosis. When calcium deficiency has advanced to the point of hypocalcemia, tetany often results.

TABLE 8-3. HEMOGLOBIN VALUES IN NORMAL CONTROLS, MODERATE EXERCISERS, AND ELITE AEROBIC ATHLETES

	Hemoglobin Values[a] (g/dL)	
	Men	**Women**
Normal controls	14.0	12.0
Moderate exercisers	13.5	11.5
Elite aerobic athletes	13.0	11.0

[a]Hemoglobin values below these levels indicate a 95% certainty of true anemia

Adapted from Eichner ER. The anemias of athletes. Physician Sportsmed. *1986; 14:122–130.*

Phosphorus

Phosphorus, in conjunction with calcium, contributes to the structure of bone and teeth. It is a constituent of RNA and DNA and the energy-transferring substances, adenosine diphosphate (ADP) and ATP. It is involved in a wide variety of chemical reactions in the body and as phosphate is an important anion within the cell. Several B vitamins are effective only when combined with phosphate in the body. Phosphorus is found in many foods, in particular, in dairy products and meats. Phosphorus deficiency is rare, but has resulted from prolonged and excessive intake of nonabsorbable antacids.[4]

HYDRATION

Maintaining adequate body fluids is perhaps the most important nutritional requirement. Almost all body processes require the maintenance of body fluids. Energy production, waste product elimination, and body temperature regulation are all processes essential to the athlete, and all require water.

In general, body fluids are lost through three routes. First, fluid is lost in feces and urine. Illness resulting in diarrhea can increase this loss. A high-protein diet may also increase urinary water losses.[39] Second, fluid is lost in exhaled air. Exercise increases water losses through this respiratory pathway. Third, fluids are lost through the skin as both "insensible perspiration" and in sweat mechanisms. The losses through sweating are the largest loss during exercise. Climate affects both respiratory and sweat mechanisms. Respiratory losses are highest in a dry environment and lowest in a humid environment. Losses due to sweat mechanisms are highest in a hot, humid environment and lowest in a cold, dry environment. Large fluid losses can cause serious effects in athletes. Dehydration decreases blood volume, which impairs the body's ability to distribute the blood and will lead to an impaired endurance performance. Research shows that a 1% decrease in body weight (induced by diuretic use) increased running times by 0.17, 0.39, and 1.57 minutes for 1500 meters, 5000 meters and 10,000 meters, respectively.[40] Dehydration also decreases the body's ability to regulate temperature. If dehydration is not reversed and exercise continues, heat exhaustion or heat stroke may occur. In the event of heat stroke, immediate medical attention is required to prevent advancement of the disorder and death.

To prevent dehydration and its possible serious consequences, adequate fluid replacement is necessary during exercise. The major goal of fluid replacement is to maintain blood volume so cardiovascular functions and sweating can allow exercise to progress at optimal levels. To be effective, a fluid used for replacement must be absorbed rapidly and be tolerated well by the athlete.

Thirst is not an effective measure of fluid needs.[41,42] During most exercise, athletes need to consume fluids on a schedule rather than letting thirst dictate their fluid consumption. Monitoring changes in body weight is an accurate method of determining fluid needs. It is usually difficult to measure body weight during exercise, but this is a practical method for determining fluid needs after exercise. The athlete should weigh nude before and after exercise. Any weight loss occurring during exercise can be assumed to be caused by fluid loss. For every pound an athlete loses, 1 pt (16 oz) of fluid is needed to replace the loss. This replacement should be achieved before the next exercise session. During exercise the athlete should drink frequently and consume enough fluid to minimize weight loss. Suggestions on fluid intake and timing vary. Clark suggests 8 to 10 oz every 20 minutes[42] and Coleman suggests 3 to 6 oz every 10 to 15 minutes.[35]

In an attempt to prevent dehydration some athletes use a technique called hyperhydration in addition to regular fluid intake during an event.[35,43] Hyperhydration is the ingestion of 14 to 20 oz of cold water 10 to 15 minutes before exercise, which helps lower the core temperature of the body and thus decreases the stress the additional heat places on the cardiovascular system.[35] For some athletes this may result in an uncomfortable feeling of fullness, although it is not a problem for most athletes.

The type of fluid to be used for replacement depends on the type of exercise. The duration of exercise is important. For nonendurance exercise, water is a good choice. Water is absorbed rapidly, is generally well-tolerated, and when consumed in adequate amounts can prevent cardiovascular and thermoregulatory problems. Cold fluids (41°F) are emptied from the stomach more rapidly than fluids at room temperature.[44] For nonendurance events, the carbohydrates and electrolytes found in many sports drinks are not necessary. It is important to note that water is effective only when adequate amounts are consumed. For some athletes "boredom" with water may result in less than appropriate intake. In these cases using a sports drink may help achieve adequate intake.

For endurance events, a carbohydrate-containing fluid may provide a source for replacing lost glycogen and lead to improved performance. One study has shown that fluids with less than a 6% carbohydrate content did not improve performance, whereas a 6% fluid did.[45] If one chooses to use a sports drink, the type and concentration of carbohydrate and electrolyte should be considered. In the past, it was suggested that an effective sports drink contain no more than 2.5% carbohydrate because a greater concentration decreased gastric emptying. More recently, researchers have taken into consideration more of the absorption process than only gastric emptying and have found that carbohydrate concentrations up to 10% were absorbed rapidly.[46]

Glucose polymers are a fairly recent addition to the sports drink industry. Glucose polymers, also called maltodextrins, are made by controlled hydrolysis of corn starch and contain a variety of polymer lengths.[35] Glucose polymers have a lower osmolality than glucose solutions of equivalent concentration.[43,47] As a result, they provide a higher carbohydrate concentration while still allowing rapid gastric emptying.

When water is lost from the body through sweat, some electrolytes are also lost. The major electrolytes found in sweat are sodium, chloride, potassium, magnesium, and calcium, with the first two found in the largest percentages.[48,49] Sweat secretion is ordinarily hypotonic relative to blood. The blood will become hyperosmotic when dehydration is caused chiefly by sweating.[48-50] Therefore, under normal exercise conditions, the addition of electrolytes to replacement fluids appears unnecessary and even counterproductive. In ultraendurance events, however, (e.g., 50-mile runs and long triathalons) intake of electrolyte-containing fluids may be essential to prevent abnormally low plasma levels of sodium and chloride.[48] Electrolyte-containing fluids may also be necessary when exercise occurs in hot, humid weather, resulting in large water losses through sweat.[43]

NUTRITION MISINFORMATION

Misinformation is common in the field of nutrition. Nutrition misinformation can be intentional or unintentional. Intentional misinformation is often the result of fraud or quackery. Generally, there is an incentive, usually financial, for the proprietor. The proprietor of this information is frequently aware that the claims will not withstand scientific scrutiny. Since prosecution is often difficult, however, the fraudulent claims continue. Unintentional misinformation results when the person does not realize the claims are false. This can result from poor research or faulty interpretation of research. Also in the area of unintentional misinformation is the uninformed person who has seen some "cure." This person firmly believes a nutritional practice caused the cure and wants others to be cured. Often, a person in this position spreads this information by word of mouth and profits very little from it.

Because many athletes are highly motivated to win, misinformation concerning nutrition and other topics abounds in the athletic population. Among common sports nutrition fallacies are the following:

1. Dairy products cause indigestion or diarrhea or both. Because of this fallacy, dairy products are forbidden before an event and sometimes in-

take is even limited in practice sessions. The sugar in the milk, lactose, is the basis for this misunderstanding. To digest lactose, the naturally occurring enzyme lactase must be present in the intestinal tract. Without lactase, lactose is not digested and often results in indigestion and diarrhea. In some athletes, but not all, emotional stress, such as pregame nervousness, decreases the amount of lactase. Also, members of many ethnic groups, such as African Americans, Orientals, and Hispanics have naturally low levels of lactase. As a result, the use of dairy products should be individualized. For the athlete with normal lactase who enjoys milk, a glass of nonfat or low-fat milk may be an appropriate pregame food. There are also dairy products in which the lactose has already been broken down, such as yogurt and cheese, which may be appropriate for lactase-deficient athletes.

2. Bee pollen: There are many claims associated with bee pollen. Among the most common claims are improved athletic performance, increased sexual function, improved digestion, and prolonged life. Several research studies have shown bee pollen to have no special effects, including no improvement in athletic performance.[51,52]

3. Protein to increase muscle: It is true that adequate protein is necessary for muscle maintenance. Once needs have been met, however, excess protein is useless and even counterproductive. Large amounts of protein can cause renal (kidney) stress and lead to dehydration. Excess protein also provides excess calories, which can result in fat deposits.

4. Honey: Honey is another food product to which many claims, especially increased energy, have been attached. Research has shown no special properties attributable to honey. Honey and sugar are very similar. Both provide disaccharides. Depending on the source of the honey, it may contain very minute amounts of minerals but these are far too small to be of any significance. Honey also contains a small percentage of fructose, which is metabolized slightly differently than sucrose, the predominant carbohydrate in table sugar.

5. Fasting to clean the body of toxins: The body's response to fasting is the same as it would be to starvation. During the initial phase of fasting, liver glycogen stores are depleted. This results in the breakdown of protein from muscles and organs to supply the brain with glucose and the breakdown of lipid causing ketone production. If food deprivation continues, plasma ketone levels rise and it becomes more difficult to maintain a normal pH. The liver and kidney must work harder to use and then eliminate the by-products of protein and fat breakdown. In some ways, fasting does not clean the body of toxins, it creates them.

REPUTABLE INFORMATION SOURCES

Accurate information concerning sports nutrition is available. The difficulty is distinguishing it from the misinformation. First, consider the information—does it sound too good to be true? Then it probably is! Claims of "melting off fat" while eating your regular diet or curing cancer by drinking a special mineralized water are obviously false. Frequently claims made about the product, diet, or program are an excellent clue to its validity. Second, examine the authors, directors, or proprietors of the item. Look for professional titles as well as the institution that awarded them. The initials "R.D." stand for registered dietitian and indicate that a person has a degree from an accredited university, has passed a national exam, and maintains continuing education hours. The initials "L.D." stand for licensed dietitian. Licensure is a state-controlled matter and requirements vary in each state. An L.D. is an indication of reputability, but one should investigate this person's qualifications a little further. Frequently an L.D. is also an R.D. or has a master's degree or doctorate from an accredited university. The lack of R.D. status does not in itself indicate a lack of quality. There are very qualified individuals who have advanced degrees from accredited universities and have chosen for one reason or another to not become a R.D. It is important that the university or college awarding the degree be examined closely. There are many sham or "mail-order" colleges and universities selling degrees in nutrition. A university or college should be accredited by an official accrediting agency recognized by the U.S. Department of Education.

CONCLUSION

In general an athlete should follow a well-balanced diet that includes a wide variety of foods. This will provide the basis of an optimal sports nutrition program. Carbohydrate is important for energy production, but lipid and protein are also essential components of an athlete's diet. Although nutrition does not offer a quick method for a magical improvement of performance, careful nutrition practices can enhance performance in a well-trained athlete.

In many ways, sports nutrition is a changing science. New research and new interpretations of old re-

search are expanding the field daily. These new findings are based on physiology, biochemistry, and basic nutrition. Application of these findings will continue to advance the field of sports nutrition and provide athletes with new methods for enhancing performance.

REFERENCES

1. Evans JE, Fischer EC, Hoerr RA, Young VR. Protein metabolism and endurance exercise. *Physician Sportsmed.* 1983; 11:63–72.
2. Dohm GL. Protein metabolism in exercise. In: Fox EL, ed. *Nutrient Utilization During Exercise. Ross Symposium.* Columbus, Ohio: Ross Laboratories; 1983:8–13.
3. Whitney EN, Hamilton EM. *Understanding Nutrition.* St. Paul, Minn: West Publishing Co; 1987:161.
4. Committee on Dietary Allowances, Food and Nutrition Board, National Research Council. *Recommended Dietary Allowances.* 9th ed. Washington DC: National Academy of Sciences; 1980.
5. Brotherhood JR. Nutrition and sports performance. *Sports Med.* 1984; 1:350–389.
6. Lemon PWR, Yarasheski KE, Dolny DG. The importance of protein for athletes. *Sports Med.* 1984; 1:474–484.
7. Laritcheva KA, Yalovaya NI, Shubin VI, Smirnov PV. Study of energy expenditure and protein needs of top weight lifters. In: Parizkova J, Rogozkin VA, eds. *Nutrition, Physical Fitness, and Health.* Baltimore, Md: University Park; 1978:155–163.
8. Celejowa I, Homa M. Food intake, nitrogen and energy balance in Polish weight lifters during a training camp. *Nutri Metab.* 1970; 12:259–274.
9. Tarnopolsky MA, MacDougall JD, Atkinson SA. Influence of protein intake and training status on nitrogen balance and lean body mass. *J Appl Physiol.* 1988; 64:187–193.
10. McGarry JD, Kuwajima M, Newgard CB, Foster DW. From dietary glucose to liver glycogen: The full circle round. *Annu Rev Nutr.* 1987; 7:51–73.
11. Stryer L. Biochemistry. 2nd ed. New York, NY: WH Freeman Co; 1981: 374–394.
12. U.S. Senate, Select Committee on Nutrition and Human Needs. *Dietary Goals for the United States.* 2nd ed. Washington DC: US Government Printing Office; 1977.
13. Sherman WM. Carbohydrate, Muscle Glycogen and Improved Performance. *Physician Sportsmed.* 1987; 15:157–164.
14. Costill DL, Sherman WM, Fink WJ, et al. The role of dietary carbohydrates in muscle glycogen resynthesis after strenuous running. *Am J Clin Nutr.* 1981; 34:1831–1836.
15. Coleman E. *Eating for Endurance.* Palo Alto, Calif: Bull Publishing Co; 1988:40–49.
16. Bergstrom J, Hermansen L, Hultman E, Saltin B. Diet, muscle glycogen and physical performance. *Acta Physiol Scand.* 1967; 71:140–150.
17. Gollnick PD, Matoba H. Role of carbohydrate in exercise. *Clin Sports Med.* 1984; 3:583–593.
18. Fielding RA, Costill DL, Fink WJ, et al. Effects of pre-exercise carbohydrate feedings on muscle glycogen use during exercise in well-trained runners. *Eur J Appl Physiol.* 1987; 56:225–229.
19. Gleeson M, Maughan RJ, Greenhaff PL. Comparison of the effects of pre-exercise feeding of glucose, glycerol and placebo on endurance and fuel homeostasis in man. *Eur J Appl Physiol.* 1986; 55:645–653.
20. Williams MH. Nutritional ergogenic aids and athletic performance. *Nutr Today.* 1989; 24:7–14.
21. Grundy S. Comparison of monounsaturated fatty acids and carbohydrates for lowering plasma cholesterol. *N Engl J Med.* 1986; 314:745–748.
22. Rogers AE, Lee SY. Chemically-induced mammary gland tumors in rats: Modulation by dietary fat. *Prog Clin Biol Res.* 1986; 222:255–282.
23. Wade AE, Dharwadkar S. Metabolic activation of carcinogens. *Prog Clin Biol Res.* 1986; 222:587–606.
24. Bieber MA. Cancer and diet interactions. *Prog Clin Biol Res.* 1986; 222:789–799.
25. Nash HL. Reemphasizing the role of exercise in preventing heart disease. *Physician Sportsmed.* 1989; 17:219–225.
26. Cohen JC, Noakes TD, Benade AJ. Hypercholesterolemia in male power lifters using anabolic–androgenic steroids. *Physician Sportsmed.* 1988; 16:49–56.
27. Hurley BF, Seals DR, Hagberg JM, et al. High density-lipoprotein cholesterol in bodybuilders v powerlifters. *JAMA.* 1984; 252:507–513.
28. American Dietetic Association. *Handbook of Clinical Dietetics.* New Haven, Conn: Yale University Press; 1981:I27.
29. Zucker P (moderator). Eating disorders in young athletes: A round table. *Physician Sportsmed.* 1985; 13:89–104.
30. Balaa MA, Drossman DA. Anorexia nervosa and bulimia: The eating disorders. *Dis Mon.* 1985; 31:1–52.
31. Weight LM, Myburgh KH, Noakes TD. Vitamin and mineral supplementation: Effects on the running performance of trained athletes. *Am J Clin Nutr.* 1988; 47:192–195.
32. Dalton K. Dalton MJ. Characteristics of pyridoxine overdose neuropathy syndrome. *Acta Neurol Scand.* 1987; 76:8–11.
33. American Dietetic Association. *Handbook of Clinical Dietetics.* New Haven, Conn: Yale University Press; 1981:A85.
34. Robinson CH, Lawler MR. *Normal and Therapeutic Nutrition.* 16th ed. New York, NY: Macmillan Publishing Co; 1982:166.
35. Coleman E. *Eating for Endurance.* Palo Alto, Calif: Bull Publishing Co; 1988:83–89.
36. Coleman E. *Eating for Endurance.* Palo Alto, Calif: Bull Publishing Co; 1988:74–77.
37. Robinson CH, Lawler MR. *Normal and Therapeutic Nutrition.* 16th ed. New York, NY: Macmillan Publishing Co; 1982:146.
38. Eichner ER. The anemias of athletes. *Physician Sportsmed.* 1986; 14:122–130.
39. McArdle WD, Katch FI, Katch VL. *Exercise Physiology: Energy, Nutrition and Human Performance.* 2nd ed. Philadelphia, Pa: Lea & Febiger; 1986:62.
40. Armstrong LE, Costill DL, Fink WJ. Influence of diuretic-

induced dehydration on competitive running performance. *Med Sci Sports Exer.* 1985; 17:456–461.

41. Sawka MN, Francesconi RP, Young AJ, Pandolf KB. Influences of hydration level and body fluids on exercise performance in the heat. *JAMA* 1984; 252:1165–1169.

42. Clark N. *The Athlete's Kitchen.* New York, NY: CBI Publishing Co; 1981:243.

43. McArdle WD, Katch FI, Katch VL. *Exercise Physiology: Energy, Nutrition and Human Performance.* 2nd ed. Philadelphia, Pa: Lea & Febiger; 1986:452–454.

44. Costill DL, Saltin B: Factors limiting gastric emptying during rest and exercise. *J Appl Physiol.* 1974; 37:679–683.

45. Davis JM, Lamb DR, Pate RR, et al. Carbohydrate-electrolyte drinks: Effects on endurance cycling in the heat. *Am J Clin Nutr.* 1988; 48:1023–1030.

46. Davis JM, Lamb DR, Burgess WA, Bartoli WP. Accumulation of deuterium oxide in body fluids after ingestion of D_2O-labeled beverages. *J Appl Physiol.* 1987; 63:2060–2066.

47. Murray R. The effects of consuming carbohydrate-electrolyte beverages on gastric emptying and fluid absorption during and following exercise. *Sports Med.* 1987; 4:322–351.

48. Lamb D, Brodowicz G. Optimal use of fluids of varying formulations to minimize exercise-induced disturbances in homeostasis. *Sports Med.* 1986; 13:247–274.

49. Costill D, Cote R, Fink W, Van Handel P. Muscle water and electrolyte distribution during prolonged exercise. *Int J Sports Med.* 1988; 2:130–134.

50. Senay L, Christensen M. Changes in blood plasma during progressive dehydration. *J Appl Physiol.* 1965; 20:1136–1140.

51. Maughan RJ, Evan SP. Effects of pollen extract upon adolescent swimmers. *Br J Sports Med* 1982; 16:142–145.

52. Mirkin G. Bee pollen: Living up to its hype? *Physician Sportsmed.* 1985; 13:159–160.

9
The Female Athlete

Karen A. Knortz

INTRODUCTION

Participation of women in organized sports is a 20th century phenomenon, and certainly one that has raised many questions with regard to social and physical issues related to the suitability of sports for women. This chapter briefly addresses historical perspectives of women's sports participation, but has its focus on physiological considerations responsible for performance limitations, injuries, and overall health of exercising women. Though much of the related literature refers to the status of women involved in organized sports, some of the aforementioned factors, particularly gynecological considerations, are relevant to recreational athletes as well.

HISTORY OF WOMEN'S SPORTS PARTICIPATION

A number of factors influenced the rise in popularity of women's involvement in sports, beginning in the early part of the nineteenth century. The Turnverein movement in Germany and advent of gymnastics in Sweden provided early opportunities for participation of women.[1] In addition, the introduction of basketball by Naismith brought about an interest in intercollegiate team competition. Surprisingly, by 1925, 22% of the colleges in the United States offered intercollegiate women's sports.[2]

During the same era, recreational sports such as tennis, golf, bowling, and archery became popular for women seeking an appropriate opportunity for social encounter. As the popularity of individual and team sports grew during the "golden era" between 1925 and 1935,[3] sports governing bodies became organized and controversy arose regarding the place of women in sports. The Victorian ideal of womanhood dictated the social thinking of the time, and this characterization of women as passive, dependent, and dainty objects of a potential husband's attraction was in conflict with women's sports participation.[3] Moreover, the prospect that vigorous physical activity might pose physical hazards such as injury to or interference with reproductive function sparked a long history of medical concern that is still apparent today.

Olympic Participation

In 1912, women were permitted to participate in Olympic tennis and swimming competition, but it was not until 1928 that Olympic track events were offered to women. In the 1928 Olympics, the 800-meter run for women seemingly validated the social and medical concerns of the time. Of the 11 participants, only 5 finished the race, with the other 6 women either dropping out or fainting in the locker room. So alarming was this occurrence that in 1930, the Olympic Congress nearly succeeded in limiting women's Olympic participation to swimming, tennis, gymnastics, and skating.[4]

Current Trends

Despite such setbacks, opportunities for women's participation in the Olympics and sports in general has grown exponentially. Eventually the social milieu changed, perhaps in part because of the women's suffrage movement and as a result of the model set by ambitious and successful women adventurers of the early part of the twentieth century.[3] The stereotype of femininity has indeed changed through these events and the spread of the equal rights movement. Now living in an achievement-oriented society, women are no longer discouraged from achieving and have a greater opportunity for reaping the social, psychological, and physical benefits of sports and exercise.

Commensurate with this increased opportunity for sports participation, however, is an increased risk for injury. Statistics for competitive intercollegiate programs reveal that injury rates for women are similar to those of men.[5] Efforts to prevent injuries to women athletes must include an adequate medical history and

examination, including a musculoskeletal screening for identification of individuals who are predisposed to injury because of biomechanical nuances, or flexibility and strength deficits. Tables 9–1 through 9–3 provide guidelines for health screenings and tests for the average healthy individual and serve as a useful guide for women who exercise regularly.[6] It should be noted that optional assessments, including dietary and fitness evaluations as well as graded exercise testing, are extremely important with respect to prevention of injuries and health disorders.

TRAINING AND CONDITIONING

Despite increased awareness and implementation of such preventative measures, inappropriate conditioning and training methods tend to increase the risk of injury to female athletes. It is well accepted that a certain amount of physical stress to the body results in improved performance, but overstressing the body causes injury as well as a decline in physical function.[7] This is illustrated in Fig 9–1, which shows that there is an optimal level of physical stress for improved performance, above which performance deteriorates. The major problem with regard to conditioning and training of female athletes is that we do not yet have a grasp of what this optimal level should be for a population of female athletes, much less for the individual woman.

The relatively high incidence of injuries among competitive female athletes has raised concern as to whether their training and conditioning programs should be different from those of their male counterparts. Training studies involving female athletes have repeatedly demonstrated, however, that the responses of men and women to training are virtually identical.[8,9] Moreover, the consensus of strength and conditioning experts is that such programs should be based upon the demands of the sport and the needs of the individual,[10] and need not be gender specific.

The most important concern regarding training and conditioning for women is the progression of intensity and duration. Although the problem of overtraining is not gender specific, it may be more apparent in women for a number of reasons. First of all, many female college athletes are simply not prepared for the physical stress of competitive training by virtue of their involvement in high school programs characterized by low demand and intensity. Secondly, inexperience with highly competitive training makes it difficult for the female athlete to differentiate between the pain and postexercise soreness associated with exertion and the pain of injury. Lastly, not having a grasp of optimal training levels for women, coaches and athletes too often succumb to the pressures of winning and overstep the line between optimal training and injurious training.

There is an unfortunate lack of research and experience in the area of training and conditioning of women athletes primarily because the history of women's participation in sports is quite short when compared to that of men. Consequently, the majority of physical training studies have examined male athletes, and al-

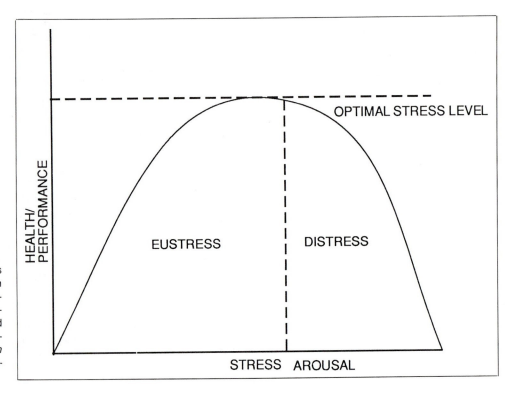

Figure 9–1. Optimal stress level: Relationship between stress arousal and health/performance. (*From Everly GS, Rosenfeld R.* The Nature and Treatment of the Stress Response. *New York, NY: Plenum Press: 1981; 7–9, with permission.*)

TABLE 9-1. GUIDELINES FOR HEALTH SCREENINGS AND TESTS FOR AGES 18-39

Age:	18	19	20	21	22	23	24	25	26	27	28	29	30	31	32	33	34	35	36	37	38	39
COMPLETE HISTORY & PHYSICAL:			•				•				•				•				•			
Blood count, Chemical Profile & Thyroid Function			•				•				•				•				•			
EKG																						
Chest X-Ray																						
Urinalysis			•				•				•				•				•		•	
Colon Screening—Occult Blood & Digital Exam			•				•				•				•				•	•		
Height, Weight & Blood Pressure	•	•	•	•	•	•	•	•	•	•	•	•	•	•	•	•	•	•	•	•	•	•
SCREENING EXAM:																						
Breast Exam—Clinical	•		•		•		•		•		•		•		•		•		•		•	
Pelvic Exam—Clinical	•		•		•		•		•		•		•		•		•		•		•	
Testes Exam	•				•						•					•					•	
Instruct self exam oral cavity, breast, skin, testes				•									•									
Health Risk Assessment[a]	•					•					•					•					•	
SCREENING TESTS:																						
Pap Smear	•		•		•		•		•		•		•		•		•		•		•	
Mammogram																						
Visual Acuity Screening			•					•					•					•				
Rubella Titer (female)																						
IMMUNIZATION:																						
Tetanus Booster						•											•					
Rubella (if necessary)				•																		
OPTIONAL OR ACCORDING TO RISK:																						
Dietary Assessment	•		•				•			•					•				•			•
Exercise Treadmill																						
Fitness Assessment[b]	•		•				•			•					•				•			•
Pulmonary Function (if smoke)																	•					
OTHER:																						

•—Circles indicate a suggested age for screenings and tests.
[a]Assessment and education about exercise, nutrition, weight, alcohol and drug abuse, smoking, stress management, etc.; projects life expectancy.
[b]Fitness assessment includes flexibility, body fat, strength and endurance, cardiovascular endurance and posture evaluation.
Information compiled by and provided courtesy of the St. Elizabeth Wellness Center, Lincoln, Neb.

TABLE 9-2. GUIDELINES FOR HEALTH SCREENINGS AND TESTS FOR AGES 40-69

Age:	40	41	42	43	44	45	46	47	48	49	50	51	52	53	54	55	56	57	58	59	60	61	62	63	64	65	66	67	68	69
COMPLETE HISTORY & PHYSICAL:	•		•		•		•		•		•		•		•		•		•		•		•		•		•		•	
Blood count, Chemical Profile & Thyroid Function	•		•		•		•		•		•		•		•		•		•		•		•		•		•		•	
EKG	•		•		•		•		•		•		•		•		•		•		•		•		•		•		•	
Chest X-Ray	•				•						•				•						•					•				
Urinalysis	•		•		•		•		•		•		•		•		•		•		•		•		•		•		•	
Colon Screening—Occult Blood &	•	•	•	•	•	•	•	•	•	•	•	•	•	•	•	•	•	•	•	•	•	•	•	•	•	•	•	•	•	•
Digital Exam	•		•		•		•		•		•		•		•		•		•		•		•		•		•		•	
Height, Weight & Blood Pressure	•	•	•	•	•	•	•	•	•	•	•	•	•	•	•	•	•	•	•	•	•	•	•	•	•	•	•	•	•	•
SCREENING EXAM:																														
Breast Exam—Clinical	•	•	•	•	•	•	•	•	•	•	•	•	•	•	•	•	•	•	•	•	•	•	•	•	•	•	•	•	•	•
Pelvic Exam—Clinical	•	•	•	•	•	•	•	•	•	•	•	•	•	•	•	•	•	•	•	•	•	•	•	•	•	•	•	•	•	
Instruct self exam oral cavity, breast, skin, testes	•										•										•									
Health Risk Assessment[a]	•		•		•		•		•		•		•		•		•		•		•		•		•		•		•	
Sigmoidoscopy	•				•						•				•						•					•				
Teach to report post-menopausal bleeding											•																			
Educate on Osteoporosis risk and prevention	•																													
SCREENING TESTS:																														
Pap Smear	•	•	•	•	•	•	•	•	•	•	•	•	•	•	•	•	•	•	•	•	•		•		•		•		•	
Mammogram	•		•		•		•		•		•	•	•	•	•	•	•	•	•	•	•	•	•	•	•	•	•	•	•	•
Visual Acuity Screening	•				•						•				•						•					•				
Tonometry	•				•						•		•		•		•		•		•		•		•		•			
IMMUNIZATION:																														
Tetanus Booster					•										•										•					
Influenza[b]																										•	•	•	•	•
Pneumococcal Vaccine—high risk grp.																														

(continued)

Age:	40	41	42	43	44	45	46	47	48	49	50	51	52	53	54	55	56	57	58	59	60	61	62	63	64	65	66	67	68	69
OPTIONAL OR ACCORDING TO RISK:																														
Dietary Assessment	•			•			•			•			•			•			•			•			•			•		
Exercise Treadmill					•					•					•					•					•					
Fitness Assessment[c]	•			•			•			•			•			•			•			•			•			•		
Pulmonary Function (if smoke)	•				•						•					•					•						•			
OTHER:																														

•—Circles indicate a suggested age for screening and tests.
[a]Assessment and education about exercise, nutrition, weight, alcohol and drug abuse, smoking, stress management, etc.; projects life expectancy.
[b]For persons older than 65 or with chronic heart, pulmonary, renal or metabolic (diabetes) disease, or chronic anemia, immunosuppressed patients.
[c]Fitness assessment includes flexibility, body fat, strength and endurance, cardiovascular endurance and posture evaluation.
Information compiled by and provided courtesy of the St. Elizabeth Wellness Center, Lincoln, Neb.

TABLE 9-3. GUIDELINES FOR HEALTH SCREENINGS AND TESTS FOR AGES 70–95

Age:	70	71	72	73	74	75	76	77	78	79	80	81	82	83	84	85	86	87	88	89	90	91	92	93	94	95
COMPLETE HISTORY & PHYSICAL:	•		•		•		•		•		•		•		•		•		•							
Blood count, Chemical Profile & Thyroid																										
Function (inc. Cholesterol)	•		•		•		•				•		•		•		•		•							
EKG	•		•		•		•		•		•		•		•		•		•							
Chest X-Ray	•					•					•					•										
Urinalysis	•		•		•		•		•		•		•		•		•		•							
Colon Screening—Occult Blood	•	•	•	•	•	•	•	•	•	•	•	•	•	•	•	•	•	•	•							
Digital Rectal Screening	•		•		•		•		•		•		•		•		•		•							
Height, Weight & Blood Pressure	•	•	•	•	•	•	•	•	•	•	•	•	•	•	•	•	•	•	•	•						
SCREENING EXAM:																										
Breast Exam—Clinical	•	•	•	•	•	•	•	•	•	•	•	•	•	•	•	•	•	•	•	•						
Pelvic Exam—Clinical	•		•		•		•		•		•		•		•		•		•							
Instruct self exam oral cavity, breast,																										
skin, testes	•										•															
Health Risk Assessment[a]	•		•		•		•		•		•		•		•		•		•							
Sigmoidoscopy	•					•					•					•										
Teach to report postmenopausal bleeding	•																									

(continued)

TABLE 9-3. GUIDELINES FOR HEALTH SCREENINGS AND TESTS FOR AGES 70-95

Age:	70	71	72	73	74	75	76	77	78	79	80	81	82	83	84	85	86	87	88	89	90	91	92	93	94	95
SCREENING TESTS:																										
Pap Smear	•		•		•		•		•		•		•		•		•		•							
Mammogram	•	•	•	•	•	•	•	•	•	•	•	•	•	•	•	•	•	•	•	•						
Visual, Auditory, Acuity Screening	•					•					•					•										
Tonometry		•		•		•		•		•		•		•		•		•		•						
IMMUNIZATION:																										
Tetanus Booster					•															•						
Influenza[b]	•	•	•	•	•	•	•	•	•	•	•	•	•	•	•	•	•	•	•	•						
OPTIONAL OR ACCORDING TO RISK:																										
Dietary Assessment	•			•			•			•			•			•			•							
Exercise Treadmill	•					•					•					•										
Fitness Assessment[c]	•			•			•			•			•			•			•							
Pulmonary Function (if smoke)	•				•						•					•										
OTHER:																										

•—Circles indicate a suggested age for screenings and tests.
[a]Assessment and education about exercise, nutrition, weight, alcohol and drug abuse, smoking, stress management, sleep habits, seat belt use, excessive sun exposure, and projects life expectancy.
[b]For persons older than 65 or with chronic heart, pulmonary, renal or metabolic (diabetes) disease, or chronic anemia, immunosuppressed patients.
[c]Fitness assessment includes flexibility, body fat, strength and endurance, cardiovascular endurance and posture evaluation.
Information compiled by and provided courtesy of the St. Elizabeth Wellness Center, Lincoln, Neb.

though general guidelines regarding sport specificity may apply equally well to women, differences in physical limitations and sport experience make it impossible to transfer precisely men's training programs to women. Clearly, more research using female athletes is required.

Because a difference in sports participation experience implies a difference in physical readiness, identification of predisposing factors to injury is a step toward prevention. Establishing individualized training programs with a focus on proper progression will also help to reduce injuries. Lastly, athletes must be monitored closely for signs of overtraining, and even the slightest hint of injury should be evaluated without delay.

PHYSIOLOGICAL CONSIDERATIONS

Morphological Factors

Structurally, men and women differ with respect to height, weight, pelvic width, adiposity, muscle mass, heart size, and skeletal growth. These factors have a definite impact upon physical capabilities and limitations. It must be noted, however, that when these variables are plotted in a frequency distribution, the resulting bell-shaped curves overlap considerably for a given variable measured on a normal population of men and women. Most of the data related to such differences compare mean values for populations of normal men and women.

In terms of height, the average adult male is taller than the average female by 5 or 6 in.[1,11] Although the leg length of men accounts for 52% of their height, it accounts for only 51.2% of the height of women,[1] and this is partially responsible for a lower center of gravity in women. Likewise, women's upper extremities are generally shorter than men's, and in throwing sports this shortened lever arm combined with smaller muscle mass make it difficult for women to swing an implement such as a ball or discus as rapidly as men.

According to the data from National Center for Health Statistics,[11] female athletes are some 32 lb

lighter than their male counterparts, with a mean weight of 128 lb for female athletes and 160 lb for male athletes. When only lean body mass is considered, however, the normal population of women is only 25 lb lighter than a similar sample of men.[1]

Pelvic width in women is generally greater than that of men,[1,12] although it has been speculated that such differences are not significant.[3] A study of Olympic athletes[13] revealed a mean difference of only 1 cm between male and female athletes, with men exhibiting a greater pelvic width. An increased pelvic width in women has often been implicated as a contributor to an increased Q-angle at the knee; therefore it may be possible that some interrelationship between pelvic width and other biomechanical factors exists.

Body composition measurement results in valuable information regarding adiposity and lean body mass. There are a number of different techniques for this assessment, including skinfold measurement, measurement of electrical impedance, hydrostatic weighing, and isotopic dilution. Although all these methods have both merits and limitations, in terms of accuracy in measurement of total body composition, the last two mentioned are considered to be best. Through a review of numerous studies involving normal adult men and women, McArdle et al[14] estimates the average percentage body fat at 25.5 for women and 13.1 for men.

Differences in skeletal growth patterns account, not only for height and limb length discrepancies, but also for differences in age at closure of epiphyseal plates. Up until the age of 10 years, skeletal growth occurs at roughly the same rate for girls and boys, with boys slightly, but not significantly taller. Because of the earlier onset of puberty in girls, by age 13 or 14, girls are usually taller than boys. Shortly thereafter, however, boys begin their growth spurt, and may continue growing up until the age of 22, generally surpassing the height of girls by some 5 or 6 inches, as the growth spurt for girls usually ends at about age 19. Closure of epiphyseal plates likewise occurs sooner in girls, occurring at roughly age 16 as compared to age 19 for boys.

Physiological Factors

Physiologically, there are more similarities than differences between men and women; however, those that have the greatest influence upon physical abilities are differences in cardiovascular capacity, fuel stores, and hormones. The average woman's heart, as measured by transverse diameter, is only 88% as large as the average man's.[1] Because heart volume, to a great extent, determines stroke volume, women generally exhibit lower stroke volumes and a lower cardiac output than men. Additionally, the smaller size of the woman results in a lower total blood volume, with approximately 6% fewer red blood cells (RBCs), and hemoglobin values some 15% less. The small thoracic and lung size of

women results in a lower tidal capacity and lung volume than men. The net result of these cardiovascular differences is a lower total oxygen carrying capacity for women as compared to men.

Short, high-intensity events require energy from creatine phosphate and adenosine triphosphate (ATP), utilized during anaerobic glycolysis. The overall size of muscles is generally smaller in women than men, and there is a proportional decrease in phosphagen stores. The presence of testosterone in men is largely responsible for the greater size of their muscles. In addition to its androgenic properties, testosterone also has a potent anabolic effect, permitting greater muscle growth in men.

Performance Factors

Characterization of women as "the weaker sex" is largely based upon the fact that, as a group, women have smaller muscles and less potential for muscle growth than men. There is, however, some controversy regarding the appropriate method of comparison of strength in the two sexes. When muscle strength is expressed relative to total body mass or lean body mass, the margin of difference decreases as a function of the generally smaller mass of women.[15] Regardless of relative strength, however, in terms of performance, the fact remains that the greater muscle mass of men permits greater force production during athletic performance.

Absolute strength in men and women also tends to differ depending upon the muscle groups compared. For example, in a comparison of absolute static strength between untrained men and women, Laubach found that, expressed as a percentage of men's absolute strength, women averaged 56% for the upper body, 64% for the trunk, and 72% for the lower extremities.[16] Although such differences in strength exist between gross muscle groups, it has also been shown that when absolute strength is defined as maximal tension development relative to the cross section of muscle, there is no strength difference between male and female muscle tissue.[17]

Many researchers have compared men and women with respect to upper body strength. Wilmore reported that upper body strength in women measured between 43% and 63% of upper body strength values for men.[18] In a review of nine studies comparing strength of untrained men and women, Laubach described a range in values from 35% to 79%, with a mean female upper body strength value equalling 56% of that of males.[16]

When upper body strength values were expressed as a percentage of body weight, mean values for women were on the order of 65% of mean values for men.[10] Moreover, when upper body strength was expressed relative to lean body mass, it was found that mean values for women were 80% to 90% of mean values for men.[10] These findings indicate that differences

in muscle mass account for strength differences between men and women.

Similar observations have been made regarding sex differences in lower body strength, although the difference appears to be less pronounced, with women generally achieving a higher mean percentage of men's strength for the lower body as compared to the upper body. Wilmore proposed that two key factors account for this observation.[18] First, women have a greater percentage of adipose tissue in their upper extremities than in their lower extremities, so that the percentage of lean body mass is greater in the lower than upper extremities. Secondly, Wilmore suggested that male and female patterns of upper extremity use differ considerably in athletics, whereas lower extremity use patterns are similar for men and women athletes.

In terms of absolute lower body strength, Cureton et al found that mean values for women were 60% to 80% of mean values for men,[10] whereas Laubach's review of studies revealed a range of 57% to 82%, with an average value of 72%.[16] When expressed relative to fat-free weight, mean values for women were 90% to 100% those of men.[10] In addition, when the covariates body mass and percentage body fat were controlled for, only 2% of the differences in lower extremity strength was attributed to gender.[15]

It should be obvious from the research related to strength differences between the sexes that differences in total muscle mass play a major role in strength discrepancies. To a great extent, this is a result of the presence of the anabolic–androgenic hormone testosterone in males. Testosterone is a tissue-building steroid that facilitates muscle hypertrophy as a result of training. This is not to say that muscle building cannot occur without testosterone, but rather that the potential for increasing muscle size and strength is increased by testosterone. Resistive training is extremely effective in increasing strength in both men and women, although the potential for muscle hypertrophy in women is limited.

Moreover, the contribution of neuromuscular mechanisms to strength improvement should not be underemphasized. Phenomena such as improved neural association, recruitment, and disinhibition are also important factors in strength acquisition, and these effects are not gender specific. This may well account for the observation that gender-specific strength differences are less apparent in trained than in untrained subjects.[18] As strength training methods become more efficient, further decreases in this discrepancy are quite likely.

Another component of fitness that exerts a major effect on performance is cardiovascular endurance. Defined as efficiency of aerobic metabolism for work performance, the most common index of cardiovascular endurance is maximum oxygen uptake (VO_2 max), or the rate of oxygen exchange during maximal work.

Quantitative differences in cardiovascular endurance between individuals certainly occur as a result of training, but gender-related factors such as heart and lung capacity, lean muscle mass, age-related development, and hematological indices account for significant differences in the potential for achieving high levels of cardiovascular endurance between men and women.

Until puberty, cardiovascular endurance is roughly equal for boys and girls.[19] Thereafter, boys exhibit VO_2 max values some 20% greater than girls until adulthood.[19] For untrained women, aerobic capacity is 15% to 30% lower than for untrained men.[20,21] When comparing endurance-trained men and women, however, the difference is somewhat less, and when expressed relative to lean body mass, the difference in VO_2 max is slight.[22,23] Again, total muscle mass accounts for differences in aerobic performance between men and women. Nonetheless, from a functional perspective this means that, in general, male athletes outperform female athletes in endurance activities, although "pound for pound" physiological differences may be minimal.

Factors other than total muscle mass have an effect on aerobic capacity, however, and among these are differences in heart and lung capacity. The smaller heart size of women limits stroke volume, and thus cardiac output, so that the rate of movement of blood through the systemic circulation is less for women than for men at a given heart rate.

Hematological parameters, including total blood volume, hemoglobin level, and hematocrit are highly correlated to VO_2 max regardless of gender.[19] Total blood volume and hemoglobin values for untrained women are some 25% lower than those of untrained men, but this discrepancy decreases to 12% with training.[24] Recently, there has been a surge of interest in the relationship between anemia and performance in women, but results are inconclusive because it is difficult to separate iron loss through sweating and menstruation from deficiency caused by inadequate dietary intake. Nonetheless, it has been suggested that female athletes are more susceptible than male athletes to iron deficiency anemia because of iron loss through menstruation and sweating, as well as decreased dietary iron intake.[25] Ultimately, the decreased oxygen-binding capacity associated with lower blood volume and hemoglobin levels in women results in women having a lesser aerobic capacity than men.

GYNECOLOGICAL AND OBSTETRIC CONSIDERATIONS

Menstruation

Premenstrual Syndrome. Of all the menstrual dysfunctions and factors that affect women, premenstrual

syndrome (PMS) is perhaps the most common, affecting some 70% to 90% of women in varying degrees of severity.[26] It has been estimated that in 5% of cases, this syndrome is accompanied by symptoms so severe that normal daily function is impaired for days or weeks.[26] Although the effects of PMS vary considerably, many of the physical and emotional signs and symptoms can exert a profound effect upon performance of the woman athlete.

Premenstrual syndrome was identified in the 1930s, and has just recently gained attention as a physiological, rather than psychological, condition. Premenstrual syndrome coincides with the luteal phase of the ovulatory cycle, when the released egg (corpus luteum) is traveling to the uterus via the fallopian tubes. This phase occurs over a period of approximately 14 days and is accompanied by the release of progesterone by the corpus luteum. By definition, PMS symptoms can occur only during the luteal phase; otherwise, symptoms may be attributed to some other dysfunction, or a combination of PMS and another dysfunction.[27]

The physical symptoms and signs of PMS are extremely variable.[28] Some women experience breast tenderness and swelling, accompanied and related to a sense of bloating, secondary to water retention.[28] Others experience backaches and headaches of unknown etiology, whereas still others report a craving for sweet and salty foods.[26] Transient weight gain is often associated with PMS, primarily as a result of water retention.[28] Perhaps the most common symptoms affecting female athletes are the onset of menstrual cramps and a general feeling of fatigue.

Although these physical signs and symptoms can certainly affect performance, the psychological and emotional changes associated with PMS can be even more important factors in athletic performance. The physical fatigue that accompanies PMS can result in a feeling of lethargy and decreased motivation for physical training or performance. Often this feeling of lethargy is accompanied by bursts of energy that sometimes leads to compulsive behavior such as excessive and harmful training. Similarly, mood swings are not uncommon, ranging from feelings of inadequacy and depression to aggression and irritability.

Premenstrual syndrome is diagnosed primarily via the medical and physical/emotional history.[28] Many treatments have been tried, including modification of dietary intake, medication, and interestingly enough, exercise.

In terms of medication, supplementation of vitamin B$_6$ (pyroxidine) has met limited success.[29] Diuretics are frequently used to offset the water retention associated with PMS. Other medications, such as bromocriptine and danazol, may decrease PMS symptoms via inhibition of prolactin, estrogen, and progesterone.[30,31] There is still a great deal of controversy regarding the effects of such medications and the indications for their use.

The physiological and psychological benefits of exercise may offset some symptoms associated with PMS. The release of endorphins in the central nervous system (CNS) may occur with aerobic exercise, and this chemical has a tranquilizing effect. Muscle relaxation has, indeed, been reported as a result of aerobic exercise.[32] In addition, psychological effects of exercise such as decreased anxiety and aggression and increased self-esteem,[7] can offset the depression and sense of frustration that may occur with PMS. It should be noted, however, that low-intensity, sustained exercise seems to be more effective in evoking such responses than high-intensity, short bursts of activity.[7]

Dietary modification can be an important adjunct in prevention or control of PMS signs and symptoms. Eating several small meals throughout the day can counter the development of low blood glucose levels which contribute to irritability and mood swings.[29] Other suggestions include limiting salt, sugar, and fat intake as well as eliminating caffeine and alcohol from the diet.[29]

In some individuals, the effects of PMS may be rather profound and may certainly interfere with athletic performance. Although modification of dietary and exercise patterns may provide some benefit, when PMS becomes disruptive to an athlete's function, medical advice should be sought. Recognition of PMS as a treatable condition has been a recent occurrence, and further research in terms of understanding PMS can only lead to more effective management.

Dysmenorrhea. Although PMS is a rather current topic of concern for many women, other menstrual irregularities such as dysmenorrhea, oligomenorrhea, and amenorrhea are well recognized and are perhaps better understood. Dysmenorrhea refers to painful menstruation and is most commonly characterized by abdominal pain and cramping several days before or during menstrual flow.[33] Primary or essential dysmenorrhea has no demonstrable cause,[34] although it has been found that increased levels of prostaglandins are associated with painful contraction of the muscles of the uterus.[35] Secondary dysmenorrhea, on the other hand, results from pelvic lesions.[34]

Although the symptoms of primary and secondary dysmenorrhea are the same, each has some distinguishing clinical characteristics. Primary dysmenorrhea occurs only during ovulatory cycles and the onset is usually before 20 years of age. It is characterized by abdominal or lower back pain or both, and usually lasts for less than 72 hours. In the case of secondary dysmenorrhea, however, the timing and duration of symptoms may be different and can be due to organic pelvic diseases such as endometriosis, inflammatory diseases, or tumors. For this reason it is extremely important that

the cause of menstrual pain be determined by a gynecologist.

The mechanism for cramping associated with primary dysmenorrhea is related to hormonal changes during the ovulatory phase. Among these changes, an increase in the production of prostaglandins appears to be a causal factor in the onset of abdominal cramps.[36] Prostaglandins are a group of naturally occurring free fatty acids (FFAs), which increase uterine muscle contractility, decrease uterine blood flow, and sensitize afferent uterine nerve endings.[36] These effects are thought to result in menstrual cramping.

Nonsteroidal anti-inflammatory drugs (NSAIDs) are often prescribed for dysmenorrhea because they are prostaglandin inhibitors. Several actions of these pharmacological agents have been proposed, including inhibition of cyclo-oxygenase, an enzyme necessary for prostaglandin synthesis, and interference with prostaglandin binding at receptor sites.[36] Nonsteroidal anti-inflammatory agents have some undesirable side effects, the most common of which is gastrointestinal irritation, and in some cases oral contraceptive therapy is an alternative. Combined progestin–estrogen agents work via inhibition of ovulation and possibly by decreasing prostaglandin production.[36] Oral contraceptive agents are a secondary measure, reserved for instances when NSAIDs are not tolerated or do not relieve symptoms, and when contraception is desired by the patient.

The recommended timing for use of antiprostaglandins is to begin at the time of onset of the symptoms and to continue for 2 or 3 days.[36] Since medications are highly variable with respect to their efficacy for individuals, it may be necessary to try several different compounds before finding one that works. Table 9–4 provides some guidelines for use of various NSAIDs for the control of menstrual cramps.

Dysmenorrhea is often accompanied by heavy menstrual bleeding, and both of these factors may exert a negative effect upon athletic performance. It should be noted that the NSAIDs described previously also tend to decrease menstrual flow. There is certainly no contraindication to physical exercise in the presence of dysmenorrhea; in fact, sustained aerobic exercise may actually decrease menstrual pain via release of endorphins in the CNS.

Amenorrhea and Oligomenorrhea. It has become apparent in recent years that high levels of athletic activity are related to the incidence of amenorrhea (absence of menstruation) and oligomenorrhea (abnormally infrequent menstruation). It has been shown that primary amenorrhea, or failure of the onset of menstruation at puberty, is more prevalent in athletes than nonathletes.[33] Moreover, female athletes also tend to exhibit a higher incidence of secondary amenorrhea,[37] or cessation of menses for at least 6 months in a woman who has previously had menstrual periods.

Recent reports have suggested that many different factors may contribute to amenorrhea, and it is interesting to note that these same factors are those to which an athlete is often subjected to during training. These include weight loss, low body weight, low body fat, dietary and nutritional deficiencies, physical and emotional stress, and acute and chronic hormonal alterations.[38]

Rapid weight loss has been cited as one of the most common causes of secondary amenorrhea.[39] Female athletes, particularly those involved in endurance training, tend to lose both weight and body fat as a result of training. It has been suggested that there exists a critical level of body fat, below which women become amenorrheic.[40] Although some studies have validated this claim,[41,42] there is still some controversy in this area, as there are many normally menstruating (eumenorrheic) athletes who demonstrate abnormally low body fat content.

There is another theory, as yet unproven, regarding the relationship between body fat content and amenorrhea. It is fairly well accepted that when an individual loses weight, the basal metabolic rate decreases. Amenorrhea may occur as a result of a protective mechanism whereby the body senses that insufficient energy exists in the form of stored fat to support pregnancy and lactation. It has been noted, however, that more specifically, loss of body fat from the lower body seems to predispose a woman to amenorrhea to a greater degree than loss of upper body fat.[43]

There is also evidence that nutritional deficiency may play a role in amenorrhea. Female athletes, especially endurance athletes, often modify their diets so that they consume fewer calories, less fat, less calcium, and less red meat.[44] In addition, it has been suggested that amenorrheic runners may not consume sufficient amounts of cholesterol to produce adequate amounts of estrogen, but there remains some controversy regarding this issue.[38]

Emotional and physical stress have also been proposed as causative factors in athletic amenorrhea. Al-

TABLE 9-4. NONSTEROIDAL ANTI-INFLAMMATORY DRUGS FOR CONTROL OF MENSTRUAL PAIN

Drug	Trade Name	Dose
Ibuprofen	Motrin, Nuprin, Advil Medipren	400 mg qid
Naproxin	Naprosyn	250 mg bid
Naproxin sodium	Anaprox	275 mg qid
Mefenamic acid	Ponstel	250 mg qid
Diflunisol	Dolobid	200 mg tid

From Chaper FK. Primary dysmenorrhea. Presented at Hawkey Sportsmedicine Symposium; April 17, 1986; Iowa City, Ia, with permission.

though there is general agreement regarding the relationship between the physical demands of training and amenorrhea,[42,45] there is some controversy with respect to the contribution of emotional and psychological stress.[45,46] Therefore, stress may play an additive role in amenorrhea, but does not appear to be an independent or primary causative factor.

There is some evidence that follicular and luteal phase lengths may be altered in athletic women. Several studies have demonstrated an inverse relationship between intensive training and length of the luteal phase.[47,48] Luteal phase deficiency has been associated with infertility,[49] although phase length tends to normalize with the cessation of intense training.[48]

The relationship between endurance exercise and amenorrhea has led to speculation that chronic hormonal changes occurring with exercise may play a role in amenorrhea. Although decreased levels of estradiol, FSH, and LH have been found in amenorrheic athletes, no consistent pattern of hormonal alteration has been identified.[50] The increase in cortisol and β-endorphin levels that occur with chronic exercise have also been implicated as contributing factors in athletic amenorrhea.[51,52] An increase in circulating β-endorphin may suppress the frequency of gonadotropin pulses and thereby alter FSH and LH production.[51,52]

The signs and symptoms of exercise-induced menstrual irregularities are often similar to those associated with pathological conditions; therefore, all dysmenorrheic, oligomenorrheic, and amenorrheic athletes should be referred for medical evaluation. Initial evaluation of oligomenorrhea and amenorrhea should include the following: (1) history, (2) physical examination including a pelvic examination, (3) thyroid function tests, (4) evaluation of prolactin, thyroid-stimulating hormone (TSH), FSH, LH, and human chorionic gonadotropin (hCG) levels, and (5) progesterone challenge test.[38] When estrogen levels are normal, treatment, which depends on the patient's desire for fertility or contraception, may include progestin therapy, use of oral contraceptives, or use of chlomibene citrate.[38] These same measures have been used in the case of hypoestrogenic amenorrhea, with some additional alternatives including cyclic estrogen therapy, weight gain, or reduction in exercise intensity.[38] Because these menstrual disorders are so diverse in symptomatology and may involve complex interactions of numerous contributing factors, gynecological referral is recommended.

Contraception

There is no evidence to indicate that contraceptive devices such as foams, sponges, diaphragms, or condoms have any negative effects upon athletic performance.[33] Low-dose oral contraceptives, or birth control pills containing less than 35 μg of ethinyl estradiol, may ac-

tually pose some benefits to athletic women, including a decrease in incidence of irregular or heavy bleeding or both as well as a decrease in incidence of benign breast tumors and endometrial and ovarian cancer.[38] Oral contraceptives, especially when taken in higher doses (35 to above 50 μg ethinyl estradiol) may have some adverse effects upon the athletic performance, including weight gain, increased blood lipid and body fat content, and water retention.[33] It has been suggested, however, that these potentially adverse effects are less likely to occur with the use of low-dose oral contraceptives, and that regular exercise tends to offset some negative effects, particularly hemolytic changes and increased blood lipid levels.[38]

Pregnancy

Although pregnancy is certainly not common among high school and intercollegiate athletes, it should be noted that 11% of all United States women between the ages of 15 and 45 years are pregnant at any given time and that 50% of American women are sexually active before age 20.[53] For this reason it is extremely important that the sports physical therapist be familiar with the effects of pregnancy upon exercise as well as the effects of exercise upon pregnancy. In addition, precautions and recommendations must be given to pregnant women athletes, and guidelines must be provided with respect to postpartum exercise. To be sure, recommendations with respect to exercise during pregnancy have changed a great deal over recent years; nevertheless, there is still some controversy regarding optimal levels of exercise during pregnancy because much of the knowledge base in this area has been derived from anecdotal reports and animal studies, as opposed to well-controlled research lending physiological data on the interaction of exercise and pregnancy.

The physiological effects of pregnancy are numerous, and many of the gestational changes that occur can affect exercise tolerance. These include musculoskeletal changes, adaptations in energy metabolism, cardiorespiratory changes, altered blood flow, and an altered ability for physical work. These physiological adaptations are discussed as they pertain to the normal pregnant woman.

In addition to the weight gain associated with pregnancy, there are some marked changes in soft tissue extensibility and posture. Ground substance and connective tissues become softer and more extensible secondary to an increase in gestational hormones.[54,55] This results in a generalized increase in joint laxity, particularly affecting the pubic symphysis and sacroiliac joints.[54] Related to this is the rather common presentation of the pregnant woman with lower back pain, muscle spasm, and difficulty with ambulation as well as other activities of daily living. Such symptoms are sometimes exacerbated by the compensatory lumbar

lordosis that results from a forward displacement of the center of gravity with pregnancy.[55,56] Additional postural changes include anterior tilt of the pelvis, thoracic kyphosis, cervical lordosis, and genu recurvatum.[53,55,56]

It has been shown that pregnant women have an increased metabolic requirement of approximately 300 kcal/d, with an even greater additional caloric requirement if they are physically active.[55–57] In addition, the pregnant woman tends to burn more carbohydrates than normal during exercise, and hypoglycemia may result from sustained or intense exercise.[55] This may be related to the finding that plasma glucose levels are depressed, especially in the third trimester, presumably as a result of fetal energy requirements.[54] This occurs in part as a result of elevated plasma insulin levels in late pregnancy, possibly in response to the anti-insulin effect of placental hormones.[54]

Most of the cardiorespiratory changes associated with pregnancy are a result of a decrease in systemic vascular resistance secondary to increased blood flow to the uterus and the effect of high progesterone levels in terms of decreasing vascular tone.[58] As a result, an increase in blood volume on the order of 30% to 50% occurs as a compensatory mechanism.[53,56,58] This increase in blood volume in turn results in a compensatory increase in stroke volume as well as cardiac output.[58] Stroke volume typically increases during early pregnancy and then decreases near term, while resting cardiac output increases 30% to 50% by 20 to 24 weeks, then levels off.[59] In addition, the heart rate increases by 10 to 15 beats per minute up until approximately 32 weeks, at which time heart rate returns to normal levels near term.[53,59] Respiration is likewise affected, with increased tidal volumes during pregnancy and an increase in respiratory minute volume up to 40%.[53,56] These adaptations are accompanied by significant decreases in expiratory reserve volume and residual volume, though they are thought to pose no problems during exercise, as the respiratory system has the ability to increase capacity up to tenfold during exercise.[53,56]

The physical increase in size of the uterus may obstruct blood flow in the vena cava in the supine position, with a reduction in cardiac output up to 50%. This has been described as the supine hypotensive syndrome, and when cardiac output is increased as a result of exercise, it is possible that positional changes may result in an increased tendency for such hemodynamic changes.[58]

The increase in fluid volume observed in pregnant women has several implications. Combined with the partial obstruction of blood flow in the iliac veins during standing, this may result in a lower-extremity edema.[53,56] In addition, increases in plasma volume are observed in all pregnant animals, and this is considered to be a significant adaptation necessary for normal pregnancy and delivery. Indeed, many complications of pregnancy are associated with failure of the maternal expansion of plasma volume.[54]

There is some evidence that energy requirements for weight-bearing tasks may be greater for pregnant women than for nonpregnant women. It has been estimated that approximately 20% more energy is required for activities such as walking or running as a result of the increased weight associated with pregnancy.[58] This has been validated through the study of oxygen uptake in pregnant versus nonpregnant women performing graded exercise tests both on a treadmill and on a stationary cycle.[60] Oxygen uptake was significantly greater for pregnant women both at rest and during treadmill running, with no significant difference between pregnant and nonpregnant groups on the cycling activity.[60] In addition, pregnant women have demonstrated lower values for maximum oxygen uptake than nonpregnant individuals during exercise.[53]

All of the aforementioned physiological adaptations to pregnancy have an effect upon exercise performance. Connective tissue laxity, which may result in joint instability, may cause a predisposition toward ligamentous injuries during athletic activity. Postural changes may place unusual stress to the lumbar spine and may inhibit mobility and balance. The decrease in blood glucose levels that accompanies the later phases of pregnancy may predispose the exercising woman to hypoglycemia during pregnancy. The increased cardiovascular demand associated with pregnancy may be related to the decreased levels of physical work capacity and a lower maximum oxygen uptake. Lastly, a lack of adrenergic activity is known to decrease vascular resistance and increase plasma volume, changes that are associated with normal pregnancy, whereas acute exercise may inhibit maternal plasma volume expansion, as it tends to stimulate adrenergic activity. Although the long-term effects of this consequence are unknown at this time, each of these factors must be considered when recommending exercise programs for pregnant women.

There is a great deal of controversy surrounding the effects of exercise on pregnancy. There is some evidence that strenuous exercise may result in heart rates as high as 200 beats per minute (bpm), with systolic blood pressure increasing by as much as 30 to 40 mm Hg.[61] Although it is not known whether these acute changes in heart rate and blood pressure are detrimental to the fetus, it has been demonstrated that training during pregnancy results in improved maximum oxygen consumption values in both pregnant women and in animals.[58]

During exercise, muscular demand for oxygen results in a diversion of blood flow from the uterus to

exercising muscles, with a net decrease in maternal uterine blood flow both immediately at the onset of exercise and throughout the exercise.[54,62] In fact, uterine blood flow may be reduced by as much as 35%, and is characterized by an inverse and linear relationship to heart rate during exercise.[63] It has been suggested, however, that despite decreased uterine blood flow, fetal oxygen consumption may be maintained via compensatory hemoconcentration or increased oxygen content in the placental exchange area so that oxygen delivery to the uterus decreases minimally during exercise as opposed to during rest.[64] On this basis, fetal hypoxia does not appear to be a significant factor in exercise.

Another consequence of exercise is an increase in maternal core temperature. There appears to be a critical teratogenic level for core temperature during early pregnancy, and elevation of core temperature during the first trimester, whether it be via fever or through exercise, may be associated with higher than normal incidences of abnormal newborns.[54] It should be noted that fetal temperature is already 0.5%C higher than maternal body temperature as a result of a higher fetal metabolic rate, and because of limitations in heat transfer from the fetus through the placental membrane.[58] This is an important concern with regard to exercise, particularly strenuous exercise undertaken in hot or humid weather conditions.

Several studies have investigated the effects of exercise on pregnancy, demonstrating an increase in physical work capacity with training, and none of these studies have come to the conclusion that exercise is detrimental to the pregnant woman.[65-67] Moreover, there is some evidence that moderate aerobic exercise during pregnancy results in a decreased duration of labor with less pain and a faster recovery.[67,68] Nonetheless, a recent study based on interviews with 336 pregnant women concluded that women who exercised regularly prior to and during pregnancy delivered newborns with weights significantly below controls and had a 38% incidence of birth-retarded newborns compared to 11% for controls.[69] This was probably one of the most detailed studies and used a large number of subjects (N = 336), but it should be noted that only 29 of these subjects had exercised both prior to and during their pregnancy. The lack of well-controlled experimental studies that are necessarily limited by ethical considerations makes it difficult to draw conclusions about the effects of exercise upon pregnancy outcome.

It seems that pregnancy outcome may depend more upon general health and level of conditioning prior to pregnancy than exercise interventions during pregnancy.[54] It is logical that if exercise promotes the tranquility associated with decreased adrenergic activity and increased plasma volumes, then exercise would have a beneficial effect upon pregnancy outcome. It is

well agreed, however, that in cases of abnormal or complicated pregnancy, including maternal hypertension or increased venous tone, strenuous exercise during pregnancy is not advisable.[54]

Understandably, most published research with respect to the effects of exercise during pregnancy err on the side of caution. Some specific suggestions relating to the aforementioned relationship between exercise and pregnancy are in order. In 1985, The American College of Obstetricians and Gynecologists published guidelines for exercise during pregnancy and postpartum (Table 9–5),[70] and in the same year Maeder[71] provided some additional recommendations as well (Table 9–6). It must be acknowledged that exercise during pregnancy is not without risk. In practice, physical therapists often use the analogy that exercise is like medicine, and

TABLE 9-5. ACOG GUIDELINES FOR EXERCISE DURING PREGNANCY AND POSTPARTUM

1. Regular exercise (at least three times per week) is preferable to intermittent activity. Competitive activities should be discouraged.
2. Vigorous exercise should not be performed in hot, humid weather or during a period of febrile illness.
3. Ballistic movements (jerky, bouncy motions) should be avoided. Exercise should be done on a wooden floor or a tightly carpeted surface to reduce shock and to provide a sure footing.
4. Deep flexion or extension of joints should be avoided because of connective tissue laxity. Activities that require jumping, jarring motions, or rapid changes in direction should be avoided because of joint instability.
5. Vigorous exercise should be preceded by a 5-minute period of muscle warmup. This can be accomplished by slow walking or stationary cycling with low resistance.
6. Vigorous exercise should be followed by a period of gradually declining activity that includes gentle stationary stretching. Because connective tissue laxity increases the risk of joint injury, stretches should not be taken to the point of maximum resistance.
7. Heart rate should be measured at times of peak activity. Target heart rates and limits established in consultation with the physician should not be exceeded.
8. Care should be taken to gradually rise from the floor to avoid orthostatic hypotension. Some form of activity involving the legs should be continued for a brief period.
9. Liquids should be taken liberally before and after exercise to prevent dehydration. If necessary, activity should be interrupted to replenish fluids.
10. Women who have led sedentary lifestyles should begin with physical activity of very low intensity and advance activity levels very gradually.
11. Activity should be stopped and the physician consulted if any unusual symptoms appear. These include pain, bleeding, dizziness, faintness, shortness of breath, palpitations, tachycardia, back or pubic pain, or difficulty walking.

From The American College of Obstetricians and Gynecologists. Exercise During Pregnancy and the Postnatal Period (ACOG Home Exercise Programs). Washington, DC: ACOG Resource Center; 1985, p 4, with permission.

TABLE 9-6. EXERCISE GUIDELINES FOR PREGNANT PATIENTS

1. Do not suddenly increase the amount of exercise undertaken.
2. Do not exceed the amount of exercise normally undertaken before pregnancy.
3. Eliminate sports in which the risk of injury is high, e.g., waterskiing.
4. Late in pregnancy, avoid excessive aerobic exercise, e.g., long-distance running.
5. Avoid exercises that require lying on the back.
6. Avoid activities where balance is of major importance.
7. In the latter part of pregnancy, avoid activities likely to cause joint strains.
8. Avoid changing positions quickly (to prevent dizziness).
9. Wear good supportive footwear and adequate breast support while exercising.
10. Do not exercise to the point of exhaustion or severe breathlessness.
11. Remember the importance of good nutrition when undertaking an exercise program.
12. Monitor pulse rate and keep within the recommended target zone.

From Maeder EC. Effects of sports and exercise in pregnancy. Postgrad Med. *1985; 77:112, with permission.*

this is certainly true with respect to pregnancy. The duration, intensity, and frequency must be carefully controlled for normal pregnant women, and exercise may not be indicated at all for individuals at risk for abnormalities or complicated pregnancies.

EATING DISORDERS

Definitions

When discussing eating disorders, it is useful to make a distinction among bulimia, bulimarexia, and anorexia nervosa. Bulimics go on binges of eating large quantities of food and then rid themselves of it by self-induced vomiting or the use of laxatives or diuretics. Bulimarexia is characterized by alternating bouts of starving and overeating. Bulimarectics may consume 15,000 to 20,000 calories in 1 day, and this may be followed by periods of starvation lasting for 4 or 5 days. Anorexia nervosa is a more general term for an eating disorder that involves self-starvation caused by a fear of becoming overweight. Anorectic behavior usually involves a combination of bulimia and bulimarexia.

Incidence

Estimates are that 1% to 5% of all women in the United States suffer from some kind of eating disorder, and these disorders are most common in women between the ages of 12 and 25.[72] Many times, eating disorders are brought on by stressful events such as parental divorce, rejection, or the expectation for a high level of performance with regard to athletics. It is interesting to note that those individuals afflicted by this disorder generally come from middle to upper class homes; they

are often good students and self-disciplined individuals who have an above average understanding of body physiology but exhibit an abnormal anxiety regarding weight gain.

Recognition

Of all the injuries and disorders identified in athletics, eating disorders are probably one of the most severe because they are potentially fatal. It is extremely important that coaches, sports physical therapists, and athletic trainers have an awareness of these syndromes because they are often the first to recognize the symptoms and are in a good position to initiate proper care for such individuals.

The cause of anorexia nervosa is unknown, but it is thought to be a disorder of psychological origin, yet many researchers believe that patients have a physiological predisposition to anorexia nervosa that is triggered by psychosocial stresses. In athletics, the preoccupation with a low percentage of body fat sometimes causes coaches to pressure their athletes to lose weight, and this may be transferred to self-imposed pressure by an athlete. Initial weight loss may cause a sense of accomplishment, often accompanied by positive reinforcement from an athlete's peers and coaches. It has been proposed that rapid weight loss via decreased food intake and increased physical activity may even be an unconscious attempt to reproduce the good feeling that accompanies compliments regarding weight loss and further serves to drive the cycle.[72] In some instances, the athlete comes from a domineering family and has little control over her life. By starving herself she takes control over her dietary intake and body weight. Family pressure to exhibit "perfect behavior" or to perform better also contributes to these other factors.

There are several behavioral aspects of this disorder that should be recognized by athletic trainers, sports physical therapists, and coaches. In general, these include emotional maladjustment, aberration in eating patterns, and manifestation of a disproportionate view of body weight status. Some of the most common signs of symptoms of such eating disorders include (1) insecurity, poor self-image, and lack of confidence in abilities, (2) organizing food on a plate, dawdling over food, (3) obsession with counting calories, (4) abnormal social isolation, withdrawal from family and friends, (5) excessive exercise in attempts to expend calories, often right before a meal, (6) bulimia, (7) overestimation of body size, (8) related disorders such as malnutrition, dental caries, amenorrhea, and general malaise, (9) obsession with measuring body weight, and (10) use of diuretics and laxatives.

Treatment

It is extremely important that any and all signs and symptoms should be recognized, and immediate treatment

should be initiated, as this can be a life-threatening disorder. The first line of action should be to notify the family physician, who is in a position to refer the patient for appropriate psychological counseling should the necessity be present. It is rather important that the athlete see someone whom she can trust, as this clinical presentation is characterized by a tendency to hide abnormal behavior and symptoms. Counseling is probably the most significant intervention, as this allows the athlete to deal with resolution of the underlying emotional problems. It is usually not productive for coaches and teammates to point out the athlete's abnormal eating habits, and the sooner psychological counseling is initiated, the better the chance of cure. In severe cases, patients do not respond to therapy, and although many patients improve considerably there is a significantly high percentage of individuals who maintain long-term vulnerability to this disorder.[73]

Prevention

It is interesting that although this is a potentially life-threatening disorder, there are no guidelines as yet for screening nutritionally deficient athletes from sports participation. In 1984, Clark proposed several guidelines with respect to identifying athletes suspected of anorectic tendencies and providing some guidelines with regard to monitoring their eating behavior.[74] These include the following requirements: (1) provide a weight and diet history, including present weight, desired weight, highest and lowest weight, and current height and weight as a child; (2) keep a log of eating and activity patterns; (3) the trainer or sports physical therapist should estimate the athlete's caloric needs; (4) the trainer or sports physical therapist should design a normal eating pattern for the athlete; and (5) the trainer or sports physical therapist should emphasize the role of food as an energizing fuel and foundation for good health.

PATELLOFEMORAL DYSFUNCTION

Definition

Patellofemoral dysfunction is common among female athletes, particularly those participating in running and jumping activities. Its widespread incidence has brought about a rehabilitative challenge to athletic trainers and sports physical therapists. Patellofemoral dysfunction is a rather broad category that refers to irritation, inflammation, or pain under or around the patellofemoral joint. The spectrum of patellofemoral disorders may be placed on a continuum ranging from relatively minor sport aches such as patellar tendonitis or peripatellar inflammation to more disabling conditions such as chondromalacia patella, medial plica syndrome, patellar dislocation and patellar subluxation.

Indeed almost any pain or dysfunction affecting the distal extensor mechanism has been referred to as patellofemoral dysfunction.

Causative Factors

Causative factors for this syndrome may be subdivided into static and dynamic factors. Malalignments and anatomic variables that may be observed statically include femoral anteversion, external tibial torsion, shallow patellofemoral groove, excessive Q angle, foot pronation, patella alta, patella baja, lateral displacement of the tibial tubercle, lateral tilt of the patella, external rotation of the patella, inferior tilt of the patella, femoral internal rotation, tight lateral retinaculam, and tight iliotibial band. Although any combination of these factors may contribute to the onset of patellofemoral dysfunction, dynamic factors that may be observed via muscle testing and observation may play an even more important role. These include tight hamstrings, tight gastrocnemius, vastus medialis obliquus insufficiency, gluteus medius weakness, and extensor mechanism weakness. It is extremely important that the physician and the sports physical therapist work together to identify such static and dynamic components, as treatment will only be effective if it is specifically directed at causative factors.

Signs and Symptoms

The static and dynamic factors mentioned above all contribute to malalignment, which may affect the orientation of the patella during activity. Most of the symptoms associated with this broad category of dysfunction are a result of abnormal mechanical stress, which leads to a sequelae of events. Often mild swelling is observable at the patellofemoral joint, and this may be a significant factor in inhibiting extensor mechanism function, particularly the vastus medialis obliquus (VMO).[75] The VMO is primarily responsible for realigning the patella medially and providing dynamic medial stability through the entire range of motion (ROM).[76,77] In the case of VMO insufficiency, the patella tends to track laterally during quadriceps activity, as no counterforce offsets the pull of the vastus lateralis. This may result in a change in the patellofemoral contact areas through the range of motion, and the abnormal stresses associated with this malalignment may be a primary factor in patellofemoral pain.[78]

The most common symptoms of patellofemoral dysfunction include a generalized pain over the anterior aspect of the knee, crepitus, stiffness after prolonged postural positions, tenderness to palpation of the patella, pain worsened by stair negotiation and squatting, buckling, clicking, or catching, and pain after activity. Swelling is usually not a hallmark of patellofemoral dysfunction, although sometimes mild swelling can be measured or observed. The clinical presentation

can be extremely varied, however, and it is important to rule out other possible dysfunctions such as bursitis or meniscal and ligamentous lesions.

Evaluation

The history and subjective assessment can provide a great deal of information at the outset of the evaluation. Often the female athlete will report a sudden increase in the quantity or intensity of her activity level that immediately preceded the onset of her symptoms. Previous injury to other lower extremity joints may also predispose the athlete to patellofemoral dysfunction, particularly in the case of previous knee surgery with incomplete rehabilitation. Sometimes young athletes will present with patellofemoral dysfunction during or after a growth spurt. Athletes involved in repetitive motor activities should be questioned with respect to athletic footwear and training surfaces. Subjective information such as when the pain occurs, where it occurs, and its nature is also an important factor in evaluation.

Radiographic assessment provides information about the presence of arthritic changes or spurs, the adequacy of the femoral trochlea groove and condyle height, superior/inferior or medial/lateral position of the patella, and presence of bone pathology such as fracture or tumor. Adequacy of the femoral trochlea groove is generally evaluated on the skyline or sunrise view, and a flattened groove or a lateral condyle height less than 4.5 mm higher than the medial condyle is an indication of a tendency for patellar subluxation or dislocation.[79] Lateral x-ray films taken at 45 to 50 degrees of flexion are helpful in evaluating a patella alta and patella baja, the former meaning that the patellar tendon is 20% or more longer than the diameter of the patella, and the latter meaning that the patellar tendon is 20% or more shorter than the patellar diameter.[80] Computed tomography, with an injection of contrast material, permits visualization of articular surfaces for assessment of the integrity of articular cartilage.[80]

With the patient in the sitting position, the sports physical therapist should visually evaluate for the presence of patella alta or baja, squinting or grasshopper eye patellae, patellar tracking during active extension, and patellar tracking or reproduction of pain during isometric extension done at flexion angles of 30, 60, and 90 degrees. When the patellae are squinting, the medial pole is more posterior than the lateral pole; when the patellae are in a grasshopper eye position, the lateral pole is more posterior than the medial pole. The presence of squinting patellae is an indication of internal femoral rotation, whereas grasshopper eye patellae indicates external rotation of the femur. As the patient performs active knee extension, it is important for the sports physical therapist to observe the tracking of the patellae, with particular attention to the orientation of

the patellae at 20 or 30 degrees of flexion, as this is the position in which patellar subluxation is most likely to occur. An increase in peripatellar pain on isometric extension done at knee flexion angles of 30, 60, and 90 degrees is not, in and of itself, diagnostic, but if the pain is relieved when the sports physical therapist applies manual pressure to the patella in a medial direction, it is likely that the tracking problem exists.[78]

Several preliminary tests are performed with the patient in the supine position. These include hip and back clearing tests, as well as tests for meniscal and ligamentous pathology. With the athlete in this position, the sports physical therapist should also evaluate hip flexor, gastrocnemius, and flexibility of the hamstrings. The orientation of the patella with respect to glide, tilt, rotation, and anterior/posterior position is also done in the supine position.

Assessment of patella orientation has been described in detail by McConnell[81] and the following methods for determining the orientation of the patella has been derived from her work. The component of static glide is determined by comparing the distance between the medial femoral condyle and the midpoint of the patella with the distance between the lateral femoral condyle and the midpoint of the patella. When the distance between the lateral femoral condyle and the midpoint of the patella is less than the distance between the medial femoral condyle and the midpoint of the patella, lateral glide is said to exist. This may also be assessed dynamically by observing the patellar movement during a quadriceps set performed very slowly. Lateral patellar glide is characterized by supralateral movement of the patella, with delayed firing of the VMO. Static tilt refers to the height of the medial patellar pole compared to the lateral patellar pole, with lateral tilt characterized by a posterior position of the lateral pole relative to the medial pole. This may be assessed statically simply by observation, but should also be assessed dynamically, by manually gliding the patella medially. If the patella scoops upward on the medial side during medial glide, the deep lateral retinacular structures are tight.

The rotational component of the patella is assessed by placing the fingers at the widest points of the medial and lateral patellar poles and comparing an imaginary line drawn between them to the long axis of the femur. The intersection of these two lines should be perpendicular, but when the patellar is externally rotated the most medial point of the patella is inferior to the most lateral point, with the opposite occurring in the case of internal patellar rotation. The static anterior/posterior component of patellar orientation is assessed via observation of tilt, inferior tilt characterized by a relatively posterior position of the inferior pole compared to the anterior pole and superior tilt characterized by a relatively posterior position of the anterior pole compared

to the inferior pole. This should also be assessed dynamically by asking the patient to perform a quadriceps set and observing any change of position in patellar orientation. If the inferior pole becomes buried in the fat pad during the quadriceps contraction, the patella is said to be inferiorly tilted.

Postural alignment is evaluated in the standing position via observation from the front, the side, and the rear. All lower extremity joints should be scrutinized for the presence of biomechanical abnormalities, which may be contributing factors to a patellofemoral dysfunction. In this position the presence of genuvalgus may be apparent, and this provides an opportunity for assessment of the amount of tibial torsion as well. Normally the tibia is externally rotated approximately 15 degrees, but more external rotation will often be observed in patients presenting with patellofemoral dysfunction. Likewise, foot position, including both fore foot and rear foot position, should be assessed with the patient in the standing posture.

Assessment of dynamic alignment via observation of gait is one of the most important components of evaluation. Again, biomechanical abnormalities for all lower extremity joints must be observed at the various phases of the gait pattern, including heel strike, stance phase, pushoff, and swing phase. It is often helpful to use videotape in assessing dynamic alignment, as this permits the sports physical therapist to view the gait pattern in slow motion, often revealing abnormalities that are not apparent upon visual observation.

McConnell[78] also describes a functional test involving negotiation of a step or repetitive unilateral squatting. These tests are performed in an attempt to reproduce the patient's pain and for the purpose of comparing function before and after treatment. It is essential that the patient perform these activities slowly, as the sports physical therapist observes for symmetry and gathers subjective information about the presence and location of pain.

Treatment

Palliative measures designed to reduce inflammation are somewhat effective in dealing with patellofemoral dysfunction. This includes ice packs or ice massage, NSAIDs, and decreased levels of activity. Although most patients respond favorably to these interventions, the aim of treatment is to remove as many causative factors as possible.

Once the assessment has been completed, and causative factors have been determined, the sports physical therapist should promote restoration of normal function in improving biomechanical abnormalities via strengthening, stretching, muscle reeducation, and use of orthotics. Sustained, low-intensity stretching should be used to increase the flexibility of the hamstrings, quadriceps, iliotibial band, and gastrocnemius mus-

cles. If hip abductors are weak, they should be strengthened, and an attempt should be made to normalize the weight-bearing pattern by strengthening of foot intrinsic musculature or use of orthotics or athletic shoe prescription. Stretching may be used to improve flexibility of lateral retinacular structures.

Strengthening of the extensor mechanism can present a dilemma to the sports physical therapist because many of the exercises that are most effective at improving strength are also extremely irritating to the patellofemoral joint. Isolated quadriceps strengthening may be done safely through straight leg raising preceded by a quadriceps set, and by submaximal isotonic and isometric leg extension within the patient's pain tolerance. Closed kinetic chain activities, done for the purpose of improving total limb strength, seem to be less irritating to the patellofemoral joint, yet provide functional strengthening with both eccentric and concentric components.

McConnell has suggested that it is important to change the timing of the VMO contraction so that the VMO fires prior to or simultaneously with the vastus lateralis.[81] Vastus medialis obliquus muscle reeducation may be done initially in the sitting position with the patient's knee slightly flexed, using manual contact for feedback as the patient attempts to fire the VMO.[78] This is followed by VMO reeducation in more functional positions such as a standing walk stance,[78] and finally during ambulation. Biofeedback can be extremely helpful in improving the timing of VMO firing.

McConnell has also suggested that taping may be used in order to control the orientation of the patella.[81] For example, if evaluation reveals lateral glide, lateral tilt, inferior tilt, and external rotation of the patella, tape may be applied in such a manner as to improve patellar orientation and decrease symptoms. This has the added benefit of providing some degree of static stretching to tight structures, and permits the patient to perform rehabilitative and reeducation activities free of pain. The technique for application of tape is beyond the scope of this chapter, but the reader is referred to McConnell's article,[81] which appeared in the *Australian Journal of Physical Therapy* in 1986.

Prevention

Many causative factors such as biomechanical malalignment are apparent in individuals before the onset of symptoms. The preseason screening examination should identify such factors and remedial measures should be taken for the prevention of patellofemoral dysfunction. Above all, in terms of quantity and quality, training must progress slowly, and it must be tailored to the individual's needs. Prevention is the key when dealing with patellofemoral dysfunction, as once the symptoms begin, this syndrome may be extremely persistent and difficult to treat.

SUMMARY

The historical perspective of women's participation in sports has been discussed, and some suggestions have been provided with regard to differences between men and women in terms of training and conditioning. Physiological considerations that have a bearing on athletic performance have been identified. Gynecological and obstetric considerations such as menstruation, contraception, and pregnancy have been discussed. Two of the most serious and common disorders afflicting women athletes, eating disorders and patellofemoral dysfunction, have been identified and suggestions made regarding recognition, treatment, and prevention.

During the time that women have been involved in sports, they have continually exceeded expectations, and have, as a group, demonstrated an ever increasing potential for physiological adaptation and improved performance. As such, training methods have become quite rigorous, and injuries are certain to result in such situations. As women continue to expand their athletic potential, it will be the challenge of sports physical therapists, athletic trainers, coaches, and physicians to identify limiting factors, and to develop appropriate preventative and treatment programs to deal with the inevitable injuries and disorders that accompany high levels of competitive training.

REFERENCES

1. Klafs CE, Lyon MJ. *The Female Athlete*. St. Louis, Mo: C V Mosby; 1973.
2. Rice EA, Hutchinson JL, Lee M. *A Brief History of Physical Education*. New York, NY: Ronald Press; 1958.
3. Gerber EW. *The Athletic Woman in Sport*. Reading, Mass: Addison Wesley; 1974.
4. Diem L. The olympic sport for women, evaluation of declarations. *Rev Anal Educ Phys Sport*. 1966; 8:1.
5. NCAA. Athletic injury rates (1982–88). *Athlet Dir Coach*. December 1988; 8.
6. St. Elizabeth Wellness Center. *Guidelines for Health Screenings and Tests*. Lincoln, Neb; 1988.
7. Everly GS, Rosenfeld R. *The Nature and Treatment of the Stress Response*. New York, NY: Plenum Press; 1981:7–9.
8. Atomi Y, Ito K, Isasaki H, Miyashita M. Effects of intensity and frequency of training on aerobic work capacity of young females. *Phys Sportsmed*. 1978; 18(1):3–9.
9. Weltman A, Moffatt R, Stamford BA. Supramaximal training in females: Effects on anaerobic power output, anaerobic capacity and aerobic power. *J Sports Med*. 1978; 8(3):237–244.
10. Cureton KJ, Gieck J, Glass B, et al. Roundtable: Strength and conditioning for the female athlete. *Natl Strength Cond Assoc J*. 1985; 7(3):10–29.
11. Abraham S, Johnson CL, Najjar MF. *Weight and Height of Adults 18–74 Years of Age*. United States Vital and Health Statistics. Washington, DC: United States Government Printing Office; 1979; 11:211.
12. Hunter-Griffin LY. Orthopedic concerns. In: Shangold M, Mirkin G, eds. *Women and Exercise*. Philadelphia, Pa: F A Davis; 1988:195–197.
13. Carter JE. Body composition of Montreal Olympic athletes. In: Carter JE, ed. *Medicine and Sport*. Basel: Karger; 1982.
14. McArdle WD, Katch FI, Katch VL. *Exercise Physiology*. Philadelphia, Pa: Lea & Febiger, 1981.
15. Morrow JR, Hosler WW. Strength comparisons in untrained men and trained women athletes. *Med Sci Sports*. 1981; 13:3.
16. Laubach L. Comparative muscular strength of men and women—Review of literature. *Aviat Space Environ Med*. 1976; 5:534.
17. Schantz P, Randall-Fox E, Hutchison W, et al. Muscle fiber type distribution, muscle cross sectional area and maximal voluntary strength in humans. *Acta Physiol Scand*. 1983; 117(219):219–226.
18. Wilmore JH. *Practice of Pediatrics*. Philadelphia, Pa: Harper & Row, 1984.
19. Berg K. Aerobic function in female athletes. *Clin Sports Med*. 1984; 3:779–789.
20. Astrand I. Aerobic work capacity in men and women with special reference to age. *Acta Physiol Scand*. 1960; 49:169.
21. Astrand PO. Human physical fitness with special reference to sex and age. *Physiol Rev*. 1956; 36:307.
22. Dill DB, Myhre LG, Greer SM, et al. Body composition and aerobic capacity of youth of both sexes. *Med Sci Sports*. 1972; 4(198):198–204.
23. Klaus EJ. The athletic status of women. In: Jokl E, Simon E, eds. *International Research in Sport and Physical Education*. Springfield, Ill: Charles C Thomas; 1964.
24. Astrand PO. Experimental studies of physical working capacity in relation to sex and age. Copenhagen: Munksgaard; 1952.
25. Siegal AJ. Medical conditions arising during sports. In: Shangold M, Mirkin G, eds. *Women and Exercise*. Philadelphia, Pa: F A Davis; 1988:226–229.
26. Havens C. Premenstrual syndrome. *Postgrad Med*. 1985; 77:7.
27. Magos AL, Studd JW. The premenstrual syndrome. In: Studd JW, ed. *Progress in Obstetrics and Gynecology*. Edinburgh: Churchill Livingstone; 1984.
28. Shangold MM. Gynecologic concerns in exercise and training. In: Shangold M, Mirkin G, eds. *Women and Exercise*. Philadelphia, Pa: F A Davis; 1988:189–191.
29. Coleman E. The premenstrual syndrome. In: McKee G, ed. *The Female Athlete—Sportsmedicine Digest Special Report*. Van Nuys, Calif: PM Inc; 1988:15–16.
30. Andersch B. Bromocriptine and premenstrual symptoms: A survey of double blind trials. *Obstet Gynecol Surv*. 1983; 38(643):657–664.
31. Day J. Danazol and the premenstrual syndrome. *Postgrad Med J*. 1979; 55(suppl 5):87–89.
32. DeVries H, Adams G. Electromyographic comparison of single doses of exercise and meprobamate as to effects on muscular relaxation. *Am J Phys Med*. 1972; 52:130.

33. McCoy J. Gynecologic and obstetric concerns in women athletes. Presented at National Athletic Trainers District V Spring Symposium, March 20, 1988; Lincoln, Neb.

34. Friel JP. *Dorland's Pocket Medical Dictionary.* Philadelphia, Pa: W B Saunders; 1977.

35. Shangold MM. The woman runner. *Runners World.* July 1981; 88–89.

36. Chapler FK. Primary dysmenorrhea. Presented at Hawkeye Sportsmedicine Symposium; April 17, 1986; Iowa City, Ia.

37. Carlberg K, Buckman MT, Peake GT. Menstrual dysfunction in athletes. In: Appenzeller O, Atkinson R, eds. *Sports Medicine—Fitness, Training, Injuries.* Urban & Schwarzenberg, Baltimore, Md: 1981:119–133.

38. Shangold MM. Menstruation. In: Shangold M, Mirkin G, eds. *Women and Exercise.* Philadelphia, Pa: F A Davis; 1988:129–144.

39. Frisch RE. Food intake, fatness, and reproductive ability. In: Vigersky RA, ed. *Anorexia Nervosa.* New York, NY: Raven Press; 1977:149–161.

40. Frisch RE. Body fat, puberty and fertility. *Biol Rev.* 1984; 59(2):161–188.

41. Shangold MM, Levine HS. The effect of marathon training on menstrual function. *Am J Obstet Gynecol.* 1982; 143:862.

42. Schwartz B, Cumming DC, Riordan E, et al. Exercise-associated amenorrhea—a distinct entity? *Am J Obstet Gynecol.* 1982; 141:862–869.

43. Brownell K. Eating disorders in the female athlete. *Perf Team Newslett.* 1988; 1(2):9–16.

44. Jaffee L, Webster M, Lutter JM. Dietary differences of amenorrheic and eumenorrheic athletes. *Melphone J.* Fall 1988: 15–19.

45. Sanborn CF, Martin BJ, Wagner WW. Is athletic amenorrhea specific to runners? *Am J Obstet Gynecol.* 1982; 143:859–861.

46. Loucks AB, Horvath SM. Exercise induced stress response of amenorrheic and eumenorrheic runners. *J Clin Endocrin Metab.* 1984; 59:1109–1120.

47. Shangold M, Freeman R, Thysen B, Gatz M. The relationship between long-distance running, plasma progesterone, and luteal phase length. *Fertil Steril* 1979; 3:130–133.

48. Prior JC, Ho Yuen B, Clement P, et al. Reversible luteal phase changes and infertility associated with marathon training. *Lancet.* 1982; 2:269–270.

49. Seegar–Jones G. The clinical evaluation of ovulation and the luteal phase. *J Reprod Med.* 1977; 18:139.

50. Chapler FK. Athletic amenorrhea. Presented at Hawkeye Sportsmedicine Symposium; April 17, 1986; Iowa City, Iowa.

51. Carr DB, Bullen BA, Skinner GS, et al. Physical conditioning facilitates the exercise-induced secretion of beta endorphin and beta lipoprotein in women. *N Engl J Med* 1981; 305:560.

52. McArthur JW. Endorphins and exercise in females: Possible connection with reproductive dysfunction. *Med Sci Sports Exerc* 1985; 17(1):82–88.

53. Varner MW. Is pregnancy a problem for the athlete? Hawkeye Sportsmedicine Symposium; April 17, 1986; Iowa City, Iowa.

54. Goodlin RC, Buckley KK. Maternal exercise. *Clin Sports Med.* 1984; 3:881–894.

55. Artal R. Exercise in pregnancy. In: McKee G, ed. *The Female Athlete—Sportsmedicine Digest Special Report.* Van Nuys, Calif: PM Inc; 1988:5–7.

56. Artal R, Wiswell RA. *Exercise in Pregnancy.* Baltimore, Md: Williams & Wilkins Co; 1986.

57. Lawrence M, Singh J, Lawrence F, Whitehead RG. The energy cost of common daily activities in African women: Increased energy expenditure in pregnancy? *Am J Clin Nutr.* 1985; 42:753.

58. Lotgering FK. Pregnancy. In: Shangold MM, Mirkin G, eds. *Women and Exercise.* Philadelphia, Pa: F A Davis; 1988:145–155.

59. Blackburn NW, Calloway DH. Heart rate and energy expenditure of pregnant and lactating women. *Am J Clin Nutr.* 1985; 42:1161.

60. Knuttgen HG, Emerson K. Physiological response to pregnancy at rest and during exercise. *J Appl Physiol.* 1974; 36:549.

61. Dressendorfer RH, Goodlin RC. Fetal heart rate responses to maternal exercise testing. *Phys Sportsmed.* 1980; 8:91.

62. Lotgering FK, Gilbert RD, Longo LD. Exercise responses in pregnant sheep: Oxygen consumption, uterine blood flow, and blood volume. *J Appl Physiol.* 1983; 55:834.

63. Clapp FJ. Acute exercise stress in the pregnant ewe. *Am J Obstet Gynecol.* 1980; 136:489.

64. Lotgering FK, Gilbert RD, Longo LD. Exercise responses in pregnant sheep: Blood gases, temperatives and fetal cardiovascular system. *J Appl Physiol.* 1983; 55:842.

65. Hutchinson PL, Cureton KJ, Sparling PB. Metabolic and circulatory responses to running during pregnancy. *Phys Sportsmed* 1981; 9:55.

66. Kulpa PJ, White BM, Vischer R. Aerobic exercise in pregnancy. *Am J Obstet Gynecol.* 1987; 156:1395–1403.

67. Shy KK, Brown ZA. Maternal and fetal well being. *West J Med.* 1984; 141:807.

68. Hall DC, Kaufmann DA. Effects of aerobic and strength conditioning on pregnancy outcomes. *Am J Obstet Gynecol.* 1987; 157:1199–1203.

69. Clapp JF, Dickstein S. Endurance exercise and pregnancy outcome. *Med Sci Sports Exerc.* 1984; 16:556–562.

70. The American College of Obstetricians and Gynecologists. *Exercise During Pregnancy and the Postnatal Period (ACOG Home Exercise Programs).* Washington, DC: ACOG Resource Center; 1985:4.

71. Maeder EC. Effects of sports and exercise in pregnancy. *Postgrad Med.* 1985; 77:112–114.

72. Katz JL. Eating disorders. In: Shangold MM, Mirkin G, eds. *Women and Exercise.* Philadelphia, Pa: F A Davis; 1988:248–263.

73. Knortz KA, Reinhart RS. Women's athletics: The trainer's viewpoint. *Clin Sports Med.* 1984; 3:851–852.

74. Clark N. How I manage athletes food obsessions. *Physician Sportsmed.* 1984; 12(7):96.

75. Spencer J, Hayes K, Alexander I. Knee joint effusion and quadriceps reflex inhibition in man. *Arch Phys Med.* 1984; 65:171–177.

76. Lieb F, Perry J. Quadriceps function. *J Bone Joint Surg.* 1968; 50A(B):1535.

77. Reynolds L, Levin T, Medeiros J, et al. EMG activity of the vastus medialis oblique and vastus lateralis in their role in patellar alignment. *Am J Phys Med.* 1983; 62(2):61–70.

78. McConnell J: McConnell Patellofemoral treatment plan. Presented at North Tustin Sports Medicine Center; April 22, 1989; Tustin, Calif.

79. Fisher SP. The patellofemoral joint: Anatomy, Surgical indications and findings. Presented at North Tustin Sports Medicine Center. April 22, 1989; Tustin, Calif.

80. Hunter–Griffin LY: Orthopedic concerns. In: Shangold MM, Mirkin G, eds. *Women and Exercise.* Philadelphia, Pa: F A Davis; 1988:195–219.

81. McConnell J. The management of chondromalacia patellae: A long term solution. *Aust J Physiother.* 1986; 32(4):215.

10

The Pediatric and Adolescent Athlete

Joseph M. Murphy

INTRODUCTION

It has been estimated that 50% of boys, and 25% of girls between the ages of 8 and 16 play competitive sports in the United States.[1] Twenty million young athletes are participating in organized community sports programs, which include regional, national, and international competition;[2] 79.1% of middle and junior high schools have sports programs;[3] and there are 7 million high school athletes in the United States who are involved in school programs.[2] It is the exception for someone to graduate from high school and not to have been involved in some organized athletic program.

This tremendous expansion in athletic participation among the pediatric and adolescent population presents a new challenge for the physical therapists and other medical professionals who are providing care for them. These athletes are a unique group within the sports medicine population because they are in the process of growth and development. It is necessary to have an understanding of how these normal developmental processes interface with athletic performance in order to provide safe and effective care and counsel for the child athlete.

This chapter addresses the maturation of the child athlete through a presentation of normal growth, musculoskeletal development, cardiorespiratory development, and thermoregulatory capacity. It also reviews the effect training has on strength, acclimatization, and the cardiorespiratory system.

GROWTH IN HEIGHT

Growth is a continuous process from conception to adulthood. The rate of growth is far from constant, however. The maximum rate occurs before birth, dur-

ing the fourth month of fetal life, when the fetus grows about 11 cm.[4] From this time on there is a rapid deceleration in the rate of growth. Nevertheless, infants increase their birth length by 50% in the first year. They double it by age 4, and triple it by the age of 13.[5] After age 3, the rate of growth plateaus, with an average annual gain of 5 to 6 cm.[6]

Boys and girls continue to grow at the same rate, with little difference in height until adolescence. Girls begin their growth spurts sooner, at age 10½ to 11 with peak height velocity occurring at 12.1 (± 0.14) years with a standard deviation of 0.87 years. Tanner et al found girls' peak height velocity to be 9.0 (± 0.16) cm/yr, because of an earlier start at the growth spurt, girls between the ages of 11 and 13 are taller than boys.[7] This is reversed when boys begin their growth spurt at age 12½ to 13, 2 years after girls. Peak height velocity occurs at 14.1 (± 0.13) years with a standard deviation of 0.93 years, and the peak height velocity of boys averages 10.3 (± 0.22) cm/yr.[7] These basic differences between the sexes account for the difference in final height achieved. Boys have two more years of preadolescent growth and are therefore 10 cm taller at the beginning of their growth spurts than girls at the same developmental stage.[2] Males will also have longer legs relative to their trunks because of this period of extended preadolescent growth. Boys also achieve a greater peak height velocity than girls, and this lasts for a longer period of time. Thus far, the average progression of height has been presented with some of the differences between boys and girls being noted. The data that provide the most valuable information, however, are those that give us some insight into the variability of onset of the growth spurt experience.

Boys experience peak height velocity at 14.1 years, with a standard deviation of 0.93 years. This means that an early maturing boy can still be going through a

normal growth pattern and experience his peak velocity for growth at age 12. Likewise, a 16-year-old boy who is just beginning his peak velocity for growth will be within the normal growth pattern. Although the pattern for growth is consistent for the population, the onset of the adolescent growth spurt is highly variable. At 14 years of age, a normal population of boys can vary as much as 5 years in bone age.[8]

GROWTH IN WEIGHT

Unlike height, the most rapid growth rate in weight occurs after birth, with the birth weight tripled after the first year and quadrupled after the second.[6] Just as the rate of growth for height plateaus, so does the rate of growth in weight, with 2 to 3 kg/yr being added until the onset of the adolescent growth spurt.

The onset for peak weight velocity follows peak height velocity. For boys the delay is 0.25 years later, and in girls it is 0.63 years later. The peak weight velocity averaged 9.8 ($\pm$ 0.30) kg/hr in boys and 8.8 ($\pm$ 0.25) kg/yr in girls.[7]

More important than total weight gained is the percentage of that weight gain that is fat. As boys go through adolescence their body fat decreases to 11% whereas that of girls increases to 25%.[9,10] With height as the reference, males gain 2.12% lean body mass for every centimeter of height gain, and females gain 1.84%. Although this pattern for peak weight velocity is consistent for the population, it can vary among normal individuals by as much as 100 lb in a population of 14 year old boys.[8]

BONE GROWTH

A child grows in height as the bones increase their length. Bone is a rigid structure and therefore unique among tissues in that it cannot expand within itself. It must grow by adding onto its surfaces. This is accomplished through two mechanisms: membranous ossification and endochondral ossification.

Membranous ossification enables the bone to widen by laying down new bone on the surface of the cortex. Osteoblastic cells within the deep layer of the periosteum carry out this function. As the bone widens through oppositional growth on the outside of the shaft, there is a concurrent widening of the bone marrow cavity within the shaft. This ensures that the ratio of the total diameter of the shaft to the thickness of its walls is maintained fairly constant throughout growth.[6]

Endochondral ossification occurs at the ends of bones within the epiphyseal plate. The epiphyseal plate can be pictured as having two zones: the zone of cartilage production where growth actually occurs, and the zone of transformation where no growth in length occurs but where cartilage is transformed to bone.[11] These zones have been further subdivided by function and divided by Brighton[12] into four zones: the zone of small cartilage cells, the zone of cell columns, the zone of hypertrophic cells, and the metaphysis.

The zone of small cartilage cells is closest to the epiphysis and firmly anchored. Chondrocytes are scattered throughout the intercellular substance of the cartilage. This is the site of active synthesis of collagen and protein.[13]

The zone of cell columns is the site of most of the longitudinal growth. Division of cells and collagen synthesis occur here. This process is aided by an abundant blood supply by vessels from the epiphyseal side of the plate.

The zone of hypertrophic cells is where the cells in columns undergo an increase to 15 times their original volume. The cells begin nuclear degeneration and the surrounding matrix begins to calcify. The cells experience complete degeneration, as they are adjacent to the metaphyseal side of the plate.

The metaphysis and the last column cell are separated by a thin transverse septum. The septum breaks down and the cell is invaded by a vascular bud that is soon followed by osteogenic cells. The walls of the columns are covered by osteoblasts and new bone is laid down on the calcified matrix. This area is gradually remodeled until it is completely replaced by trabeculae of lamelar bone.

A very similar growth process occurs at the apophyses. This growth does not contribute to bone length but does accommodate the increase in tendon size and required area for insertion. Children's bones are different than mature bones by virtue of the growth process and therefore account for the unique types of musculoskeletal injuries seen in the young athlete.

Children's bones are softer, more pliable, and more porous, with a greater proportion of Haversian canals and therefore able to tolerate greater deformation without fracture.[14] When fractures do occur, there are some unique possibilities for the skeletally immature. A growing bone, particularly the radius and ulna, can bend as the result of microfractures without the loss of bone continuity.[15] This may be misdiagnosed because of a lack of clinical signs without a countralateral comparison by radiograph.

Greenstick fractures occur in normal bone only in childhood. The younger the child, the more likely a greenstick fracture will occur.[14] The bone cortex fails on one side with bony continuity remaining on the opposite side.

When a complete fracture does occur in a child it is common for the periosteum to remain intact, simplifying reduction and preventing excessive displacement.[14]

Because of the mechanisms of bone growth, some fractures and overuse injuries are also unique to the growing child. Epiphyseal plate fractures usually occur through the zone of hypertrophic cells, where the trabecular are thin and composed of poorly calcified cartilage,[11] but may also occur through the metaphysis, which is weakened because of the remodeling process with the laying down of new bone.

Fortunately, the vascular supply to the growing cells is not compromised during fracture through the zone of hypertrophic cells, since this arises from the epiphyseal side of the plate. The dividing cells are susceptible to crushing, however, which can be a component of any epiphyseal injury and cannot be recognized radiographically.[11] This makes follow-up radiographic and clinical comparisons necessary in the management of these types of fractures.

In growing bone, the epiphyseal plate is the weak link and will succumb to stress before the ligamentous and capsular structures. This is commonly seen at the knee when a varus or valgus stress is sustained, and the result is epiphyseal fracture as opposed to ligament sprain. The same applies to the distal fibular epiphyseal plate with an inversion sprain.

The apophyseal centers of growth are common areas for trauma for the young athlete. As an adult would strain a muscle, a child may possibly pull the apophyseal center off the bone where that muscle attaches. This would represent the apophyseal line of growth as the site of least tolerance for stress. These avulsion fractures are the result of acute high-level stress. The pelvis is a common site for avulsion fracture because of the powerful muscles that originate here. The apophyses are also susceptible to repetitive low levels of stress. The most common examples of apophysitis would be Osgood Schlatter's disease of the tibial tubercle and Seiver's disease of the calcaneus. Both are overuse syndromes that are the result of chronic microtrauma to the apophyseal plate.[16-22]

STRENGTH GAINS

As children grow they become stronger. This increase in strength has been correlated to a few physical growth characteristics. Strength gains have been directly related to growth in height, with a linear relationship occurring until the age of 13,[23] increases in height and weight,[24] and increases in girth measurements.[25] Skeletal muscle accounts for a larger part of the overall increase in body size that a child and adolescent experiences.[5] At birth, skeletal muscles account for 25% of total body weight, and this gradually increases to 40% with maturity.[6] As the child's body size increases, so does his or her strength.

In addition to physical growth, age plays a role in strength development. It has been found that when height is held constant older children are slightly stronger.[23] This may be explained by neuromuscular development or simply the opportunity to practice the skills necessary to perform certain strength tests for a longer period of time.

The pattern of strength development is consistent for both boys and girls, with boys being slightly stronger, especially in upper body strength, until the advent of secondary sex characteristics. Strength differences become more pronounced following puberty, as boys become significantly stronger. These differences can be correlated to quantitative differences in muscle mass. Boys experience a 14-fold increase from birth to maturity whereas girls undergo a 10-fold increase.[6] During puberty significant differences exist between the sexes in terms of muscular development. By measuring the amount of creatinine excreted in the urine, the total mass of muscle in the body can be estimated. This is possible because the conversion of creatine to creatinine occurs only in the muscle.[6] Significant intersex variations in creatinine excretion have been found between the ages of 11 and 17, most prominently at age 13.[26]

These differences in strength are related to the androgenic stimulation associated with the development of secondary sex characteristics. Peak increases in strength occur approximately 1 year following both peak height and peak weight velocity. Considering the variability of onset for both growth spurt and puberty there exists the potential for great variance in strength for children of the same age.

CARDIORESPIRATORY DEVELOPMENT

Cardiorespiratory development has been directly related to body growth. As body size increases so does cardiorespiratory capacity. With an increase in body size there is an accompanying increase in cardiac dimensions which in turn leads to a greater stroke volume and VO_2 max.[27] This basic mechanical principle establishes the strong relationship between body size and cardiorespiratory capacity. For each centimeter of height increase between 100 and 180 cm there is a 1 beat per minute (bpm) decrease in submaximal heart rate at a given power output.[28] The most commonly accepted measure of cardiorespiratory capacity is VO_2 max or the highest attainable oxygen uptake rate in exhaustive exercise and is usually described in terms of milliliters of oxygen per kilogram of body weight per minute. VO_2 max has been measured to increase at the same rate for both sexes, with boys having slightly higher values.[29-31] Although VO_2 max continues to increase for boys through their adolescent years, there is little development beyond early adolescence in girls.[32]

Another study found a decrease in VO_2 max with age for girls. This was most evident beyond early adolescence.[33] These sex-related differences may be explained by the relatively larger amounts of body fat in females compared to males after puberty. These differences almost disappear once maximal O_2 uptake is related to the muscle mass that performs the activity.[34]

Boys also experience a peak VO_2 max velocity that is closely related to peak height velocity. VO_2 max velocity is delayed approximately 4 months behind peak height velocity and occurs simultaneously with an increase in testosterone. This relationship is a proven factor in the development of muscle strength, increased hemoglobin, and red blood cells.[35]

THERMOREGULATORY CAPACITY

Children have less efficient thermoregulatory capacity than adults. This becomes most apparent with extremes in temperature, whether of heat or cold. This can be explained by the following characteristics: larger surface area per kilogram of body weight, high oxygen cost of walking and running, lower cardiac output at a given oxygen uptake, and lower sweating rate.[32]

When an 8-year-old child was compared to a 20-year-old adult, the child was found to have 36% greater surface area per unit mass in spite of having a smaller absolute surface area.[32] This places the child at a great disadvantage in extremes of temperatures. When it is hot, the child has relatively more surface area to gain heat, and in a cold environment to lose heat.

Exposure to the cold certainly involves potential risks, particularly given children's propensity for heat loss. With participation in sports, however, there is generally enough heat generated through increased metabolic rate that this does not present a problem. The exception to this is with water sports. Water is 25 times greater a thermal conductor than air. This is a liability for everyone, but particularly so for the child because of the relatively larger surface area. A greater risk presents itself for the child with a very low percentage of body fat since subcutaneous fat can act as an insulator. Exposure to heat places the child at risk because of a number of physiological limitations. Children expend more chemical energy per unit mass for locomotion,[29,36,37] and since 75% to 80% of the chemical energy required for muscle contraction is converted to heat, the thermoregulatory system will be further stressed when locomotion occurs in a hot environment. Children also have a lower stroke volume, higher heart rate, and lower cardiac output at each metabolic level when compared to adults.[38,39] A problem arises when the circulatory system is called upon to meet the demands of the increased metabolic rate and the need of blood flow to the skin to dissipate heat.

It has been found that such demands cannot be fully met and therefore limit the capacity for exercise in the heat.[40] This factor may place a greater intolerance for exercise in the heat for girls because their stroke volume is somewhat lower than that of boys.[41,42]

Children perspire less than adults.[43,44] Adults can perspire at rates exceeding 500 to 600 mL/m² of skin per hour, whereas the child's rate seldom exceeds 350 mL/m²/hr when exposed to identical conditions.[43] Although children have a proportionally greater number of active sweat glands, the output per gland is decreased, with adults excreting 2.5 times more sweat per gland than children.[40] This decreased potential for cooling by evaporation is also affected by children requiring a greater increase in core temperature before they start perspiring.[43]

ACCLIMATIZATION

In addition to children's limitations for tolerance of environmental extremes, they also differ in the rate and manner in which they acclimate to exercise in the heat. When compared to adults, they respond slower. This process is characterized by a decrease in body temperature and heart rate for a given metabolic rate as well as an increase in sweating rate and a decrease in salt in the sweat. A child may require five to six exposures to achieve the same level of acclimatization that an adult will achieve in two to three.[40] This makes the initial period of exposures for children the time when they are more vulnerable to heat-related injuries. The total acclimatization period requires 7 to 10 days.[45]

Another difference in children is their perceived rate of exertion. Children subjectively report a faster declining exertional rate than adults. This presents a potential hazard for a child who is physiologically slowly adapting to the environment and yet subjectively experiences a more rapid decline in exertional level.

STRENGTH TRAINING

A commonly accepted myth has been that prepubescent children who trained for strength through some form of resistance were wasting their time because of a lack of circulating androgens.[46,47] Recent studies, however, have proved that prepubescent children do increase muscle strength with training.[47-51] Concerns about strains, tendonitis, epiphysitis, avulsions, fractures, and vertebral injuries[52-56] have led to suggestions that weight training be avoided in the preadolescent population.[9] Other authors have found, however, that with proper supervision and with submaximal resistance there has been no incidence of injury.[47,57] The American Academy of Pediatrics,[46] the National

Strength and Conditioning Association,[58] and the American Orthopaedic Society for Sports Medicine[59] have condoned strength training for prepubescents. They have, however, made a number of recommendations for this age group:[59]

Program Considerations

1. A preparticipation physical exam is mandatory.
2. The child must have the emotional maturity to accept coaching and instruction.
3. There must be adequate supervision by coaches who are knowledgeable about strength training and the special problems of prepubescents.
4. Strength training should be a part of an overall comprehensive program designed to increase motor skills and level of fitness.
5. Strength training should be preceded by a warmup period and followed by a cool-down period.
6. Emphasis should be on dynamic concentric contractions.
7. All exercises should be carried through a full range of motion.
8. Competition is prohibited.
9. No maximum lift should ever be attempted.

Prescribed Program

1. Training is recommended two or three times per week for 20- to 30-minute periods.
2. No resistance should be applied until proper form is demonstrated. Six to fifteen repetitions equal one set, and one to three sets per exercise should be done.
3. Weight or resistance is increased in 1- to 3-lb increments after the prepubescent does 15 repetitions in good form.

CARDIOVASCULAR TRAINING

Before puberty, it is inconclusive if training will have an effect on maximum oxygen uptake. Some studies have shown no increase in VO_2 max with training.[60–66] Others have found a less than 10% improvement.[67,68] No explanation for this lack of physiological response to training in the prepubescent population has been found. One possibility is that VO_2 max is not a valid indicator of aerobic capacity in the prepubescent population.[69] One indication for the validity of this suspicion is that prepubescent athletes have an improvement in long-distance running with training in spite of their lack of improved VO_2 max. Many questions remain unanswered in this area of research on the prepubescent athlete.

Some researchers have considered adolescence as a critical period for the development of a high VO_2 max. When active adolescent boys were compared to an inactive control group, it was found that the active group experienced a greater increase of VO_2 max immediately following the age of peak height velocity. This increase was also extended for a longer period of time.[70] Kobayashi et al[65] found that aerobic training in the year prior to peak height velocity resulted in an increase in VO_2 max that exceeded expectations for the predicted adolescent growth spurt.

The research on this adolescent age group is conflicting, as another study uncovered no critical stage for aerobic trainability.[71] Even the issue of the stage in the developmental process at which aerobic trainability reaches the level of the young adult is unresolved.

Normal growth and development occur in a predictable sequential pattern, with dramatic acceleration of these processes occurring during adolescence. During this growth spurt, increases in height, weight, strength, and cardiorespiratory function reach peak velocities. The age at which the growth spurt begins varies greatly, however. Adolescents can begin the growth spurt anytime between the ages of 12 and 16 and still be well within normal limits. This fact makes the practice of matching competitors by age inappropriate for this age group. It creates the opportunity for increased incidence of injury, and denies the athlete the opportunity to compete with others who are at the same physiological level.

Bone growth is a necessary component of normal growth and development. Because of the unique characteristics of growing bone, there are also a unique set of musculoskeletal injuries. Beyond the normally occurring improvements in the physiological functions, which are necessary for successful participation in sports, children can reap the benefits of training. Their response is limited, however, in comparison to adults, for acclimatization and cardiorespiratory improvement.

REFERENCES

1. Shaffer TE. The uniqueness of the young athlete: Introductory remarks. *Am J Sports Med.* 1980; 8:370.
2. Smith NJ. Children and parents: Growth, development and sports. In: Strauss RH, ed. *Sports Medicine.* Philadelphia, Pa: W B Saunders; 1984; 207–217.
3. Thornburg HD, Clark DC. Middle school/junior high school research needs questionnaire. National Middle School Association Symposium; 1980.
4. Smith DW. *Growth and Its Disorders.* Philadelphia, Pa: W B Saunders; 1977; xv.
5. Lowrey GH. *Growth and Development of Children.* Chicago, Ill: Year Book Medical Publishers Inc; 1973.
6. Sinclair D. *Human Growth After Birth.* London: Oxford University Press; 1978.
7. Tanner JM. Standards from birth to maturity for height, weight, height velocity, and weight velocity: British children. *Arch Dis Child.* 1966; 41:454.

8. Smith NJ. Sports related problems of late maturing young males: In: Smith NJ, ed. *Common Problems in Pediatric Sports Med.* Chicago, Ill: Year Book Medical Publishers Inc; 1989.

9. Goldberg B. Pediatric sports medicine. In: Scott WN, Nisonson B, Nicholas J, eds. *Principles of Sports Medicine.* Baltimore, Md: Williams & Wilkins Co; 1984:403–426.

10. Penny R, Goldstein I, Frasier S. Gonadotropin excretion and body composition. *Pediatrics* 1978; 61:294.

11. Moseley CF. Growth. In: Lovell WW, Winger RB, eds. *Pediatric Orthopaedics.* Philadelphia, Pa: J B Lippincott Co; 1978.

12. Brighton CT. Clinical problems in epiphyseal plate growth and development. *AAOS Instruc Course Lect.* 1974; 23:105.

13. Kuhlman RE. A microchemical study of the developing epiphyseal plate. *J Bone Joint Surg.* 1965; 42A:457.

14. Sharrard WJW. *Pediatric Orthopaedics and Fractures.* Oxford: Blackwell Scientific Publications; 1979; 1484.

15. Wilkins KE. The uniqueness of the young athlete: Musculoskeletal injuries. *Am J Sports Med.* 1980; 8:377–382.

16. Kitiyakara A, Angevine DM. A study of the pattern of post-embryonic growth of the *M Gracilis* in mice. *Dev Biol.* 1963; 8:322–340.

17. Goldspink G. Sarcomere length during the post-natal growth of mammalian muscle fibers. *J Cell Sci.* 1968; 3:539–548.

18. Rowe RWD, Goldspink G. Muscle fibre growth in five different muscles in both sexes in mice. *J Anat.* 1969; 104:519.

19. Montgomery RD. Growth of human striated muscle. *Nature* 1962; 195:194–195.

20. Williams PE, Goldspink G. Longitudinal growth of striated muscle fibres. *J Cell Sci.* 1971; 9:751–767.

21. Mackay B, Harrop TJ, Muir AR. The fine structure of the muscle tendon junction in the rat. *Acta Anat.* 1969; 73:588–604.

22. Enesco J, Puddy D. Increase in the number of nuclei and weight in skeletal muscles of rats of various ages. *Am J Anat.* 1964; 114:235–244.

23. Asmussen E. Growth in muscle strength and power. In: Rarick GL, ed. *Physical Activity: Human Growth and Development.* New York, NY: Academic Press; 1973:60.

24. Carron AV, Bailey DA. Strength development in boys from 10 through 16 years. *Monogr Soc Res Child Dev.* 1974; 39:4.

25. Lamphier DE, Montoye JT. Muscular strength and body size. *Human Biol.* 1976; 48:147.

26. Clark LC, Thompson HL, Beck FI, et al. Excretion of creatine and creatinine by children. *Am J Dis Child.* 1951; 86:774.

27. Blimkie CJR, Cunningham DA, Nichol PM. Gas transport capacity and echocardiographically determined cardiac size in children. *J Appl Physiol.* 1980; 49:994–999.

28. Godfrey S. The growth and development of the cardiopulmonary responses to exercise. In: Dobbing J, Davis JA, eds. *Scientific Foundations of Paediatrics.* Philadelphia, Pa: W B Saunders; 1974:271–280.

29. Astrand PO. *Experimental Studies of Physical Working Capacity in Relation to Sex and Age.* Copenhagen: Munksgaard; 1952.

30. MacDougall JD, Roche PD, Bar-Or O, Moroz JR. Oxygen cost of running in children of different ages, maximal aerobic power of Canadian school children. *Can J Appl Sports Sci.* 1979; 4:237. Abstract.

31. Shephard PJ, Allen C, Bar-Or O, et al. The working capacity of Toronto school children. *Can Med Assoc J.* 1969; 100:560–566.

32. Bar-Or O. *Pediatric Sports Medicine for the Practitioner.* New York, NY: Springer-Verlag; 1983.

33. Rutenfranz J, Anderson KL, Selinger V, et al. Maximum aerobic power and body composition during the puberty growth period: Similarities and differences between children of two European countries. *Eur J Pediatr.* 1981; 136:123–133.

34. Davies CTM, Barnes C, Godfrey S. Body composition and maximal exercise performance in children. *Hum Biol.* 1972; 44:195–214.

35. Mirwald RL, Bailey DA, Cameron N, Rasmussen RL. Longitudinal comparison of aerobic power in active and inactive boys aged 7.0 to 17.0 years. *Ann Hum Biol.* 1981; 8:405–414.

36. Daniels J, Oldridge N, Nagle F, White B. Differences and changes in VO_2 among young runners 10 to 18 years of age. *Med Sci Sports* 1978; 10:200–203.

37. MacDougall JD, Roche PD, Bar-Or O, Moroz JR. Maximal aerobic capacity of Canadian school children: Prediction based on age-related oxygen cost of running. *Int J Sports Med.* 1983; 4:194–198.

38. Bar-Or O, Shephard RJ, Allen CL. Cardiac output of 10 to 13 year old boys and girls during submaximal exercise. *J Appl Physiol.* 1971; 30:219–223.

39. Eriksson BO, Gollnick PD, Saltin B. Cardiac output and arterial blood gases during exercise in pubertal boys. *J Appl Physiol.* 1971; 31:348–352.

40. Bar-Or O. Climate and the exercising child—A review. *Int J Sports Med.* 1980; 1:53–65.

41. Cumming GR. Hemodynamics of supine bicycle in "normal" children. *Am Heart J.* 1977; 93:617–622.

42. Godfrey S, Davies CTM, Wozniak E, Barnes CA. Cardiorespiratory response to exercise in normal children. *Clin Sci.* 1971; 40:419–431.

43. Araki T, Toda Y, Matsushita K, Tsujino A. Age differences in sweating during muscular exercise. *Jpn J Phys Fitness Sports Med.* 1979; 28:239–248.

44. Davies CTM. Thermal responses to exercise in children. *Ergonomics.* 1981; 24:55–61.

45. American Academy of Pediatrics. *Sports Medicine: Health Care of Young Athletes.* Evanston, Ill: AAP; 1983.

46. American Academy of Pediatrics. Weight training and weight lifting: Information for the pediatrician. *Physician Sportsmed.* 1983; 11(3):157–161.

47. Sewall L, Micheli LJ. Strength training for children. *J Pediatr Orthop.* 1986; 6:143–146.

48. Hettinger T. *Physiology of Strength.* Springfield, Ill: Charles C. Thomas; 1961.

49. Schneid D, Vignos PJ, Archibald KC. Effects of brief maximal exercise on quadriceps strength in children. *Am J Phys Med.* 1962; 41:189.

50. Pfeiffer R, Francis RS. Effects of strength training on muscle development in prepubescent, pubescent, and postprepubescent males. *Physician Sportsmed.* 1986; 14(9):134–143.

51. Sailors M, Berg K. Comparison of response to weight training in pubescent boys and men. *J Sports Med Phys Fitness.* 1987; 27:30–37.

52. Troup J. The risk of weight training and weight lifting in young people. *Br J Sports Med.* 1970; 5:27.

53. Aggrawal ND, Kaur R, Kumer S, et al. A study of changes in the spine in weight lifters and other athletes. *Br J Sports Med.* 1979; 13:58.

54. Kulund DN, Dewey JB, Brubaker CE, et al. Olympic weight lifting injuries. *Physician Sportsmed.* 1978; 6:111.

55. Ryan JR, Salciccioli GG. Fractures of the distal radial epiphysis in adolescent weight lifters. *Am J Sports Med.* 1976; 4:26–27.

56. Jesse JP. Olympic lifting movements endanger adolescents. *Physicians Sportsmed.* 1977; 5:61–67.

57. Servedio FJ, Bartels RL, Hamlin RL, et al. The effects of weight training, using olympic style lifts on various physiological variables in pre-pubescent boys. *Med Sci Sports Exerc.* 1985; 17:288. Abstract.

58. National Strength and Conditioning Association. Position statement on prepubescent strength training. *Natl Strength Cond J.* 1985; 7:27–31.

59. Duda M. Prepubescent strength training gains support. *Physician Sportsmed.* 1986; 14(2):157–161.

60. Bar-Or O, Zwiren LD: Physiological effects of increased frequency of physical education classes and of endurance conditioning on 4 to 10 year old girls and boys. In: Bar-Or, ed. *Pediatric Work Physiology IV.* Natanya, Israel: Wingate Institute; 1973.

61. Yoshida TI, Ishiko I, Muraoka I. Effect of endurance training on cardiorespiratory functions of 5 year old children. *Int J Sports Med.* 1980; 1:91–94.

62. Mocellin R, Wasmund U. Investigations on the influence of a running-training programme on the cardiovascular and motor performance capacity in 53 boys and girls of a second and third primary school class. In: Bar-Or O, ed. *Pediatric Work Physiology IV.* Natanya, Israel: Wingate Institute; 1973.

63. Stewart KJ, Gutin B. Effects of physical training on cardiovascular fitness in children. *Res Q Am Assoc Health Phys Ed* 1976; 47:110–120.

64. Gilliam TB, Freedson PS. Effects of a 12 week school physical fitness program on peak VO$_2$, body composition, and blood lipids in 7- to 9-year-old children. *Int J Sports Med.* 1980; 1:73.

65. Kobayashi K, Kitamura K, Miura M, et al: Aerobic power related to body growth and training in Japanese boys: A longitudinal study. *J Appl Physiol.* 1978; 44:666.

66. Hamilton P, Andrew GM. Influence of growth and athletic training on heart and lung functions. *Eur J Appl Physiol.* 1976; 36:27.

67. Ekblom B. Effect of physical training in adolescent boys. *J Appl Physiol.* 1969; 27:350–355.

68. Rotstein A, Dotan R, Bar-Or O, et al. Effect of training on anaerobic threshold, maximal aerobic power and anaerobic performance of preadolescent boys. *Int J Sports Med* 1986; 7:281–286.

69. Mayers N, Gutin B. Physiological characteristics of elite prepubertal cross-country runners. *Med Sci Sports Exerc.* 1979; 11:172–176.

70. Mirwald RL, Bailey DA, Cameron N, Rasmussen RL. Longitudinal comparison of aerobic power in active and inactive boys aged 7.0 to 17.0 years. *Ann Hum Biol.* 1981; 8:405–414.

71. Anderson B, Froberg K. Circulatory parameters and muscular strength in trained and normal boys during puberty. *Acta Physiol Scand.* 1980; 105:D36. Abstract.

11

The Older Athlete

Arnold T. Bell

INTRODUCTION

Impact of the Older Adult on Society

Our society is today undergoing many changes with regard to population, particularly population demographics. A segment of the population on which much attention has been focused recently is the elderly or aging population. Technological advances in medicine and science are increasing the longevity of the geriatric population, even in the presence of disease and disability. The data and statistics on longevity are startling.

According to Saldo, an estimated 25.5 million elderly Americans comprised about 11% of the US population in 1980.[1] Guccione acknowledged that the chronological criterion used to distinguish the elderly or old persons in America is usually the age of 65.[2] The proportion of the US population aged 65 or over will continue to increase into the 21st century,[3] and some researchers project that by the year 2030, persons age 65 and older will comprise about 20% of the US population.[4]

With increased longevity, many older adults are remaining active in sports, on both a recreational and competitive level. To allow for efficient and effective exercise training, as well to prevent injuries, the sports physical therapist should understand how the basic principles of sports medicine are applied to the elderly and what modifications are necessary.

Geriatric Sports Medicine: A Variation From the Traditional

Being an older adult today is not synonymous with being plagued with numerous and complex disabilities. Older adults are often physically active, employing basic principles of physical training to bring about or maintain a certain level of physical fitness. Although individuals reach their normal physiological peak in their mid to late twenties, the rate of decline in physiological functions may be reduced or postponed by physical exercise.[5]

With increasing age, physical activity patterns may change. Aging persons may choose to remain active or to become inactive. Both alternatives may present problems, as there are risks associated with inactivity, but the older adult who exercises must be cautious and use proper training principles to avoid injury. An increasing percentage of the older adult population has chosen to remain physically active by means of recreational activities and even, in some instances, competitive sports. It is very important to have a knowledge and understanding of physical activity in the older population.

Specific physical fitness needs, exercise guidelines, and precautions, injury trends and prevention, and potential complications of exercise and sport in our older population are a few areas that need to be addressed. We know that with advancing age, many body functions decline.[3,6] Despite reaching many physiological peaks in the mid to late twenties, many individuals in later decades of life are capable of performing physical feats far beyond what they were capable of in earlier decades of life.

We witness older adults engaging daily in group and individualized physical fitness programs, such as aerobics, jogging, racquet sports, and so on, as well as participating in local, national, and international competitions in sports. It is not uncommon to see magazine articles on older adults who have challenged the aging process and performed miraculous feats in activities and sports usually dominated by younger participants. George Blanda and Satchel Paige are examples of older adults who competed successfully in professional sports against much younger individuals. Clarence Demar, the famous marathoner, ran marathons of 25 and 26 miles well into his sixties and ran his last 15-kilometer race at 68 before dying of cancer at age 70.

Despite the process of aging, there are physiological benefits of training, such as improved muscle function, posture, flexibility, joint range of motion, en-

durance, physical working capacity,[7,8] and exercise may retard symptoms of aging and disease effects.[9] The active older adult or older athlete may seek the services of the sports physical therapist or general practitioner for treatment of exercise-induced injuries or advice regarding exercise programs. With an older patient population, the physical therapist must be cognizant of age-related physiological changes to allow for modification of exercise regimens to adopt to those changes,[9] and must apply an alteration of clinical expertise for this population to promote and insure quality patient care. This chapter focuses upon the older competitive and recreational athlete, as well as the exercising older adult.

ANATOMIC AND PHYSIOLOGICAL CHANGES WITH AGE

A discussion of the effects of the aging process on human body systems is necessary for the sports physical therapist to modify treatment programs for the older adult or athlete. Aging is characterized by a normal decline and gradual deterioration in many physiological functions.

It has been suggested that aging begins early in life and that attempts to alter the rate of decline in body systems need to begin equally early. It is acknowledged also that the physiological aging process is not necessarily congruent with chronological age and significant individual variation is possible.[6]

Aging and the Nervous System
It is important for the physical therapist to have a keen appreciation and understanding of some of the neural effects of aging, as the effects can influence gross motor tasks (Table 11–1). A major consequence of aging on the nervous system is loss of neurons, as they are postmitotic cells, incapable of replication.[10] There is a net

TABLE 11-1. CHANGES IN THE NERVOUS SYSTEM WITH AGE

Loss of neurons
Reduction in brain weight and size
Vulnerability to wear and tear of neurons
Decreased cerebral blood flow
Decreased brain functioning
Increased cerebral vascular resistance
Decreased cerebral oxygen consumption
Decreased sensory and motor nerve conduction
Appearance of lipofuscins in the inner neuron structure
Decreased reflex responses
Decreased sensory acuity
Reduction of alpha waves
Decreased reaction time
Decreased coordination of motor skills

reduction of the weight of the brain between the second and ninth decades of life by approximately 10% to 20%.[9] Lewis[11] attributes the decrease to the lack of replication and vulnerability of the neurons to wear and tear.

Frolkis[12] reported a change in cerebral blood flow, usually a net decrease resulting in a decrease in most functions of the brain with aging. With this decrease, there is an increase in cerebral vascular resistance and a decrease in cerebral oxygen consumption.[13]

Additional changes in the human nervous system include a decrease in sensory and motor nerve conduction starting at age 35,[9,14] changes in the inner structure of the nerve cell, such as accumulation of waste products known as lipofuscins,[11,15] decreases in the rate and magnitude of reflex responses,[9] decreased sensory acuity, and reduction of alpha waves in cycles per second.[12] With the many cellular changes, as well as systemic changes in the nervous system, there are consequences reflected in activity.

With increasing age there is a decrease in speed of movement and a slowing of reaction time.[16] Additionally, we see decreased coordination in motor skills and ability to maintain balance. These functional changes with regard to neuronal aging have definite implications for types of activities selected for recreation by the older adult and enlighten us about the need for equalization in competition in certain activities for the older competitive athlete.

Aging and the Cardiovascular System
The cardiovascular system is vital in the maintenance of a state of total body homeostasis, especially in the presence of different types of stress on the body. With aging this homeostatic mechanism becomes less efficient, resulting in inefficiency in achieving homeostasis, less efficient functioning of homeostasis, or a failure to adapt to the occasion or imposed demands. Age-related and concomitant disease-related changes in the cardiovascular system may influence the functioning of every component of the human organism. Thus, familiarity with some of the changes in the cardiovascular system with aging is very important.

Among the reported changes at the cellular and tissue levels are myocardial darkening with presence of lipofuscin pigment, increased collagen content, and altered elasticity of blood vessel walls.[11,17-19] The presence of lipofuscin is believed possibly to lead to mitochondrial damage.[20] In the aging heart, especially one that suffers from arteriosclerosis, there is a reduction in the cross-sectional area of the coronary artery lumen with age.[21] Hypokinetic existence may complicate this process even further.

The changes in tissue structure of the cardiovascular system are the basis for functional changes with age.

The maximum attainable heart rate at rest and in

exercise remains a subject of controversy, with much support for a slight to significant decrease with aging.[16,22-25]

There is considerable agreement that there is decreased efficiency in certain parameters of cardiac hemodynamics. There is a decrease in stroke volume, especially with regard to exercise, which begins a steady decline after age 20,[26] and in maximum efforts the decrease in stroke volume can be quite significant in the older individual.[27] Cardiac output (heart rate × stroke volume) also has been found to decrease with the aging process.[9,22,27,28]

Factors possibly influencing stroke volume, and thus cardiac output, include ventricular pre-ejection blood volume, forcefulness of the ejection contraction, and amount of arterial pressure resisting blood ejection from the ventricle.[29] With aging, these factors may show less efficiency.[29] The combination of decreased cardiac reserve,[9] decline in the strength of the myocardium,[30] and additional changes mentioned previously often leads to diminished cardiac reserve with a decreased ability to make the appropriate physiological responses to emotional, physical, and psychological stresses.

Among other changes in the cardiovascular system in the presence of aging are increased systolic and diastolic blood pressure,[9,11,31] venous problems such as varicosities and distention of veins,[19] rigid and tortuous blood vessel walls,[17] loss of muscle cells in the sinoatrial node with an increase in fibrous tissue,[32] and age-related decreases in the effectiveness of adrenergic stimulation in the heart and smooth muscle of vascular tissue.[9,33]

The major changes in the cardiovascular system with regard to the aging process are found in Table 11-2.

Of course, there may be cases where there are exceptions to the aging cardiovascular system, such as the case of Clarence Demar mentioned earlier. There is much variability in this system in the older adult, and one may see a continuum ranging from the deconditioned patient to the patient who runs triathalons. According to Lewis,[11] the heart of the older adult free from pathology or disease often appears to resemble a younger heart, and it is the combination of injury and disease, as well as disuse, that produces decreased function in the older adult.

Aging and the Pulmonary System

The aging process has a definite impact on the pulmonary system and our mechanics of breathing as well as gaseous exchange. The anatomic disadvantage of the older adult is a less efficient gas delivery and exchange system and a poor lung–thoracic pump mechanism.[11]

Reddan[34] has reported reduction of maximum voluntary ventilation by 50% between the ages of 25 and 85, resulting from increased airway resistance, and reductions in vital capacity, and chest wall compliance. It has been firmly established that aging results in a decrease in vital capacity and an increase in residual volume.[35] Age differences in lung volumes and capacities have their basis in hypomobility of the chest wall with increasing age.

Certain lung and chest wall tissues are known to have a property known as elasticity that enables normal inspiration and expiration to occur. Compliance or elastic force per unit stretch of the thorax is important in the normal mechanics of respiration.[16] Lung tissue, as well as the wall of the thoracic cage, provide elastic resistance in respiration. It has been shown that lung compliance increases with age, whereas thoracic compliance decreases.[36-38]

Additional changes in pulmonary function with aging include decreases in pulmonary diffusion capacities during work and exercise,[39] decreases in partial pressure of arterial oxygen,[40] and decreases in the number of pulmonary capillaries, resting arterial oxygenation, and maximum oxygen uptake.[41] With the problems presented by decreases in the efficiency of gaseous exchange, arterial oxygenation, and mechanics of breathing producing poor ventilation, breathing often becomes harder and exercise capacities are reduced in the older adult.[11] A summary of normal pulmonary changes with aging is presented in Table 11-3.

TABLE 11-2. CARDIOVASCULAR SYSTEM CHANGES WITH AGE

Decreased stroke volume and cardiac output

Increased systolic and diastolic blood pressure

Increased resting heart rate

Decreased cardiac reserve to respond to stress

Decreased maximal attainable resting and exercise heart rate

Increased blood vessel wall rigidity

Loss of elasticity of blood vessel walls

Increased arterial pulse pressure

Presence of venous complications (varicosities, vein distention)

Decreased efficiency as a homeostatic mechanism

Decreased myocardial strength

Lipid accumulation on arterial walls with vessel narrowing

TABLE 11-3. PULMONARY SYSTEM CHANGES WITH AGE

Decreased thoracic wall compliance

Decreased vital capacity and increased residual volume

Decreased pulmonary diffusion

Increased airway resistance

Decreased arterial oxygenation at rest and exercise

Decreased partial pressures of arterial oxygen

Decreased number of pulmonary capillaries

Decreased maximum oxygen consumption

Musculoskeletal Changes With Aging

A variety of changes ensues in the musculoskeletal system with the aging process. The changes affect a variety of structures and have the potential of interfering with joint and muscle function, which are vital components for performance in the older athlete and normal function in the exercising older adult.

The aging adult is predisposed to joint pathology (e.g., arthritides) due to changes in joint surfaces, ligaments, tendons, and connective tissue.[42] Despite the wide variety of life-styles in older adults, where a definitive age of onset of decline cannot be pinpointed due to aging, evidence is available that regressive changes in tissues of diarthrodial joints begin to occur after 20 years of age.[43] Lewis[44] identified the change in the collagen structure of the older adult as a major culprit in musculoskeletal aging.

There is loss of elasticity of joint cartilage, ligaments, and periarticular tissue. Characteristics of altered collagen in the older adult include irregular shaping due to cross linking, lack of parallel formation of the fibers, and reduced mobility, with a slower response to stretch than occurs in the younger person.[44] Decreased mobility of body tissues has also been attributed to a closer meshing, with a decreased linear pull relationship in collagen tissue.[45] These changes may compromise joint functions and joint range of motion (ROM) in the older adult or older athlete.

Although decreases in joint ROM in the older individual are a reality,[11] there are only a limited number of studies on normative joint ROM values in adults over 60 years of age.[46,47] Walker et al[48] found that active ROM measurements did not differ significantly in older individuals of different age groups, and that clinicians may expect to find decreased ROM in healthy older individuals. It should also be remembered that pain and muscle weakness may also limit joint ROM, and that the limitation can be compounded by disuse, which will also produce decrements in muscle function.

Many changes in muscle structure and function with regard to aging continue to be discovered. Some discussion continues to evolve regarding whether losses in muscle function in older individuals are more a disuse phenomenon than a true age effect.[49] Despite this discussion, age-related changes in muscle are evident and well documented.

The presence of muscle atrophy is a primary concomitant of the aging process due to loss of number and size of muscle fibers.[16,50–52] Due to loss of contractile elements in aging, we do see some losses in muscle strength. The amount of strength lost per decade of life as we age remains a subject of controversy. A decline in muscle strength of the human has been identified as early as the third and fourth decades of life;[53] however, the decline has been found to occur slowly during this period, with a greater rate of decline after the fifth dec-

TABLE 11-4. MUSCULOSKELETAL CHANGES WITH AGE

Joint Changes
  Decreased resilience in elasticity of joint cartilage
  Decreased range of motion
  Altered collagen formation
  Decreased collagen mobility with slower response to
    stretch
  Predisposition to joint pathology and malfunction
  Pain and increased incidence of joint discomfort
Muscle Changes
  Muscle atrophy and declining muscle strength
  Decreased enzymatic activity in mitochondria
  Decreased muscular endurance and respiratory capacity
    of muscle
  Decreased capacity for exercise recovery
  Decreased ATP and creatine phosphate resynthesis
  Decreased volume of red and white muscle fibers
  Greater amounts of fibrous tissue in muscle
  Slowing of movement and decreased muscle coordination
  Altered contraction times of red and white fibers

ade of life.[16] With the decline in muscle strength with aging, movements tend to be slower and there is accompanying deficit in motor coordination.[51,52] There is evidence that aging affects certain muscles more than others,[51] and greater incidences of muscle weakness occur due to replacement of an increased proportion of skeletal muscle by fibrous tissue.[54]

Additional cellular changes in muscle with aging also affect function of muscle. There are changes in the mitochondria characterized by decreases in enzyme activity leading to impaired energy supply and tension development in muscles.[9,52] Related to this are decreases in respiratory capacity of muscle, which accounts for decreased muscle endurance and capacity for recovery.[55] Evidence has also been presented that there are decreased concentrations of adenosine triphosphate (ATP) with creative phosphate resynthesis.[51] The loss of human muscle tissue with aging has also been found to account for the downward trend in basal metabolism as we age.[56] The result of combining the cellular and tissue changes of aging with the phenomenon of disuse are decreases in function of muscle, most notably muscle strength and endurance. The older individual must be advised to be as active as possible within certain guidelines to retard this process. Muscle strength and aging and the effects of disuse are discussed further below. A summary of musculoskeletal changes with the aging process is presented in Table 11–4.

PROBLEMS POTENTIALLY COMPROMISING HUMAN PERFORMANCE IN THE OLDER ADULT/OLDER ATHLETE

The sports physical therapist should remember that despite the high activity profile presented by older competitive and recreational athletes, typical problems

seen in older adults are still capable of being present. Specifically, disease processes in many of the aforementioned systems and other debilitating effects of aging are still present, although possibly to a lesser degree despite the high activity profile. Other problems are presented in the older competitive and recreational athlete potentially compromising exercise tolerance and human performance such as age-related changes in physical working capacity, motivation, and psychological problems, metabolic disease processes, pain, and nutritional imbalances. A knowledge of some of the basic characteristics of these problems and their potential for impeding performance is imperative for the sports physical therapy clinician who rehabilitates or conditions the older athlete.

Cardiovascular Problems

Arteriosclerotic Heart Disease. Much attention has been focused in recent years on arteriosclerotic heart disease, also known as coronary heart disease, ischemic heart disease, and atherosclerotic heart disease. There has been much research on the effects of exercise in retarding or reversing this process with inconclusive results. The death of author and avid runner, Jim Fixx, several years ago provided evidence that this disease process can debilitate and kill older individuals who are very active and athletic, despite their seemingly excellent physical condition.

An attempt to discuss the extensive, fine, intricate details of the pathophysiology is beyond the scope of this section. The purpose of the section is to elaborate briefly on arteriosclerotic cardiovascular disease, present some clinical manifestations of the disease that may occur in the exercising older adult, and discuss the benefits of physical conditioning in patients with this problem. Hopefully, this approach will provide guidelines and safety precautions for the clinician to consider when working with a patient with this problem.

Arteriosclerotic heart disease is a progressive disease characterized by a series of changes involving the intima of the arterial wall. The changes involve a laying down of arteriosclerotic plaque and necrosis of the vessel, leading to alterations in arterial structure and function.[57] With the progressive disease process there is a decrease in the elasticity of the arterial walls and a gradual narrowing of the artery.

With the progressive occlusion of the artery lumen, blood flow decreases, and, if the coronary arteries are involved, the decreased blood flow results in inadequate oxygenation of the myocardium. The imbalance between myocardial oxygen supply and demand is known as ischemia. Ischemia is characterized by insufficient blood flow to the cell to meet cellular needs.[58] When this occurs there may be clinical manifestations that may interfere with, impede, or terminate physical activity of the older individual. Clinical manifestations include angina pectoris, myocardial infarction, and sudden cardiac death.

Angina pectoris, a clinical manifestation of the ischemic process, results from the arterial changes caused by arteriosclerosis of the coronary arteries. Due to insufficient blood flow, myocardial oxygen demand exceeds myocardial oxygen supply. The symptoms of angina pectoris include a retrosternal feeling of a squeezing or pressure, referred pain to different parts of the face and neck, and shortness of breath (dyspnea). The chest pain is often facilitated by exercise, unusual exertion, or consumption of large amounts of food. Various types of angina pectoris have been described, such as stable and unstable angina pectoris. The latter is more severe than the former, with greater frequency, and often indicates an impending myocardial infarction.[58-60]

Myocardial infarction is characterized by a localized necrosis of part of the myocardium due to a progressive and prolonged myocardial ischemia. With the necrosis, blood cannot get through to supply the heart muscle. Severe chest pain ensues, often progressively worsening until it is unbearable. The myocardial infarction victim may also experience feelings of weakness, dyspnea, nausea, vomiting, and cool, clammy skin. He or she often loses consciousness. The condition is emergent and requires that the physical therapist institute appropriate emergency procedures, whether in the clinic or while covering an athletic event outside the clinic.

Sudden cardiac death is a phenomenon that continues to baffle the medical community. It occurs often in apparently healthy individuals engaged in normal activities, in some cases exercise, without any warnings. The phenomenon is not characteristic of older adults only, and is occurring at an increasingly alarming rate. Often significant pathology is uncovered in its victims (e.g., Jim Fixx, Pete Maravich). The cause of sudden cardiac death is unknown; however, it is theorized to be precipitated by ventricular fibrillation or quivering.[58]

All the above clinical manifestations are capable of interfering with or preventing physical activity in older recreational and competitive athletes. Many older individuals embark upon exercise programs without a knowledge of the extent of disease present, participate in cardiac conditioning programs for rehabilitative or preventive purposes, or use exercise for conditioning programs for successful participation in recreational and competitive sport. Proper exercise testing is essential to ascertain the physiological responses to exercise in all these types of patients. Regardless of the scenario, there are benefits of aerobic exercise in the individual with coronary heart disease and those are presented in Table 11–5.

TABLE 11-5. BENEFITS OF AEROBIC EXERCISE CONDITIONING IN PATIENTS WITH ARTERIOSCLEROTIC HEART DISEASE

Decreased heart rate and blood pressure at any given submaximal work load

Increased coronary perfusion

Greater myocardial oxygen supply and less myocardial oxygen demand

Greater usage of oxygen by peripheral muscles

Quicker return of heart rate to pre-exercise level

Reduction in plasma catecholamine levels

Increased work capacity

Improved psychological status

Modification of blood chemistry

Weight reduction

Modification of certain coronary risk factors

Improved efficiency of the oxygen transport system

Hypertension. Hypertension, or elevation of resting systolic and diastolic blood pressure, remains an enormous health problem and intriguing anomaly of the cardiovascular system of unknown origin, often leading to disastrous consequences. It is estimated that the disorder affects 37 million Americans, most of whom receive inadequate or no treatment for the disorder.[61] It is often discovered accidentally (e.g., insurance physicals, yearly physical examinations, preseason evaluations of athletes) and, if left untreated, can reduce the average life expectancy of its victims by 20 years.[62]

The most common type of hypertension treated by physicians is "primary" or "essential" hypertension, which is characterized by an unstable or continuous elevation of resting blood pressure above the normal range due to unknown causes.[63] Equally undetermined is the boundary between the upper range of normal blood pressure and the point at which a diagnosis of hypertension is established, as many different values have been given in the literature.[63–66] Many of us have been taught that the upper normal level of resting blood pressure is a reading of 140/90 mm Hg. Although the origin or pathogenesis of this disorder has not yet been clearly defined, we do know that untreated essential hypertension contributes to major cardiovascular complications later in life.

Asymptomatic elevation of blood pressure often begins in the second and third decades of life and does not manifest itself until decades later, with gloomy results. Some of the problems presented include atherosclerotic heart disease, stroke, congestive heart failure, kidney dysfunction and disease, left ventricular dysfunction, and cerebral hemorrhage.[62,63] Young people with high blood pressure have a greater likelihood of having hypertension with advancing age,[67] and hypertensive diastolic blood pressure at rest has been identified as a known risk factor for atherosclerosis.[68] This disorder, with its potential complications and consequences, has many implications for the older athlete,

competitive and recreational, as well as the exercising older adult.

An older adult, especially the habitually sedentary individual, should not consider exercise training for competitive or recreational pursuits before undergoing a thorough physical examination by a physician, including an exercise test. It has been reported that several older people who died suddenly during athletic competition or recreational activity, whose deaths were ascribed to coronary heart disease, often had a history of hypertension.[69,70] Important clinical data can be obtained from resting and exercise blood pressure readings, and they are determined by age, overall health status, especially of the cardiovascular system, physical fitness status, and effects of medication.

The normal blood pressure response to exercise involves an increase in systolic blood pressure proportional to the work load, with little or no change in diastolic blood pressure.[16] An exaggerated blood pressure response in exercise may be seen in older healthy individuals, and inadequate responses in blood pressure may occur in the sedentary individual.[60] The body usually adapts to the increased systolic blood pressure with exercise, as the increased oxygen demand of tissues requires that cardiac output be increased.

The hypertensive individual often displays an excessive blood pressure response to exercise, and marked increases of systolic blood pressure are common in hypertensive patients at relatively low work loads.[63] A persistent increase in diastolic blood pressure (greater than 20 mm Hg above the resting value) has been found to be an indicator of the presence of coronary artery disease,[71] as well as contraction abnormalities of the left ventricle.[63] These factors reveal the need for monitoring of exercise blood pressure response in older individuals with hypertension prior to undertaking an aerobic conditioning program. The older athlete or exercising adult with a history of hypertension should be cautious in the selection of exercises to increase muscular strength and endurance.

Weight training using a variety of resistive exercise devices, such as various commercial exercise machines and free weights, is an integral part of conditioning programs of many sports and involves isometric (static) types of exercise. Static exercise increases systolic and diastolic blood pressure, increases cardiac output and pulse rate, and causes slight changes in arterial resistance in normal subjects,[72] and these adverse responses are intensified in hypertensive individuals.[73] Extensive periods involving activities requiring strenuous static isometric contractions (e.g., lifting, pushing, holding, hanging) should be discouraged by the health professional because they consume large oxygen supply requirements for the heart, compress blood vessels, and elevate blood pressure.[74,75]

The prospective older athlete with hypertension should initially be cleared by a physician for compet-

itive or recreational activities, and the conditioning program should be closely monitored by an appropriate health professional. Characteristics of the exercise conditioning program should include vital sign monitoring, especially during new activities, proper (gradual) warmup before exercise, a gradual increase in exercise intensity, and avoidance of isometric forms of exercise. The health professional supervising the conditioning program should also be cognizant of the patient's medication plan and pharmacological influences on exercise responses.

Venous Problems. It is important to discuss venous problems as a complication that may hinder exercise capacity or performance in the older athlete, especially with reference to age-related changes in venous circulation and veins mentioned earlier in this chapter. The sports physical therapist must use basic evaluation skills in evaluation of vascular problems, such as venous incompetency, as many vascular system problems are actually of a musculoskeletal nature.[76] Two disorders or diseases of the venous circulatory system that may be seen in the older athlete are varicose veins and thrombophlebitis.

Varicose veins occur due to dilation and tortuosity, causing impairment of function of small valves in the veins and limiting backflow. Individuals with varicosities are often asymptomatic and are capable of physical activity; however, some individuals with symptoms will complain of feelings of aching, heaviness, cramps, and excessive swelling of the feet and lower legs usually at the end of the day, as well as itching and burning.[77] Varicose veins can be treated with exercise to increase muscle pumping action and venous return, use of different types of elastic stockings, and elevation of the lower extremities.

Thrombophlebitis is a venous disorder characterized by the clotting of blood, with consequent obstruction of a vein in which there has been inflammation, or where inflammation of the vein appears to result during the formation of a clot. It may occur in superficial or deep vessels of the lower extremities and often occurs in older individuals involved in exercise programs.[77] Treatment for this disorder may involve a variety of approaches, including anti-inflammatory antibiotic and anticoagulant medications prescribed by a physician, elastic stockings, exercise, and elevation of the extremity.[77] Prior to a return to full physical activity, especially in the very active older individual, there should be appropriate serial diagnostic evaluations (e.g., venogram).

Compromises in Physical Working Capacity—Human Performance

Cardiovascular Endurance—Aerobic Power. It is generally agreed that cardiovascular endurance and aerobic capacity decline with increasing age, and that the oxygen transport and delivery system become less efficient. Many studies have documented a decrease in cardiovascular function with increasing age.[23,78] A consequence of the decreased function is a decreased aerobic exercise capacity. Longitudinal as well as comprehensive studies have revealed a steady decline in maximum oxygen consumption with aging.[79-84]

The classic work in this area was done by Robinson,[85] and corroborated by Noble,[86] where the findings were startling. An investigation of 93 subjects between the ages of 6 and 91 years revealed that aerobic power increased until 17.4 years, where it reached 30 L/min, and experienced a steady decline thereafter. Subsequent studies in this area have revealed significant decreases in aerobic power per year as we age and by percentages across the lifespan.

Several studies have revealed the decline in aerobic capacity from the twenties or thirties to the sixties, seventies, and beyond to approximate about 40%,[78,79,81,87] with some studies reporting values as high as 50%.[88] Most estimates of average annual loss in maximum oxygen consumption approximate 1.2%.[78,84,89-92] The age-related decline in performance and aerobic capacity has been attributed to different theories of causative factors, such as cardiac system deficits and decreased arterial venous oxygen concentrations,[93] possibility of decreased muscle mass,[86] and decreased energy production and circulatory delivery of oxygen regardless of activity history.[9]

In recent years a key concern has been whether the deterioration in cardiovascular function in the aging person results more from the aging process or a sedentary life-style.[94] Although a longer period of time is required for the older person to achieve maximum fitness from almost any starting point,[95] elderly individuals who are active have been shown to cut the average decrease in aerobic power attributed to aging by as much as 50%.[90,92] Aging and disuse do have similar characteristics, with each suggested to be responsible for close to 50% of the functional decline that occurs between the ages of 30 and 70.[89,96] Exercise training, cardiovascular function, and aerobic capacity in the older individual are discussed later in the chapter.

Flexibility—Joint Range of Motion (ROM). It is essential for the older athlete, competitive or recreational, to combat traditional declining flexibility with age, as normal flexibility and efficient joint motion are needed for warmup activities prior to exercise, and to execute movements required in the respective motor activity in which the athlete is involved. Flexibility involves exposing the contractile unit to active or passive movement, with appropriate positioning of the joint spanning the respective muscle–tendon unit.[97]

A decrease in flexibility and joint ROM may be the result of changes in collagen formation, effects of dis-

ease processes (e.g., arthritis), decreased physical activity or a combination of these factors.[11,44] The states of muscle tissue, joints, tendons, and ligaments are probably integrated to determine the extent of flexibility,[98] and when soft tissue around a joint shortens there is restriction of movement.[97]

Decreased flexibility increases the difficulty of functional movements and activities involved in the aforementioned recreational and competitive sport endeavors. Due to pain, discomfort, and associated muscle weakness, which can all restrict amplitudes of motion, joint aging may be a big hindrance for older individuals contemplating an exercise program.

Decreases in flexibility may also be accompanied by decreases in stability, mobility, power, and resistance to load or muscle strength.[44,99] A decrease in flexibility may also limit enthusiasm or motivation for exercise, as the limited motion may not allow for proper exercise execution, producing more pain or muscle soreness, thus discouraging the participant. Maintenance of flexibility is crucial and enhances both specific and general body movements for activities in which the older athlete might be engaged.[100] Flexibility may possibly be the most difficult component of muscular efficiency to regain after it has declined significantly.[98]

Body Composition. The older individual should be encouraged to attain and maintain a body weight recommended by his or her physician. The consequences of excessive weight gain in the adult years are myriad, and directly related to many adult onset disorders and illnesses. It is important for the clinician to have an understanding of the adverse effects of excessive weight on the patient with whom he or she is working, as it can have an adverse effect on performance.

Excessive weight places many burdens on many body systems, especially the ciculatory system, and is associated with promoting poor exercise tolerance when the body is stressed. Furthermore, excessive weight is also related to the prevalence of hypertension, atherosclerosis, high cholesterol levels, and the onset of diabetes in the adult.

Excessive weight often becomes a problem in the later part of the early adult years and progresses steadily to a maximum point, usually in the fifth or sixth decade, at which point weight starts to decline again.[101] Due to the inverse relationship between excess weight and exercise performance, the older athlete should be very concerned about maintaining proper body weight and body composition (relationship of body fat and lean body mass).

It is often difficult to estimate the percentage of body fat because of alterations in characteristics of tissues, especially in elderly individuals.[102] Examples include changes in skin texture, muscle atrophy, and decreases in bone density.[102] There have been several attempts over the last several years to develop standard approaches for evaluating percentage of body fat, with considerations for differences in age as a major factor.[103-106]

Muscular Strength-Endurance. In the presence of increasing age, muscle function, as well as physical activity patterns, may change. The life expectancy of the American population is increasing, and the elderly are remaining physically active in recreational and competitive sports, necessitating an understanding of muscle function in older adults. It has been acknowledged that muscle strength reaches its maximum somewhere between the ages of 20 and 30, after which it decreases gradually.

After the fifth decade of life, strength tends to decrease at a greater rate, with the loss in muscle strength being greater in women than in men.[16] Both sexes tend to have a greater decline in strength in lower extremity and trunk muscles as opposed to upper extremity muscles.[86,107] It is postulated that humans tend to become less adaptable to muscle–strength training in presence of the aging process.[108] There is still some discrepancy in the literature regarding the cause of waning muscle strength with increasing age. The decline has been linked to cell death and changes within the muscle contractile system,[98] as well as changes in muscle mass.[86] Small losses of muscle strength with aging have also been hypothesized to be caused by disuse rather than representing a true aging effect.[16]

It is well documented that isometric and dynamic muscle strength decreases with age[109,110]; however, research on muscle endurance effects with aging continues to get much attention. The literature has presented no conclusive evidence about the effects of aging on isometric and dynamic muscle endurance. Continuous evidence regarding maintenance and even increase of isometric and dynamic muscle endurance in the presence of aging has refuted some earlier studies regarding muscle endurance loss with aging.[110-112]

Altered muscle strength may be a reality in the older athlete and a factor limiting optimal performance. With this knowledge of the age-related limitations of muscle strength, caution and discretion should be used in selecting strengthening activities for conditioning and rehabilitation of older athletes.

Musculoskeletal Problems

Osteoarthritis. Degenerative joint disease can pose a significant hindrance to the older competitive or recreational athlete because of its painful and debilitating symptoms. It is a common disorder of aging that affects one or more joints and is characterized by a progressive pathological degeneration of articular cartilage, formation, remodeling, and hypertrophy of subchondral

bone, and secondary synovial membrane inflammation.[113,114]

Weight-bearing joints are chiefly involved and it is fairly common in individuals over the age of 50.[115] Certain characteristics of the disease are related to progressive wear and tear of joints through the lifespan, with characteristic appearance of symptomatology during the later years of life.

Symptoms of the disorder include pain, loss of joint motion, crepitus, joint swelling, and weakness and spasm of muscles surrounding the affected joint. These symptoms often influence the type of exercise training mode the older individual uses for conditioning purposes, and whether traditional forms of exercise can be used to prepare the older athlete for competition.

Delayed Muscle Soreness. Older individuals returning to physical conditioning after an extended period of inactivity (e.g., months, years, decades) may experience severe muscular discomfort a few days after exercising. The problem may also be seen in sporadic exercisers, or individuals undertaking new or different forms of exercise, and is known as "delayed onset muscle soreness."[116]

Many older individuals display this trend upon returning to physical activity for recreation, as well as when training for competitive events. The physical activity often represents a new activity to which the individual is not accustomed, thus producing the soreness, and if the exercise is not of a continuous nature, the problem also arises frequently. Eccentric exercises have been identified in the literature as a major culprit in the onset of this phenomenon.[117-119] Different models or theories of delayed onset muscle soreness have been presented, the two most readily accepted of which include tearing and rupturing of muscle fibers with exercise (torn tissue theory) and delayed postexercise muscle pain as a result of muscle elastic components overstretching in the fibrils and fibers (connective tissue damage theory).[116]

Psychological Problems

Motivational Problems. Older individuals often need encouragement to become involved in physical activity, not only for rehabilitation, but also for recreational as well as health purposes. There are many faulty perceptions about activity and aging in our youth-oriented and weight-conscious society that potentially interfere with successful and positive attitudes about physical activity in this population. Among these false notions are the unwarranted emphasis on slowing down and resting in the elderly, the belief that the need for energy expenditure through exercise diminishes with aging, the exaggeration of the risks of vigorous exercise after middle age, and the belief that exercise requires a significant effort in the aged.[99] Additionally, many older individuals tend to underrate the abilities and capacities they possess for efficient execution of physical tasks. A problem that may interfere with the willingness of the elderly to exercise or engage in competition with their peers is the negative comparison of their current capabilities to former capabilities.

The media pay little attention to competitive events in older athletes, especially those capable of enormous physical feats. The reality is that there are many benefits of exercise physically and psychologically in older individuals utilizing exercise to train for competition or for recreational endeavors. The older athlete should realize that a gradual increase of physical fitness is desirable and that fitness cannot be attained immediately. The understanding that benefits of exercise training are attained at a slower rate in aging might help to reduce motivation problems in the elderly.

Hypochondriasis. The hypochondriacal older athlete may place undue emphasis on aches or discomforts, exaggerating the symptoms and seeing a variety of physicians despite assurances that there is no injury. The condition may interrupt the individual's exercise program and promote sedentary living.

Depression. Depression affects a significant portion of the elderly population. It is characterized by feelings of gloom, negative self-image, hopelessness or despair, despondency, discouragement, dejection, unhappiness, pessimism, and a sense of aloofness. The problem may become apparent in the older athlete when a sense of reaching a plateau in training is sensed, upon failure to reach individual goals in training or competition, upon illness that interferes with training, and as a reaction to injury. The sports physical therapist should be cognizant of the problems associated with depression, especially when rehabilitating the injured older athlete. In both animal[120] and human[121] studies, the effects of exercise have been found to have a favorable effect on preventing or treating depression by increasing brain levels of serotonin and norepinephrine.

The Stress of Athletic Career Termination. The termination of a competitive or recreational athletic career in an older athlete may produce a psychological stressor for which the athlete is not prepared. Chronological age, compounded by health problems interfering with safe and successful competition, has a profound effect on the athlete trying to maintain his or her career. Physiological changes in the body potentially hampering performance may present problems for the older athlete who must face the reality of competing against younger, stronger, quicker, more durable, and

often superior athletes. The older athlete who has retired from professional sport usually faces a period of adjustment laden with dilemmas and identity crises, which should be managed by an appropriate professional.

Additional Problems Potentially Influencing Exercise Response

Medications. Medications used to treat problems may also create problems for the elderly. This group takes a large variety of prescription as well as nonprescription medications, increasing the likelihood of adverse drug reactions and toxicity.[122,123]

The sports physical therapist working with an older athlete should be familiar with common medications taken by older patients, frequently for different reasons. The *Physicians Desk Reference* (PDR) should be consulted regarding different or unfamiliar medications and their effects. It should be remembered that medications also have many side effects and adverse reactions that may influence or even interfere with a conditioning or rehabilitation program in active older individuals.

Medications can have such adverse side effects as drowsiness, fatigue, alteration of exercise response, muscle cramps and weaknesses, and claudication, among others, that would have a definite influence on an exercise program. Particular attention should be given to patients taking cardiac medications that may influence heart rate, both for the side effects of the medication and the symptoms of the underlying pathology. The major classifications of cardiac medications are antiarrhythmics, antihypertensives, β-adrenergic blockers, calcium antagonists, vasodilators, and cardiotonic glycosides.[124]

The older athlete should be encouraged to ask his or her physician or pharmacist about individual medications, especially with regard to how they influence exercise. Medications must be used properly, with adequate understanding of dosage, desired effects, side effects, and method of taking the medication. Fewer problems would ensue if medications were treated with more respect.[125]

Pain. In older athletes, pain can hinder performance, exercise training, and rehabilitation programs. Any complaint of discomfort or pain should receive serious, meticulous scrutiny from the clinician. Lewis[19] cites several reasons for difficulties in assessing pain in older adults including altered or decreased pain sensitivity, difficulty localizing pain, hypochondriasis, and tendencies to focus on pain when depressed.

Pain that appears to be musculoskeletal in origin may in fact have a cardiopulmonary, neurological, or even an oncological etiology. Therefore, pain complaints must be evaluated thoroughly, and if the source cannot be detected, further medical intervention may be indicated. The cause of underlying pain should be treated properly before the individual resumes physical activity.

Nutritional Problems. Older athletes should eat properly to ensure that they have the proper fuel for meeting energy requirements in recreational as well as competitive activities. The older individual needs to find a happy medium for nutrition and diet, as a poor diet may induce premature senility, whereas a diet that exceeds human needs may lead to obesity and produce symptoms associated with degenerative diseases.

Similar nutritive essentials are required in adequate quantities to nourish the body throughout a lifetime, and an insufficiency in any of the essentials can be harmful at any age.[101] The older person needs diet planning, with more frequent but smaller meals being better suited to the diminished digestive and absorptive capacity.[101] Additional considerations may include the person's income, social situation, cooking and activity of daily living (ADL) abilities, refrigeration facilities, and tendencies in food faddism.

The older athlete might want to have the guidance of a registered dietitian in helping him or her to design a menu tailored to individual needs. Clark[126] recommends this for athletes of any age, especially for athletes with eating disorders or food obsessions. Included in the dietary consultation should be a diet history, estimation of body composition and daily caloric needs, comparison of eating and energy expenditure needs, and promotion of healthy eating practices. The dietitian should also realize that nutritional needs may be different between the 80-year-old marathoner and the 80-year-old individual confined to bed in a nursing home.

Hearing and Visual Problems. Acuity of various body senses tends to diminish with aging. Our senses of hearing, sight, feeling, and smell are affected to a great degree. Two senses declining in function with age that may adversely affect motor performance, especially in competition, are hearing and visual problems.

Among problems presented by elderly individuals with regard to hearing are failure to hear, slower reaction to sounds, distortion of high-frequency sounds, difficulty in discrimination between essential and nonessential sounds, and sound distortion.[127] A lack of hearing and hearing distortions may leave the older athlete at the starting line of a swimming meet or leave him or her stranded in the track blocks, creating a potentially embarrassing situation and psychological problem. Failure to hear the whistle of an official may mean the difference between stopping or continuing momentum, possibly exposing the individual or others to injury.

Visual acuity loss can also create problems for the

older athlete. Misjudging of distances, distortion of images, inability to see or follow an object (e.g., visual tracking), color distortion, poor depth perception, and visual field abnormalities are realities in the older adult. The problem can manifest itself by affecting reaction time and affecting the ability to react properly. A split-second misperception might mean the difference between getting injured and not getting injured. Examples of this might include dodging a softball, quickly returning a tennis stroke, or reacting to a volleyball. Older athletes are advised to have regular examinations of the eyes and ears to evaluate their intactness for normal function and whether they are capable of reacting in pressure situations.

Balance. Normative data on balance abilities according to age do not exist. It is generally agreed that balance tends to diminish as one ages, and this has been documented in evaluations such as the Romberg test.[128,129] Reports of inability to maintain balance on one leg with the eyes closed has also been reported with progressive aging.[130]

Balance problems also have implications for the older athlete in both competitive and recreational activities. With balance difficulties, the potential of falling is presented in the older individual,[131] with a danger of pathological fractures in this population. This has some implications for the activities the older individual selects for recreational and competitive purposes. Activities requiring good balance, such as skiing, martial arts, gymnastics, and certain types of dance activities, would present problems for the elderly. Older athletes have also suffered injuries due to loss of balance in common activities such as playing tennis, golf, and running. Ideally, prospective older athletes should have their balance evaluated to determine whether it is adequate to meet the demands of the desired competitive or recreational activity.

Menopause. The cessation of menstrual function in the older women brings about many physiological and psychological changes. The changes may affect the older female athlete and have unfavorable effects on performance. Associated problems include osteoporosis, cardiovascular disease, and depression, which may be from estrogen deficiency or may result from the aging process itself.[121] Because exercise is beneficial in combatting these problems, the women approaching menopause should be encouraged to stay as active as possible.

Osteoporosis. Osteoporosis continues to be a major problem in the elderly and receives much attention due to its sequelae. It has been defined in many ways, reflecting its different characteristics. Osteoporosis may involve a reduction in bone mass, with subsequent increased susceptibility to fracture,[132] a net loss of mineralized bone mass due to an imbalance between bone resorption and formation during the remodeling cycle,[133] or a loss of bone matrix and mineral.[134] Osteoporosis has become a significant area of interest due to increased longevity among the geriatric population and increasing participation in recreational sports by female athletes.[135] With the increase in society of the elderly population, the incidence of cases of older patients with osteoporosis will increase.[136]

The sports physical therapist may treat the older athlete who already has osteoporosis or who is at high risk for developing it. Many risk factors for osteoporosis have been identified, such as nutritional status, hormonal level activity, and physical activity history.[137-139] The lack of dietary calcium has been reported to be a cause of osteoporosis,[121,136] along with estrogen deficiency, especially after menopause.[121,140,141] Although osteoporosis is usually linked more to women, especially petite Caucasian women of Northern European descent,[121,136] it can occur in men,[135] and its incidence seems to be greater in white than black women.[142] Other contributing factors are a positive family history, alcoholism, and tobacco abuse. In the presence of osteoporosis, bone becomes more susceptible to fracture and often has a decreased ability to withstand normal load or stress placed on it,[144] increasing the likelihood of a pathological fracture to certain areas of the body (e.g., vertebrae, wrist, and hip) after an abnormal body movement or a fall.[139] Lack of exercise or sedentary life-style due to imposed immobility is known to have a devastating effect on osteoporosis by accelerating the process of bone loss.

Exercise and stress on bone is necessary for preventing or retarding the onset of osteoporosis, as lack of stress has been attributed to breakdown of bone tissue.[140] Bone atrophy and loss of skeletal mass along with losses of calcium have been reported during periods of inactivity,[136] and periods of immobility or bed rest due to disease or injury in the elderly often produces "disuse osteoporosis." The immobilization period leads to loss of calcium and demineralization of bone, accelerating the process of osteoporosis.[143] Weight-bearing exercises in particular are essential in maintaining bone mass and stressing bone,[140] and several studies have provided conclusive evidence that bone mineralization is enhanced by exercise, and that exercise is a vital modality in preventing and treating involitional bone loss.[145-147]

What then are the implications of osteoporosis for the older athlete? Despite varying activity levels, ranging from the recreational to the highly competitive participant, the reality remains that the demineralization process still occurs. The bone quality of a 60- or 70-year-old individual is not the same as that of one who is 20 or 30. Activities in which the older athlete chooses to participate must be carefully selected. Osteoporosis, along with loss of balance in an activity, can have im-

mediate and dire consequences, turning an active independent person into an inactive convalescent. During periods of immobility of the entire body or immobilization of a body part, the older athlete should be quickly started on a rehabilitation program to counteract the adverse effects of prolonged recumbency or immobilization. This would apply from the individual immobilized in a cast for a fracture to the individual who may be bedridden for an illness. It is apparent also that bone loss occurring naturally with age can be accelerated by a pathological fracture and subsequent immobility and more bone loss in a vicious cycle. This cycle is depicted in Fig 11–1.

Diabetes Mellitus. The sports physical therapist should have a clear understanding of the relationship between diabetes and exercise, including the necessary precautions and proper foot and skin care, when dealing with an older athlete who is diabetic. The clinician may come into contact with the diabetic athlete in one of several ways. The individual may be a patient with diabetes mellitus of a longstanding nature who is referred for another problem, a patient with adult-onset

type of diabetes referred for an exercise training program to lose weight and help regulate the condition, or an older diabetic athlete participating in a sports event, most likely a marathon race that the sports physical therapist is covering. The clinician may also encounter a healthy diabetic older athlete seeking advice about exercise.

Regular physical activity, diet, and insulin therapy are usually the basic methods of proper management of the diabetic patient.[148] Exercise may be favorable or highly risky to diabetic patients depending upon the circumstances. There must be evidence of good clinical control of blood glucose levels through diet and medication.[149] Moderate prolonged and sustained aerobic exercise decreases the need for insulin.[148,150-152] Insulin and diet are more efficiently managed if the patient exercises daily and consistently, as this usually reduces insulin needs.[148] Exercise training assists in increasing cellular sensitivity to insulin, helping to overcome insulin resistance, and improves glucose tolerance, especially in adult-onset diabetes.[151] Following a regimen of regular exercise training, the insulin-dependent diabetic who is well controlled will improve glucose toler-

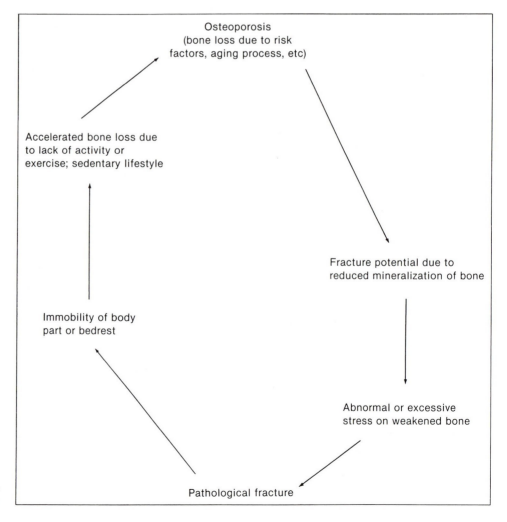

Figure 11–1. The osteoporosis–immobility–osteoporosis cycle.

Osteoporosis
(bone loss due to risk factors, aging process, etc)

Accelerated bone loss due to lack of activity or exercise; sedentary lifestyle

Fracture potential due to reduced mineralization of bone

Immobility of body part or bedrest

Abnormal or excessive stress on weakened bone

Pathological fracture

ance, with resultant reduction in daily insulin need due to this enhanced tissue sensitivity to insulin, especially in skeletal muscle.[153] In addition to inducing changes in glucose tolerance and increasing the ability of cells to use glucose, exercise has been found to lower plasma triglycerides, increase levels of high-density lipoproteins, and increase mobilization and utilization of free fatty acids at the cellular level in diabetic individuals.[151] Aerobic exercise by the diabetic has also been linked to provision of a more efficient oxygen exchange by reducing thickened capillary membranes and decreasing stress with promotion of relaxation.[152]

Certain precautions must be taken with the exercising diabetic athlete or patient. A meticulous balance must be maintained among diet, insulin, or medication, and the exercise program. The exercising diabetic with insufficient insulin levels is in danger due to increasing levels of blood sugar levels, potentially leading to hyperglycemia. Thus, exercise by the uncontrolled diabetic is not advisable and may be more harmful than helpful to the individual.[149] It is also important for the individual to coordinate exercise and meal schedules properly, and to know times of peak insulin levels to avoid potential hypoglycemic episodes with exercise. The diabetic individual should not choose an injection site on an extremity that will be involved in exercise (e.g., thigh injection if bicycling) due to a greater chance of hypoglycemia resulting from increases in peripheral circulation and muscle sensitivity to insulin.[151] The respective clinic or field situation where diabetic exercisers are present should have sources of glucose present and be conveniently located for use by patients in case of hypoglycemic reactions. These sources should include items such as orange juice or hard candy.

Higher heart rates and greater blood pressure responses to submaximal exercise indicative of greater myocardial oxygen consumption and a stressful load on the exercising diabetic heart have been reported,[154] and the exercising diabetic with cardiovascular disease must be monitored carefully. The importance of proper footwear, foot inspection daily, and proper skin and foot hygiene is paramount to the exercising diabetic.[152] The diabetic distance runner must have some active insulin available for facilitation of glucose uptake in muscle for normal metabolism, and it is recommended that a portion of the daily insulin dosage be administered the evening before (long-lasting insulin) or 2½ to 3 hours before exercise in the arm or abdomen.[148] Most authors also recommend a light carbohydrate meal about 2 hours before running. Glucose supplements are also often recommended during sustained strenuous exercise at hourly intervals.[151]

Exercise precautions that should be taken by the older diabetic athlete are several and should include use of proper footwear, carrying extra carbohydrates, and

TABLE 11-6. BENEFITS OF EXERCISE IN DIABETIC PATIENTS

Decreased insulin requirement

Improvement of glucose tolerance

Lowered plasma glucose levels

Decreased thickening of capillary membranes

Decreased stress and promotion of relaxation

Increased storage of glycogen in exercising muscle cells

Increased sensitivity of muscle tissue to insulin, thus decreased need for insulin in muscle

Increased HDL levels

Lowered plasma triglycerides

Increased free fatty acid usage

Decreased need for oral hypoglycemic agents

knowledge of medication and meal schedules, among others. Exercise benefits for the diabetic are listed in Table 11–6; precautions for exercising diabetics are presented in Table 11–7. Increasing numbers of people with diabetes are embarking upon exercise programs and desire information about diabetes and exercise. The sports physical therapist may encounter the older athlete who is diabetic and must be prepared to answer questions appropriately regarding diabetes and exercise to the best of his or her ability.

Postural Problems. Postural abnormalities are very common with aging. These abnormalities may result from weakness of muscles or muscle groups, poor flexibility, pain, postural fatigue, or pathology. They can limit performance by producing pain in the malalignment area (e.g., foot) and referring pain elsewhere.

In evaluation of the older athlete, a postural analysis should be done to look for potential areas or sources of concern. Areas commonly evaluated in routine evaluations of posture should be scrutinized carefully for any deviations from the normal.

TABLE 11-7. SOME EXERCISE PRECAUTIONS IN DIABETES

Know adverse symptoms of hyperglycemia and hypoglycemia.

Carry extra carbohydrates (e.g., hard candy).

Wear proper footwear with loose-fitting clothing.

Exercise with a partner.

Carry diabetic emergency identification.

Inspect feet after each exercise session.

Know times of insulin peaks.

Use a familiar, enjoyable activity.

Use caution with injection sites if using insulin.

Carry change for telephone call in case of emergency.

Increase exercise intensity gradually.

Make sure diabetes is controlled prior to exercise.

EXERCISE TRAINING—CONDITIONING OF THE RECREATIONAL AND COMPETITIVE OLDER ATHLETE

Training may be needed for older individuals who are exercising for recreational purposes, preparing for competition, or undergoing rehabilitation. The scenario may range from the older competitive athlete training for a marathon to the recreational runner who jogs daily to the individual exercising to lose weight or regulate diabetes.

Age-related changes in different body systems that potentially affect exercise, as well as additional problems possessed by older athletes, have been presented. Despite these problems, exercise can be beneficial in older people. Several benefits of exercise are discussed, especially with regard to the older individual. Prior to participation in activity there should be a medical examination along with an evaluation of physical fitness level, preferably including an exercise test. Older athletes also need to take special precautions in activity, especially in cases where there may be concomitant disease processes. Finally, some attention must be focused on precautions and considerations when treating and rehabilitating the older athlete with an injury.

Benefits of Exercise Training in Older Adults

We must remember that our focus in this chapter is both the recreational and the competitive older athlete. The competitive older athlete has a higher likelihood of having been active most of his or her life, whereas the recreational older athlete may have only recently decided to initiate an exercise program. Whether exercising for conditioning, for competition, or for recreation, exercise is advantageous to the older adult.

Physical conditioning of previously sedentary older adults is known to produce important health and physical fitness benefits. These include a more efficient oxygen transport system and aerobic capacity, lowered blood pressure, improved breathing capacity, improved mobility of joints, and reduction of osteoporotic changes.[16] Middle-aged and older individuals appear to have a great capacity to be trained.[86,155] Although benefits of physical conditioning have been found to have favorable effects on most human performance parameters, certain parameters have been investigated more.

A component commonly investigated in elderly athletes is cardiovascular endurance or aerobic power. Several studies have demonstrated that significant cardiovascular adaptations are possible in older individuals as a result of regular physical training.[156-158] Along with these benefits come increases in aerobic power of varying degrees. Higher maximum oxygen consumption values have been found in middle-aged and older men participating in physical fitness programs, as opposed to their sedentary counterparts of similar ages.[156,159,160-165] The improvements have been found to be in different increments, and there is little doubt that this component of physical working capacity or human performance can be significantly improved with exercise training.

Studies focusing on effects of exercise on skeletal muscle strength and endurance are lacking. Changes in muscle strength, reflecting a net increase in strength are often seen in the older individual; however, they usually are not congruent with muscle hypertrophy as seen in younger subjects.[166] The increased strength seen in the elderly is related more to an increase of neural activation than muscle hypertrophy.[86,166] Age-related differences in isometric and dynamic strength and endurance have also been investigated and findings indicate that endurance seems to remain the same in the older population.[110]

Other benefits of exercise training in the older individual may include improved psychological outlook,[167] improved joint mobility and flexibility,[168,169] and increases in bone mineral content.[170] Balance exercises can improve balance and posture and have been shown to decrease the incidence of falling in the elderly.[131]

Assessing Physical Fitness in the Older Athlete

A thorough medical workup and evaluation of physical fitness components is vital as a precautionary measure before the older individual embarks upon a program of physical conditioning. The medical examination should include a detailed medical history and a thorough physical examination, preferably with an exercise test[16] to monitor cardiorespiratory physical fitness. The exercise test is important, especially for the prospective older athlete who has not been extensively involved in physical activity or has been sedentary for a period of time. A variety of professionals are now becoming involved in the physical fitness assessment in different situations. Many physicians are now getting involved in office evaluation of physical fitness of the athlete,[171] and exercise physiologists are often involved also in different settings. The sports physical therapist working with patients of all ages may also be involved in the evaluation of physical fitness and needs to have some guidelines for evaluation of physical fitness parameters.

Cardiorespiratory Endurance/Aerobic Power. Ideally, there should be evaluation of physiological response to exercise on a treadmill or bicycle ergometer, with close scrutiny of heart rate, blood pressure, electrocardiogram, and symptomatic response to the progressively imposed stress. We know that among the purposes of exercise testing is determination of levels of physical fitness. If equipment is not available to mea-

sure oxygen consumption, endurance capability can be assessed from time to exhaustion during treadmill walking.[102] The specifics of exercise stress testing to determine physiological responses to exercise are beyond the scope of this chapter; however, the reader is referred to excellent sources on the topic.[172,173] Field tests such as the 12-minute run or 1.5-mile run are often used as fitness tests to evaluate cardiorespiratory endurance, as proposed by Cooper.[174] Caution should be taken, however, and only individuals who have been active in aerobic activities previously should be tested, with close supervision. These tests demand an all-out effort by the older athlete and can be dangerous.[102] Laboratory monitoring of cardiorespiratory endurance is preferable, as it allows prescription of exercise on an individual basis where test data serve as baseline values for the individual, and he or she does not have to work against or toward established norms.

Muscular Strength—Endurance. A variety of techniques can be employed to assess muscle strength and endurance of the older athlete. Some major considerations prior to testing might include integrity of the musculoskeletal system, presence of musculoskeletal pathology with exercise-related symptoms, and integrity of the cardiovascular system. Isometric exercises should be avoided if possible, and if done on isokinetic devices, the athlete should be encouraged to breathe during the effort. Isokinetic evaluation of strength and endurance is probably the safest method of evaluating muscle strength and endurance in this population, due to the ability of many isokinetic devices to accommodate to pain, fatigue, and changes in skeletal leverage. It should be remembered that physiological response to isokinetic exercise can be extreme during certain types of protocols (e.g., velocity spectrum), and the older patient needs to be carefully monitored for heart rate and blood pressure.[175]

Flexibility. Flexibility is a human performance parameter that is vital in the prevention of injury, and assessment of flexibility of major muscle groups is an absolute necessity in the older athlete. The athlete should be given a battery of flexibility tests to evaluate the ability of muscles and muscle groups to respond to elongation. Flexibility testing should involve muscles and muscle groups of the upper and lower extremities, as well as the trunk. Areas that are often problems in the older population, such as the lower back and hamstrings, should be scrutinized closely. It should be remembered that the older athlete may have some limitations in flexibility that tend to occur with advancing age.

Body Composition. Assessment of percentage of body fat is desirable, especially when an overweight

recreational middle-aged or older athlete might be initiating a physical fitness program to promote weight loss. Caution should be exercised when using conventional techniques of body fat assessment with the older population because of the previously mentioned problems with testing. Among these problems are changes in characteristics of different body tissues (e.g., skin, muscle, etc.), which can lead to considerable amounts of error in estimation of the percentage of body fat when using the techniques of skinfold measurements and hydrostatic weighing in this population.[102]

Other Fitness Parameters. The major physical fitness parameters have been identified and the older athlete will frequently have programs implemented to increase or maintain some of these parameters. Motor ability components are also related to physical fitness and should be tested in the older competitive athlete because they may be needed in a sport in which the athlete competes.[5] Included in this classification are coordination, agility, speed, power, and balance. Many recreational sports require these motor ability components for successful execution of the sport and may need to be tested in the older athlete to determine whether an adequate level of the component is present to execute the sport.

The Exercise Program

Although both the competitive and recreational athlete are considered in this chapter, the majority of the older population who will seek the services of a sports physical therapist for treatment or consultation on an exercise program will fall in the latter category. A very small percentage of older adults can be classified as competitive athletes, and the majority of others can benefit greatly from an appropriate, supervised program of physical activity.[99] The exercise prescribed should be completely individualized and based on the functional testing.[176] There is no evidence that vigorous exercise can injure a healthy older individual.[16]

The primary concern for the older recreational athlete or exercising adult is usually maintenance of function rather than athletic performance. Factors motivating the older adult to exercise are quite different from those motivating a younger individual. Three key components of physical fitness discussed previously in the chapter that are influenced by aging and changes in life-style (e.g., decreased activity or sedentary living) are flexibility, muscular strength and endurance, and cardiorespiratory endurance (aerobic power). The major objectives of exercise programs for the elderly, then, should be to combat decreasing flexibility, maintain muscle strength and endurance, and challenge and improve the cardiovascular system.[96,98]

Enhanced flexibility is beneficial for specific and general body movements necessary for daily activities,

such as bending and reaching.[100] Improved flexibility would also enhance component movements of sport in which the older recreational or competitive athlete might be involved. Stretching exercises of various types have been recommended for maintenance of flexibility in older athletes.[98]

Deficits in flexibility are capable of being rectified in older adults with traditional flexibility routines,[19] but caution, as well as special attention, should be exercised when stretching musculature affected by injury, postimmobilization, or crossing joints affected by pathology (e.g., arthritis). Care should be taken also to ensure that the flexibility routine is executed properly, as improperly performed stretching exercises may produce muscle soreness due to stress on connective tissue. Lewis[19] has reported that providing long, slow stretching is vital in increasing flexibility in the older population, and that an older person will require a longer time to achieve a stretch than a younger person. Flexibility exercises as a vital part of warmup, prior to muscular strengthening or cardiovascular endurance exercises, have also been found to increase flexibility, augment joint motion, and decrease the incidence of injury.[177]

Maintenance of muscle strength and endurance remains a big challenge for the older athlete, as it must often be done using nonconventional techniques. The older athlete should not be interested in how much strength can be displayed at a given time or individual effort; the concern should shift to adequate muscle function to execute exercise tasks in which he or she participates, normal activities of daily living (which may require minimum muscle strength), and occasional above-average exertion when necessary.

Weight training, especially awkward heavy forms of weight training, as well as isometric exercise, is not advisable and should be avoided. Older athletes using weight training for conditioning or rehabilitation should confine their efforts to muscular endurance training protocols using low weight and high repetitions. With endurance training, it is known that there can be maintenance and improvements in muscle strength.[16,107] As previously noted, isometric exercise may be dangerous, due to energy costs and the efforts of the associated Valsalva maneuver. Athletes using isotonic or isokinetic muscle loading must be instructed in proper breathing patterns. Many different forms of isokinetic exercise are used in rehabilitating older patients[44]; however, caution must be exercised and vital signs monitored due to acknowledged energy demands.[175]

Exercise of muscle groups for muscle strength and endurance should be done two or three times per week, with emphasis placed on areas where muscle weakness commonly occurs in older adults, such as the thigh, back, abdominal, and arm muscles.[100] Calisthenics have been recommended for maintenance of muscular

strength and endurance[98]; however, these exercises must be checked to ensure that they are biomechanically sound and do not have the potential for injury. Innovative and creative techniques may need to be used for development of strengthening and endurance exercise for this population. Some common techniques include use of rubber-tubing exercises, water-resistive exercises in a pool, and straight leg raising in different positions.

Challenging the cardiovascular system to improve its efficiency and ability to adapt to the stress of exercise or emergency situations should be a major concern of the older individual. The prospective older athlete should have an exercise test in order to identify any potential risks of exercise, provide baseline values for determination of exercise prescription, and detect any particular potential limitations or restrictions of exercise that should be imposed. The older individual able to finish an exercise test without disease symptoms (e.g., angina pectoris, dyspnea) at, near, or past the predicted maximum of the test can often be trained with parameters similar to those of a healthy younger population, but often the older individual has to stop due to symptom limitation.[176] The exercise test data will determine the work capacity and the specific individualized guidelines upon which the individual exercises should be based. Sports physical therapists working with fitness and conditioning programs for new exercisers or higher-risk individuals should have access to the stress test data and good communication with the physician, exercise physiologist, or cardiopulmonary physical therapist who performed the test if any questions arise. Exercise programs seeking to improve cardiovascular endurance and aerobic power are often successful when the exercise training parameters have been based on individual performance in exercise testing. Included in these parameters are mode of exercise, proper warmup and cool-down techniques, and intensity, frequency, duration, and progression of exercise.

The mode of exercise selected should allow rhythmic, continuous exercise using large muscle groups for an extended period of time capable of stimulating heart and lung function. Some factors to consider with selection of exercise mode include geographic location, access to facilities, and availability of equipment.[176] Some common types of exercise modes used for exercise conditioning with special consideration for the older adult are discussed below and examples of these exercise modes are shown in Figs 11–2 through 11–5.

Walking. A walking program may be the best option for deconditioned adults initially starting a fitness program. For those individuals with musculoskeletal problems, a walking program is best for a gradual training mode toward more strenuous exercise.[178,179] Walking has been shown to be a beneficial mode of exercise

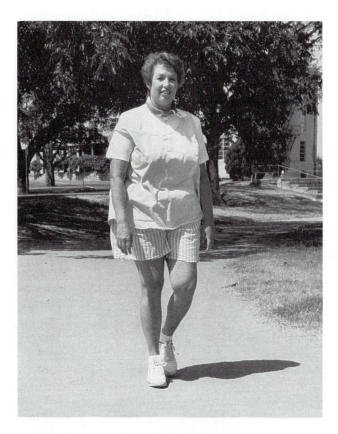

Figure 11-2. Walking.

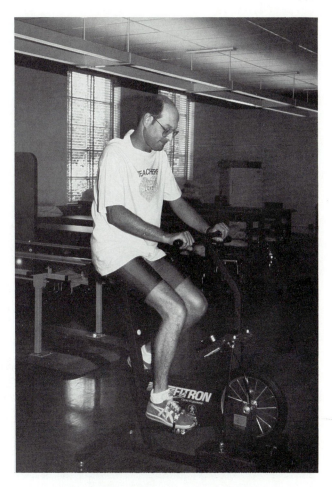

Figure 11-3. Stationary isokinetic bicycle.

training, definitely exerting a training effect.[180,181] Variations of surface, grade, and amount of weight carried may have some influence on exercise response and conditioning effect[182]; however, walkers are not subjected to the musculoskeletal hazards of other exercise modes. A variation of walking, especially in the presence of musculoskeletal problems, is walking in a swimming pool, which has been found to be beneficial in weight reduction and rehabilitation programs.[183-185] Walking programs can also be designed for use on the treadmill and isokinetic weight-bearing devices (e.g., Kinetron) if desired.

Stationary Bicycle. Exercise bicycles are a popular form of exercise and are capable of improving physical fitness when the exerciser uses the bicycle with proper frequency, duration, and intensity. Care must be taken in selection of stationary bicycles, especially ensuring that devices on the bicycle allow quantification of exercise work load.[186] Exercise bicycles may be used when cycling is a preferred mode of activity, when an injury precludes an older competitive athlete from performing his or her high-intensity activity for exercise training, or as a general conditioner. Lower-extremity exercise bicycles may aggravate some musculoskeletal abnormalities in the lower extremities as well as cause localized fatigue and cramping in the thighs and legs. Con-

sideration of past and present musculoskeletal history and conditions is imperative before an exercise program with a stationary exercise bicycle is instituted. Upper extremity cycle ergometers are also becoming very popular in sports medicine and fitness facilities. The sports physical therapist should exercise caution when recommending use of these devices for older adults due to energy requirements of upper-extremity exercise, especially in the presence of possible underlying heart disease.

Running/Jogging. Many older recreational and competitive athletes use short-, middle-, and long-distance running or jogging to maintain or improve cardiovascular fitness. If this activity is selected as an exercise mode, the older athlete should have an exercise test with periodic retesting to determine the appropriateness of the activity and his or her responses to training. Proper footwear is essential to prevent injury.[187] Despite preventive measures, such as good footwear and a stretching program, running-related injuries do occur. Running or jogging can be devastating to the musculoskeletal system of the older athlete, especially a new

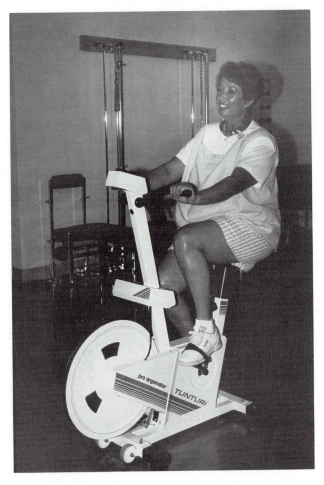

Figure 11-4. Stationary isotonic bicycle.

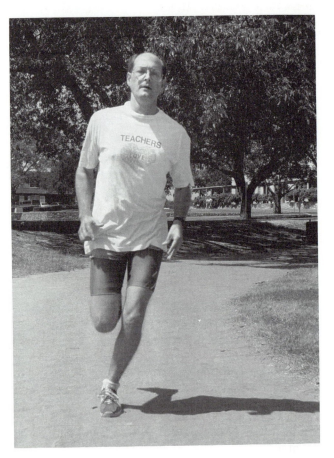

Figure 11-5. Running–jogging.

athlete, in whom underlying pathologies surface, overuse syndromes are promoted, and old injuries are aggravated. The prospective older jogger should have a thorough musculoskeletal examination of past and present problems, as well as a complete musculoskeletal evaluation as part of the evaluation for running.

Swimming. Swimming is an excellent conditioner and may serve as an adjunct to the exercise program. A major problem with swimming is difficulty monitoring the individual while swimming. Older participants must exercise caution when walking on the edges of the swimming pool, which are slippery, as well as when getting into and out of the pool.

Cross-Country Skiing. Cross-country skiing is an excellent exercise conditioner and is used by many older individuals. The principal problem with this form of exercise is the risk of a fall, which could result in injury due to decalcification of bones.[102] Good balance is therefore essential in persons wishing to attempt cross-country skiing. Poorly conditioned persons and individuals with heart disease should be aware of the high en-

ergy demands of this aerobic activity. The oxygen cost of cross-country skiing is affected by factors such as variations in efficiency, arm exercise, snow surface, cold temperatures, inclines, altitude, and skiier misperception of exercise effort and energy cost.[188]

Rebound Exercise. Exercise rebounders (Fig 11–6), which resemble mini-trampolines without as much

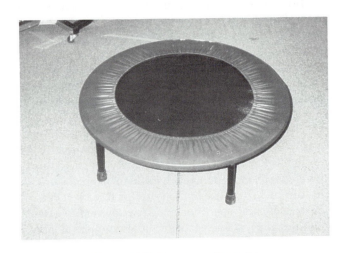

Figure 11-6. Exercise rebounder.

spring and a larger jumping area, are becoming popular in the health fitness industry. They are relatively new and untested in scientific arenas for their benefits and risks, however. Many sedentary individuals use them in initiating fitness programs; however, they require good balance and the older individual must become thoroughly accustomed to them prior to using them as an exercise mode.[186]

Rope Skipping. There are many benefits of rope skipping, including increasing endurance and coordination. It is a strenuous exercise that increases heart rate quickly with high aerobic and anaerobic demands.[189] Additionally, it requires efficient balance, coordination, and agility, which the older individual often does not have. It is not advised for poorly conditioned people who need precise monitoring and control of exercise intensity.[190]

Competitive Sports. It is recommended that competitive sports be used as an adjunct to the primary aerobic mode of exercise if desired. Partners and opponents for recreational sports, such as tennis, badminton, or golf, should be chosen to ensure a tempo of play appropriate to the individual's physical condition.[102] When sufficient cardiovascular and muscular endurance has been regained or developed, sports activities can be used for maintenance of physical fitness if done on a regular basis.[98]

Proper warmup and cool-down activities are important components of exercise training in an older person to decrease the risk of musculoskeletal injuries and cardiac dysrhythmias.[191] Warmup is also beneficial in the prevention of muscle soreness when done correctly using static stretching techniques.[16] Postural, flexibility, and other warmup techniques are valuable in the exercising older adult or before competition for the older athlete to decrease injury frequency, improve range of motion, and prepare muscles for activity. Cool-down techniques allow physiological systems stressed with exercise to return to normal, adjustment of circulation, and prevention of venous pooling. The individual is advised to walk around and do some stretching exercises after the aerobic aspect of exercise. The older athlete may also need a longer warmup and recovery period.

Recommendations regarding optimal intensity of exercise have been based on percentages of maximum heart rates on exercise tests, on age, on a percentage of maximum oxygen consumption, or on a formula. The two important considerations here are that the intensity of exercise should take into account the results of the exercise test and the individual's effort. Training should begin with low-intensity exercise, especially in the person who has been inactive, and be allowed to increase gradually in intensity.[192] It is not uncommon

to witness excessive heart rate evaluation with low levels of exercise in this population, especially due to deconditioning effects.[176] With a decreased ability to adapt to exercise, more time may need to be spent at a given exercise level for better adaptation prior to increasing the exercise intensity. Higher levels of exercise intensity when the older individual is not prepared for it may aggravate cardiovascular, musculoskeletal, or neuromuscular problems and increase the individual's susceptibility to injury and fatigue.[96,192]

Frequency and duration of exercise are important exercise conditioning concepts and are dependent on the individual's condition and exercise test results. The typical exercise program recommended is 20 to 30 minutes at least three times per week for minimal conditioning results.[173,193] This may have to be modified for the older adult who is severely deconditioned. The individual who cannot exercise continuously for 20 to 30 minutes may have to exercise intermittently or use an interval-training type exercise program to attain the minimum exercise time. Once the ability to exercise for 30 minutes is attained, clinicians may have to work on increasing exercise intensity, especially if the intensity of exercise is low.

Patient monitoring during the exercise conditioning, especially in the clinic, is imperative and the patient should be taught to monitor the pulse for exercise heart rate range. The older individual capable of training at high intensities should be advised to exercise three to four times a week, which often produces good physiological benefits.[177] Although daily aerobic exercise is desirable, it may increase the incidence of musculoskeletal problems.[194] The older individual who is a new exerciser should be advised to do the higher-intensity aerobic exercise three times a week on nonsuccessive days, and do stretching and calisthenic exercises on the other days if daily exercise is desirable.

SPECIAL PRECAUTIONS IN EXERCISE CONDITIONING FOR OLDER ATHLETES

The older athlete, both recreational and competitive, needs to be cautious about physical activity and exercise conditioning, as it can be hazardous to the health if certain precautions are not taken to prevent potential injury. The sports physical therapist needs to be aware of these precautions and share them with the older athlete under his or her care for exercise conditioning or rehabilitation of injury. Some of the areas that need to be discussed include general precautions about exercise, isometric exercise, proper attire for exercise, medications and exercise, overtraining, and exposure to environmental extremes.

Some general precautions about exercise really involve common sense and include recommendations

about the exercise program, such as stopping exercise upon signs of distress (e.g., chest pain), buddy exercise or exercising in pairs, regularity of exercise, pacing and gradually increasing exercise levels, avoiding too much exercise too soon, and adhering to individualized exercise programs. If exercise is begun after a prolonged layoff or sedentary existence, it should be started in moderation, with gradual progression to a desired level of intensity,[25] only after appropriate testing. The dangers of exceeding exercise intensity can be minimized by teaching the athlete to monitor his or her pulse using the carotid or radial artery.[195]

As stated earlier, isometric exercise is a hazard for the older adult. The isometric contraction produces closure of the glottis and involves a sustained pressure in the thoracic and abdominal areas, with a constriction of blood vessels and a restriction of venous return to the heart.[16,98] Although some recent evidence indicates that isometric exercise is less hazardous than traditionally presumed, and that everyone may not respond adversely the same way to isometric exercise,[196] one should be cautious when teaching traditional isometric setting exercises to orthopedic patients due to the potential dangers associated with the Valsalva maneuver.

Proper attire for thermal extremes and proper footwear are imperative for the older athlete. The sports physical therapist should give the patient advice, especially on proper footwear, as improper footwear increases the risk of injury and exposure to overuse, especially in aerobic exercise programs.[187] Overuse syndromes may occur in the older athlete who uses improper footwear or who departs radically from prescribed exercise programs. As mentioned previously, medications can also be a problem with exercise programs, especially in the older exercising athlete who may take one or more medications for a variety of problems. Medications may influence heart rate and exercise response, deplete tissue of vital electrolytes often needed for muscle contraction, or cause problems such as fatigue or drowsiness.[125]

Environmental extremes also adversely affect the elderly, especially hot environments. There is ample documentation of heat-related deaths in the elderly,[197,198] and older individuals, especially those past the fifth decade of life, seem to be at a higher risk in hot environments.[199-201] Although the cause of thermoregulation problems with heat is unclear, some studies have implicated the sweating mechanism, namely inadequate sweat response and diminished cardiovascular fitness in the older individual.[201,202]

The Masters Athlete. Throughout this chapter, continuous reference has been made to the competitive and recreational athlete. A description of the competing older athlete known as the masters athlete will be attempted, as these individuals exercise continuously to compete in various activities. Most masters athletes are 40 years or older and compete in events according to age categories, established by decades. Most male athletes are well trained, as well as highly motivated, and afford the scientific community opportunities to study middle-aged and sometimes older athletes who continue to train vigorously.[203] Older masters athletes compete into the sixth, seventh, and eighth decades of life, but the majority of participants are much younger.

The unavoidable effects of aging, extent of training, and rigor of competitive selection are often determinants in the physical condition of the masters athlete.[102] Some of these athletes participate in an attempt to break records, others for the social interaction, and others to set personal goals. The training program of the masters athlete depends upon his or her particular goal. The percentage of body fat and serum lipid levels of these athletes have been lower as compared to their sedentary counterparts.[203] Some of these well-trained individuals have a tendency to overtrain, exposing themselves to injury, and fail to acknowledge that limitations are placed on different body systems with aging. Masters competitors often sustain exercise training-related injuries that may temporarily or permanently halt training and competition.[204] The sports physical therapist needs to be familiar with some of the characteristics of this well-motivated, highly trained individual who might be encountered clinically for a variety of reasons.

Treating the Older Athlete When Injury Occurs

Specific guidelines need to be followed when treating the competitive or recreational athlete. The sports physical therapist must realize that he or she is not dealing with the young, well-trained, highly fit athlete of both competitive and recreational situations. The older athlete may thrive on activity, and interference with the activity may produce a depressed or highly aggressive type of personality. The clinician should get to know the older athlete and understand the effects of injury with interruption of activity patterns on him or her. Good communication is essential between the therapist and the older athlete. A promise of recovery of injury or exact length of treatment should never be made to the older athlete, as processes of healing and responses to treatment may be different in the presence of aging.

When treating the older athlete in the clinic, several things must be taken into consideration. Many contraindications for modalities and certain exercise learned in our education apply to the older individual. There may be decreased sensation or increased sensitivity to heat and cold that may necessitate extra layers of toweling, shorter treatment times, and positioning modifications.[205] It may take an individual more time

TABLE 11-8. CONSIDERATIONS IN PRESCRIBING EXERCISE FOR THE ELDERLY

Medical–Physiological Factors
  Reduced cardiorespiratory capacity
  Less ability to perform moderate- and high-intensity exercise
  Decreased ability to adapt to and recover from exogenous physiologic stimuli (e.g., exercise, heat, cold)
  Muscle weakness and increased fatiguability
  Degenerative bone, joint, and tendon problems
  Increased susceptibility to soreness and injury
  Impaired balance and neuromuscular coordination
  Impaired vision and hearing
  Senile gait disorders and foot problems

Psychological Factors
  Lack of encouragement to be active
  Inaccurate perception by young and old of how active the elderly are, can be, or should be
  Increased inhibitions and depression
  Negative attitudes toward physical activity
  Distorted self-image

From Skinner JS. Importance of aging for exerice testing and exercise prescription. In: Skinner JS, ed. Exercise Testing and Exercise Prescription for Special Cases: Theoretical Basis and Clinical Application. *Philadelphia, Pa: Lea & Febiger; 1987, with permission.*

to stretch and do flexibility routines, and strength training modes may have to be modified for this population. New activities, such as head-down tilting done traditionally for management of low-back disorders, have excessive requirements on the cardiovascular system[206] and may not be able to be used in this population. The therapist must be vigilant for other limitations, such as symptom-related exercise response in older athletes with some manifestations of disease processes. The older athlete is a completely different individual from the young athlete, and is often different from his or her sedentary counterpart. These factors must be considered when treating the older athlete. Skinner[96] has identified several factors that must be considered when prescribing exercise for the aged (Table 11–8).

CONCLUSION

Physical fitness and sport competition in the older adult are now realities in society. People are living longer and individuals over 65 years of age will constitute a significant portion of the American population by the beginning of the twenty-first century. Many of these individuals will continue to participate in exercise and sport, will become injured, and will seek the services of the sports physical therapist for treatment and advice about exercise programs.

It will not be uncommon to rehabilitate a 75-year-old woman who sustained a fractured forearm in a tennis match, the geriatric softball player, or the 80-year-old marathon runner with an overuse syndrome. The sports physical therapist needs to become aware of characteristics of the older athlete described in this chapter, as the older athlete will comprise a considerable portion of the sports physical therapist's clientele in the near future.

REFERENCES

1. Saldo BJ. America's elderly in the 1980s. *Pop Bull.* 1980; 35:1–48.
2. Guccione A. Needs of the elderly and politics of health care. *Phys Ther.* 1988; 68:1386–1390.
3. Jette AM. The graying of America. *Phys Ther.* 1987; 36:1537–1541.
4. Brody SJ, Margel JR. DRG: The second evolution in health care for the elderly. *J Am Geriatr Soc.* 1984; 32:676–679.
5. Melograno VJ, Klinzing JE. *An Orientation to Total Fitness.* Dubuque, Iowa: Kendall/Hunt Publishing Co; 1974.
6. Kuroda Y. Sport and physical activities in older people. In: Dirix A, Knuttgen HG, Tittel K, eds. *The Olympic Book of Sports Medicine.* Boston: Blackwell Scientific Publications; 1988.
7. Pollack MF, Miller HS, Ribish PM. Effects of physical fitness on the aging process. *Phys Sports Med.* 1978; 6:45–48.
8. Smith EF, Serfass RC, eds. *Exercise and Aging.* Hillside, NJ: Enslow Publishing; 1981.
9. Payton OD, Poland JF. Aging process: Implications for clinical practice. *Phys Ther.* 1983; 63:41–48.
10. Frolkis J, Barzuou V. Aging of the central nervous system. *Human Physiol.* 1978; 4:478–479.
11. Lewis CB. *Aging: The Health Care Challenge.* Philadelphia, Pa: F A Davis Co; 1985.
12. Frolkis W, Martynenko OA, Zamostyan VP. Aging of the neuromuscular apparatus. *Gerontology.* 1976; 22:244–279.
13. Katy SS. Aging in the nervous system. *J Chron Dis.* 1956; 3:478–479.
14. Norris AH, Shock NW, Wagman JH. Age changes in the maximum conduction velocity of motor fibers of human ulnar nerves. *J Appl Physiol* 1953; 5:589.
15. Diamond M. The aging brain: Some enlightening and optimistic results. *Am Sci.* 1968; 66:1–9.
16. deVries H. *Physiology of Exercise for Physical Education and Athletics.* Dubuque, Iowa: William C Brown Co; 1980.
17. Golden A. *Pathology: Understanding Human Disease.* Baltimore, Md: Williams & Wilkins; 1982.
18. Strehler BF. Rate and magnitude of age pigment accumulation in the human myocardium. *J Gerontol.* 1959; 14:43–435.
19. Lewis CB. Modifying treatment programs for the elderly. *Clin Manage.* 1985; 5:14–17.
20. Koobs DH, Schultz RZ, Jutzy RV. The origin of lipofuscin and possible consequences to the myocardium. *Arch Pathol Lab Med.* 1978; 102:66–68.

21. Simonson E. Changes of physical fitness and cardiovascular functions with age. *Geriatrics*. 1957; 12:28–39.

22. Bradfonbrenner M, Landowne M, Shock NW. Changes in cardiac output with age. *Circulation*. 1955; 12:557–566.

23. Astrand J. Aerobic work capacity in men and women with special reference to age. *Acta Physiol Scand*. 1960; 49:1–92.

24. Carre KA, Cho H, Barnard RJ. Maximum exercise heart rate reduction with maturation in the rat. *J Appl Physiol*. 1976; 40:741–744.

25. Morehouse LE, Miller AT. *Physiology of Exercise*. St Louis, Mo: C V Mosby; 1976.

26. Rockstein M, Sussman I. *Biology of Aging*. Belmont, Calif: Wadsworth Inc; 1979.

27. Becklake MR, Frank H, Dagenais GR. Influence of age and sex on exercise cardiac output. *J Appl Physiol*. 1965; 20:938–947.

28. Granneth A, Johnson B, Strandell T. Studies on the central circulation at rest and during exercise in the supine and sitting body positions in old men. *Acta Med Scand*. 1964; 176:425–430.

29. Montoye HJ. Cardiac pre-ejection period: Age and sex comparisons. *J Gerontol*. 1971; 26:208–210.

30. Starr J. An essay on the strength of the heart and on the effect of aging upon it. *Am J Cardiol*. 1984; 14:771–783.

31. Jones RL, Overton JR, Hammerlindl DM. Effects of age in regional residual volume. *J Appl Physiol*. 1978; 44:195–199.

32. Davies MJ, Pomerance Q. Quantitative study of aging changes in the human sinoatrial node and internodal traits. *Br Heart J* 1972; 34:150–152.

33. Lakatta EG. Age-related alterations in the cardiovascular response to adrenergic related stress. *Fed Proc*. 1980; 39:3173–3175.

34. Reddan WG. Respiratory system and aging. In: Smith EF, Serfass RC, eds. *Exercise and Aging: The Scientific Basis*. Hillside NJ: Enslow Publishing; 1981.

35. Norris AH, Shock NW, Landown M. Pulmonary function studies: Age differences in lung volumes and bellows function. *J Gerontol*. 1956; 11:379–387.

36. Turner JM, Mead J, Wohl ME. Elasticity of the human lungs in relation to age. *J Appl Physiol*. 1968; 225:664–671.

37. Mittman C, Edelman NH, Norris AH. Relationship between chest wall and pulmonary compliance and age. *J Appl Physiol*. 20:1211–1216.

38. Rizzato G, Mazzini F. Thoracoabdominal mechanisms in elderly men. *J Appl Physiol*. 1970; 28:457–460.

39. Donovan RE, Palmer WH, Varvis CJ, Bates DV. Influence of age on pulmonary diffusing capacity. *J Appl Physiol*. 1959; 14:483–492.

40. Sorbini CA. Arterial oxygen tension in relation to age in healthy subjects. *Respiration*. 1968; 25:3–6.

41. Zadai C. Pulmonary physiology of aging: The role of rehabilitation. *Top Geriatr Rehabil*. 1985; 1:1.

42. Adrian MJ. Flexibility in the aging adult. In: Smith EF, Serfass RC, eds. *Exercise and Aging: The Scientific Basis*. Hillside, NJ: Enslow Publishing; 1981.

43. Tipton CM, Matthes RD, Martin RK. Influence of age and sex on strength of bone-ligament junctions in knee joints of rats. *J Bone Joint Surg*. 1978; 60:230–234.

44. Lewis CB. Musculoskeletal changes with age. *Clin Man*. 1984; 4:12–15.

45. Bick EM. Aging the connective tissues of the human musculoskeletal system. *Geriatrics*. 1971; 11:445–447.

46. Boone DC, Azen SP. Normal range of motion of joints in male subjects. *J Bone Joint Surg*. 1979; 61:756–759.

47. Smith J, Walker JM. Knee and elbow range of motion in healthy older individuals. *Phys Occupat Ther Geriatr*. 1983; 2:31–38.

48. Walker JM, Debbie S, Miles-Elkousy N, et al. Active mobility of the extremities in older subjects. *Phys Ther*. 1984; 64:919–923.

49. Petrofsky JS, Lind AR. Aging isometric strength and endurance, and cardiovascular responses to static effort. *J Appl Physiol*. 1975; 38:91–95.

50. McCarter R. Effects of age on contraction of mammalian skeletal muscle. In: Kalkor G, Di Battista WJ, eds. *Aging in Muscle*. New York, NY: Raven Press; 1978.

51. Gutman E, Hanzlikova V. Fast and slow motor units in aging. *Gerontology*. 1976; 22:280–300.

52. Larsson F. Morphological and functional characteristics of the aging skeletal muscle in man: A cross sectional study. *Acta Physiol Scand* 1978; 457:1–36.

53. Raven PB, Mitchell J. The effects of aging on dynamic and static exercise. In: Weisfelt MF, ed. *The Aging Heart*. New York, NY: Raven Press; 1980.

54. MacLennan WJ, Hall MR, Timothy JI. Postural hypotension in old age: Is it a disorder of the nervous system or of blood vessels? *Age Aging* 1980; 9:25–32.

55. Ermini M. Aging changes in mammalian skeletal muscle. *Gerontology*. 1976; 22:301–316.

56. Tzankoff SP, Norris AH. Effect of muscle mass decrease on age-related basal metabolic rate changes. *J Appl Physiol*. 1977; 43:1001–1006.

57. Ross R, Glosmet JA. The pathogenesis of atherosclerosis, Part I. *N Engl J Med* 1976; 295:369–375.

58. Brannon FJ, Geyer MJ, Foley MW. *Cardiac Rehabilitation: Basic Theory and Application*. Philadelphia, Pa: F A Davis; 1988.

59. Tannenbaum RP, Sohn CA, Cantwell R, et al. Angina pectoris: How to recognize, how to manage it. *Nurs 81*. 1981; 11:9.

60. Irwin S. Clinical manifestations and assessment of ischemic heart disease. *Phys Ther*. 1985; 65:1806–1811.

61. American Heart Association. *Heart Facts*. Dallas, Tex: American Heart Association; 1981.

62. Wilkins RW, Hollander W, Chobanian AV. Evaluation of hypertensive patients. *Ciba Clin Symp*. 1972; 24(2):5–30.

63. Watchie J. Hypertensive heart disease. *APTA Cardiopul Sect Q*. 1984; 5(3):2–4.

64. Recommendations of the task force on blood pressure control in children. *Pediatrics* 1977; 59 (Suppl):797–820.

65. The 1984 report of the joint national committee on detection, evaluation, and treatment of high blood pressure. *Arch Intern Med*. 1984; 144:1045–1057.

66. Horan MJ, Sinaiko AR. Synopsis of the report of the second task force on blood pressure control in children. *Hypertension.* 1987; 10:115–121.

67. Rabkin SW, Mathewson FA, Tate RB. Relationship of blood pressure in 20- to 39-year-old men to subsequent blood pressure and incidence of hypertension over a 30-year observation period. *Circulation.* 1982; 65:291–330.

68. Kannel WB. Some lessons in cardiovascular epidemiology from Framingham. *Am J Cardiol.* 1976; 37:269–282.

69. Cantwell JF, Fletcher GF. Sudden death and jogging. *Phys Sportsmed.* 1978; 6(3):93–98.

70. Walther RJ, Tiftt CP. High blood pressure in the competitive athlete: Guidelines and recommendations. *Phys Sportsmed.* 1985; 13(5):93–114.

71. Sheps DS, Ernest JC, Briese FW. Exercise-induced increase in diastolic pressure: Indicator of severe coronary artery disease. *Am J Cardiol.* 1979; 43:708–712.

72. Nutter DO, Schlant RC, Hurst JW. Isometric exercise and the cardiovascular system. *Mod Concepts Cardiovasc Dis.* 1972; 41(3):11–15.

73. Fixler D, Laird P, Brown R. Response of hypertensive adolescents to dynamic and isometric exercise stress. *Pediatrics.* 1979; 64:579–583.

74. Tipton CM. Exercise and hypertension: Management concepts for coaches and educators. *Sports Sci Exchange.* 1988; 1(4):1–4.

75. Tipton CM. Exercise, training and hypertension. *Exerc Sports Sci Rev* 1984; 12:245–306.

76. McCullough JM. Examination procedure for patients with vascular system problems. *Clin Man.* 1981; 1(3):17–19.

77. Steingard PM. How I manage varicose veins and thrombosis in athletes. *Phys Sportsmed.* 1984; 12(6):97–101.

78. Hodgson JF, Buskirk ER. Physical fitness and age with emphasis on cardiovascular function in the elderly. *J Am Geriatr Soc.* 1977; 25:385–392.

79. Robinson S, Dill DB, Robinson RD. Physiological aging of champion runners. *J Appl Physiol.* 1976; 41:46–51.

80. Dill DB, Robinson S, Ross JC. A longitudinal study of 16 champion runners. *J Sports Med Phys Fit.* 1973; 7:1–27.

81. Amussen E, Mathiason P. Some physiological functions in physical education students reinvestigated after 25 years. *Am Geriatr Soc J.* 1962; 10:379–387.

82. Anderson KF, Hermanson F. Aerobic work capacity in middle-aged men. *J Appl Physiol.* 1965; 20:432–436.

83. Astrand I. The physical work capacity of workers 50–64 years old. *Acta Physiol Scand.* 1958; 42:73–86.

84. Dehn MM, Bruce RA. Longitudinal variations in maximal oxygen intake with age and activity. *J Appl Physiol.* 1972; 33:805–807.

85. Robinson S. Experimental studies of physical fitness in relation to age. *Arbeitsphysiologie* 1938; 10:251.

86. Noble BJ. *Physiology of Exercise and Sport.* St Louis, Mo: Times Mirror/Mosby College Publishing; 1986.

87. Plowman SA, Drinkwater BF, Horwath SM. Age and aerobic power in women: A longitudinal study. *J Gerontol.* 1979; 34:512–515.

88. Shephard RJ. The cardiovascular benefits of exercise in the elderly. *Top Geriatr Rehabil.* 1986; 2(1):10–16.

89. Smith EF. Age: The interaction of nature and nurture. In: Smith EF, Serfass RC, eds. *Exercise and Aging: The Scientific Basis.* Hillside, NJ: Enslow Publishing; 1981.

90. Astrand I, Astrand PO, Hallback O. Reduction in maximum oxygen uptake with age. *J Appl Physiol.* 1973; 35:649–654.

91. Frontero WR, Evans WJ. Exercise performance and endurance training in the elderly. *Top Geriatr Rehabil* 1966; 2(1):17–31.

92. Fitzgerald PF. Exercise for the elderly. *Med Clin N Am.* 1985; 69:186–196.

93. Pirchardo S. Normal aging of the cardiovascular system. *Cardiopulm Rec.* 1987; 2(1):2–6.

94. Kasch FW, Wallace JP, Van Camp SP, et al. A longitudinal study of cardiovascular stability in active men aged 45 to 65. *Phys Sportsmed.* 1988; 16(1):117–123.

95. Ryan A, Meyer B, Paffenberger R, et al. Exercise and the cardiovascular system: A roundtable discussion. *Physician Sportsmed.* 1979; 7(9):55–71.

96. Skinner JS. Importance of aging for exercise testing and exercise prescription. In: Skinner JS, ed. *Exercise Testing and Exercise Prescription for Special Cases: Theoretical Basis and Clinical Application.* Philadelphia, Pa: Lea & Febiger; 1987.

97. Gould JA, Davies GJ. *Orthopedic and Sports Physical Therapy.* St Louis, Mo: C V Mosby Co; 1985.

98. Lersten KC. *Physiology and Physical Conditioning: Theory to Practice.* Palo Alto, Calif: Peek Publications; 1971.

99. Sager K. Senior fitness: For the health of it. *Phys Sportsmed.* 1983; 11(10):31–36.

100. Smith EF, Gilligan C. Physical activity prescription for the older adult. *Phys Sportsmed.* 1983; 11(8):91–101.

101. Bogert J, Briggs G, Calloway D. *Nutrition and Physical Fitness.* Philadelphia, Pa: W B Saunders Co; 1973.

102. Shephard RJ. Physical training for the elderly. *Clin Sports Med.* 1986; 5(3):515–533.

103. Durnin JV, Womersly J. Body fat assessment from total body density and its estimation from skinfold thickness: Measurements on 481 men and women aged 16 to 72 years. *Br J Nutr.* 1974; 32:77–97.

104. Jackson AS, Pollack MF. Generalized equations for predicting body density of men. *Br J Nutr.* 1978; 40:497–504.

105. Jackson AS, Pollack MF, Ward A. Generalized equations for predicting bone density of women. *Med Sci Sports Exerc.* 1980; 12:175–181.

106. Lohman TG. Body composition methodology in sports medicine. *Phys Sportsmed.* 1982; 10:47–58.

107. Astrand PO, Rodahl K. *Textbook of Work Physiology.* New York, NY: McGraw-Hill Book Co; 1970.

108. Liemohn WP. Strength and aging: An exploratory study. *Int J Aging Hum Dev.* 1975; 6:347–357.

109. Murray MP, Gardner GM, Mollinger FA. Strength of isometric and isokinetic contractions: Knee muscles of men aged 20 to 86. *Phys Ther.* 1980; 60:412–419.

110. Johnson T. Age-related differences in isometric and dynamic strength and endurance. *Phys Ther.* 1982; 62:985–989.

111. Larsson F, Karlsson J. Isometric and dynamic endurance as a function of age and skeletal muscle characteristics. *Acta Physiol Scand.* 1978; 104:129–136.

112. Aniasson A, Grimby G, Hedberg M. Muscle function in old age. *Scand J Rehabil Med.* 1978; 56:43–49.

113. Rodman G. Primer on rheumatic diseases. *J Am Geriatr Soc.* 1973; 224:5–7.

114. Salter RB. *Textbook of Disorders and Injuries of the Musculoskeletal System.* Baltimore, Md: Williams & Wilkins Co; 1970.

115. Goldthwait JC. Bone, joint and muscle disorders. In: Myers, J. ed. *An Orientation to Chronic Disease and Disability.* New York, NY: Macmillan Co; 1965.

116. Francis KT. Delayed muscle soreness: A review. *J Orthoped Sports Phys Ther.* 1983; 5(1):10–13.

117. Talag TS. Residual muscular soreness as influenced by concentric, eccentric, and static contractions. *Res Q.* 1973; 44:458–469.

118. Abraham WM. Factors in delayed muscle soreness. *Med Sci Sports* 1977; 9:11–20.

119. Abraham WM. Exercise-induced muscle soreness. *Phys Sportsmed* 1979; 7:57–60.

120. Brown B, Payne T, Kim C. Chronic responses of rat brain norepinephrine and serotonin levels to endurance training. *J Appl Physiol.* 1979; 46:19–21.

121. Shangold M. Gynecologic concerns in the woman athlete. *Clin Sports Med.* 1984; 3:869–879.

122. Smith JW, Seidl FG, Cluff LE. Studies on the epidemiology of adverse drug reactions. *Ann Intern Med.* 1966; 65:629–640.

123. Melmon KF. Preventable drug reactions: Causes and cures. *N Engl J Med.* 1971; 284:1361–1368.

124. Ice D. Cardiovascular medications. *Phys Ther.* 1985; 65:1845–1855.

125. Simonson W. Medication of the elderly: Effect on response to physical therapy. *Phys Ther.* 1978; 58:178–179.

126. Clark N. How I manage athletes' food obsessions. *Phys Sportsmed.* 1984; 12(7):96–103.

127. Lewis CB. Hearing loss and communication with the aged. *Clin Man.* 1983; 3(2):36–37.

128. Sheldon JH. The effect of age on the control of sway. *Gerontol Clin.* 1963; 5:129–138.

129. Thyssen HH, Brynskov, Jansen EC. Normal ranges in reproducibility for quantitative Romberg's Test. *Acta Neurol Scand.* 1982; 66:100–104.

130. Bohannon R, Larkin P, Cook A, et al. Decrease in timed balance test scores with aging. *Phys Ther.* 1987; 67:1067–1075.

131. Overstall PW. Prevention of falls in the elderly. *J Am Geriatr Soc.* 1980; 28:481–484.

132. Chestnut CH. Treatment of postmenopausal osteoporosis. *Comp Ther.* 1984; 10:41–47.

133. Ericksen EF, Mosekilde F, Melsen F. Effects of sodium fluoride, calcium phosphate, and vitamin D_2 on trabecular bone balance and remodeling in osteoporotics. *Bone.* 1985; 6:381–389.

134. Browse NF. *The Physiology and Pathology of Bed Rest.* Springfield, Ill: Charles C Thomas Publishers; 1965.

135. Circulla JA. Osteoporosis. *Clin Man.* 1989; 9:15–19.

136. Ainsenbry JA. Exercise in prevention and management of osteoporosis. *Phys Ther.* 1987; 67:1100–1104.

137. Coldwell F. Light boned and lean athletes: Does the penalty outweigh the reward? *Phys Sportsmed* 1984; 12:139–149.

138. Cummings SR. Epidemiology of osteoporosis and osteoporotic fractures. *Epidemiol Rev.* 1985; 7:178–208.

139. Riggs BF, Melton JF. Involitional osteoporosis. *N Engl J Med* 1986; 314:1676–1684.

140. MacKinnon JF. Osteoporosis: A review. *Phys Ther.* 1988; 68:1533–1539.

141. Richelson FS, Wahner HW, Melton FJ. Relative contributions of aging and estrogen deficiency to postmenopausal bone loss. *N Engl J Med.* 1984; 311:1273–1275.

142. Cohn SH, Abesagamis C, Yasumura S. Comparative skeletal mass and radial bone mineral content in black and white women. *Metabolism* 1977; 26:171–178.

143. Graham BA, Gleit CJ. Osteoporosis: A major health problem in postmenopausal women. *Orthoped Nurs.* 1984; 3(6):19–26.

144. Frost HM. The pathomechanics of osteoporosis. *Clin Orthoped.* 1985; 200:198–225.

145. Aloia JF, Cohn SH, Ostuni, JA. Prevention of involitional bone loss by exercise. *Ann Intern Med.* 1979; 89:356–358.

146. Smith EF, Reddan W, Smith PE. Physical activity and calcium modalities for bone mineral increase in aged women. *Med Sci Sports Exerc.* 1981; 13:60–64.

147. Brewer V, Meyer BM, Keele MS. Role of exercise in prevention of involutional bone loss. *Med Sci Sports Exerc.* 1983; 15:445–449.

148. Costill DF, Miller JM, Fink WJ. Energy metabolism in diabetic distance runners. *Phys Sportsmed.* 1980; 8(10):64–71.

149. Jette DU. Physiological effects of exercise in the diabetic. *Phys Ther.* 1984; 64:339–341.

150. Berger M, Haag S, Ruderman MB. Glucose metabolism in perfused skeletal muscle: Interaction of insulin and exercise on glucose uptake. *Biochem J.* 1975; 146:231–238.

151. Ryan A, Leon AF, Zinman B, et al. Roundtable discussion: Diabetes and exercise. *Phys Sportsmed.* 1979; 7(3):49–60.

152. Frantz S, Lawton R, Schmagel C, et al. The physical therapist's role in the treatment of diabetes. *Clin Man.* 1987; 7:30–31.

153. Wallberg–Henriksson H, Gunnarsson R, Henriksson J. Increased peripheral insulin sensitivity and muscle mitochondria enzymes but unchanged blood glucose control in type I diabetics after physical training. *Diabetes* 1982; 31:1044–1050.

154. Wahren J, Hagenfeldt F, Felig P. Splanchnic and leg exchange of glucose, amino acids, and free fatty acids during exercise in diabetes mellitus. *J Clin Invest.* 1975; 55:1303–1314.

155. Raven PB, Wilson JR. Exercise and the elderly. *Sports*

Med Dig. 1988; 10(6):1–2.

156. Saltin B, Grimby G. Physiological analysis of middle-aged and former athletes. *Circulation.* 1968; 38:1104–1113.

157. Bassey JE. Age, inactivity, and some physiological responses to exercise. *Gerontology.* 1978; 24:66–77.

158. Sidney KH, Shephard RJ. Frequency and intensity of exercise training for elderly subjects. *Med Sci Sports Exerc.* 1978; 10:125–131.

159. Miyashita M, Haga S, Mizuta T. Training and detraining effects on aerobic power in middle-aged and older men. *J Sports Med Phys Fit.* 1978; 18:131–135.

160. Pollack MF, Dawson GA, Miller HS. Physiologic responses of men 49 to 65 years of age to endurance training. *J Am Geriatr Soc.* 1976; 24:97–101.

161. deVries HA. Physiological effects of an exercise training regimen on men aged 52 to 88. *J Gerontol.* 1970; 25:325–336.

162. Sidney KH, Shephard RJ. Activity patterns in elderly men and women. *J Gerontol.* 1977; 32:25–32.

163. Yerg JE, Seals DR, Hagberg JM. Effect of endurance exercise training on ventilatory function in older individuals. *J Appl Physiol.* 1985; 58:791–794.

164. Seals DR, Hagberg JM, Hurley BF. Endurance training in older men and women. *J Appl Physiol.* 1984; 57:1024–1029.

165. Adams GM, deVries HA. Physiological effects of an exercise training regime upon women aged 52 to 79. *J Gerontol.* 1972; 28:50–55.

166. Moritani T. Training adaptations in the muscles of older men. In: Smith EF, Serfass D, eds. *Exercise and Aging: The Scientific Basis.* Hillside, NJ: Enslow Publishing; 1981.

167. Young RJ, Ismail AH. Personality differences of adult men before and after a physical fitness program. *Res Q.* 1976; 47:513–519.

168. Chapman EA, deVries HA, Swezey R. Joint stiffness: Effects of exercise on old and young men. *J Gerontol.* 1972; 27:218–221.

169. Frekany GA, Leslie DK. Effects of an exercise program on selected flexibility measurements of senior citizens. *Gerontologist.* 1975; 15:182–183.

170. Smith EF. Bone changes in the exercising older adult. In: Smith EF, Serfass D, eds. *Exercise and Aging: The Scientific Basis.* Hillside, NJ: Enslow Publishing; 1981.

171. Ryan A. Office examination of the athlete. *Physician Sportsmed.* 1976; 4(10):86–105.

172. Jopke T. Choosing an exercise test protocol. *Phys Sportsmed.* 1981; 9:141–146.

173. American College of Sports Medicine. *Guidelines for Exercise Testing and Prescription.* Philadelphia, Pa: Lea & Febiger; 1986.

174. Cooper K. *The New Aerobics.* New York, NY: Bantam Books; 1977.

175. Negus RA, Rippe JM, Freedson P, et al. Heart rate, blood pressure and oxygen consumption during orthopedic rehabilitation exercise. *J Orthoped Sports Phys Ther.* 1987; 8:346–350.

176. Zadai CC. Prescribing exercise for geriatric individuals. *Cardiopulm Rec.* 1987; 2(1):16–20.

177. Shephard RJ. *Physical Activity and Aging.* London: Croom Helm Publishers; 1978.

178. Schultz P. Walking for fitness: Slow but sure. *Phys Sportsmed.* 1980; 8(9):24–27.

179. Schultz P. Walking for rehabilitation: The first step. *Phys Sportsmed.* 1980; 8(10):109–112.

180. Pollock MF, Miller HS, Janeway R. Effects of walking on body composition of adult men. *J Appl Physiol.* 1971; 30:126–130.

181. Pollack MF, Dimmick J, Miller HS. Effects of mode of training on cardiovascular function and body composition of adult men. *Med Sci Sports Exerc.* 1975; 7:139–145.

182. Givoni B, Goldman RF. Predicting metabolic energy cost. *J Appl Physiol.* 1971; 30:429–433.

183. Evans BW, Cureton KJ, Purvis JW. Metabolic and circulatory responses to walking and jogging in water. *Res Q.* 1978; 49:442–449.

184. Kindl MM, Brown P. Successful treatment of obesity. *Mod Med.* 1977; 45(9):49–51.

185. Pease W, Flentje W. Rehabilitation through underwater exercise. *Phys Sportsmed.* 1976; 4:143.

186. Dunn K. Exercising at home: Hard work is good work. *Phys Sportsmed.* 1981; 9(10):110–114.

187. Falkel JE. Guidelines for running shoe selection to prevent running injuries. *Cardiopulm Rec.* 1986; 1(1):3–7.

188. Oldridge NB, MacDougall JD. Cross-country skiing: Precautions for cardiac patients. *Phys Sportsmed.* 1981; 9(2):64–70.

189. Quirk JE, Sinning WE. Anaerobic and aerobic responses of males and females to rope skipping. *Med Sci Sports Exerc.* 1982; 14:26–29.

190. Town GP, Sol N, Sinning W. The effect of rope skipping on energy expenditure of males and females. *Med Sci Sports Exerc.* 1980; 12:295–298.

191. Barnard RJ, MacAlpin RM, Kattuss AA, et al. Ischemic response to sudden strenuous exercise in healthy men. *Circulation.* 1973; 48:936–942.

192. Lewis CB. Effects of aging on the cardiovascular system. *Clin Man.* 1984; 4(4):24–29.

193. American College of Sports Medicine. The recommended quantity and quality of exercise for developing and maintaining fitness in healthy adults. *Phys Sportsmed.* 1978: 6(10):39–41.

194. Orava S, Ala-Ketola F, Puranen J. Stress fractures caused by physical exercise. *Acta Orthop Scand.* 1978; 49:199–27.

195. Couldry W, Corbin CB, Wilcox A. Carotid vs radial pulse counts. *Physician Sportsmed.* 1982; 10(12):67–72.

196. Fardy PS. Isometric exercise and the cardiovascular system. *Physician Sportsmed.* 1981; 9(9):43–56.

197. Levine J. Heart stroke in the aged. *Am J Med.* 1969; 47:251–255.

198. Wheeler M. Heat stroke in the elderly. *Med Clin N Am* 1976; 60(6):1289–1290.

199. Henschel A, Cole MB, Lyczkowskyj J. Heat tolerance of elderly persons living in a subtropical environment. *J Gerontol.* 1968; 23:17–22.

200. Wagner JA, Robinson S, Tzankoff SP, et al. Heat tolerance and acclimatization to work in the heat in relation to age. *J Appl Physiol.* 1972; 33:616–622.

201. Drinkwater BF, Horwath SM. Heat tolerance and aging. *Med Sci Sports Exerc.* 1979; 11:49–55.

202. Lind AR, Humphreys PW, Collins KJ, et al. Influence of age and daily duration of exposure on responses of men to work in the heat. *J Appl Physiol.* 1970; 28:50–56.

203. Barnard RJ, Grimditch GK, Wilmore JH. Physiological characteristics of sprint and endurance Masters runners. *Med Sci Sports Exerc.* 1979; 11:161–171.

204. Kavanaugh T, Shephard RJ. The effects of continued training on the aging process. *Ann NY Acad Sci.* 1970; 301:656–670.

205. Kauffman T. Thermoregulation and use of heat and cold. In: Jackson OF, ed. *Therapeutic Considerations for the Elderly: Clinics in Physical Therapy.* New York, NY: Churchill Livingstone Inc; 1987:14.

206. Sobush DC, Nosse F, Davis AS. Influence of aerobic fitness on cardiovascular responses during slow head-down tilting. *Phys Ther.* 1986; 66:524–530.

12

The Disabled Athlete

A. Lynn Millar

INTRODUCTION

In discussions of coaching or treating athletes, the disabled athlete is frequently overlooked. Although the disabled athlete may have injuries that are similar to those of other athletes, occasionally there are special variables that must be considered. This chapter considers the types of disabled athletes with whom a physical therapist may be working, any physical differences that the therapist must consider, and additional sources of information about each group.

Each of the major disability classifications for which there is nationally recognized competition is introduced, with associated pertinent information. At the end of the chapter is a list of contact addresses for some of the national level sport groups that might provide specific information regarding rules and regulations regarding the athletes and competitions for their respective group.

The number of athletes entering disabled competitions is increasing yearly, and new sports have been added for the various athlete groups. Every year approximately 11,000 persons become paraplegic or quadriplegic as a result of disease or injury.[1] Add to that number 100,000 mentally retarded babies born each year in the United States, as well as the thousands who join the other disability classifications, and one can see that the pool of potential participants is growing.[2] The Special Olympics alone has over one million children and adults who have participated in their annual competitions since 1968. Not only is sport competition for the disabled becoming more common, it is also being noticed. Competitions are held starting at the local level and for many groups, all the way through the international level. The Olympic Games of 1984 and 1988 had wheelchair demonstration competitions that were televised internationally.

SPORT ORGANIZED BY DISABILITY

The Amputee Athlete

In 1977 there were 385,000 amputees in the United States, with 43,000 new amputees each year.[3] If only 1% of these join competition for the disabled, that would represent an additional 430 new athletes per year. Amputee athletes are classified by level of amputation, using the system of the United States Amputee Athletic Association. This system follows guidelines set by the International Sports Organization for the Disabled (ISOD)[3] Classifications (Table 12–1), using a letter and number system: A = Amputee, 1 = Above knee, both limbs; to 9 = Any combo of lower and upper limb involvement. Athletes in classifications A1 through A3 use wheelchairs for competition, whereas those in A4 use a prosthesis. Specially organized competitions may include wheelchair basketball, fencing, track and field, and skiing among many other possibilities. It is important, however, to realize that many of the athletes may be able to compete in open competitions if they so desire. Some of the new prosthetic devices allow for more rapid locomotion and increased jumping ability than did the older devices, thus expanding the potential for use in competition by the amputee athlete.

The therapist working with an amputee athlete must be aware of several health-related concerns. The first is recognized immediately by most therapists, namely pressure sores to the residual limb. Edelstein identified three areas for below-the-knee amputations that were pressure-sensitive areas: the anterior distal stump, the crest of the tibia and tibial tubercle, and the head of the fibula.[4] Other areas of the stump are more pressure tolerant, and thus the prosthesis should be fitted to alleviate pressure on the sensitive areas. Pressure-sensitive areas on above-the-knee amputees include the

TABLE 12-1. CLASSIFICATION OF AMPUTEE ATHLETES

Class	Description
A1	Amputation of both legs above or through the knee joint.
A2	Amputation on one leg above or through the knee.
A3	Amputation of both legs below the knee.
A4	Amputation of one leg below the knee.
A5	Amputation of both arms above or through the elbow.
A6	Amputation of one arm above the elbow.
A7	Amputation of both arms below the elbow, but through or above the wrist.
A8	Amputation of one arm below the elbow, but through or above the wrist.
A9	Combined lower plus upper limb amputation.

pubic ramus, lateral distal femur, adductor longus tendon, and ischial tuberosity. The physical therapist can help the prosthetist by evaluating both the athlete's walking gait and the biomechanical forces that might be altered during the athlete's competitive event. The therapist should not attempt to make changes in the prosthetic appliance, as this is the province of the prosthetist. The therapist should also make sure that the athlete is checking for pressure-sensitive areas, changes in residual limb size, and general health of the limb on a regular basis. For those competing in wheelchair, proper fit of the chair is of extreme importance. Abrasions are a primary problem for the wheelchair athlete. These can be decreased by proper wheelchair fit, wearing of nonabrasive clothing, and the use of vaseline over areas that are prone to abrasion (such as under the arms).

A second source of concern for the amputee athlete is usually that of muscular tightness (contractures) and contralateral overuse injuries. Most rehabilitation therapists are aware of the potential for contractures following amputation; however, the therapist's focus frequently turns toward acute or musculoskeletal injuries once the patient starts to exercise on a regular basis and compete. the athlete should be educated regarding the importance of a balanced training program, which includes strength training, stretching, and aerobic activity.

The third topic of concern for the amputee athlete is that of aerobic fitness. Murray and Fisher cite research that found increased oxygen consumption values during ambulation, ranging from 9% for transtibial amputees to 300% for bilateral transfemoral amputees.[5] As ambulation with a prosthesis or propulsion with a wheelchair takes more aerobic energy than does normal ambulation; proper training is essential to prevent unnecessary fatigue. Following the theories of specificity of training, the athlete's program should in-

clude a significant portion of ambulatory training (or wheeling) at a sufficient intensity to stimulate cardiovascular training effects. Due to the increased oxygen cost, this intensity will be reached at a comparatively low level of activity.

The Blind Athlete

In 1977 Dickman reported that the National Society for the Prevention of Blindness (NSPB) estimated there would be approximately 519,000 legally blind persons in the United States by the year 1980.[6] Rainbolt and Sherrill, however, report that less than 1% of eligible blind persons participate in competitive activities sponsored by the United States Association for Blind Athletes (USABA).[7] They did note that increasing numbers were participating in competition, and if their statistics are analyzed, it is found that approximately 38% of blind athletes frequently competed with nondisabled persons. In fact, Buell offers many examples of blind athletes who compete successfully with nondisabled athletes.[8] A notable example that he gives is that more than 5000 blind athletes compete each year in wrestling. Buell's main contention is that many blind persons can and should participate in sports activities with able-bodied counterparts. It is not the purpose of this section to argue this issue, but it is important to realize that most of the physical capabilities of the blind athlete are the same as athletes with normal vision.

Competitive classification for blind athletes is based upon vision, and includes three classes (summarized in Table 12–2).[9]

Physical limitations or differences (other than vision) between the blind and those with normal vision are limited, but it is important for the therapist to be cognizant of them. Equilibrium depends upon information from the vestibular apparatus, proprioceptive receptors, and vision. Because of lack of vision, it was hypothesized that blind subjects would not perform as well as sighted subjects on balance tests. Ribadi et al tested this hypothesis with a group of 17 congenitally blind subjects and 34 sighted subjects.[10] As hypothesized, the sighted subjects performed significantly better than the blind subjects for both static and dynamic

TABLE 12-2. CLASSIFICATION OF BLIND ATHLETES

Class	Description
B1	Sightlessness ranges from no light perception to ability to perceive light, but unable to recognize objects or contours at any distance.
B2	Recognizes objects or contours up to and including 2/60, or field limited to less than 5 degrees.
B3	Visual acuity is greater than 2/60 and up to 6/60 (20/200); Visual field limitation ranges from 5 to 60 degrees.

balance. Interestingly, the blind subjects were superior in dynamic balance when compared to blindfolded sighted individuals. The authors suggested that the blind subjects had learned how to adapt to the lack of visual input, and pointed out the importance of initiating training as early as possible to facilitate the adaptation of blind individuals and development of their equilibrium mechanism.

Running patterns of blind athletes reflect the changes in balance, resulting in mechanical inefficiency. In 1984 Pope et al analyzed the running gait of 48 blind students (29 male, 19 female) during a 50-yard dash.[11] They noted that stride length and hip joint range of motion were predictive of velocity, as they are with sighted athletes. Importantly, the head-neck angle correlated negatively to velocity and was typical of the class B1 subjects. The authors concluded the athletes should be taught to lean forward from the neck to improve running velocity.

Arnhold and McGrain expanded the previous research and examined the gait of 27 blind students.[12] Not only did they analyze the mechanical variables, they also compared these variables between classification groups. Interestingly, the gait cycle of the class A subjects was one-half the length of the class B subjects (i.e., they had shorter strides). Class A subjects were slower, attaining 50% of the velocity of the other two groups. In addition, the authors noted, "visually impaired students, especially Class A students, demonstrated a lack of muscle activity at the hip joint."[12] These kinematic studies illustrate the need for those coaching visually impaired athletes to be aware of efficient mechanics for that sport and to work with the athlete to improve body mechanics.

A second physical difference arising from the loss of vision is reflected in an increased physiological cost for activity. Peake and Leonard conducted a series of experiments that examined the stress of locomotion upon blind subjects.[13] They used heart rate as a simple indicator of the physical stress that the blind subject was feeling during guided or unguided walking, with cane during guided and unguided walking, and over a simple or complex route during unguided walking. Heart rates were significantly higher ($p < 0.025$) for unguided walking than for guided walking, and, were significantly higher ($p < 0.025$) over complex routes as compared to simple routes, even though the terrain was similar. Thus any measures that might reduce the uncertainty of the athlete will reduce the physical stress, and allow those physical reserves to be better used during training or competition. Familiarity with surroundings is extremely important in the reduction of uncertainty.

Kobberling et al commented on the importance of normal vision for "efficient locomotion," and proceeded to hypothesize that blind subjects would have a higher metabolic cost for locomotion than sighted individuals using the same speeds.[14] They compared 30 sighted and 30 legally blind adolescents on oxygen consumption parameters elicited by treadmill walking and running and found that the blind subjects had a significantly higher energy cost than the sighted subjects for both walking and running. They suggested that this difference could not be attributed to systematic physical differences but might be due to differences in stride length, prolonged ground time, and greater braking and accelerating forces (i.e., decreased mechanical efficiency). From these data it might be concluded that blind subjects would fatigue earlier, and thus will have to work harder to reach the same physical levels as sighted individuals. These data also explain the low oxygen consumption values for blind children found by Jankowski and Evans,[15] who tested 20 blind children (age range = 4 to 18) for oxygen consumption as elicited by a modified Balke treadmill test. The average maximal oxygen consumption was 29.0 mL/kg/min ±6.3, which was 58% of normal for this age range. Although these low scores are not caused by any limitations in the cardiovascular system, they reflect a sedentary life-style or limited training opportunities. Aerobic training is essential to improve the cardiovascular status of blind persons, and even more important for those wishing to compete in sports. An aerobic training program can be designed following American College of Sports Medicine or other established guidelines.[16]

In sports where vision or equilibrium is an integral part of the sport it may be necessary to modify rules or participation method. The typical modification is a sound device to identify direction. Any type of sound signal produced at regular intervals will suffice. The National Beep Ball Association (NBBA) has made a few adjustments in softball rules, as well as modifications to equipment to promote participation by blind individuals. The two major modifications are the use of a 16-inch softball with a sound-emitting device and the use of bases that have sound-emitting devices. In road racing, verbal cues are used, not only to give the athlete a sense of orientation, but to also give the athlete information about upcoming physical changes in the landscape. Another modification that is often used with track or running is that of a guide runner or guidewire for short distances. It is important to realize that the United States Association for Blind Athletes tries to adhere to NCAA rules where possible, and that physical contact for track races is illegal. Legal contact with the guide runner is through any flexible material not more than 50 cm long.

There are really no differences regarding types of injuries or treatment for the blind athlete and the sighted athlete. More important in predicting injury will be the specific athletic event in which the athlete is competing.

The Athlete With Cerebral Palsy

Sports participants with cerebral palsy are numerous, and range from persons who are ambulatory and with few physical symptoms to wheelchair-dependent persons with severe symptoms. As noted by Nelson, cerebral palsy encompasses a conglomerate of neuromuscular dysfunctions.[17] There are a variety of causes, but the result is an insult to the developing central nervous system that results in a disorder of posture control and movement. The characteristic movement patterns associated with cerebral palsy include spasticity, athetosis, hypotonicity, and ataxia. Each of these movement patterns responds to slightly different stimuli, and a sports therapist should be aware of stimuli that may be counterproductive to training and performance. It is strongly recommended that the therapist review the athlete's health record prior to working with an athlete who has cerebral palsy, in order to identify any potential risks associated with the cerebral palsy.

The United States Cerebral Palsy Athletic Association (USCPAA) currently sponsors competitions in a wide variety of sports (Table 12–3) and has a membership of approximately 2,500.[18] Classification of athletes with cerebral palsy is complex, in that it is not only based upon functional capabilities, but may differ between sports. Sherrill et al presented an excellent synopsis of classification and the issues which are involved in classification at the 1984 Olympic Scientific Congress.[19] As they noted, most with cerebral palsy have more than one dysfunction. Dysfunctions that accompany movement disorders often include mental retardation, visual problems, seizures, perceptual disorders, hearing deficits, and reflex problems. The classification system attempts to take the myriad of dysfunctions into consideration on an individual basis. The current classification system used by the USCPAA is summarized in Table 12–4.

Little research is available regarding the fitness status or training potential of persons with cerebral palsy. In 1984, Short and Winnick presented the results from fitness testing of 396 adolescents with cerebral palsy and 1192 able-bodied adolescents.[20] Tests measured factors of body composition, muscular strength/endurance, speed, agility, flexibility, and cardiorespiratory endurance. The authors noted that some of the subjects with cerebral palsy could not participate in all

TABLE 12-3. USCPAA-RECOGNIZED SPORTS

Archery	Horseback riding	Soccer
Boccie	Powerlifting	Swimming
Bowling	Shooting	Table Tennis
Cycling	Slalom	Track/Field/Cross Country
Wheelchair Team Handball		

TABLE 12-4. SPORT CLASSIFICATION OF ATHLETES WITH CEREBRAL PALSY

Class	Description
Class 1	Uses motorized wheelchair because of poor functional use of upper extremities. Severe involvement in all four limbs with limited trunk control and inability to grasp softball. Only 25% ROM.
Class 2	Propels chair with feet and/or very slowly with arms. Severe to moderate quadriplegic with poor functional strength and control of the upper extremities. Approximately 40% ROM.
Class 3	Propels chair with arms with impaired control. Moderate quadriplegic with fair functional strength and control of the upper extremities. Approximately 60% ROM.
Class 4	Propels chair with arms with control. Only lower limb involvement with good trunk and upper extremity strength. Approximately 70% ROM.
Class 5	Ambulates with or without aids. Moderate to severe hemiplegia or paraplegia. Approximately 80% ROM.
Class 6	Ambulates without aids, but balance and coordination problems. Moderate to severe quadriplegia with greater upper extremity problems. Approximately 70% ROM in dominant arm.
Class 7	Ambulates well with slight limp. Moderate to mild hemiplegia or quadriplegia. Ninety percent ROM in all limbs with quadriplegia and 90% to 100% ROM in dominant arm with hemiplegia.
Class 8	Runs and jumps well. Mild hemiplegia with minimal coordination problems. Normal ROM.

of the tests, due to inappropriateness of the test. The able-bodied subjects scored significantly higher ($p < 0.01$) than the subjects with cerebral palsy on all of the tests, with the exception of body composition. It was suggested that cerebral palsy individuals might have a greater metabolic cost than able-bodied individuals during simple movement, thus explaining the similar body composition in conjunction with a low fitness level. In addition, no improvements in performance were found with increasing age, contradictory to findings with able-bodied and other disabled groups. The authors proposed that failure to improve with maturation might be a result of "educational and/or therapeutic approaches that do not emphasize the development of physical fitness."[20] It is important, however, to realize that individuals with cerebral palsy do respond to training. This was demonstrated in 1967 by Lundberg et al in children,[21] and again in a similar study in adolescents by Ekblom and Lundberg.[22]

Recently, McCubbin and Shasby examined the effects of isokinetic training or repetitive nonresistive movement on 20 individuals with cerebral palsy.[23] The majority of subjects had spastic-type cerebral palsy, though classification levels ranged from 1 through 7. Movement time and torque produced during elbow ex-

tension were the dependent variables. Both groups had significantly ($p < 0.05$) decreased movement times and increased torques as compared to a control group. Importantly, the isokinetic treatment group had significantly ($p < 0.05$) better scores than the repetitive treatment group. Changes in strength and speed occurred during the first 3 weeks and were due to neurological adaptations. The authors noted that further research is required to corroborate these findings with larger groups, variations of training speed, and other classification levels of cerebral palsy.

Modifications of equipment or sport technique is diverse for those with cerebral palsy and sport specific. An example of modification is floatation devices for swimming (with slightly warmer water temperatures) or the use of headgear during ambulatory competitions for athletes with severe spasticity. The reader is referred to the USCPAA handbook for more detailed information regarding modifications.[18]

Training programs must be individualized because of the diversity of symptoms and confounding factors, such as mental retardation. Similar to a therapeutic program, attention must be given to present symptoms, such as spasticity, so the condition will not be exacerbated, although it may be desirable to allow for a slightly greater muscle tone because of the psychological benefits of competition. Sports physical therapists working with athletes with cerebral palsy should consider current therapy modes, such as proprioceptive neuromuscular facilitation and exteroceptive stimulation, to address muscle control. They should also consider whether those will meet the training needs, however, and if they might be used supplementary to a more traditional training program. Contracture prevention is a constant concern with the disabled and a proper stretching program will help address this problem. Temperature regulation is often poor for athletes with cerebral palsy and should be monitored frequently.

Hearing-Impaired Athletes

Hearing impairment includes persons who are deaf or hard-of-hearing. In 1974 it was estimated that there were 13.4 million hearing-impaired persons in the United States,[24] of whom 1.8 million were deaf. Hard-of-hearing is defined as defective hearing, although some functional hearing may be achieved with the use of a hearing aid. This definition may be narrowed to be defined as a hearing loss ranging from 27 to 90 dB. Deafness is defined as nonfunctional hearing ability with or without the use of a hearing aid and a resultant impairment in processing linguistic information. This may be narrowed to stipulate hearing loss greater than 91 dB in the better ear.

The American Athletic Association for the Deaf is the national organization for deaf athletes and sponsors competitions in track and field, swimming, wrestling, and basketball, among other sports. The primary modification necessary for competitive events is the use of light signals or physical cues. In general, there are few limitations to participation in competitive activities, although damage to the vestibular apparatus may restrict involvement in tumbling and students who have had a fenestration operation are usually disqualified from swimming.[25] Butterfield points out that many deaf children have poor static and dynamic balance, but that researchers have not been able to clearly establish a causative factor.[26] Thus, precompetitive testing might aid the sports physical therapist to ascertain motor skill and balance ability.

Butterfield attempted to ascertain level of motor skill and balance skill by age, sex, and etiology of hearing loss.[26] Subjects were 132 hearing-impaired children; age range, 3 to 14 years. As with hearing subjects, age was a significant factor in development of motor skills. Performance for static and dynamic balance was also significantly correlated to age ($p < 0.01$) and there were no differences in performance between men and women. Only one significant difference was attributable to etiology, with the genetic group performing significantly better ($p < 0.05$) than the idiopathic group in static balance. Importantly, this study confirmed previous findings of poor balance skills for deaf children and the relation between balance and motor skill development. The author suggested that increased opportunities to practice balance and motor skills is extremely important.

Pertinent to the topic of training, Winnick and Short examined the physical fitness status of 686 hearing and 1,045 hearing-impaired, including 153 hard-of-hearing and 892 deaf adolescents.[27] Items tested included body composition, hand grip and abdominal strength, low back-hamstring flexibility, 50-yard dash, and cardiorespiratory endurance. Relatively few differences were found between the hearing-impaired and the hearing adolescents. The authors concluded that the hearing-impaired were capable of normal fitness levels, given proper training.

Special concerns when training a hearing-impaired person are limited to those already identified—abnormal equilibrium and the necessity for visual or physical cues. Musculoskeletal injuries may occur with any athlete and are thus related to the competitive sport.

Mentally Retarded Athletes

The American Association on Mental Deficiency defines mental retardation as "subaverage general intellectual functioning existing concurrently with deficits in adaptive behavior, and manifested during the developmental period" (as cited in ref. 28). There are currently 7 million individuals in the United States who

are mentally retarded and more than 1 million have participated in the Special Olympics.[2] Competitions are held at every level from the school to international games. The Special Olympics sponsors a winter and a summer program, including a wide variety of sports. Table 12–5 lists sports that are currently approved for inclusion in the two programs, as well as demonstration sports. Within each sport the athletes are classified by disability, which includes intellectual status, mode of movement (ambulation, wheelchair, etc.), and gender.

Mental retardation is usually accompanied by a variety of physical impairments, some caused by the defect that caused the mental retardation and others with unrelated etiologies. When training regimens are being developed these impairments must be considered, as they may be performance-limiting. Comparative/descriptive studies are the most common method of studying the physical capabilities of mentally retarded individuals. Popular topics have included the relationship between intelligence and physical fitness, gross motor development, and general physical fitness. In general, the mentally retarded population has a lower life expectancy, lower cardiovascular endurance, and a higher percentage of body fat than nonretarded persons.[29–31] Francis and Rarick were among the first to test physical fitness parameters in a large sample of mentally retarded children.[32] They concluded that the developmental pattern was the same for mentally retarded children as normal children but that mentally retarded children were consistently lower at all stages. Roswal et al reached similar conclusions in their analysis of the fitness data of 887 mentally retarded individuals and suggested that comparison of test results for this group should be to normative data for other Special Olympians and not to test percentiles for general populations.[33] The American Association for Health, Physical Education, and Recreation developed a fitness test battery for use with mentally retarded children that is a modification of the battery of tests used with normal children.[34] Norms were established using a sample of 4200 educable mentally retarded girls and boys, thus making the fitness battery pertinent to the retarded population. The test battery includes a flexed arm

hang, situp test, shuttle run, standing broad jump, 50-yard dash, softball throw, and 300-yard run-walk. In 1977 a revision of the tests was published.[35] In 1985, Winnick and Short developed Project UNIQUE, for the purpose of testing a variety of disabled persons, including individuals with cerebral palsy or mental retardation.[36]

Three important fitness variables of a training program for a mentally retarded individual are (1) coordination, (2) body composition, and (3) aerobic capacity. Although other variables, such as strength, are not unimportant, these variables are often performance-limiting. As already stated, the motor performance of mentally retarded individuals is lower than nationally established norms, but the developmental curve is similar. Thus, when establishing a training program, the sports physical therapist can still follow traditional skill progressions. Both Special Olympics and Project UNIQUE identify suggested skill progressions for some sports.[36,37] In addition, the level of retardation has an effect on motor skill development. Drowatzky found that Down's syndrome children tested lower than other trainable retarded children on a battery of motor skill tests.[38] Similar findings have been reported among individuals from different classifications of retardation.

Increased body fat can be performance-limiting because of the increased energy that is required to produce the same movement when a greater body mass must be moved. Rarick and Dobbins found that mentally retarded children had greater amounts of fat than nonretarded children.[39] These findings were corroborated by Chumlea and Cronk in a study of children with Down's syndrome[40] and elaborated upon by Fox and Rotatori in a study of 1152 mentally retarded individuals.[30] An aerobic training program might aid weight loss while simultaneously improving an individual's aerobic capacity, another performance-limiting factor. In order for any program to result in weight loss, however, it is recommended that dietary intake be monitored. Millar found that an aerobic training program with 14 Down's syndrome adolescents failed to result in the expected changes in body composition, (normally, training would have resulted in a decrease in body fat) and noted that many of the subjects had increased their dietary intake during the time of the study.[41]

Aerobic capacity in mentally retarded individuals is typically below age-related norms but can be improved through regular training. Fernhall et al present an excellent review of the literature about the cardiovascular status of mentally retarded individuals.[42] In prior studies, cardiovascular fitness levels of mentally retarded individuals ranged from 10% to 45% below those of nonretarded individuals. Furthermore, not all studies were able to document improvements in VO_2

TABLE 12–5. RECOGNIZED SPECIAL OLYMPIC SPORTS

Official Summer Sports

Aquatics	Equestrian	Soccer
Athletics	Gymnastics	Softball
Basketball	Roller Skating	Volleyball
Bowling		

Official Winter Sports

Alpine Skiing	Floor Hockey	Poly Hockey
Figure Skating	Nordic Skating	Speed Skating

Demonstration Sports

Canoeing	Table Tennis	Tennis
Cycling	Team Handball	Weightlifting

max with aerobic training, although the majority were able to find some positive training effects.

Aerobic training should follow established guidelines.[16] A few helpful points for training programs may be culled from some of the research. In general, mentally retarded individuals require constant motivation to continue any activity beyond the point of slight fatigue (or of sufficient intensity to stimulate a training effect). With a lower coach-to-student ratio, the coach will have more time to work with each individual, thus increasing the motivation. Some type of a reward system, even as simple as daily mileage marked on a chart in a conspicuous place, can be a very effective motivator. An interval training program might be more successful with some individuals, as it is less monotonous, and the attention span of many of these individuals is short.

All athletes competing in the Special Olympics must have a physical prior to competition, but it is important that the sports physical therapist be aware of some specific problems that might occur with Down's syndrome individuals. It is well known that individuals with Down's syndrome have a high incidence of heart malformations, and although most have been identified, it is wise to check the status of each individual and if strenuous activity has been approved. The most common cardiac defects include atrial septal defect, ventricular defect, persistent common atrioventricular canal, and patent ductus arteriosis. These, as well as other defects, cause the mortality of Down's syndrome individuals to be extremely high (>45%), although modern surgical techniques have greatly improved the survival rate. Stressful activity for those with congenital defects may be contraindicated.[43]

All individuals with trisomy 21 are also required to have a cervical x-ray if they will be competing in gymnastics.[37] Research has shown an increased incidence of atlantoaxial instability for individuals with Down's syndrome, with a potential complication of dislocation, especially during extreme flexion.[44] Thus, the Special Olympics has identified atlantoaxial instability as a disqualifer for participation in gymnastics. In a similar, though different category, joint laxity is another problem often encountered with Down's syndrome individuals.

In 1988, McCormick presented data from preparticipation screening and injury records from area games in Galveston, Texas.[45] He suggested that a properly designed questionnaire would detect 71% of significant findings. Two of the more common problems found were a history of seizures and ophthalmological abnormalities. Furthermore, he advocated the use of physical therapists to do musculoskeletal evaluations, due to their training and experience with injuries. The injury rate was extremely low—less than 0.05 per 100 participant hours—and the majority of the problems were medical illnesses. As might be surmised from previous paragraphs, Down's syndrome athletes had a 3.32 greater chance of injury than the other mentally retarded athletes. M. Lord, Director of the Capital Area Games in Austin, Texas identified heat-related illnesses as the major concern for most of the games in the southern regions. She noted that most of the athletes had to be told to drink water and stay in the shade, the older athletes and those in wheelchairs seemed especially susceptible to heat illness.

Sports physical therapy with mentally retarded athletes requires knowledge of the individual's health history, specific disability, and, if possible, the etiology of the mental retardation. In addition, patience is essential, especially when working with the more severely retarded. The Special Olympics Foundation has outlined the qualifications necessary to be certified as a coach for a Special Olympics team, as well as some ideas for year-round training.[37] This has been done in order to help ensure qualified coaching for the athlete and thus increase safety.

Athletes With Spinal Cord Injuries

Spinal cord injuries include not only traumatic injuries but also victims of polio, spina bifida, and any other process that impairs the function of the spinal cord. Statistics from the National Spinal Cord Injury Data Research Center estimate that 11,000 new cases of traumatic spinal cord impairment occur annually, with more than half of this group being in the 15- to 24-year-old age group.[1] Nontraumatic spinal cord injuries are believed to comprise 30% of all spinal cord injuries. At one time, the longevity for patients with spinal cord injuries was extremely short, but medical advances have resulted in substantial increases in longevity. Sport participation offers a means of increasing the quality of life by improving the health status and increasing the self-esteem of patients with spinal cord injuries.

Persons with spinal cord injuries compete in wheelchairs, and competitions are regulated by such governing bodies as the National Wheelchair Athletic Association (NWAA), International Foundation for Wheelchair Tennis (IFWT) and the National Wheelchair Basketball Association (NWBA).[46] Sanctioned competitions include swimming, track and field, basketball, tennis, and skiing. There are currently two major classification systems for wheelchair athletes, the first through the NWAA and the second through the NWBA. Tables 12–6 and 12–7 list the various classifications, including those for amputees who are competing with wheelchair athletes. This is one area in which some controversy exists, as Class V amputees have a physiological advantage over athletes with spinal cord injuries, as the former usually have intact sympathetic systems.

TABLE 12-6. CLASSIFICATION OF WHEELCHAIR ATHLETES—NWAA

Class	Description
Wheelchair Events	
Class 1A	Cervical lesions with complete or incomplete quadriplegia; involvement of both hands, weakness of triceps (≤ grade 3); severe weakness of trunk and lower extremities interfering significantly with trunk balance and ability to walk.
Class 1B	Cervical lesions with complete or incomplete quadriplegia; involvement of upper extremities, normal or good triceps (grades 4–5); generalized weakness of trunk and lower extremities interfering significantly with trunk balance and ability to walk.
Class 1C	Cervical lesions with complete or incomplete quadriplegia; involvement of upper extremities, normal or good triceps (grades 4–5); normal or good finger flexion and extension, but without intrinsic hand function; generalized weakness of trunk and lower extremities interfering significantly with trunk balance and ability to walk.
Class II	Complete or incomplete paraplegia below T1 to and including T5, or comparable disability; total abdominal paralysis or poor strength (grades 0–2); no useful trunk sitting balance.
Class III	Complete or incomplete paraplegia or comparable disability below T5 to and including T10; upper abdominal and spinal extensor musculature sufficient to provide some element of trunk sitting balance, but not normal.
Class IV	Complete or incomplete paraplegia or comparable disability below T10 to and including L2; without quadriceps or very weak (≤ grade 2); gluteal paralysis.
Class V	Complete or incomplete paraplegia or comparable disability below L2; quadriceps grades 3–5.
Swimming Events	
Class V	Complete or incomplete paraplegia or comparable disability below L2; quadriceps grades 3–5 up to and including 39 points.
Class VI	Complete or incomplete paraplegia or comparable disability below L2; with 40 points or above on point scale.

Because of the major involvement of the central nervous system, athletes with spinal cord injuries have a wide variety of concomitant physiological disabilities. These are generally directly related to the level of injury in the spinal cord, possible involvement of autonomic neurons, muscular atrophy, and decreased weight-bearing. This section addresses the following topics in relation to persons with spinal cord injuries: (1) respiratory capacity; (2) autonomic disability; (3) long-term effects of non-weight bearing; (4) fitness variables in wheelchair athletes; (5) response to training of wheelchair athletes; and (6) wheelchair performance variables. For additional literature on traumatic spinal cord injury, see Schmitz's excellent review of general information and physical therapy requirements for patients with spinal cord injuries.[47]

Respiratory capacity ranges from greatly diminished in high-level quadriplegics to normal in low-level paraplegics. This is due to the loss of primary and secondary respiratory musculature as the injury progresses from lumbar to cervical levels. Hullemann et al reported vital capacities of trained athletes ranging from 3.913 to 4.858 L for classes II and V, respectively.[48] They noted that the increase between class II and class III was statistically significant ($p < 0.02$) for maximal expiratory flow rate, which illustrates the effect of loss

TABLE 12-7. CLASSIFICATION OF WHEELCHAIR ATHLETES—NWBA

Class	Description
Class 1	Complete motor loss at T7 or above or comparable disability. Poor to absent sitting balance and trunk control.
Class 2	Complete motor loss T8 through and including L2; may be some motor strength in hips and thighs. Fair to good sitting balance and trunk control. Includes bilateral hip disarticulations.
Class 3	All other paralysis originating at or below L3. All lower extremity amputees, except above class 2. Good to normal sitting balance and trunk control.

TABLE 12-8. CLASSIFICATION OF WHEELCHAIR ATHLETES—AMPUTEES

Class	Description
Class IV	Unilateral amputee
Class IV	Bilateral above knee (amputations above level of greater trochanter)
Class V	Bilateral below knee (amputations below level of greater trochanter)
Class V	Above knee/below knee
Class VI	Bilateral below knee

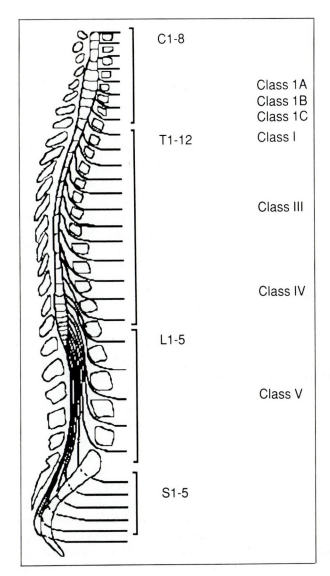

Figure 12-1. Wheelchair classification related to spinal cord levels.

of some of the muscles of expiration for the class II athletes. Furthermore, they recognized that these values were higher than those that had been reported for sedentary paraplegics. Zwiren and Bar-Or found slightly higher values for forced vital capacity in a group of wheelchair athletes (4.96 L).[49] Interestingly, they found no significant difference between the wheelchair athletes and wheelchair or normal sedentary subjects. This study contained only paraplegic subjects, however. In an excellent review of the cardiorespiratory status of individuals with spinal cord injuries, Hoffman concluded that vital capacity progressively reduced with higher lesion levels.[50]

Dynamic pulmonary function, or ventilation equivalent during exercise, is affected for the same reasons as static pulmonary function. It has been theorized that maximal ventilatory equivalent ($\dot{V}_{E\,max}$) would be decreased by a greater amount than vital capacity, due to the loss of expiratory musculature not normally used during ventilation at rest. Hulleman et al were not able to find significant differences between athletes of different class for $\dot{V}_{E\,max}$,[48] however, Coutts et al were able to document statistically significant ($p < 0.01$) differences for $V_{E\,max}$ when comparing athletes from each classification.[51] They found maximal ventilation equivalents ranging from 49.0 to 107.0 $l\cdot min^{-1}$ for athletes from class 1a and class V, respectively. Similar findings were made by Hoffman[50] and Gass and Camp.[52]

The autonomic system is often involved in spinal cord injuries because of the close proximity of the sympathetic trunk to the spinal cord and the presence of autonomic system cell bodies within the spinal cord itself. A review of neuroanatomy will aid the sports physical therapist in identifying the distribution of autonomic segmental innervation. The implications of autonomic involvement become greater with higher spinal cord injuries, not only because of impairment of sympathetic innervation to organs such as the heart, but also because of the complications inherent in loss of autonomic control of the vascular system. Impairment of sympathetic control of the heart is noticeable in quadriplegics, especially during exercise. Coutts et al noted a significantly ($p < 0.01$) lower maximal heart rate for class 1a when compared to class V athletes (100 bpm vs. 188 bpm, respectively).[51] It has been suggested that the lack of increased heart rate is a reflection of the small muscle mass being used, but such a differentiation may need to be made on an individual level. A major complication that is also noticeable during exercise is the reduction or complete lack of sweating, an important mode of heat regulation. Thus, the sports physical therapist must regularly monitor the athlete with a spinal cord injury, especially one with high lesion levels. In addition, competition in the heat might be contraindicated, depending upon the individual's tolerance.

There are several side effects from spinal cord injury and non-weight bearing, such as loss of sensation, muscle atrophy, and osteoporosis. Loss of sensation may seem an obvious result of spinal cord injury, but it is important to realize that this means the athlete will not feel chronic pressure areas or acute injuries. All persons with spinal cord injuries are taught self-checks to monitor tissue status of pressure-sensitive areas. With increased activity or participation in a new activity, however, new pressure areas may develop, and it is necessary that athletes check their entire body for tissue viability. Acute trauma, such as fractures, may occur more easily due to the increased frailty of the bones. It is therefore important to perform a thorough check after even the most minor of falls or bumps.

As already noted, there are several changes in the respiratory system that occur as the result of a spinal cord injury. These changes and the changes in the func-

tional muscle mass result in decreased aerobic capacity. As noted by Zwiren and Bar-Or, wheelchair athletes perform significantly ($p < 0.01$) better than wheelchair sedentary individuals of similar classifications.[49] They found maximal oxygen consumption (VO_2 max) values of 35.0 ± 7.6 mL/kg/min for wheelchair athletes, as compared to 19.6 ± 5.5 ml·kg·$^{-1}$min^{-1} for sedentary wheelchair subjects. Although these values are significantly below those that might be found with able-bodied athletes on a treadmill test, the authors found no significant differences when the able-bodied athletes were tested using arm ergometry. Coutts et al found similar values for 21 wheelchair subjects and noted that the VO_2 max was progressively lower with higher lesion levels, similar to previously noted differences in ventilation capacity.[51] Gass and Camp studied 16 national class male wheelchair athletes and found slightly higher VO_2 max values (20.0 to 49.0 ml/kg^{-1}/min^{-1}).[52] They also found a correlation between the level of the spinal cord lesion and oxygen consumption.

In order to assess the potential, some researchers have conducted case studies of exceptional wheelchair athletes. In 1979, Gandee et al tested a male elite wheelchair marathoner.[53] They found a VO_2 max of 65 ml·kg·$^{-1}$min^{-1}, the highest VO_2 reported at that time. In a similar study, Francis and Nelson examined a nationally classed wheelchair marathoner.[54] The subject had a VO_2 max of 52 mL/kg/min and a stroke volume of 62 mL. Millar and Ward found slightly higher values for a group of four elite wheelchair track athletes and suggested that upper body musculature and intensity of training were correlated to oxygen consumption values.[55] Coutts and Stogryn reported peak VO_2 max values ranging from 16.9 to 50.7 mL/kg/min and found peak anaerobic power values ranging between 31 and 148 W, which was similar to values reported by other authors.[56]

Upon identifying the existing range of physiological values for wheelchair athletes, the question then becomes, how do wheelchair subjects respond to training? McDonell et al addressed this question in their 1981 study with 13 wheelchair athletes. The subjects were tested for VO_2 max prior to and following 2 months of aerobic training.[57] Significant ($p < 0.01$) increases in VO_2 max values were found in the experimental group as compared to the control group. In addition, the study included a group of elite athletes who had significantly ($p < 0.01$) greater slow and fast twitch diameter area than the experimental group. In a review of the benefits of aerobic exercise for spinal cord injured, Cowell et al noted that inspiratory muscles increased in strength and endurance capacity, thus reducing ventilatory fatigue during exercise.[58] Other improvements they cited included dynamic strength, cardiovascular function ($\dot{Q}$), and power output. Glaser identified the need for aerobic training as of primary importance, especially considering the energy cost of wheelchair locomotion.[59] He noted that mechanical efficiency for wheelchair locomotion was as low as 5% as compared to over 20% for walking and 10% for arm ergometry. Thus, wheelchair exercise is extremely demanding, and the better the cardiorespiratory system, the more resistant the athlete will be to fatigue.

The majority of the research has focused upon aerobic training for the wheelchair athlete, with little having been done to identify changes that might occur with strength training. Cooney and Walker examined the changes in VO_2 max and strength that resulted from 9 weeks of resistance training with a hydraulic system.[60] Ten subjects trained three times per week using a circuit type program, following which they were retested for VO_2 max, power output, and strength. The subjects significantly ($p < 0.01$) improved all scores, with a mean improvement for VO_2 max of 28.1%. Importantly, the same type of improvements were found for the quadriplegic and paraplegic subjects. Gairdner notes that some exercises can be used in a home circuit program for athletes without nearby training facilities.[61]

The sports physical therapist working with wheelchair athletes will benefit from becoming knowledgeable about other performance variables. One extremely important variable is that of racing technique and the influence of chair and rim modifications upon performance. Ridgway et al found that cycle time, distance, and rate were correlated to competitive classification, with the lower lesion levels displaying faster cycle velocities.[62] They noted that leg and trunk positioning, also a function of lesion level, were related to control. VanDerWoude et al examined the effects of rim diameter on propulsion and physiological costs.[63] They found highly significant ($p < 0.001$) effects of hand rim diameter or velocity on oxygen cost of propulsion, with the smaller rims correlated to lower O_2 costs. In fact, they noted that five of the eight subjects were unable to propel the wheelchair beyond a specific velocity with the largest handrims. This has direct implications toward the use of smaller handrims, especially for endurance events, although the authors also note that caution should be used in extrapolating from kinematic analysis to competitive performance.

The physical complications of spinal cord injuries are outlined by Schmitz, and these complications hold true for the wheelchair athlete as well.[47] Sports participation should decrease some of the potential complications due to improvements in the circulatory system and better awareness of health practices. Among the most common injuries for wheelchair athletes, Gairdner lists muscle strain, tendonitis, hand blisters and cuts, and skin irritation.[61] Curtis and Dillon conducted a survey of 128 wheelchair athletes for common injuries and found similar types of injuries among their list.[64]

The most commonly reported injury was soft tissue injury such as strains and pulls (33%), followed by blisters (18%), and skin abrasions (17%). Most of the injuries were associated with track, basketball, or road racing. The authors suggested that many of the injuries could have been prevented by proper training techniques, taping fingers, or use of gloves, proper equipment, and adequate cushioning, among others. In addition, they implicated the overuse phenomenon as a contributor to many of the soft tissue injuries.

SUMMARY

The number of disabled athletes is increasing steadily, and it is important that the sports physical therapist be aware of major physiological differences that might influence training. In general, the types of injuries that the disabled athletes incur are similar to those of nondisabled athletes; thus, treatment is the same. Pretraining fitness levels should be established to provide a baseline for monitoring training changes. As with any fitness program, the components include flexibility, strength, body composition, and anaerobic and aerobic power. It is possible to test all these components for the disabled athlete, with some modifications to testing protocols and procedures. Several manuals with adapted testing procedures have been referred to for specific populations, as well as sources for more information regarding training program suggestions. It is hoped that this chapter will serve as a reference base and an introduction to disabled athletes.

REFERENCES

1. Young JS, Northrop NE. *Statistical Information Pertaining To Some of the Most Commonly Asked Questions About SCI* (Monograph). Phoenix, Ariz: National Spinal Cord Injury Data Research Center; 1979.
2. *Facts on Mental Retardation.* Special Olympics International Inc; 1988.
3. *United States Amputee Athletic Association Guidelines.* USAAA; 1987.
4. Edelstein JE. Prosthetic assessment and management. In: O'Sullivan SB, Schmitz TJ, eds. *Physical Rehabilitation: Assessment and Treatment.* 2nd ed. Philadelphia, Pa: F A Davis; 1988:407–433.
5. Murray D, Fisher FR. Normal gait. In: *Handbook of Amputations and Prostheses.* Ottawa, Ontario: University of Ottawa; 1982:28–31.
6. Dickman IR. *Living with Blindness.* New York, NY: Public Affairs Committee Report; 1977.
7. Rainbolt WJ, Sherrill C. Characteristics of adult blind athletes, competition experience, and training practices. In: Berridge ME, Ward GR, eds. *International Perspectives on Adapted Physical Activity; Proceedings of the Fifth International Symposium on Adapted Physical Ac-*

tivity. Champaign, Ill: Human Kinetics Publishers Inc; 1985:165–172.
8. Buell CE. Blind athletes who compete in the mainstream. In: Berridge ME, Ward GR, eds. *International Perspectives on Adapted Physical Activity; Proceedings of the Fifth International Symposium on Adapted Physical Activity.* Champaign, Ill: Human Kinetics Publishers Inc; 1985:173–178.
9. United States Association of Blind Athletes Rule. USABA; 1988.
10. Ribadi H, Rider RA, Toole T. A comparison of static and dynamic balance in congenitally blind, sighted, and sighted blindfolded adolescents. *Adapted Phys Act Q.* 1987; 4:220–225.
11. Pope CJ, McGrain P, Arnhold RW. Running gait of the blind: A kinematic analysis. In: Sherrill C, ed. *Sport and Disabled Athletes; The 1984 Olympic Scientific Congress Proceedings.* Champaign, Ill: Human Kinetics Publishers Inc; 1984; 9:173–177.
12. Arnhold RW, McGrain P. Selected kinematic patterns of visually impaired youth in sprint running. *Adapted Phys Act Q.* 1985; 2:206–213.
13. Peake P, Leonard JA. The use of heart rate as an index of stress in blind pedestrians. *Ergonomics.* 1971; 14(2):189–204.
14. Kobberling G, Jankowski LW, Leger L. Energy cost of locomotion in blind adolescents. *Adapted Phys Act Q.* 1989; 6:58–67.
15. Jankowski LW, Evans JK. The exercise capacity of blind children. *Vis Impair Blind.* 1981; 75:248–251.
16. American College of Sports Medicine. *Guidelines for Exercise Testing and Prescription.* 3rd ed. Philadelphia, Pa: Lea & Febiger; 1986.
17. Nelson CA. Cerebral palsy. In: Umphred DA, ed. *Neurological Rehabilitation.* St Louis, Mo: C V Mosby Co; 1985:165–183.
18. United States Cerebral Palsy Athletic Association. *Rules—Classification Manual.* USCPAA; 1989.
19. Sherrill C, Adams-Mushett C, Jones JA. Classification and other issues in sports for blind, cerebral palsied, les autres, and amputee athletes. In: Sherrill C, ed. *Sport and Disabled Athletes; The 1984 Olympic Scientific Congress Proceedings.* Champaign, Ill: Human Kinetics Publishers Inc; 1984; 9:113–130.
20. Short FX, Winnick JP. The performance of adolescents with cerebral palsy on measures of physical fitness. In: Sherrill C, ed. *Sport and Disabled Athletes; The 1984 Olympic Scientific Congress Proceedings.* Champaign, Ill: Human Kinetics Publishers Inc; 1984; 9:239–244.
21. Lundberg A, Ovenfors E, Saltin B. Effect of physical training on school children with cerebral palsy. *Acta Paediatr Scand.* 1967; 56:182–188.
22. Ekblom B, Lundberg A. Effect of physical training on adolescents with severe motor handicaps. *Acta Paediatr Scand.* 1968; 57:17–23.
23. McCubbin JA, Shasby GB. Effects of isokinetic exercise on adolescents with cerebral palsy. *Adapted Phys Act Q.* 1985; 2:56–64.
24. Schein JD, Delk. *The Deaf Population of the United States.* Silver Spring, Md: National Association of the Deaf; 1976.

25. *Physical Education, Recreation and Sports for Individuals With Hearing Impairments*. Washington, DC: Physical Education and Recreation for the Handicapped: Information and Research Utilization Center; 1976.

26. Butterfield SA. The influence of age, sex, hearing loss, etiology and balance ability on the fundamental motor skills of deaf children. In Berridge ME, Ward GR, eds. *International Perspectives on Adapted Physical Activity; International Symposium on Adapted Physical Activity*. Champaign, Ill: Human Kinetics Publishers Inc; 1985:43–51.

27. Winnick JP, Short FX. Physical fitness of adolescents with auditory impairments. *Adapted Phys Act Q.* 1986; 3:58–66.

28. Arnheim DD, Auxter D, Crowe WC. *Principles and Methods of Adapted Physical Education and Recreation*. 3rd ed. St Louis, Mo: C V Mosby Co; 1977:352–375.

29. Beasley CR. Effects of a jogging program on cardiovascular fitness and work performance of mentally retarded adults. *Am J Ment Defic.* 1982; 86:609–613.

30. Fox R, Rotatori AF. Prevalence of obesity among mentally retarded adults. *Am J Ment Defic.* 1982; 87:228–230.

31. Thase ME. Longevity and mortality in Down's syndrome. *J Ment Defic Res.* 1982; 26:177–192.

32. Francis RJ, Rarick GL. Motor characteristics of mentally retarded. *Am J Ment Defic.* 1959; 63:792–811.

33. Roswal GM, Roswal PM, Dunleavy AO. Normative health-related fitness data for Special Olympians. In: Sherrill C, ed. *Sport and Disabled Athletes; The 1984 Olympic Scientific Congress Proceedings*. Champaign, Ill: Human Kinetics Publishers Inc; 1984; 9:229–238.

34. *Special Fitness Test Manual for the Mentally Retarded*. Washington, DC: American Association for Health, Physical Education, and Recreation; 1968.

35. *Special Fitness Test Manual for the Mentally Retarded*. Washington, DC: American Alliance for Health, Physical Education, Recreation, and Dance; 1977.

36. Winnick JP, Short FX. *Physical Fitness Testing of the Disabled: Project UNIQUE*. Champaign, Ill: Human Kinetics Publishers Inc; 1985.

37. *Official Special Olympics Summer Sports Rules*. Special Olympic International Inc; 1988.

38. Drowatzky JN. *Physical Education for the Mentally Retarded*. Philadelphia, Pa: Lea & Febiger; 1971.

39. Rarick GL, Dobbins DA. Basic components in the motor performance of educable mentally retarded children: Implications for curriculum development. (project No. 142714). Washington, DC: US Department of Health, Education, and Welfare; 1972.

40. Chumlea WC, Cronk CE. Overweight among children with Trisomy 21. *J Ment Defic Res.* 1981; 25:275–280.

41. Millar AL. *Effects of Endurance Training on Down's Syndrome Adolescents and Young Adults*. Tempe, Ariz: Arizona State University; 1985. Thesis.

42. Fernhall B, Tymeson GT, Webster GE. Cardiovascular fitness of mentally retarded individuals. *Adapted Phys Act Quart.* 1988; 5:12–28.

43. Rehder H. Pathology of Trisomy 21—with particular reference to persistent common atrioventricular canal of the heart. In: Burgio GR, Fraccaro M, Tiepolo L, Wolf U, eds. *Trisomy 21—An International Symposium*. Berlin, West Germany: Springer-Verlag; 1981:57–74.

44. Peuschel SF, Scola FH. Atlantoaxial instability in individuals with Down syndrome. *Pediatrics.* 1987; 80:555–560.

45. McCormick D. Preparticipation physical examination and injury surveillance for Special Olympics athletes. Presented at the Annual Conference on Innovations in Sports Medicine; June, 24, 1988; Galveston, Tex.

46. *National Wheelchair Athletic Association Medical Guidelines*. Colorado Springs, Colo: USWA; 1987.

47. Schmitz TJ. Traumatic spinal cord injury. In: O'Sullivan SB, Schmitz TJ, eds. *Physical Rehabilitation: Assessment and Treatment*. 2nd ed. Philadelphia, Pa: F A Davis; 1988:545–588.

48. Hullemann K-D, List M, Matthes D, et al. Spiroergometric and telemetric investigations during the XXI International Stoke Mandeville Games 1972 in Heidelberg. *Paraplegia.* 1975; 13:109–123.

49. Zwiren LD, Bar-Or O. Responses to exercise of paraplegics who differ in conditioning level. *Med Sci Sports Exerc.* 1975; 7(2):94–98.

50. Hoffman MD. Cardiorespiratory fitness and training in quadriplegics and paraplegics. *Sports Med.* 1986; 3:312–330.

51. Coutts KD, Rhodes EC, McKenzie DC. Maximal exercise responses of tetraplegics and paraplegics. *J Appl Physiol Respir Environ Exerc Physiol.* 1983; 55:479–482.

52. Gass GC, Camp EM. Physiological characteristics of trained Australian paraplegic and tetraplegic subjects. *Med Sci Sports Exerc.* 1979; 11:256–259.

53. Gandee R, Winningham M, Deitchman R, et al. The aerobic capacity of an elite wheelchair marathon racer. *Med Sci Sports Exerc.* 1980; 12:142. Abstract.

54. Francis RS, Nelson AG. Physiological and performance profiles of a world class wheelchair athlete. *Med Sci Sports Exerc.* 1981; 13:132. Abstract.

55. Millar AL, Ward GR. Physiological monitoring during intensive training of Canadian national track wheelchair athletes. *Med Sci Sports Exerc.* 1983; 15:181–182. Abstract.

56. Coutts KD, Stogryn JL. Aerobic and anaerobic power of Canadian wheelchair track athletes. *Med Sci Sports Exerc.* 1987; 19:62–65.

57. McDonell E, Brassard L, Martin P, et al. The effects of arm ergometer endurance training on physiological parameters of paraplegic wheelchair subjects. *Recherches Actuelles en Activité Physique Adaptée, Actes du Symposium*. Montreal; 1981:58–78.

58. Cowell LL, Squires WG, Raven PB. Benefits of aerobic exercise for the paraplegic: a brief review. *Med Sci Sports Exerc.* 1986; 18:501–508.

59. Glaser RM. Exercise and locomotion for the spinal cord injured. In: Terjung RL, ed. *Exercise and Sport Science Reviews*. New York, NY: Macmillan Publishing Co; 1985; 15:263–303.

60. Cooney MM, Walker JB. Hydraulic resistance exercise

benefits cardiovascular fitness of spinal cord injured. *Med Sci Sports Exerc.* 1985; 18:522–525.

61. Gairdner J. *Fitness for the Disabled: Wheelchair Users.* Toronto, Canada: Fitzhenry & Whiteside Ltd; 1983.

62. Ridgway M, Pope C, Wilkerson J. A kinematic analysis of 800-meter wheelchair-racing techniques. *Adapted Phys Act Q.* 1988; 5:96–107.

63. VanDerWoude LH, Veeger HEJ, Rozendal RH, et al. Wheelchair racing: Effects of rim diameter and speed on physiology and technique. *Med Sci Sports Exerc.* 1988; 20:492–500.

64. Curtis KA, Dillon DA. Survey of wheelchair athletic injuries—common patterns and prevention. In: Sherrill C, ed. *Sport and Disabled Athletes; The 1984 Olympic Scientific Congress Proceedings.* Champaign, Ill: Human Kinetics Publishers Inc; 1984; 9:211–216.

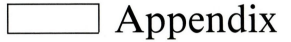 # Appendix

National Governing Organizations for Disabled Sports

USAAA
149-A Belle Forest Circle
Nashville, TN 37221
(615) 662-2323

USABA
33 N. Institute St.
Brown Hall
Colorado Springs, CO 80903
(719) 630-0422

USCPAA
34518 Warren Rd., Suite 264
Westland, MI 48185
(313) 425-8961

NWAA
3617 Betty Drive, Suite S
Colorado Springs, CO 80907
(719) 635-9300

13

Flexibility for Sports*

James E. Zachazewski

INTRODUCTION

To be successful in a given sport the athlete requires coordination, endurance, speed, strength, and flexibility. Depending upon the specific physical requirements of each particular sport, the importance of each of these characteristics will differ. The purpose of this chapter is to provide the therapist with an understanding of the role that flexibility plays in athletics. Normal physiology, pathophysiology, and clinical intervention are presented and explored.

DEFINITIONS/TERMINOLOGY

According to deVries, "Flexibility may be most simply defined as the range of motion available in a joint, such as the hip, or a series of joints, such as the spine."[1] The "flexibility" of any individual is dependent upon two distinct components: (1) the joint's range of motion (JROM), which is the motion available at any single joint based on the ability of the periarticular connective tissue to deform and that particular joint's arthrokinematics; and (2) muscle flexibility (MF), or the ability of muscle to lengthen, allowing a single joint or a series of joints to move through their full available range of motion (ROM). The total flexibility or ROM available is the sum of JROM plus that allowed by MF.

In athletics, flexibility is specific to the individual, the activity in which he or she is involved, and the joint or joints involved in that particular activity.[1–5] For example, the gymnast requires greater flexibility than does the basketball player.

Joint's range of motion is also dependent upon the shape and orientation of the joint surfaces,[6] whereas both JROM and MF are dependent upon the various physiological and neurophysiological characteristics of the body's tissues.[7–13]

During stretching all structures in the line of elongation have the potential to be deformed. Therefore any of these structures (muscle, joint capsule, ligament, tendon, skin etc.) that contain receptors could be the source of stimulus for reflex effects of elongation. Muscle spindles signal increased length. Golgi tendon organs signal tension increases (both active tension generated by muscle contraction and passive tension generated by lengthening). Receptors in the joint capsule, ligaments, and skin may also be deformed toward the end of physiological JROM. The reflex connections of most of these receptors are still being debated.

We know that the group Ia from the muscle spindle makes facilitory connections with alpha motoneurons to the agonist and its synergists, Group Ia is not only sensitive to length change but also the rate of change of length. Therefore, at least in theory, a high-velocity stretch would tend to facilitate contraction of the muscle being stretched. This is demonstrable in people with central nervous system (CNS) damage but may not be a consistent feature in normals. High-velocity stretching may facilitate active resistance to elongation. The effect of this increased resistance may not only be from motoneuron input but also from the effect of velocity on the physical and mechanical properties of muscle. As an example, in the neurologically impaired patient the stiffness and therefore the passive resistance to elongation is increased as a function of decreased mobility totally separate from a change in reflex sensitivity.[14] One might presume that in the patient with an intact nervous system who has decreased JROM and MF due to decreased activity, the effect of velocity on stiffness is at least as important if not more so than the velocity sensitivity of the muscle spindle. Even less well understood is the reflex sensitivity of the muscle spindle. Its

*Portions of this chapter have been reprinted with permission from Zachazewski JE, Reischl SR. Flexibility for the runner: Specific program considerations. *Top Acute Care Trauma Rehabil.* 1986; 1:9–27.
Zachazewski JE. Flexibility. In: Scully R, Barnes ML, eds. *Physical Therapy.* Philadelphia, Pa: J B Lippincott Co; 1989.

function varies depending upon the intactness of the animal preparation being studied. In other words, its function is different in animals with an intact cerebral spinal connection than decerebrate animals. This information does not help us understand the reflex functions in intact humans, however.

The Golgi tendon organ makes inhibitory connections with alpha motoneurons to the agonist. From this one could hypothesize that combining passive tension (passive stretch) with muscle contractions, such as in the "hold–relax" technique, would create the desired inhibition of muscle being stretched.

In summary, passive and active tension probably work to inhibit the muscle stretched. The velocity of stretch is an important consideration both mechanically and neurologically.

The sports physical therapist must be specific in determining what the requirements are and where the limitations lie. The requirements and limitations may vary between the normal athlete and the athlete who has suffered from an injury or other type of movement dysfunction.

Joints range of motion and muscle flexibility play an integral role in human movement. The individual must be able to move through a large ROM with ease and efficiency. Good JROM and MF will allow the tissues to move easily to accommodate the stress imposed upon them, dissipate the impact, and improve the efficiency and effectiveness of movement. All of these factors will assist in the prevention or minimization of injury.[7,8,15]

Flexibility, especially in sports, requires both static and dynamic components. Good static and dynamic

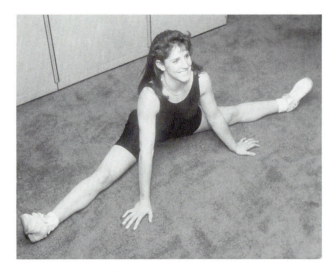

Figure 13-1. Demonstration of static flexibility.

flexibility are characteristics of the healthy athlete. In the athlete who suffers from some type of movement dysfunction or chronic recurring injury (such as a muscle strain) one or both of these characteristics may be compromised.

deVries defines static flexibility as the measured ROM available about a joint or series of joints (Fig 13–1) and dynamic flexibility as a measure of the resistance to active motion about a joint or series of joints.[1] As dynamic flexibility decreases, the resistance to motion (the ease by which that motion may be accomplished) increases. As a rule, good static flexibility is a prerequisite for good dynamic flexibility; however,

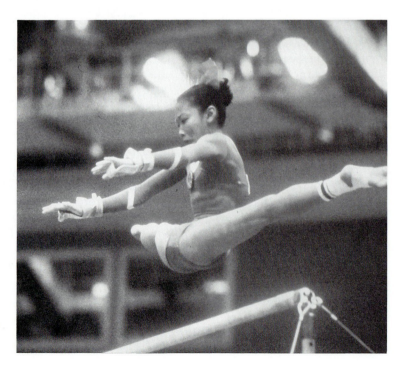

Figure 13-2. Demonstration of dynamic flexibility. *(Tony Duffy/Sports Illustrated)*

good static flexibility does not ensure good dynamic flexibility.

The velocity of normal human motion, and especially athletics, varies from slow methodical activity such as walking to high-velocity, explosive activity such as gymnastics (Fig 13–2). It is for high-velocity activities such as gymnastics, sprinting, and hurdling that good dynamic flexibility is most important for the individual to maximize performance efficiency and minimize injury. Muscle and periarticular connective tissue surrounding that joint *must* be able to deform in the time required for that activity to take place. Dynamic flexibility is limited by the ability of the connective tissue to deform quickly and easily, and by the integration of the neuromuscular system (contractile element of muscle and its innervation).

The sports physical therapist must analyze the athlete's needs. Does the athlete require JROM or MF? In which of these areas does the movement dysfunction exist if pathology or poor performance is evident? Is static or dynamic flexibility the problem?

LIMITING STRUCTURES

In the normal joint, the available JROM is dictated primarily by that joint's arthrokinematics and alignment of articular surfaces.[1,6] For example, elbow extension is ultimately limited by the olecranon fossa, whereas lateral rotation of the hip is limited when anteversion of the hip is present. In a very muscular athlete it is also possible for ROM to be limited by muscle bulk, with the bulk preventing the joint from going through its full available motion.[1]

If bony architecture and articular alignment are normal the connective tissue structures that surround the joint are the principal factors that limit normal JROM. The specific connective tissue structures that

TABLE 13-1. CONTRIBUTION OF TISSUE RESISTANCE TO JOINT DEFORMATION—MID POSITION[a]

	At Extension −0.5 radian		At Flexion, 0.5 radian[b]		Peak to Peak 0.5 radian[c]	
	g·cm	% total	g·cm	% total	g·cm	% total
Skin	−58	19	−50	−38+	8	2
Muscles	−133	43	49	37	182	41
Tendons	−25	8	17	13	42	10
Capsule	−92	30	117	88	209	47
TOTAL[c]	−308	100	133	100	441	100

Note: [a]Frequency of rotation 0.1 cycle/sec.
 [b]Skin reduced the torque required to flex the joint.
 [c]Torque in the intact joint.
From Johns RJ, Wright V. Relative importance of various tissues in joint stiffness. J Appl Physiol. 1962; 17:824–828, with permission.

TABLE 13-2. CONTRIBUTION OF TISSUE RESISTANCE TO JOINT DEFORMATION—END RANGE

Tissue	Extension −48°		Flexion +48°	
	Torque Required		Torque Required	
	Gram Cm	% Total	Gram Cm	% Total
1. Skin	−70	11.2	−45	−8.7
2. Extensors	−35	42.4	0 }	36.9
3. Flexors	−230		190 }	
4. Tendon	−70	11.2	170	33.0
5. Joint Capsule	−220	35.2	200	38.8
Total	625	100	515	100

From deVries A. In: deVries HA. Physiology of Exercise for Physical Education and Athletics. 3rd ed. Dubuque, Iowa: William C. Brown Co; 1980; 462–472. Calculated from data of Johns PJ, Wright V. Relative Importance of Various Tissues in Joint Stiffness. J Appl Physiol. 1962; 17:824–828.

provide the greatest limitation to JROM vary dependent upon the joint's position in space. Limitation of JROM in the mid range has been primarily attributed to the joint capsule. Further limitation is then provided by surrounding musculature and fascial sheath and finally the tendon (Table 13–1).[16]

At the end of the available ROM, however, it appears that the primary limitation is provided by muscle and fascial sheath, followed by the capsule and then the tendon (Table 13–2).[1] This information deserves the particular attention of the sports physical therapist working with athletes who have problems concerning MF and JROM. Through appropriate assessment the therapist should be able to determine if the limitation exists in accessory motion (involving periarticular connective tissue) or physiological motion (involving MF and periarticular connective tissue).

The therapist has the ability to influence the manner in which connective tissue limits JROM and MF. In order to accomplish this task safely and effectively the therapist must first have a sound working knowledge of the composition, anatomy, and physiology of the limiting structures. Secondly the therapist must know how to affect the physical and mechanical properties of the limiting structures.

COMPOSITION OF CONNECTIVE TISSUE

All connective tissues within the body are composed of the same basic structural elements (Table 13–3).[17–19] Fibrocytes synthesize the proteoglycans and extracellular fibers that comprise the connective tissue. In hyaline cartilage this function is performed by chondrocytes.[18,19]

Collagen and elastin are the two extracellular fi-

TABLE 13-3. STRUCTURAL COMPONENTS OF CONNECTIVE TISSUE

Water
Proteoglycans
Extracellular fibers
Elastin
Collagen
Reticular fibers
Fibrocytes/chondrocytes

TABLE 13-4. COLLAGENS OF CONNECTIVE TISSUE

Tissue	Collagen Type[a]
Skin	I, III
Bone	I
Hyaline cartilage	II
Perichondrium	I, II
Basement membrane	IV
Granulation tissue	I, III
Annulus fibrosis	I, II
Nucleus polposus	II, I
Muscle	
Epimysium	I, III, IV
Perimysium	I, III, IV
Endomysium	I/III, IV, V
Tendon	
Bundles	I
Endotendinium	III, IV
Joint capsule	I, III
Fascia	I

[a]Type listed first constitutes the most abundant collagen present.

bers that warrant the consideration of the physical therapist. These fibers complement each other functionally. Collagen is a fibrous protein and provides the skeletal structure that holds the connective tissue together, enabling the tissue to resist mechanical forces and deformation.[10,20,21] Elastin assists in the recovery of a tissue from deformation.[10,18,21] Collagen is the primary building block of connective tissue, providing connective tissue with its high tensile strength and the ability to withstand load and deformation. Overall, collagen may be compared to a fibrous suspension bridge. Its load-bearing ability depends upon its structural properties. The structural properties of this fibrous suspension bridge are dependent upon the material properties of the collagen (physical and mechanical properties), the size of the collagen fibril (area and length), and the organization of the fibrils (Fig 13-3).[22] Therefore, collagen should be the prime target when attempting to improve JROM and MF in the individual with movement dysfunction.[10,11,23]

Although collagen is the common building block of the soft tissues, the types of collagen that constitute the tissue varies (Table 13-4).[20,24-26] Types I and III collagen are the most abundant forms of collagen found in connective tissue. Type I collagen tends to be a more mature form of collagen with greater tensile strength than type III collagen. These types are usually found in association with one another, their relative proportions varying with pathological condition and age.

The biosynthesis of collagen is a complicated intracellular and extracellular process (Fig 13-4).[20,27-29] Regardless of its genetic type, collagen contains certain amino acids. These amino acids form a chain of repeating tripeptides with the composition glycine-X-Y, where X is frequently proline and Y hydroxyproline. Each collagen chain also characteristically contains lysine and hydroxylysine, the ratio varying with genetic type. This single chain of amino acids is termed *protocollagen*. During the intracellular process, three chains

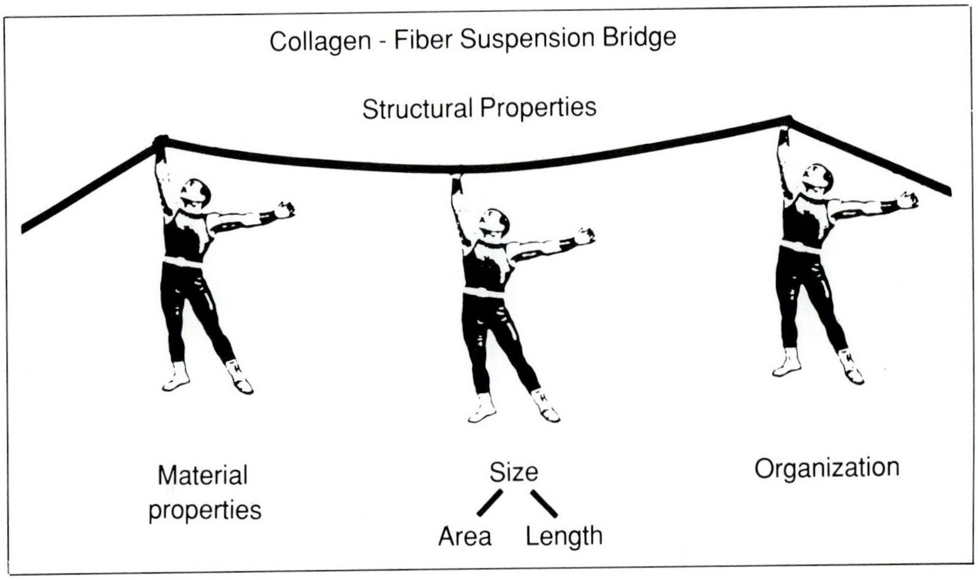

Figure 13-3. Collagen–fiber suspension bridge. Collagen act as a fibrous suspension bridge because of its structural, physical, and mechanical properties. *(From Akeson WH, Woo SLY, Amiel D, et al. The chemical basis of tissue repair: The biology of ligaments. In: Hunter LY, Funk FJ, eds. Rehabilitation of the Injured Knee. St. Louis, Mo: C V Mosby Co; 1984;93–148, with permission.)*

Collagen - Fiber Suspension Bridge

Structural Properties

Material properties   Size — Area Length   Organization

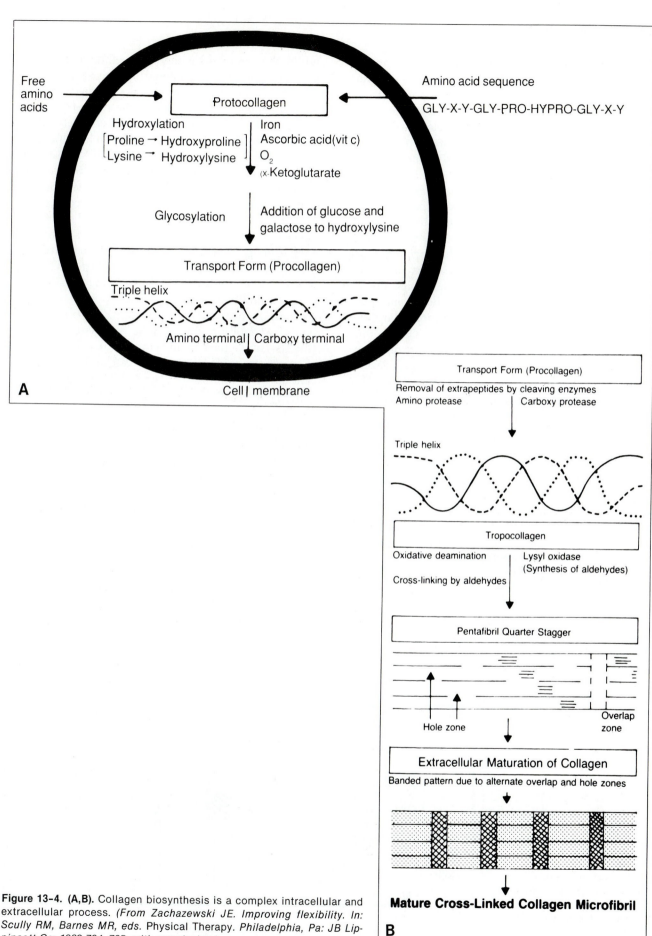

Figure 13–4. (A,B). Collagen biosynthesis is a complex intracellular and extracellular process. *(From Zachazewski JE. Improving flexibility. In: Scully RM, Barnes MR, eds.* Physical Therapy. *Philadelphia, Pa: JB Lippincott Co; 1989;704–705, with permission.)*

of protocollagen are synthesized individually and simultaneously. Specific proline and lysine residues within the protocollagen tripeptide chains are hydroxolated to form hydroxyproline and hydroxylysine. In the presence of the enzyme transferase, select hydroxylysines are then glycosylated. By these two steps the three protocollagen chains are spontaneously bound together in the form of a right-handed triple helix, stabilized by intramolecular hydrogen bonds, thus forming the molecule procollagen. This triple helix of procollagen is then transported outside the cell membrane. Once outside the cell membrane, extra peptides are removed from the ends of the procollagen, transforming it into tropocollagen. Intermolecular crosslinks are then formed between the tropocollagen molecules. Present knowledge suggests that five tropocollagen molecules come together, held together by intermolecular crosslinks, in a quarter staggered array.[20,27,28] The intermolecular crosslinks that are usually present are dihydroxylysinonorleucine (DHLNL), hydroxylysinonorleucine (HLNL), and histodonohydroxymerodesomine (HHMD).[30] The intramolecular and intermolecular crosslinks are quite strong and resistant to external load. It is the intramolecular and intermolecular crosslinks which provide collagen with its stability and tensile strength.

Tropocollagen molecules band together in a characteristic pattern to form a microfibril. Microfibrils come together to form subfibrils and subsequently the collagen fibril, which is the basic load-bearing element of connective tissue. In the relaxed state collagen has a characteristic crimp structure on the microfibrillar level (Fig 13-5).[31] The strength and integrity of the fibril is dependent upon its intramolecular and intermolecular crosslinks (Fig 13-6).[6,17,27,28,32] An analogy that might be used is the formation of a rope in which strand upon strand comes together to form the rope and give it strength.

The collagen fibrils of any tissue are embedded within the ground substance (intracellular matrix). The ground substance is composed of glycosaminoglycans (GAG) and water. Glycosaminoglycans are responsible for holding and binding water in the ground substance. The principal GAGs associated with connective tissue are chondroitin 4-sulfate, chondroitin 6-sulfate, hyaluronic acid, and dermatan sulfate.[17,19] These GAGs are macromolecules with elastic properties that are present in the ground substance of a variety of tissues. In normal tissue this ground substance is a viscous gel that probably serves to provide lubrication and spacing between the collagen fibers at intercept points where they cross. The space provided between collagen fibrils may prevent excessive crosslinks between fibrils that could serve to decrease tissue mobility and deformation.[33]

The ability of a collagen fibril to withstand stress is primarily the result of its crosslinks. The fibrils' direction of orientation must also be considered, however (Fig 13-7).[21] Collagen is able to tolerate a great amount of tensile stress but is not capable of supporting significant shear or compressive stress.[9] Therefore collagen tends to be oriented along its lines of stress.[19]

Tendon, ligament, capsule, fascia, and aponeurosis are all classified as dense regular connective tissue.[18,19] The collagen fibrils of tendon have the most parallel orientation; therefore tendon is primarily resistant to tensile stress. A less distinct parallel orientation is evident with ligament and capsule. Fascia and apponeurosis are arranged in multiple sheets or lameli. Although following a parallel and slightly wavy course within each layer, the direction of orientation of the various layers may differ.[9,10,21,34] Therefore, the fibril orientation of these tissues allows some stress tolerance in a greater number of directions, but still primarily along the collagens lines of orientation. Loose connective tissue, with its abundant, highly hydrated ground substance, is commonly found between muscles and in other sites where mobility is advantageous.[18,19]

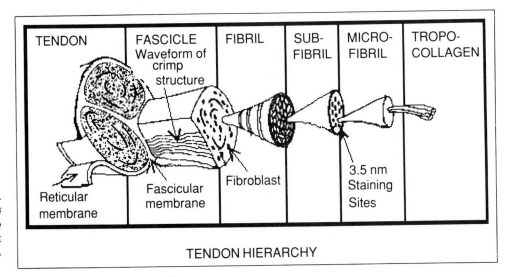

Figure 13-5. Formation of tendon. (From Kastelic J, Galeski A, Baer E. The microcomposite structure of tendon. Connect Tissue Res. 1978;4:283-348, with permission.)

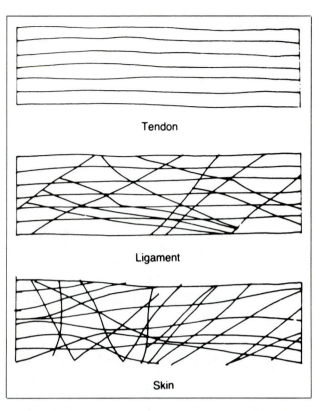

Figure 13-7. Direction of fibril orientation. *(From Nordin M, Frankel VH. Biomechanic of collagenous tissue. In: Frankel VH, Nordin M, eds.* Mechanics of the Skeletal System. *Philadelphia, Pa: Lea & Febiger; 1980;87–109, with permission.)*

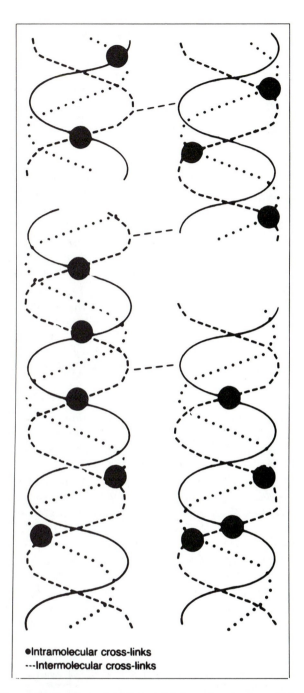

•Intramolecular cross-links
---Intermolecular cross-links

Figure 13-6. Intramolecular and intermolecular crosslinks. *(From Donatelli R, Owens-Burkhardt H. Effects of immobilization on the extensibility of periarticular connective tissue.* J Orthop Sports Phys Ther. *1981;3:67–72, with permission.)*

HOMEOSTASIS

Normal JROM and MF are required for optimal function to be maintained. Connective tissue is a metabolically active substance that is undergoing constant change. The deformation of connective tissue, facilitated by motion, is necessary for homeostasis.[35,36] The response of the tissue may be broken down into three components—cellular modeling, ground substance, and collagen response. These three components comprise the total tissue response (Fig 13–8).[37]

Cellular Modeling

The stresses and forces imposed upon the tissues by motion throughout the range cause the fibroblasts to modulate collagen and GAG synthesis[35,36] while enzymatic degradation removes collagen and GAG, which are no longer needed.[38–40] The rate of turnover or change for GAG is much faster than for collagen.

Ground Substance/Collagen Response

The GAG (synthesized by the fibroblasts) binds with water, forming the ground substance that in turn serves to lubricate the collagen fibrils and minimize excessive crosslinking by maintaining fibril distance. Motion prevents the development of anomilous crosslinks.[35] Stress and motion influence the deposition of newly formed collagen by orienting it along lines of tensile stress.[19,35,36]

Tissue Response

Joint range of motion and muscle flexibility are maintained for the range through which the body part normally moves. The connective tissue maintains its integrity and strength, enabling it to appropriately resist the stresses imposed upon it.

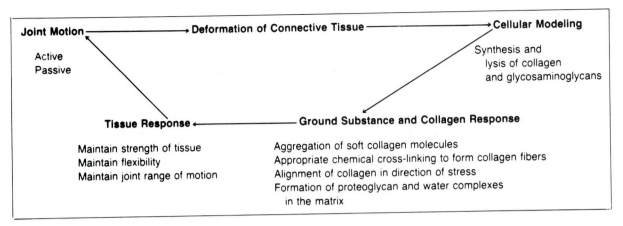

Figure 13–8. Periarticular connective tissue homeostasis. *(From Burkardt S. Tissue Healing and Repair. National Athletic Trainers Association Professional Preparation Conference, Nashville, Tenn; 1979, with permission.)*

MECHANICAL AND PHYSICAL PROPERTIES OF COLLAGEN

Collagen exhibits various mechanical and physical properties when undergoing deformation. These properties allow it to respond to load and deformation appropriately, giving the tissue the ability to withstand high tensile stress. The three mechanical properties exhibited by collagen are elasticity, viscoelasticity, and plasticity.[10] The physical properties exhibited are force relaxation, creep, and hysteresis.[9]

Mechanical Properties

Elasticity is a springlike behavior where elongation, which is produced by tensile load, is recovered after the load is removed. This property may be best symbolized by a spring (Fig 13–9A).

Viscoelasticity is a property that allows slow deformation with an imperfect recovery once the deforming force has been removed. The recovery is the result of

the elasticity and the imperfection is the result of the viscosity. This change is not a permanent one. The property of viscoelasticity may be best symbolized by a spring and dash pot in parallel, with the spring representing the elastic response and the dash pot the viscous response (Fig 13–9B).

The final mechanical property is plasticity, by which residual or permanent change due to deformation is maintained. Plastic change, which is difficult to achieve, may be best symbolized by the Coulomb element of dry friction (Fig 13–9C). It is the viscous property of tissues that permits permanent plastic deformation.[10] (Viscosity may be defined as the resistance offered by fluid to change of form or relative position of its particles due to attraction of molecules to one another.)

These mechanical properties do not occur separately in the tissues. All three properties are affected when the tissue is deformed and are best symbolized by Fig 13–9D.

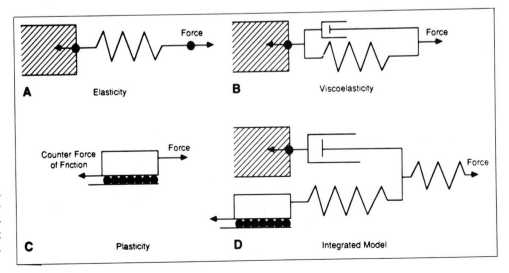

Figure 13–9. Mechanical properties of collagen. *(From Viidik A. Functional properties of collagenous tissue. Rev Connect Tissue Res. 1973;6:127–215, with permission.)*

Physical Properties

Butler and associates have extensively reviewed the physical properties of collagen.[9] The physical properties exhibited by connective tissue are force relaxation, creep, and hysteresis. The three physical properties are time dependent.

Force relaxation is defined as the decrease in the amount of force required to maintain a tissue at a set amount of displacement or deformation over time (Fig 13–10). The rate at which the force is applied will affect the resulting relaxation of the tissue. Generally speaking the more rapid the rate of deformation, the larger the peak force, and the greater the tissues' subsequent relaxation. Therefore less force is required to maintain the tissue at a set displacement. One potential problem exists in attempting to influence the force relaxation response. Time is required to facilitate viscoelastic and plastic deformation. The greater the velocity of deformation, the shorter the amount of time available for change, and the greater the chance of exceeding that tissue's ability to undergo viscoelastic and plastic change. If the capacity for viscoelastic and plastic change are exceeded, injury may occur.

In contrast to force relaxation, the creep response of the tissue is the ability of the tissue to deform over time while a constant force is being imposed upon it (Fig 13–10). This constant force causes the tissue to lengthen over time. Use of the creep response allows viscoelastic and plastic change to occur in the tissue.

The hysteresis response is the amount of relaxation a tissue has undergone during any single cycle of deformation and relaxation (Fig 13–10). It is an indication of the viscous property of the tissue.

Load-Deformation (Stress–Strain) Curve

The physical and mechanical properties of any tissue have a direct impact on the tissue's ability to tolerate load and to deform without a loss of integrity. The curve developed is termed the load-deformation curve (Fig 13–11).[9] To assist the reader in understanding the relationship of the physical and mechanical properties of collagen, the properties that are affected in each portion of the curve have been added to the normal load-deformation curve of collagen.[9]

In zone I, or the "toe" region of the curve, the crimp structure or wavy pattern normally found in collagen fibrils changes to a more parallel arrangement. Little force is required to do this; it involves an elastic type of response. The further the elongation in this region the greater the stiffness and the force required to attain or maintain this elongation. This region accounts for 1.5% to 4% of the total collagen elongation possible. Unloading the collagen within this region restores the crimp structure and resting length.[9] The mechanical property of elasticity is affected in this portion of the curve.

In zone II, or the linear region, collagen has lost its crimp structure and is now parallel in its orientation. The load required to produce further deformation increases in a linear manner. (In resting muscle that is stretched passively, the greater the muscle length becomes, the greater the force required to hold that stretch.) All mechanical and physical properties of collagen are affected within this zone. The specific velocity at which force was applied, or the length of time that the force was applied, may determine which specific property is affected. Although all of these proper-

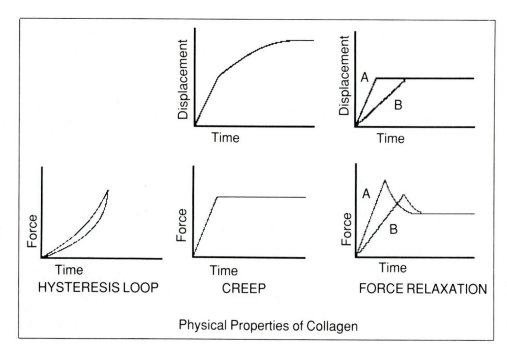

Physical Properties of Collagen

HYSTERESIS LOOP   CREEP   FORCE RELAXATION

Figure 13-10. Physical properties of collagen. *(From Butler DL, Grood ES, Noyes FR. Exercise and sports sciences review. Bio Lig Tend. 1979;6:126–282.)*

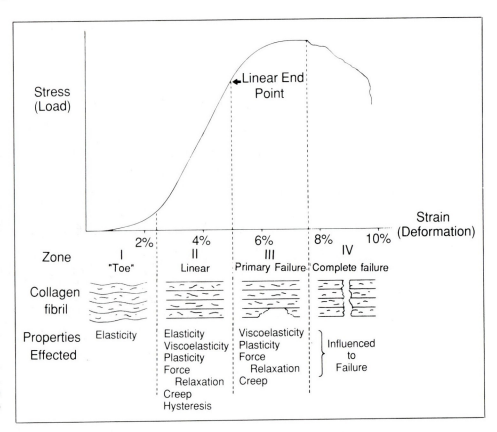

Figure 13-11. Load-deformation curve. *(From Butler DL, Grood ES, Noyes FR. Exercise and sports sciences review.* Bio Lig Tend. *1979;6:126–282.)*

ties are time dependent, force relaxation is also influenced by the velocity of the deformation. A group of collagen fibrils that are being tested will tolerate a deformation of 2% to 5%. The end of the linear zone is characterized by the linear end point that is the starting point for zone III.

Zone III is the region of primary failure. Once the linear end point has been reached, isolated collagen fibrils begin to fail. Failure occurs in an unpredictable manner. In this region if the load has been applied too quickly, not allowing for viscoelastic and plastic change, the force relaxation response is affected in such a manner that the collagen fibril fails. Excessive viscoelastic and plastic change may cause collagen failure by allowing too much deformation via the creep response. Once the maximum tolerable load is reached, complete failure occurs. This occurs when the collagen fibril has been deformed by 6% to 10% of its total resting length. In the most recent investigation the maximum strain at failure of collagen fiber bundles in human patellar tendon, lateral collateral ligament, anterior cruciate ligament, and posterior cruciate ligament have been demonstrated to range from 13% to 15%. This is thought to be a result of organization of the fiber bundles within the whole structure and the support that they provide for one another.[41]

MUSCLE

The joint capsule, ligament, fascia, and aponeurosis are all composed of collagen and may be considered passive restraints to the limitation of JROM. Tendon, as distinct from muscle, may also be considered to be a passive restraint. Only muscle has active components that may limit JROM and MF. These components are the contractile elements, actin and myosin. When discussing muscle flexibility one must consider both the connective tissue component and the neuromuscular component. Therefore the question arises, to what extent does each of these structures limit muscle flexibility?

Anatomically, muscle is a complex arrangement of contractile and noncontractile protein filaments. This arrangement complicates the task of describing muscles' ability to deform and recover from deformation.[42,43]

Muscle has a large quantity of connective tissue associated with it (Fig 13–12). The connective tissue associated with skeletal muscle can be divided into three levels of organization: (1) the endomysium, which represents the association of connective tissue with the individual muscle cells and interconnects to the perimysium; (2) the perimysium, which consists of collagenous septa that surrounds the fasicles and intercon-

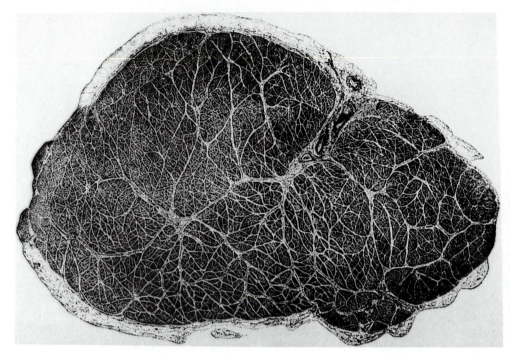

Figure 13-12. Connective tissue of muscle. Cross section through human sartorius muscle, showing the connective tissue of the epimysium surrounding the entire muscle, and the perimysium enclosing muscle fiber bundles of varying size. *(From Fawcett DW. Textbook of Histology. 11th ed. Philadephia, Pa: W B Saunders Co; 1986;136–173, with permission.)*

nects to the epimysium; and (3) the epimysium, the layer of connective tissue that surrounds the entire muscle fiber.

The endomysium, a delicate connective tissue sheath that invests and separates each individual muscle fiber, possesses three components: (1) myocyte–myocyte connectives; (2) myocyte–capillary connectives; and (3) a weave network associated with the basal laminae of the myocytes.[43] The endomysium, found external to the basal lamina and the sarcolemma, is formed primarily of two different sized filaments, neither of which penetrates into the basal lamina or sarcolemma. (Fig 13–13).[44] The thicker of the filaments (50 μm in diameter) is composed of typical collagen fibers that are arranged predominantly in a longitudinal direction. This orientation may reflect the endomysium's role in providing mechanical support for the fibers' surface and acting as an elastic device for contraction–relaxation cycles. The thinner filaments (20 μm in diameter) intermingle with the thicker filaments and represent immature forms of collagen.[44] Figures 13–13A through 13–13D show the collagenous fibrils that comprise the endomysium. These fibers run not only in a parallel direction, but in a variety of directions over and between muscle fibers. The course and distance between the fibrils varies dependent upon the degree of stretch or contraction of the muscle. When the muscle is contracted the fibrils are close together and at right angles to one another, and when the muscle is stretched they are parallel to the muscle fibers. This arrangement

of the connective tissue permits easy displacement of the muscle fibrils and offers increasing resistance to deformation at extreme lengthened ranges.[44,45] The endomysium, arranged as a weave network intimately associated with the basal lamina, could be an important factor in the passive series elastic component of muscle.

Each group of 10 to 20 muscle fibrils, which collectively form a fasicle, is surrounded by a thicker coating of connective tissue called the perimysium. The perimysium may be oriented in either a parallel or circumferential direction to the fasicle. The perimysium is composed of varying amounts of collagenous, elastic, and reticular fibers and fat cells.[45] The collagen of the perimysium consists of tightly woven bundles of fibers, 600 to 1800 μm in diameter, that interconnect with the fasicles. During passive stretch the amount and arrangement of the connective tissue in the perimysium may be more important than the endomysium. The work of Nagel, as summarized by Borg and Caulfield stated that the perimysium, which is arranged in a spiral fashion during relaxation of the muscle, was wavy during muscle contraction, indicating little tension.[43] This report allowed Borg and Caulfield to conclude that the perimysium could be a major component of the parallel elastic component of muscle, being important in maintaining proper position of the muscle bundles and distributing the stress associated with passive stretch. The fasicles of individual muscle are then grouped together and surrounded by the epimysium.

The amount of elastin and collagen in a muscle's

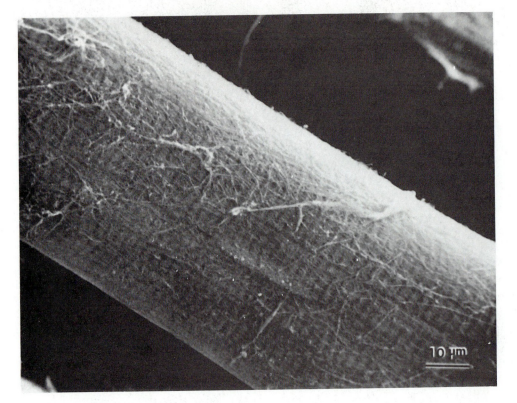

A

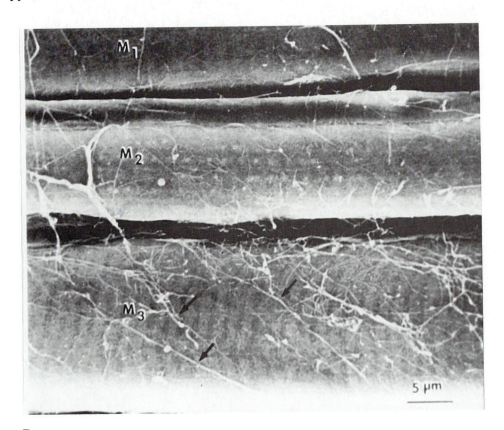

B

Figure 13-13. A. Fibrous endomysium. Frog sartorius muscle fiber. Fiber surface is covered by a fibrous layer, through which cross striation are visible. **B.** Skeletal muscle fibers (M1, M2, M3) appear as cylindrical units aligned in parallel bundles. Faint cross striations are visible along individual fibers. Coarse collagenous fibers of the endomysium run in various directions over and between muscle fibers (*arrows*). Teased preparation of frog sartorius muscle fixed with tannic acid—OsO₄ (*continues*)

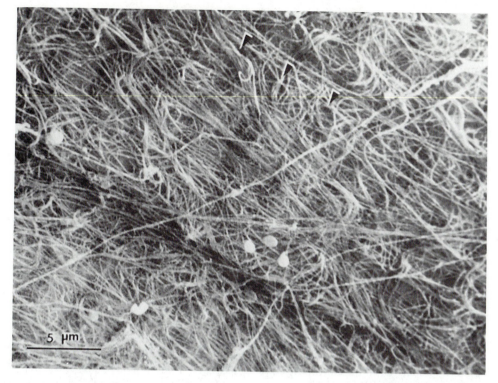

C

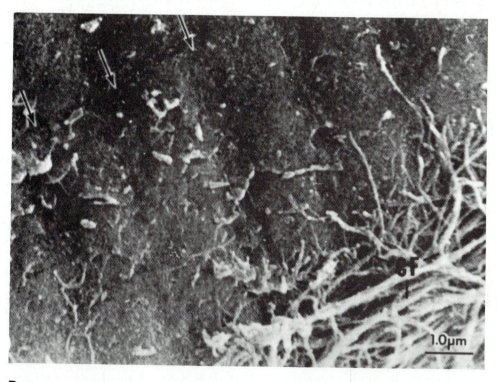

D

Figure 13-13. C. Fibrous connective tissue of muscle. Fibrous layer on surface of frog sartorius muscle fiber. Collagenous fibrils densely cover muscle fiber and take a predominantly longitudinal course. Cross striations can be seen through fibrous layer (*arrowheads*). **D.** Fibrous connective tissue of muscle. Outer aspect of basal lamina of frog sartorius muscle fiber by use of low-power SEM. Basal lamina is exposed where fibrous layer (CF) is stripped off. Cross striations (*arrows*) can be seen more clearly through the lamina than through the fibrous layer. (*From Ishikawa H, Sawada H, Yamada E. Surface and internal morphology of skeletal muscle. In: Peachey LD, Adrian RH, Geiger SR, eds.* Skeletal Muscle. Baltimore,Md: *American Physiological Society; 1983; 1-22, with permission.*)

connective tissue appears to vary with the function of the muscle. Continuously active muscles, such as the muscles of the eye or diaphragm, have a high percentage of elastic fibrils in the endomysium. In the extremities the elastic fibrils are more exclusively limited to the septa between fasiculi in the perimysium.

Muscle fibers can exist in three states: relaxed, activated, and rigor.[46] Each of these three states is characterized by tension and stiffness (the change in force or tension produced by a change in length). In a relaxed state muscle does not generate active force and therefore does not possess a high degree of stiffness. The amount of passive tension that muscle does demonstrate is more or less constant in a relaxed state. The level of this passive tension varies in direct proportional to the muscle's length. It is not known, however, to what the passive resting tension is attributed.

Six anatomic elements are possible contributors to muscle stiffness (or resistance to elongation):[47] (1) adhesion of one fibril to another or between muscle and overlying subcutaneous tissue; (2) the epimysium; (3) the perimysium and endomysium; (4) the sarcolemma; (5) contractile elements within the muscle fiber; and (6) the associated tendons and their insertion.

Opinion varies as to the exact contribution of each of these elements to passive tension. A large portion of the passive resting tension of the muscle is due to the connective tissue that lies in parallel with the muscle fibers, although some tension may be attributable to a small proportion of crossbridges between actin and myosin filaments. These crossbridges have been demonstrated to resist deformation in skinned muscle fiber (muscle fibers in which all connective tissue and innervation has been removed). The amount of stiffness or resistance to deformation provided by the crossbridges increases as the velocity of the deforming force increased.[48,49] According to Hill, these crossbridges are very stable and may have a "long life."[50]

In summary it appears that both the contractile and noncontractile elements of muscle resist deformation when we attempt to lengthen muscle. The percentage that each contributes to the muscle stiffness is unknown. The contribution supplied by the contractile elements to muscle while in the resting state appears to be related to the velocity of deformation. The farther a muscle is stretched the greater the contribution of the noncontractile element to the resistance to deformation. Although the therapist may not be able to chance the resistance of muscle to deformation (which is provided by crossbridge attachment in the contractile element) the therapist does have the ability to modify and change the resistance provided by the passive connective elements. Before the therapist can affect the structures limiting JROM and MF, however, he or she must have a sound working knowledge of the physiology of each.

The basic neurophysiology of muscle stretching has been well summarized by Stanish et al.[51] The two characteristic structures of muscle important in the neurophysiology of stretching are the intrafusal and extrafusal fibers. The primary contractile fibers of any muscle are the extrafusal fibers, innervated by alpha motoneurons. Signaling length change and the rate of change in length the intrafusal fibers may be considered the sensory elements of muscle deformation. A part of the muscle spindle, the intrafusal fibers are innervated by gamma motoneurons. Afferent impulses are perceived and transmitted by the type Ia and II sensory nerves. The perception of these afferent signals may activate alpha motoneurons supplying the extrafusal fibers. Contraction of extrafusal fibers relieves the stretch or deformation of the spindle, decreasing the afferent discharge.

The Ia and II afferent impulse rate is a function of muscle length, movement, and efferent fusimotor activity, all of which may be modified by higher CNS commands or spinal activity. Fusimotor activity via gamma efferents, which innervate the spindle, assist in resetting the spindle during muscle contraction so that it may continue to respond to length and velocity changes during muscle shortening.

Located near the muscle tendon junction the Golgi tendon organs (GTOs) or type Ib afferent fibers are sensitive to force production via muscle contraction, Golgi tendon organs activity inhibits alpha motoneuron activity to the active muscle (agonist) while facilitating activity to the antagonistic muscle.

Reflex activity may be modified by muscle activity in a number of ways. Myosynaptic reflex activity is inhibited by strong agonist contraction by recurrent inhibition of alpha motoneurons. This in turn, after relaxation, decreases the response of the agonist to subsequent stretching. There are reports in the literature however that strong agonist contraction may actually facilitate subsequent muscle contraction and actually increase the stretch reflex response. Reflex inhibition of the agonist occurs via contraction of the antagonistic muscle group.

PATHOPHYSIOLOGY

Area of Injury

When a muscle strain occurs it is because the tension generated exceeds the tensile capability of the weakest structural element.[52] The weakest portion of the muscle tendon unit and the area most often injured is the muscle tendon junction (Fig 13–14).[53,54]

PROCESS OF INJURY AND REPAIR

The process of injury and repair for muscle is similar to that of other collagenous tissues.[55,56] Initially hemor-

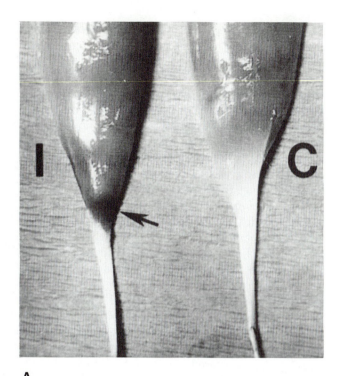

A

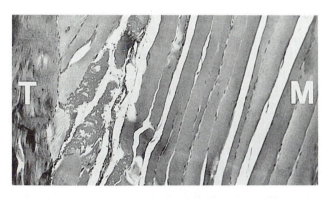

B

Figure 13–14. Location of injury during muscle strain. **A.** Gross appearance of tibialis anterior of rabbit following controlled strain injury. A small hemorrhage (*arrow*) is visible at the distal tip of injured muscle at 24 hours. I, injured; C, control. **B.** Histological appearance of tibialis anterior immediately following strain injury showing limited rupture of the most distal fibers near the musculotendinous junction along with hemorrhage. T, tendon; M, intacat muscle fibers. Massons stain (100x). *(From Nikolaou PK, MacDonald BL, Bilsson RR, et al. Biomechanical and histological evaluation of muscle after controlled strain. Am J Sports Med. 1987; 15:9–14, with permission.)*

rhage and edema occur. Soon after injury degenerative changes are noted within the muscle. Phagocytosis is then initiated to clear debris from the area. At approximately the same time satellite cells become activated. These cells are transformed into myoblastic cells, which will become myotubes and subsequently new muscle fibers. Scarring and fibrosis are evident a few days after injury as repair progresses. The connective tissue structures are disrupted and the resulting space is filled with proliferating cells and extracellular matrix. This healing process sets up two competing events, the regeneration of muscle and the production of connective tissue scar.[57,58] These events are summarized in Table 13–5.[53,55,59,60]

After healing has been initiated the scar and tissue formed does not have the same tensile strength as the original. Normal intramuscular collagenous tissue has a greater amount of type I collagen than type III collagen.[57] After injury the rapid increase in granulation tissue is primarily a result of increased levels of type III collagen. It is thought that type III collagen may establish the basic latticework for repair and that the proportion of type III to type I collagen is increased during the active phase of repair in order to accommodate the change required during the healing process. As the tis-

TABLE 13-5. SEQUENCE OF MUSCLE REGENERATION AFTER INJURY

	Muscle Regeneration				
Event/Time	15 Min.	3 Hr.	8 Hr.	16–24 Hr.	3–6 Days
Hemorrhage	+	+	+	+	
Pyknosis		+	+		
Sarcolemma breakup		+	+		
Mitochondria disruption		+	+		
Sarcoplasmic reticulum disruption		+	+		
Interrupted sarcolemma		+	+		
Phagocytosis				+	+
Satellite cell activation				+	+
Myotubes evident					+

Adapted from Carlson BM, Faulkner JA. The regeneration of skeletal muscle fibers following injury: A review. Med Sci Sports Ex. 1983; 15: 187–198. Snow M. Myogenic cell formation in regenerating rat skeletal muscle injured by mincing. Anat Rec. 1977; 188:181–200.

sue stabilizes, matures, and gains strength, the proportion of type I collagen to type III returns to normal. The type of crosslinks present appear to parallel these changes.[57]

Influential Factors in Repair

Age. As age increases the capacity for repair decreases, resembling that seen in immobilized muscle. The work of Jarvinen is summarized in Table 13–6.[61]

Immobilization. Jarvinen[61] and Lehto et al[58] studied the effect of mobilization and immobilization on muscle repair in animals. Jarvinen demonstrated that immobilization after injury results in a significant loss of breaking strength, elongation, and energy absorbed to failure. Early mobilization, on either day 1 or after 2 days of immobilization, appeared to be followed by a rapid elevation of tensile properties to the level of the uninjured control muscles (Fig 13–15). If the mobilization is overly vigorous or occurs too early in the healing sequence, rerupture may occur. Fibrosis must begin to occur if healing is to take place, and immature collagen is less tolerant of stress than mature collagen.

RESPONSE TO AGE, IMMOBILIZATION, AND REMOBILIZATION

With an understanding of the neurophysiology of stretching and the normal physiology of collagen and

its response to stress, it is appropriate to present changes that may take place with aging, immobilization, and remobilization.

Aging

Aging is a normal and continual process of the human body. The principal concern regarding mobility with respect to the connective tissue structures is aging of collagen and elastin because these comprise the tendon, capsule, muscle, fascia, and aponeurosis. These elements influence the response of the tissue to stress, the amount of deformation possible, the ability of the tissue to return to its original length after deformation, and the method of transfer of force within the tissue.

During the aging process there is an increase in the total collagen content of tendon,[62] capsule,[63] and muscle,[64] along with collagen fibril diameter,[62] increasing the stability of the collagen fibril.[62,65,66] The increased stability of the fibril is also a result of the maturation and development of stable and more complex intermolecular crosslinks between the tropocollagen molecules.[65-67] The increased maturation of these crosslinks also increases the thermal stability of the collagen.[65,66,68] Elastin also shows an increase in the number of crosslinks present,[67] but a decrease in the total number of elastin fibers.[62]

Changes are also evident in the ground substance. With age the components of the ground substance decrease. These decreases have been shown in tendon[62] and in muscle.[64] The loss of these components reduces the gel–fiber ratio. A high gel–fiber relationship assists in keeping the collagen fibrils separated. A low gel–fiber ratio may allow some binding between the collagen and GAG molecules that envelop the fiber. This may explain in part the increase in stiffness with age (Table 13–7).[62,67]

The physical properties of the crimp structure of the collagen fibril also change with development and age. With increasing age the wavelength of the crimp increases whereas the wave-crimping angle decreases.[69] Changes such as these allow the collagen fibril to reach the linear zone of the load-deformation curve sooner, resulting in a steeper curve. Clinically this translates into the tissue reaching its available limits of deformation sooner.

During the aging process the stiffness of a tissue, its resistance to deformation, may result in a loss of

TABLE 13–6. EFFECT OF AGE ON MUSCLE REGENERATION AND REPAIR[a][b]

	Young (Under 2)	Old (Over 2)
Day 2		
Hematoma	+ +	+
Inflam cells	+ +	+
Myotubes	0	0
New capill.	0	0
Day 5		
Hematoma	Decreased	Decreased
Inflam. cells	Decreased	Decreased
Day 10		
Hematoma	0	0
Inflam. cells	0	0
Necrotic tissue	+	+ +
Fibroblasts	+ +	+
Myoblasts/tubes	+ +	+
Collagen fibrils	+ +	+
Capill. sprout.	+ +	+
Day 21		
Myotube matur.	+ +	+
Collagen scar	+	+ +
Area of neo-vasc.	+	+ +

[a]Decreased repair capacity resembles immob.
[b]Response to injury decreases with age.
Adapted from Jarvinen M, Aho AJ, Lehto M, et al. Age dependent repair of muscle rupture: A histological and morphological study in rates. Acta Ortho Scand. *1983; 54:64–67.*

TABLE 13–7. AGE RELATED CHANGES IN CONNECTIVE TISSUE

Increased	Decreased
Total Collagen Content	
Collagen Fibril Diameter	Water
Collagen Crosslink Maturation	Elastin
Collagen Crosslink Stability	Glycosaminoglycans
Number of Elastic Crosslinks	

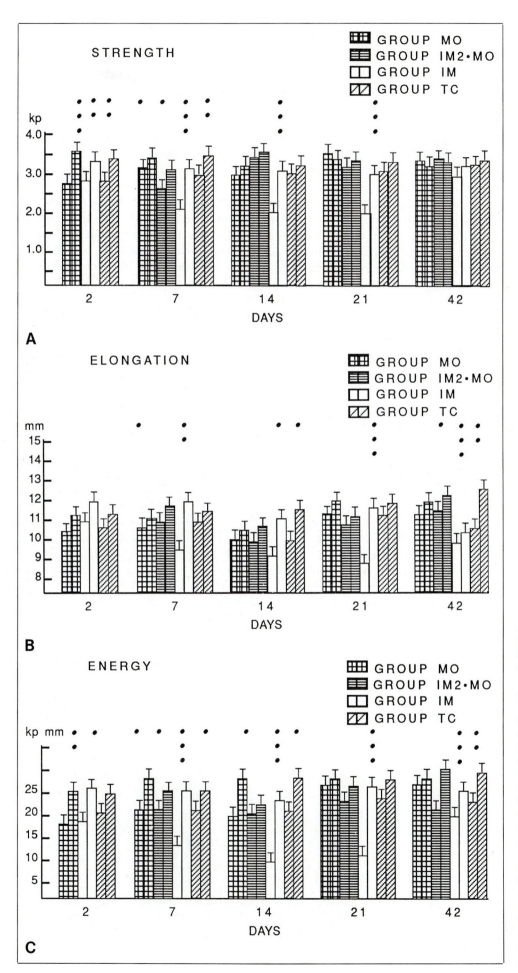

Figure 13-15. Effect of immobilization on strength of muscle repair. **A.** Breaking strength, Fmax of the left (L) and right (R) gastrocnemius muscles in relation to the healing time (days). The means with their standard errors (vertical range bars) are given ($N=8$–10). The significance of differences between left and right muscles are indicated with asterisks (***$P<0/0001$, *$P<0.05$). **B.** The elongation of gastrocnemius muscles at the breaking strength point in relation to healing time. **C.** The energy required to reach breaking strength of gastrocnemius muscle in relation to healing time. *(From Jarvinen M. Healing of a crush injury in rat striated muscle.* Acta Chir Scand. *1976; 142:47–56, with permission.)*

JROM (via capsular contracture) or a change in the static or dynamic flexibility of muscle, resulting in movement dysfunction.

Aging and JROM. With aging, there is a tendency to lose JROM and MF.[2,70-76] The JROM changes occur not only with respect to age but also with respect to the specific joint. A comparison of the average male JROM values reported by Walker and associates (ages 60 to 85 years)[76] with those reported by Boone and associates (ages 0 to 19 and 20 to 56 years)[77] reveals that JROM decreases as age increases (Table 13–8). The results of these studies are also in general agreement with studies conducted by Smith and Walder[75] and Tucker.[74] No studies presently in the literature make a similar comparison on women.

Aging and MF. Studies on MF use composite scores of an individual's ability to move through an ROM in which a two-joint muscle, such as the hamstring or gastrocnemius, are put on stretch. One of the largest stud-ies ($N = 5115$) of normal MF according to age was done by Kendall and Kendall.[72] Muscle flexibility was measured by the ability to toe touch in the long sitting position. As age increased there was a large decline in the number of subjects, both male and female, who were able to touch their toes up until the age of 12. After age 12 the ability to toe touch in the long sitting position again increased (Fig 13–16).

Hunter and associates tested the MF of the hamstrings and gastrocnemius on 2774 subjects aged 12 to 18.[71] Measurements made with a standard goniometer revealed a large decrease in hamstring and gastrocnemius MF for males between the ages of 12 and 13. Flexibility scores increased and were consistent thereafter. No trend is visible from the data presented on the women.

It appears that both men and women gradually lose MF upon reaching adulthood.[2] Though MF decreases with age it has been demonstrated that it may be regained through the use of a specific exercise program.[78]

TABLE 13-8. COMPARISON OF ESTIMATED RANGE OF MOTION AS MALES AGE

Degrees of Motion	0–19 yr N = 53		20–54 yr N = 56		60–85 yr N = 30	
	Mean	SD	Mean	SD	Mean	SD
Shoulder						
Abduction	185.4	3.6	182.7	9.0	155	22
Flexion	168.4	3.7	165.0	5.0	160	11
Extension	67.5	8.0	57.3	8.1	38	11
Medial Rotation	70.5	4.5	67.1	4.1	59	16
Lateral Rotation	108.0	7.2	99.6	7.6	76	13
Elbow						
Beginning Flexion	.8	3.5	.3	2.7	6	5
Flexion	145.4	5.3	140.5	4.9	139	14
Forearm						
Pronation	76.7	4.8	75.0	5.3	68	9
Supination	83.1	3.4	81.1	4.0	83	11
Wrist						
Flexion	78.2	5.5	74.8	6.6	62	12
Extension	75.8	6.1	74.0	6.6	61	6
Radial Deviation	21.7	4.0	21.1	4.0	20	6
Ulnar Deviation	36.7	3.7	35.3	3.8	28	7
Hip						
Beginning Flexion	3.5	4.3	.7	2.1	11	3
Flexion	123.4	5.6	121.3	6.4	110	11
Abduction	51.7	8.8	40.5	6.0	23	9
Adduction	28.3	4.1	25.6	3.6	18	4
Medial Rotation	50.3	6.1	44.4	4.3	22	6
Lateral Rotation	50.5	6.1	44.2	4.8	32	6
Knee						
Beginning Flexion	2.1	3.2	1.1	2.0	2	2
Flexion	143.8	5.1	141.2	5.3	131	4
Ankle						
Plantar Flexion	58.2	6.1	54.3	5.9	29	7
Dorsi-flexion	13.0	4.7	12.2	4.1	9	5

Adapted from Boone DC, Azen SP. Normal range of motion of joints in male subjects. J Bone Joint Surg. 1979; 61A 756–759. Walker JM, Sue D, Miles-Elrousey N. et al. Active mobility of the extremities in older subjects. Phys Ther. 1984; 64:919–923.

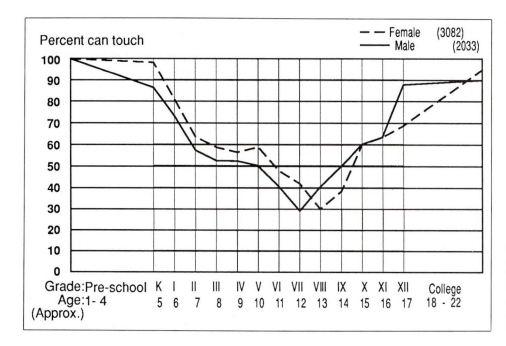

Figure 13-16. Ability of normal subjects (age 1–22 years) to toe touch. *(From Kendall HO, Kendall FP. Normal flexibility according to age groups. J Bone Joint Surg. 1948;30A:690–694, with permission.)*

Whenever JROM and MF are discussed in relation to age, the activity pattern of the subjects involved in the study must be investigated. Only two studies have examined the relationship of physical activity and JROM. Neither study demonstrated any consistent relationship between the two.[75,76] Both of these studies may have had a biased subject sample, however, as a number of the subjects were recruited from recreation centers and geriatric community centers. Samples such as this may not be representative of the typical individual who suffers from hypokinesis and movement dysfunction.

Questions can be raised regarding whether certain changes, seen in the composition and physiology of connective tissue associated with aging may be secondary to decreased physical stress. According to Viidik "Connective tissues have a capacity to react to physical exercise by a retardation of the normal temporal changes. Moderate life-long training keeps the connective tissues "younger"; the retardation is achieved in the time period before maturity and in the years thereafter. The age changes seem to occur with the same speed in training as in sedentary individuals, all the time at a parallel but "younger" level."[65]

In summary age-related changes in the connective tissue result in a tendency to decrease the ROM. There is a loss of the normal gel–fiber ratio, which may result in an increased binding between collagen fibrils. The crosslinks present become more stable, causing a steeper load deformation curve and a tissue that is more resistant to deformation. It is the physical therapist who as the primary clinician involved with movement dysfunction is able to assist an aging population to maintain optimal health, well-being, JROM, and MF.

IMMOBILIZATION

Immobilization causes many changes on the tissue level. These may be seen in both the joint and the muscle and are a result of a lack of deformation of the connective tissue. Contracture of both muscles and the capsule may be responsible for restriction of motion.[79] Changes in JROM may also be a result of proliferation of fibro fatty tissue within the joint space.[79–81] Numerous investigations examined the effect of rigid immobilization on the periarticular connective tissue (tendon, capsule, fascia, and associated capsular ligaments).[35,36,80,82–89] These changes may be divided into those that occur on a cellular level, the response within the ground substance and collagen, and the response on a tissue level. These changes are summarized in Fig 13–17.[37] Clinically it appears that the changes seen do not need rigid immobilization from internal or external fixation but will also take place if the joint does not move through a full normal ROM, stretching periarticular connective tissue and muscle to its fullest extent.

Cellular Modeling

The total collagen content measured from immobilized periarticular connective tissue shows no significant change after 9 weeks.[80,82,83–86] These results would lead one to believe that no change occurs in the rate of synthesis of new collagen. A recent investigation demonstrated, however, an increase in collagen turnover with immobilization caused by both increased synthesis and degradation.[84] These changes were demonstrated in the medial collateral ligament and patellar tendon of rabbits. It is not known at this time if other components of the periarticular connective tissue react differently.

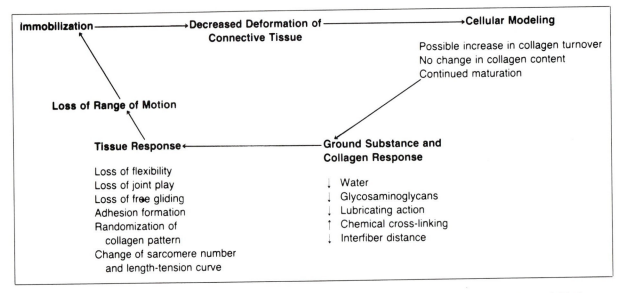

Figure 13-17. Changes from immobilization. *(From Burkhardt S. Tissue Healing and Repair. National Athletic Trainers Association Professional Preparation Conference; Nashville, Tenn; 1979, with permission.)*

It is important to emphasize that a difference exists because ligament and periarticular connective tissue react differently to immobilization. With immobilization, ligament loses stiffness whereas periarticular connective tissue gains stiffness.[17] The loss of ligamentous stiffness produces a weaker ligament, which is less able to tolerate stress imposed upon it.

The failure to demonstrate a significant increase in collagen indicates that mechanisms more subtle than fibroplasia and scar formation are involved in the contracture process.[35] No alteration occurs in the type of collagen produced during immobilization if no inflammatory process is present. With an active inflammatory response type III collagen is also produced.[57,87]

Ground Substance and Collagen Response

The response within the matrix or ground substance to immobilization is profound. A significant decrease is found in the water and GAG. The loss of GAG and water from the ground substance causes a change in the gel–fiber ratio and a decrease in the tissue's viscosity.[80,83–85] This change allows a decrease in the lubrication action and the interfiber distance. The loss of GAG is significantly correlated to joint stiffness. The loss of this GAG buffer between collagen fibrils facilitates the synthesis of increased crosslinks at strategic points between adjacent collagen fibrils (Fig 13–18).[33,36,80,83,85] As time passes, the crosslinks become more stable and mature. These mature crosslinks and collagen provide the tissue with strength and resistance to tensile deformation.[35] It is important, however, that motion take place to maintain the GAG buffer between collagen fibrils, as otherwise hypomobility and dysfunction will occur. The biochemical change in the gel–fiber ratio and the

increased crosslinks between fibrils affect the biomechanics of the tissue.

Resistance to joint motion after immobilization has been demonstrated to be due to muscle and skin as well as capsular restriction. A significant percentage of the restriction has been demonstrated to be from muscle and skin.[35,79] As both Johns and Wright[16] and deVries[1] have stated, skin provides little resistance to deformation when compared to muscle.

The biochemical and biomechanical changes described generally result in a *qualitative* rather than a *quantitative* change of the collagen structure within the connective tissue. The qualitative change in the collagen is attributable to a quantitative and qualitative change in the number and maturity of crosslinks.

Tissue Response

As time passes, formation and accumulation of new collagen, regardless of how small, is important.[83] Without motion the fibril may be laid down haphazardly, interfering with proper joint mechanics and tissue deformation.[35,36,80] This haphazard arrangement allows the formation of adhesions within the connective tissue.

One of the most profound changes that can occur on the tissue level is the change in muscle length. The changes that may occur with muscle shortening or lengthening have been researched by numerous authors. Gossman and associates provide a review of this literature and a discussion of how these length-associated changes may be prevented and corrected.[90] The majority of the following information regarding anatomic changes of muscles immobilized in lengthened and shortened positions has been summarized from Gossman and associates.[90]

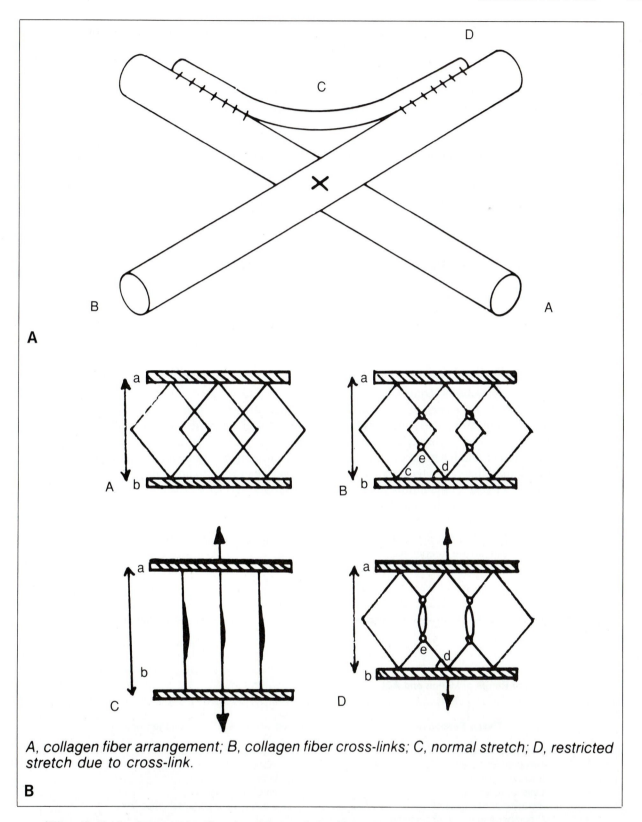

A, collagen fiber arrangement; B, collagen fiber cross-links; C, normal stretch; D, restricted stretch due to cross-link.

Figure 13–18. A. Intercept bending. A and B, preexisting fibers; C. newly synthesized fibril; D, crosslink as the fibril joins the fiber; X, nodal point where the fibers normally slide past one another freely. *(From Akeson WH, Amiel D, Woo SLY. Immobility effects of synovial joints: The pathomechanics of joint contracture. Biorheology. 1980; 17–95, with permission.)* **B.** Restriction of excessive crosslinking. A, collagen fiber arrangement; B, collagen fiber crosslinks; C, normal stretch; D, restricted stretch due to crosslink. *(From Woo SLY, Matthew JV, Akeson, WH. Connective tissue response to immobility: Correlative study of the biomechanical and biochemical measurements of normal and immobilized rabbit knees. Arthritic Rheum. 1975; 18: 257–264, with permission.)*

Immobilization With Muscle Lengthened—Anatomic Changes. Muscular adaptation to a lengthened position may begin within 24 hours of immobilization. This adaptation involves an increase in the number of sarcomeres in series found at the end of a muscle fibril, with a concurrent decrease in the length of each sarcomere. This adaptive response seems to be related to age. In the adult animal model the muscle adapts as described. In the young animal it is not muscle, but tendon that elongates. This in effect places the muscle in a shortened position. This shortened position then causes a reduction in the number of sarcomeres. The chronology of these events depends upon age. Muscle will adapt to meet the length changes imposed upon it.

Immobilization With Muscle Shortened—Anatomic Changes. Fixation of a muscle in a shortened position causes a decrease (up to 40%) in the number of sarcomeres. In conjunction with this there is a decrease in the length of the sarcomeres. The imposition of immobilization by active means (electrical stimulation or spasticity) may result in a change in as little as 12 hours. With passive immobilization the change in the length and number of sarcomeres requires approximately 5 days. These changes have been demonstrated with both prolonged immobilization and with muscles that continue to function while in chronically shortened positions.[91] The number and length of sarcomeres return to normal after immobilization is terminated. As in lengthened muscle the change in the number of sarcomeres is also related to age in the shortened muscle. In the young animal model there is a decrease in the rate of addition. In the adult there is an absolute loss. The shortened muscles demonstrate steeper passive tension curves when compared to controls. These curves may be a reflection of connective tissue loss occurring at a slower rate than muscle tissue loss, resulting in a relative increase in connective tissue and a reduction in the extensibility of muscle. The thickness of the endomysium and perimysium may also increase. An absolute proliferation of connective tissue has also been noted in denervated muscle.[92]

All of the changes on a cellular, matrix, or tissue level result in a loss of MF and JROM. These changes lead to movement dysfunction. If uncorrected this movement dysfunction may cause further immobilization, leading the individual in a vicious never-ending cycle.

REMOBILIZATION

The changes resulting from immobilization are reversible (Fig 13–19).[37]

Cellular Modeling
Synthesis and lysis of collagen continues to occur while the production of GAG is stimulated by motion.[36,86]

Matrix and Collagen Response
The ground substance, which suffered a loss of water and GAG during immobilization, now regains these two valuable components. These gains in turn return the gel–fiber ratio to normal, which increases the lubrication and interfiber distance of the collagen fibrils.[36] The rate recovery is faster than the rate at which fiber lubrication and interfiber distance were lost. The biochemical and biomechanical results show a good correlation, as the GAG and water increase the joint stiffness decreases.

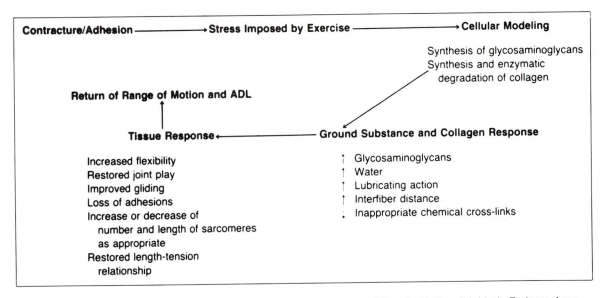

Figure 13-19. Remobilization. *(From Burkhardt S. Tissue Healing and Repair. National Athletic Trainers Association Professional Preparation Conference; Nashville, Tenn; 1979, with permission.)*

Tissue Response

With motion new collagen fibrils are now oriented along their lines of stress.[35,36,86] Previously formed collagen fibrils are reoriented along their proper lines of stress. The correct length–tension relationship is reestablished by the addition or deletion of sarcomeres as appropriate. Because of these changes JROM is increased and the joint mechanics return to normal. The negative cycle is broken and normal movement and function are restored.

THERAPEUTIC FACTORS AFFECTING CONNECTIVE TISSUE

The principal factors influencing the deformation of connective tissue are the amount, duration, and velocity of the applied force. The therapist may also use temperature and physical activity or exercise in a therapeutic manner to assist in the deformation of connective tissue.

Temperature

Temperature may have a profound effect on the physical and mechanical properties of collagen. Animal studies using in vitro preparations have demonstrated that the mechanical properties of collagen are temperature independent below a certain temperature (37°C in one animal model).[93] Above this temperature, changes occur in the mechanical properties of collagen and its crosslinks, with crosslinks breaking more easily and rapidly. The temperature at which the most profound changes are capable of occurring is 40°C.[93-95]

Numerous investigators have also explored the effects of therapeutic temperatures (which have an upper limit of 45°C) and load on the extensibility of collagen.[96] All these researchers have demonstrated that elevating the tissue temperature is beneficial when attempting to deform connective tissue.[96-98]

When considering the effect temperature has on collagen the clinician must keep the following key points in mind: (1) the amount of force required to attain or maintain a desired deformation decreases as temperature increases (Fig 13–20); (2) the time required to deform collagen to the point of failure is inversely related to temperature (Fig 13–21A); (3) the higher the temperature the greater the load collagen is able to tolerate prior to failure (Fig 13–21B); and (4) the higher the temperature the greater the amount of deformation possible prior to failure (Fig 13–21C). Less damage occurs at higher tissue temperatures. Experimental observations attribute this to an enhanced ability of viscoelastic and plastic change to occur at higher temperatures.

In the absence of a deforming force, heat alone will not cause a change in collagen deformation. A de-

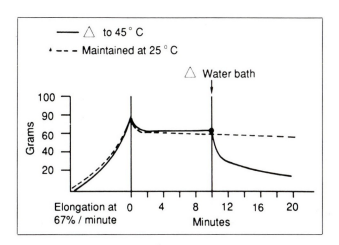

Figure 13–20. Effect of temperature on force relaxation response. (From Lehmann JF, Masock AJ, Warren CG, et al. Effect of therapeutic temperatures on tendon extensibility. Arch Phys Med Rehab. 1970; 51:481–487, with permission.)

forming force in the absence of heat will cause a change in collagenous length, however.[96]

Questions must now be raised regarding the amount of load to apply, the total time of load application, and whether it is best applied during the heating process or after. The greatest amount of residual change in the length occurs with the use of low-load, long-duration forces that are applied to the tissues while they are at their highest therapeutic temperatures.[96-99] This type of loading is thought to have a greater impact on the viscous elements of the collagen than the high-load, short-duration stress used to affect the elastic elements.[98]

Along with using therapeutic modalities to increase tissue temperature, intramuscular temperature may also be raised by active exercise (Fig 13–22).[100,101] Temperature increases to approximately 39°C are close to the "critical" temperature for collagen deformation, as discussed earlier.[93-95] This increase in temperature has implications on the design of a "warm-up" and flexibility program for any individual suffering from movement dysfunction caused in part by a lack of JROM or MF.

The effect of temperature must also be considered regarding the innervation of the muscle tendon unit. Fukami and Wilkinson concluded that the sensitivity to tension varies among different GTOs and appears to be inversely correlated with the mechanical stiffness of the muscle tendon unit in which it lies.[13] The stiffer or less flexible the muscle tendon unit, the less sensitive the GTO. Therefore a tight or inflexible muscle will be more resistant to the recruitment and firing of the GTO. It is the strain or deformation of the GTO that is perhaps most important, not the amount of applied force. In the same experiment the authors found that the sensitivity of the GTO to sustained stretch increased with increasing temperatures.

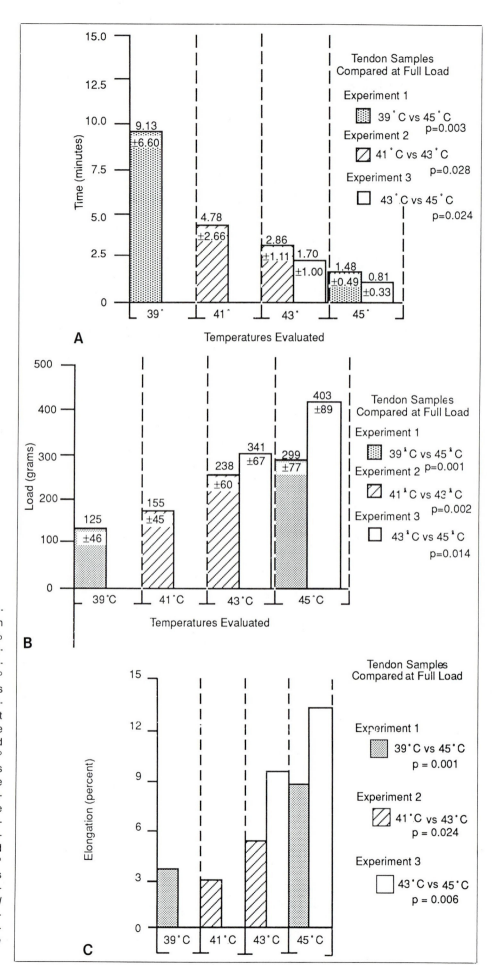

Figure 13-21. A. Effect of temperature on time of elongation to failure. Time to achieve 2.6% strain with treatment procedures using full load and comparing the temperatures of 39° vs. 45°, 41° vs 43° and 43° vs 45° C. **B.** Maximum load at rupture subsequent to treatment procedures incorporating the application of full load and temperatures compared at 39° vs 45°, 41° vs 43°, and 43° vs 45°C. **C.** Effect of temperature on percent elongation to failure. Maximum strain at rupture subsequent to treatment procedures incorporating the application of full load and temperatures compared at 39° vs 45°, 41° vs 43°, and 43° vs 45°C. *(From Lehmann JF, Koblanski JN: Elongation of rat tail tendon: Effect of load and temperature.* Arch Phys Med Rehab. *1971; 52:465–474, with permission.)*

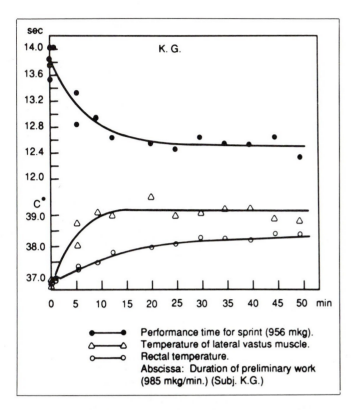

Figure 13-22. Effect of exercise on intramuscular temperature. *(From Asmussen E, Boje OVE. Body temperature and capacity for work. Acta Phys Scand. 1945; 10:1–22, with permission.)*

The combination of heat and stretching would appear from these reports to be the treatment indicated when an increase in the length of connective tissue is desired. This combination will allow the greatest deformation of the tissue using the lowest and safest deforming force possible. The time required to obtain change in the tissue length would be shorter. This combination would maximize the amount of residual gain from elongation. The residual gain may also be enhanced by allowing the tissue to "cool" while in the elongated or deformed state.

Application of the principles of heat plus deformation as just described for isolated tissue preparations has also been explored with human subjects by Henrickson et al,[102] with results similar to those of Lehmann et al.[96] Heat alone had no effect on muscle flexibility and the combination of heat plus stretching produced a greater increase in the range of motion than the change elicited by stretching alone.[102] This change was not significant, however. As the source of heat was an external heating pad, one must question whether the depth of penetration of the heat was sufficient to encourage tissue change. Little evidence exists for any temperature elevation beyond 36° to 37°C in the depths of large muscle groups during external conductive heating.[103]

Although it would appear that the application of

cold would have the opposite effect of heat on connective tissue, according to Rigby and associates no effect occurs on tendon below 37°C.[96]

Prolonged application of ice has been shown to decrease hypertonicity.[104–107] Therefore, perhaps the most beneficial use of cold would be to decrease the sensitivity of the muscle afferents and the contribution of the contractile elements to the resistance to deformation.

The use of a cryostretching technique has been advocated by Knight.[108] Cryostretching is used whenever a need exists to reduce low-grade muscle spasm. This type of spasm is often associated with muscle strains and postexercise muscle soreness. Cryostretch consists of a combination of cold application in conjunction with the use of PNF stretching techniques.

Cold and static stretching are more effective than heat and static stretching in reducing muscle pain and electrical activity in injured muscle within 24 hours of injury.[109] Application of cold at this point in time would appear to be appropriate to decrease pain and allow stretching to maintain the available painfree ROM. Once healing and scarring begin it appears that heat would be of greater value to increase the extensibility of the scar. This would allow the immature collagen fibrils to tolerate a greater amount of deformation without reinjury through enhanced viscoelastic and plastic change.

The brief application of cold cutaneous stimuli through the use of vapocoolants has been reported with differing results. Although the investigators used similar techniques, Halkovich and associates[110] reported a significant increase in hamstring flexibility and resultant passive hip flexion but Newton[111] and Koury and associates[112] did not. No concise conclusion is yet possible.

Physical Activity

The use of resistive exercise was discouraged prior to World War II by many coaches who reasoned that the athlete would become muscle bound and lose flexibility.[113] Over time this idea has been disproved.[114,115]

Exercise may have a positive effect on the strength, integrity, and organization of the collagen that is found in all types of connective tissue.[8–10,17,116–118] Although the majority of studies report on changes in ligament,[9,10,17,116–118] others discuss tendon[8,9,119] and muscle.[120]

The two critical goals of any JROM and MF program are to develop a tissue that will elongate over the required distance and to develop a tissue that is sufficiently strong to resist the forces placed upon it and thus minimize the chance of injury. A balance is required between tissue strength and extensibility.

The changes in the strength and stiffness of a tissue that has undergone elongation, without a change in its integrity, are summarized in Fig 13–23.[9] There is no

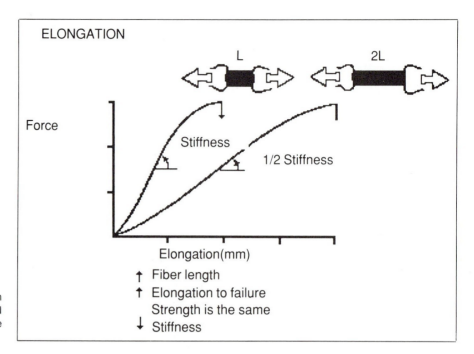

Figure 13-23. Effect of elongation on collagen. The influence of original length of tissue fibers on the shape of the load deformation curve.

decrease in the ability of this tissue to tolerate the stress placed upon it. Because the tissue has longer fibers it has less stiffness and is more easily deformable. These characteristics, an advantage in the muscle tendon unit, could pose potential problems in other tissues such as ligament and joint capsule, which are the primary restraints to joint injury and hypermobility.

Through the use of a regular exercise program of an endurance nature, an increase in collagenous strength and hypertrophy has been demonstrated in ligament[116] and tendon.[119] Although these changes are much more apparent after a ligament has been immobilized than in a "normal" ligament, there is speculation by noted authors that similar changes are possible in normal ligament.[17] Tendon also demonstrates an increase in strength and hypertrophy with active exercise.[119] The clinician must remember that these changes take a period of months. The effects of mobilization (movement) and immobilization on injured muscle in rats has been studied by Kvist and Jarvinen.[120] With mobilization, scar formation and muscle regeneration were more rapid, the orientation of new muscle fibers was more parallel with surrounding fibers, and tensile properties of the muscle were greater. Again, because of the rate of turnover of collagen it should be remembered that all of the potential changes in collagenous strength and hypertrophy take a period of many months.[17]

The changes in connective tissue strength with hypertrophy of collagen fibers are summarized in Fig 13–24.[9] With hypertrophy of collagen or a broader collagen mass the tissue is stronger. Although it does not lose ability to deform because of the increase in strength, it becomes stiffer and more resistant to deformation.

Greater collagenous strength would be a benefit for all tissues (especially ligament) in order to avoid injury, provided normal mobility is maintained. The connective tissue in and around muscle must have strength but it must also have the ability to elongate readily and easily if dynamic flexibility is to be preserved.

CLINICAL APPLICATIONS

Between 30% and 50% of all sports injuries are of musculotendinous origin,[121-123] the majority being acute muscle strains.[124] They are often considered "minor" in comparison to major joint injuries because they are rarely career threatening. Nevertheless, because they occur frequently and can prevent an athlete's participation, the most common "minor" injury—the muscle strain—warrants as much attention from the sports physical therapist as a joint injury.

Causative Factors

Muscle strain follows excessive intrinsic force production, excessive extrinsic stretch, or both. The muscle undergoes an eccentric lengthening type of contraction (intrinsic force) to counteract the excessive extrinsic stretching force applied to the point of injury.

Several factors that contribute to muscle strain include inadequate flexibility, inadequate strength or endurance, dyssynergic muscle contraction, insufficient warmup, and inadequate rehabilitation from previous injury.[124,125]

Good flexibility enhances the tissue's ability to accommodate stress, dissipate impact shock, and improve performance.[126] A muscle that can contract strongly

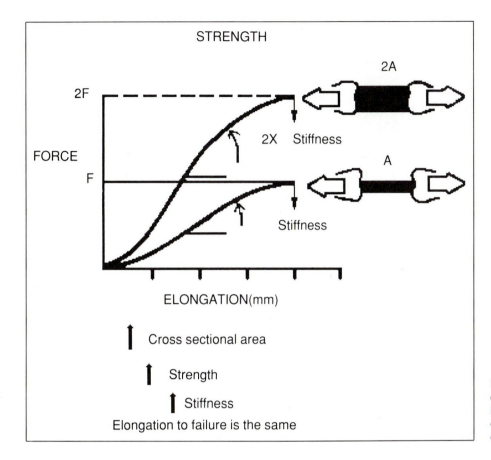

STRENGTH

2A

2F

FORCE

2X   Stiffness

A

F

Stiffness

ELONGATION(mm)

Cross sectional area

Strength

Stiffness

Elongation to failure is the same

Figure 13-24. Effect of increased collagenous strength. The effects of increasing tissue cross-sectional area on the shape of the load-deformation curve.

and effectively is well-equipped to absorb force and deformation and has a reduced risk of injury.[124]

The dual innervation of some muscles such as the semitendinous and biceps femoris may contribute to asynchrony of firing and muscle fatigue, and can increase the probability of injury.[56] Pregame warmup will increase intramuscular temperature and tissue compliance and improve the synchronization of muscular action. This will prepare the musculotendinous unit for repeated deformation in its fully lengthened position.[126]

Inadequate rehabilitation often leads to insufficient tissue maturation and excessive scarring.[55,58] This can result in a suboptimal load tolerance and can initiate a chronic cycle of injury, inflammation, suboptimal repair, and reinjury.

IMPORTANT QUESTIONS

What Is the Best Method of Stretching?

Although enhanced flexibility achieved through stretching promotes greater compliance of the muscle–tendon unit, therapists must determine which is the best method of stretching to gain the desired compliance. Three common methods of stretching are generally used in the attempt to gain an increase in flexibility. These methods are static stretching, ballistic

stretching, and stretching through the use of various proprioceptive neuromuscular facilitation techniques.

Static stretching is a method of stretching in which a stationary position is held for a period of time during which specified joints are locked into a position that places the muscles and connective tissues at their greatest possible length. Ballistic stretching involves quick motions characterized by bobbing or jerky movements imposed upon the muscles and connective tissue structures to be stretched.[1,127] These movements are initiated by active contraction of the muscle groups that are antagonistic to those which are being stretched. Although these methods have been shown to be equally effective in producing an increase in flexibility, there are advantages and disadvantages to each.[127,128]

Static stretching offers three distinct advantages: (1) there is less danger of exceeding the extensibility limits of the tissues involved; (2) energy requirements are lower; and (3) muscle soreness is less likely and may in fact be relieved.[127] These advantages are quite reasonable since connective tissue has a very high tensile resistance to a suddenly applied tension of short duration, while demonstrating viscoelastic and plastic elongation when placed under prolonged mild tension.[99] Static stretching also has the advantages of minimizing any impact of the Ia and II spindle afferent fiber stimulation and maximizing the impact of the GTO.

Although the use of ballistic stretching has not

been widely supported in the literature, one study questioned whether ballistic static stretching is being used in instances where ballistic stretching would be the better therapy.[129] Ballistic stretching *is* an effective modality, and it is the therapist's responsibility to determine when it is most appropriate. The therapist can make this judgment only after having an understanding of the normal physiology and pathophysiology of the structures involved and the particular patient and associated activities. The stretching program must be tailored to the particular individual. The program prescribed by the therapist for the athlete will be very different than that prescribed for the sedentary individual or the geriatric patient who suffers from movement dysfunction.

Ballistic stretching exercises are usually not appropriate for the sedentary individual or geriatric patient but may play a vital role in the conditioning and training of the athlete. Athletic activities are predominantly ballistic in nature.

Static stretching should predominantly be used early in the season. The proportion of ballistic stretching to static stretching should be increased as the athlete's level of fitness and conditioning increases.[129] If ballistic stretching exercises are used, they should be preceded by static stretching and confined to a small ROM, perhaps no more than 10% beyond the static range of motion.[3,129] Ballistic stretching may be used to assist in the development of dynamic flexibility at the end of the athlete's available range.

Whenever ballistic stretching is considered, the program prescribed should be of a progressive nature. A Progressive Velocity Flexibility Program (PVFP) should be used (Fig 13–25, Table 13–9). The PVFP requires the muscle group being stretched to undergo a transition from antagonist to agonist. It is this transition and potential dyssynergic contraction that have been implicated in muscle strain.[125,130] The athlete must work on his or her neuromuscular coordination through this type of activity. A motor learning response may be

set up as the athlete stretches at a higher and higher velocity over time, simulating and integrating functional activity necessary for sport.

The PVFP is preceded by warmup and static stretching. Depending upon the athlete and his or her activity and physical status (postinjury or prophylactic stretching program), the PVFP is instituted for a period of days or weeks. The PVFP takes the athlete through a series of stretching exercises in which the velocity and range of lengthening are combined and controlled on a progressive basis. The athlete progresses from an environment of control to activity simulation, from slow-velocity methodical activity to high-velocity functional activity. After static stretching, slow short end range (SSER) ballistic stretching is initiated. The athlete then progresses to slow full range stretching (SFR), fast short end range (FSER) and fast full range (FFR) stretching. Control and range are the responsibility of the athlete. *No* outside force is exerted by anyone else.

The sedentary individual and the geriatric patient do not engage in high-velocity activities in their daily life-styles, and therefore do not need the high degree of dynamic flexibility required by the athlete. In most instances, static stretching exercises are more appropriate for this patient population.

The three techniques of proprioceptive neuromuscular facilitation (PNF) for increasing JROM and MF are the contract–relax (CR), hold–relax (HR), and contract relax with agonist contraction (CRAC) techniques. These techniques seek to facilitate the GTO to inhibit the muscle in which it lies, and to use the principle of reciprocal inhibition.[131]

Various authors and studies have concluded that PNF stretching techniques are effective in increasing flexibility. There appears to be no consensus regarding which is the *single* best technique.[128,131–139] CRAC stretching has been shown to be significantly better than CR stretching ($p < 0.05$),[133,140] CR was significantly better than HR ($p < 0.05$),[135] and CR or HR was demonstrated to be significantly better than static or

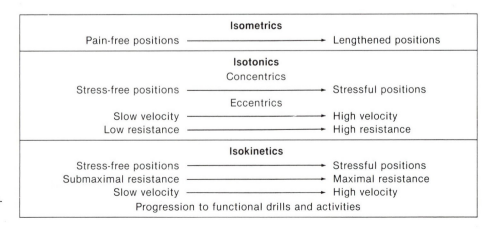

Figure 13–25. Progressive velocity flexibility program.

Isometrics		
Pain-free positions ⟶		Lengthened positions

Isotonics		
	Concentrics	
Stress-free positions ⟶		Stressful positions
	Eccentrics	
Slow velocity ⟶		High velocity
Low resistance ⟶		High resistance

Isokinetics		
Stress-free positions ⟶		Stressful positions
Submaximal resistance ⟶		Maximal resistance
Slow velocity ⟶		High velocity
Progression to functional drills and activities		

TABLE 13-9. PROGRESSIVE VELOCITY FLEXIBILITY PROGRAM

STATIC STRETCHING
↓
SSER —Slow, Short End Range Stretching
↓
SFR—Slow Full Range Stretching
↓
FSER—Fast Short End Range Stretching
↓
FFR—Fast Full Range Stretching

ballistic stretching $(p < 0.05)$.[132,134,135,138,139] Only Moore and Hutton have demonstrated no significant difference between static stretching and CRAC or CR stretching.[137]

When considering the results of these studies the reader must be aware that in most cases the amount of force used in stretching was not controlled.[132–136] Only Moore and Hutton provided controlled stretching forces.[137] The amount of force used to stretch with the CRAC, CR, and HR techniques may be greater than the force imposed by static or ballistic stretching, which may be a possible source of error in the studies.

A paradox exists in the report of Moore and Hutton, however. Although the premise behind stretching through the use of PNF techniques is to decrease the extrafusal muscle fiber activity, some research has shown the opposite to be true. Moore and Hutton have stated that "recent experiments reveal that a static contraction preceding muscle stretch facilitates contractile activity through lingering after discharge in the afferent limb of the stretch reflex. Contrary to traditional views a muscle is initially more resistant to change in length after a static contraction." Experimentally, Moore and Hutton then demonstrated that CR and CRAC conditions produce median values of 300% and 710% more hamstring activity, respectively, over static stretch EMG levels.

Within the same experiment the greatest change in the ROM was seen with CRAC. Contract relax with agonist contraction techniques also produced the greatest perception of discomfort. In an effort to explain the paradox of greater ROM using CRAC over static stretching [although not to a significant level $(p > 0.05)$], despite a greater amount of EMG activity and perception of discomfort by the subject, Moore and Hutton hypothesized that in CRAC stretching the voluntary contraction of the antagonist to the muscle group being stretched masks discomfort and allows a greater stretch.

In a follow-up study, Condon and Hutton examined integrated EMG (IEMG) and motor pool excitability of the soleus in relation to the effectiveness of stretching techniques. Significantly reduced motor pool excitability levels (using the Hoffman's reflex) in the so-

leus were observed during contraction of the tibialis anterior during CRAC stretching.[141] These results support previous findings.[137] Again, however, the IEMG of the muscle group being stretched, using surface electrodes, during activity of the antagonistic muscle group was higher than with passive stretching.

Results of the two previously mentioned studies[137,141] have been challenged by Entyre and Abraham,[142] who demonstrated that tracings from surface electrodes that gave the appearance of activity between antagonistic muscles were actually crosstalk between the electrodes. No activity was observed from fine-wire electrodes. This study supports the use of antagonistic muscle contraction during stretching to inhibit contraction of the muscle being stretched.

How Long Must a Stretch Be Held?

There appears to be no consensus among therapists regarding how long a stretch should be held. In a study assessing abduction ROM and muscle flexibility Madding et al demonstrated that holding a stretch for 15 seconds is as effective as 2 minutes for increasing muscle flexibility.[143]

How Long Does it Take to Cause an Increase in Muscle Flexibility?

No studies to date have documented the minimum amount of time which a flexibility program must be followed to cause change. Clinical experience dictates that the response time is a function of the individual. Change that is maintained takes a greater length of time rather than a shorter length of time to achieve.

How Long Does an Increase Remain After Stopping a Stretching Program?

Once gained, MF must be maintained. How long a gain in flexibility will last after the cessation of a flexibility program remains unknown. Once a flexibility program is stopped the gain made will be lost over time (unless the range gained is maintained through use). After a 6-week flexibility training program, using static, ballistic or modified PNF stretching, Zebas and Rivera have demonstrated a significant increase in MF about the ankle, shoulder, hip, trunk, and neck.[128] Significant gains occurred for all groups $(p < 0.05)$. A statistically significant loss $(p < 0.05)$ of MF occurred in all muscle groups 2 weeks after the cessation of the program. A further gradual loss was measured at the end of 4 weeks. Even with flexibility losses over this 4-week period, however, the flexibility retained was greater than prior to the start of the stretching program.

How Often Must One Stretch?

The study by Wallin and associates suggests that pursuing a flexibility program one time per week may be sufficient to maintain the flexibility gained, while engag-

ing in a program three to five times per week will increase flexibility.[132]

In summary, static, ballistic, and PNF stretching techniques have been demonstrated to increase MF. Ballistic stretching may pose the greatest potential for microtraumatic injury. PNF stretching, although potentially the most effective, requires time and expertise and may lead to subject discomfort. PNF stretching appears to be most valuable when the patient requires one-on-one intervention on the part of the therapist. Once properly instructed, the individual may engage in static stretching on his or her own, making this modality the most desirable from the standpoint of results, time, expertise, and subject comfort. To improve flexibility, a stretching program should be pursued at least three times per week. In order to maintain flexibility gained the patient should engage in his program at least one time per week. Once a stretching program is discontinued the MF gained will gradually be lost.

The ultimate goal of any MF program is to increase the ability of the muscle to lengthen through the necessary ROM in the most efficient manner. Regardless of the type of individual for whom the therapist is developing a MF program, the *basic* components of the sequence are the same: (1) a general warmup; (2) participation in an exercise or stretching program; and (3) a cool-down or postparticipation period. The number and complexity of each of these steps will vary with the individual, the type of activity in which he or she is involved, and the type of movement dysfunction. The following sections provide suggestions for the two principal patient populations.

The Athlete. The most efficient sequencing of five activities to improve the athlete's muscle flexibility is (1) general warmup, (2) preparticipation stretching, (3) neuromuscular warmup, (4) participation, and (5) postparticipation stretching. The time required for this sequence will differ depending upon the athlete and his or her specific needs.

General Warmup. As muscle contracts, heat is produced as a by-product and the intramuscular temperature increases. An increase in the intramuscular temperature should make stretching safer and more effective. Physiological warming (preconditioning) in the animal model has been demonstrated to prevent muscular injury by increasing the force of failure, length to failure, and elasticity of the muscle tendon unit.[145] The general warmup should consist of repetitive nonfatiguing exercise of the muscle groups to be stretched and should be approximately 10 to 15 minutes in duration to allow for the increase in intramuscular temperature to occur. This exercise should occur in the athlete's readily available ROM. The increase in intramuscular temperature from this activity will allow the

tissue to deform with greater ease and minimize the chance of microtrauma. A secondary purpose may be to begin to condition the connective tissue to allow it to withstand the stress that will be imposed upon it. Examples for the runner would be cycling, a very brisk walk, or a very easy jog.

The effect of a warmup period of cycling on MF has been studied.[140-144] Wilktorsson–Moller and associates have studied the effects of warmup, massage, and stretching on lower extremity range of motion.[140] After warming up, there was significant change only in dorsiflexion ($p < 0.02$). A combination of warming up and stretching produced a significant change in hip, knee, and ankle range of motion ($p < 0.02$ to $p < 0.001$). Hubley et al studied the effects of stationary cycling and static stretching on hip ROM.[144] They concluded that both static stretching and stationary cycling were equally effective for increasing hip ROM and retaining the increase for a 15-minute period independent of activity. Unfortunately they did not evaluate the effect of stretching after warming up on a stationary cycle when intramuscular temperature would have been the highest, and perhaps been able to cause the greatest change.

Massage may also be beneficial during the general warmup period; significant change has been reported in dorsiflexion ($p < 0.005$) and for the hamstrings ($p < 0.05$) following massage. No long-term carryover was evident, however.[140,146]

An initial cyclic phase or building up process of deformation within the connective tissues' tolerable limits of deformation may be most efficient prior to the addition of a residual stationary stretch. In this cyclic phase the connective tissue is deformed within its readily available limits. The deformation is progressively increased as discomfort decreases. This is similar to what was proposed by Vidik for experiments involving isolated tissue preparation.[10] This process influences the hysteresis response and readily available elastic and viscoelastic deformation. After all the readily available deformation is achieved a stretch of long duration is required to further increase the length of the tissues by influencing the creep response. Control must be exercised by the athlete in this phase to ensure that the tissues' available amount of deformation is not exceeded, causing injury.

Preparticipation Stretching. Following warmup and its concurrent increase in tissue temperature, slow, static stretching should begin. This slow, static stretching may decrease facilitation of the spindle afferents and assist in the facilitation of the GTO. Maintenance of the stretch will influence the viscoelastic and plastic properties of the connective tissue by influencing the tissue's creep response. After slow static stretching, ballistic stretching (using a slowly progressing controlled velocity) may be done at the end of the athlete's avail-

able ROM if indicated. Caution and control must be exercised with ballistic stretching to ensure that no microtraumatic injury occurs.

Neuromuscular Warmup. The purpose of the neuromuscular warmup is to begin to simulate the athlete's actual activity. The velocity of the activities chosen and the ROM through which they are carried out should be progressively increased over a series of repetitions. This progressive increase in velocity and ROM will influence connective tissue (hysteresis and force relaxation responses) by further conditioning it to tolerate the stress to be imposed at the velocity and deformation necessary for training and competition. The repetition of activity at increasing velocities will also improve motor learning and skill necessary for competition. It is during this neuromuscular warmup that the PVFP may be incorporated.

It is important that this activity not be started until the tissues have gone through a general warmup and preparticipation stretching program, which helps them to tolerate the stress imposed during the neuromuscular warmup. These activities will further increase the intramuscular temperature and the ability of the tissues to tolerate stress without injury.

During this stage the therapist may use PNF stretching techniques to assist the athlete in gaining flexibility.

Participation. The athlete is now ready to participate in his or her chosen activity. At this time the highest intramuscular temperatures will be reached.

Postparticipation Stretching. After participation or training the tissues are at their highest temperature. Slow stretching should again be done. Stretching at this time has two effects. First, it will assist in further improving flexibility. Secondly, postparticipation stretching will assist in decreasing or preventing muscular soreness commonly present after strenuous activity.[147,148] When stretching after participation the muscle or muscle groups to be affected should be maintained in an elongated position as the athlete "cools down."[97,98] This static stretch may assist in maintaining the flexibility gained. For maximum gain after participation the muscle group or groups being stretched should not be fatigued. Fatigue has been demonstrated to facilitate the muscle spindle and inhibit the GTO.[149,150]

The Sedentary Individual and Geriatric Patient.
The programs that the therapist prescribes for sedentary individuals and geriatric patients will be very similar, as both groups have a great need for good general static flexibility in order to minimize the amount of stress imposed upon the tissues during their daily activities. Based upon their activity patterns, neither of these

groups has a great need for dynamic flexibility. The stretching sequence for these groups will be similar to the athlete except that it is not usually necessary to include ballistic stretching or the neuromuscular warmup phases.

General Warmup. As with the athlete, this warmup is an important preparatory step for any stretching activity that is to follow. The goals are the same—to increase the intramuscular temperature and to obtain all of the readily available elastic and viscoelastic deformation that is possible through a cyclic process. As with the athlete these activities are carried out in the readily available ROM. Individuals increase the range through which they are exercising as they see fit. Although modalities may be used as indicated to assist in increasing the tissue temperature, the progressive cyclic activity in which the individual participates must be accomplished. Activities such as stationary cycling and walking are appropriate for the lower extremities. For the upper extremities, general exercise and activity along with the use of an arm ergometer are appropriate. The key consideration in this phase is not to exceed the tissues' available deformation and cause injury.

Flexibility Exercises. The flexibility exercises prescribed by the therapist for sedentary individuals or geriatric patients usually consist of the activity in which the patient will be involved. Slow static stretching should be prescribed for these individuals to be done on an independent basis. Proprioceptive neuromuscular facilitation (PNF) stretching activities may be used by the therapist if one-on-one intervention is needed. Joint mobilization techniques should be used during this stage if indicated.

"Cool Down." Following the stretching exercises and the treatment provided by the therapist, patients in this group may "cool down" by maintaining a position of stretch. If felt to be appropriate by the therapist, the "cool down" may be further enhanced by the application of ice. The ice may assist in the retention of deformation and may reduce any inflammatory response caused by the activity.

REHABILITATION PRINCIPLES

The sports physical therapist should be able to develop an intervention program for any type of muscle strain based upon certain principles. These principles are developed from having a sound working knowledge of the physiology and pathophysiology of muscle.

Prevention Is Easier Than Treatment
One of sports physical therapist's principal roles is patient education. Athletes and coaches should be edu-

cated in proper stretching techniques and program construction. Proper use of warmup and preventive flexibility programs should be stressed. Appropriate prophylaxis and self-intervention in the early stages of injury are imperative.

Intervention Depends Upon the Healing Stage

Muscle, like any structure that contains connective tissue goes through four phases of healing[53,55,59,60,150-152]:

1. Inflammatory response—characterized by hemorrhage and hematoma formation, pyknosis (with third-degree strains), and phagocytosis. This response initiates the repair process.
2. Ground substance proliferation—fibroblasts begin to produce a gellike matrix that surrounds the collagen fibrils. Phagocytosis continues, but at a slower rate. An attempt to limit the inflammatory process should be made. The length of time devoted to repair and rehabilitation should be contingent upon the extent of the inflammatory response.
3. Collagen protein formation—collagen is produced by the fibroblasts in the area. Initially a high proportion of this collagen is soluble or immature because of the lack of crosslinks between collagen molecules. The inflammatory response must be halted by this phase because the soluble collagen is susceptible to enzymatic breakdown.
4. Final organization—collagen fibrils begin their maturation process. Motion is important, as these fibrils react as stated in Wolff's law and reorient themselves in accordance with the tension placed upon them.

The length of time for each phase varies with the severity of injury. The following offers a rough guideline for third-degree strains or muscle tears: phase 1—1 to 3 days; phase 2—3 to 6 days; phase 3—6 to 18 days; and phase 4—18 days onward. For first- and second-degree strains, the time required for each phase is the same but the amount of damage is less. Estimations should be based on the athlete's symptoms. Recommended treatment during each phase is summarized in Table 13–10.

Controlled Mobility Rather Than Immobility

Collagen formation is the best example of Wolff's Law. An excellent example of this is a study by Kvist and Jarvinen that compared mobilization to immobilization in treating muscle and tendon injuries in rats.[120] Controlled mobilization was found to be superior for scar formation, revascularization, muscle regeneration, metabolic processes, and orientation of muscle fibers and tensile properties. They concluded that healing is

TABLE 13–10. MUSCLE STRAIN INTERVENTION

Treatment	Healing Stage			
	1	2	3	4
Rest				
Absolute	X	X		
Controlled	X	X	X	
Modalities				
Cryotherapy	X	X	A	A
Thermotherapy		B	B	B
Elec Stim	X	X	X	
Medication				
NSAIDS	X	X	X	
Phono (Pulsed)	X	X	X	
Phono (Cont.)		?	X	X
Exercise				
Maintenance	X	X		
Stretching			X	X
Strength			X	X
External Supports	X	X	X	X

A = After treatment; Prophylactic
B = Before treatment to warm tissue

accelerated by mobilization. Caution must be exercised by the sports physical therapist, however, when extrapolating and applying animal studies to humans. Kvist and Jarvinen noted that the reparative process is twice as fast in the rat as it is in humans. The sports therapist must base the athlete's treatment progression on symptoms exhibited.

Rest is important in the early stages of healing. Absolute immobilization is only necessary in the most severe cases. Progressive muscle flexibility and joint ROM programs should be developed starting within the athlete's painfree range. Pain is the guiding factor. As healing progresses increased activity is allowed.

Medications and Modalities—Important Adjuncts

Almekanders and Gilbert state that nonsteroidal anti-inflammatory drugs can delay muscle regeneration if taken during the early phases of healing.[153] Careful review of their data, however, leads one to the opposite conclusion (Fig 13–25). In their experiment after controlled strain the tibialis anterior (rat model) was immobilized. The group on proxicam (Feldene) demonstrated a greater maximum load to failure at days 2 and 11. No significant difference was demonstrated at day 4. An interesting fact to note from Fig 13–25 is the effect of immobilization on the sham control group. Again, immobilization decreases the maximum load to failure of muscle.

Topical steroids may also be used in the management of muscle strain through the use of phonophoresis and iontophoresis. No research has been completed, however, to assist the therapist in determining the actual effect of these agents on muscle strength and healing.

Ice should be used initially to limit pain, inflammation, swelling, and hematoma formation. In later phases of healing, ice is used as a prophylactic measure to prevent inflammation caused by microtrauma. It must be remembered that cold may also reduce spindle response and decrease spasm associated with pain.

Various forms of heat may be used to increase circulation and facilitate the repair response. Heat should not be used, however, if an active inflammatory response exists.

In the early stages, high-voltage galvanic electrical stimulation may be applied to minimize the inflammatory response.[154] In the later stages, it can be used to facilitate a muscle pump action to reduce the size of the hematoma and extent of the tissue edema.

In phases 3 and 4 deep heating modalities, e.g., ultrasound, can be used to raise intramuscular temperature. This will increase the tissues' compliance to stretching force and reduce the possibility of microtraumatic injury. The effect of temperature on the GTO must also be considered.[13]

Develop a Flexible Tissue

A flexible tissue will have an increased elongation to failure and a decreased stiffness. No loss of tissue strength will take place (Fig 13–23).[9] This is critical in muscle that must undergo a large range of deformation and high-velocity changes. An effect on performance may also be seen by increasing the efficiency of movement and improving dynamic flexibility.

In first- and second-degree strains the athlete should be encouraged to maintain flexibility within the painfree range almost immediately. Third-degree strains are usually prescribed absolute rest immediately after injury. During the ROM maintenance period, pain should be the athlete's limiting factor.

Develop a Strong Tissue

A strong tissue will exhibit greater strength to failure and increased stiffness (Fig 13–24).[9] There will be no change in its elongation to failure provided that the ROM is also maintained. The beneficial effects of exercise on connective tissue have been amply demonstrated, as previously discussed. The potential protective effect of muscle activation and strength has been demonstrated by Garret et al.[145]

Strengthening exercises should be initiated when they can be done without pain. An outline for a possible exercise program progression is presented in Fig 13–26.

"SAID" Principle Is Vital

The "SAID" principle (specific adaptation to imposed demands) is vital for any athlete in any sport. Just as specific training programs must be designed to assist the athlete to meet the demands of his or her sport, specific flexibility programs must be designed by the sports physical therapist to assist the athlete to meet the flexibility requirements of his or her sport. Consideration of the static and ballistic flexibility demands must be taken into account. Programs emphasizing static or ballistic stretching must change as the athlete's condition and needs change.

Although basic principles and concepts are constant, treatment programs from the onset of injury to the return to activity should be individualized in all cases.

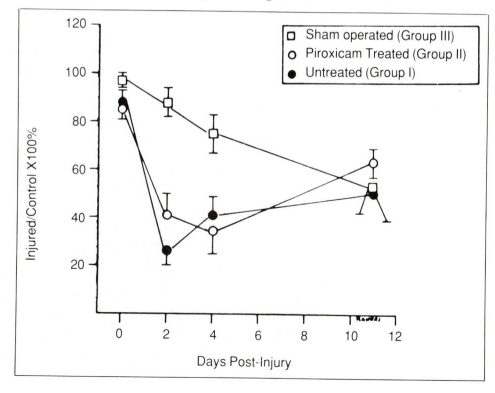

Figure 13-26. Effect of nonsteroidal anti-inflammatories on muscle load to failure. Percentage of maximum failure load in injured muscle compared to uninjured side. *(From Almekinders LC, Gilbert JA. Healing of experimental muscle strains and the effects of nonsteroidal anti-inflammatory medication. Am J Sports Med. 1986;14:303–308, with permission.)*

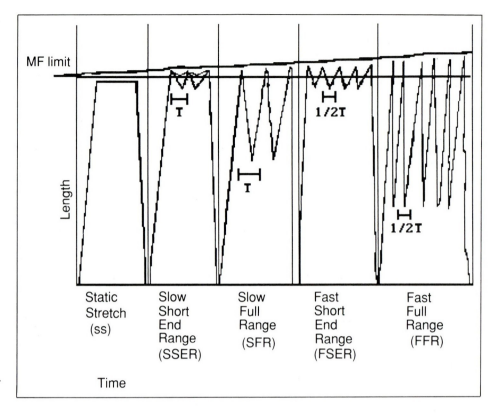

Figure 13-27. Exercise program progression.

Use Progressive Velocity Flexibility Program (PVFP)

The majority of athletic activity in which a muscle strain is likely to occur is ballistic in nature. Use of the PVFP as previously described allows the sports physical therapist to develop a flexibility program that progressively stresses the muscle and muscle–tendon junction in a manner similar to functional activity (Fig 13–27). The speed with which the injured athlete progresses through the PVFP will be affected by the severity of injury and demands of the sport. Progress through the stages of the PVFP, when used as a prophylactic program in the noninjured athlete, will be quicker.

Pain Is the Guiding Factor

Subjective feedback is always the guiding factor of the sports physical therapist when dealing with a muscle strain.

No "Quick Fix" Is Possible

Immature collagen cannot tolerate excessive stress and strain. If progressed too quickly the injury may become chronic, thus prolonging recovery time. The greater the severity of injury the longer the expected recovery time.

REFERENCES

1. deVries HA. Flexibility. In: deVries HA, ed. *Physiology of Exercise for Physical Education and Athletics.* 3rd ed. Dubuque Iowa: William C Brown; 1980: 462–472.
2. Harris ML. Flexibility. *Phys Ther.* 1969; 49:591–560.
3. Klafs CE, Arnheim DD. *Modern Principles of Athletic Training.* 3rd ed. St. Louis, Mo: C V Mosby Co; 1980: 65–66, 75–79.
4. Nicholas JA. Risk factors; sports medicine and the orthopaedic system: An overview. *J Sports Med.* 1976; 3:243–259.
5. Marshall JL, Johanson N, Wickiewicz TL, et al. Joint looseness: A function of the person and the joint. *Med Sci Sports Exerc.* 1980; 12:189–192.
6. Norkin CC, LeVangie PK. *Joint Structure and Function: A Comprehensive Analysis.* Philadelphia, Pa: Davis Co; 1983:67–84.
7. Ciullo J, Zarins B. Biomechanics of the musculotendinous unit: Relationship to athletic performance and injury. *Clin Sports Med.* 1983; 2:71–86.
8. Curwin S, Stanish W. *Tendinitis: Its Etiology and Treatment.* Lexington, Mass: Collamore Press, 1984:1–67.
9. Butler DL, Grood ES, Noyes FR, et al. Biomechanics of ligaments and tendons. *Exerc Sports Sci Rev.* 1979; 6:126–282.
10. Viidik A. Functional properties of collagenous tissue. *Rev Connect Tissue Res.* 1973; 6:127–215.
11. Sapega AA, Quedenfeld TC, Moyer RA, et al. Biophysical factors in range of motion exercises. *Phys Sportsmed.* 1981; 9:57–65.
12. Ganong WF. *The Nervous System.* Los Altos, Calif: Lange Medical Publications; 1977:67–74.
13. Fukami Y, Wilkinson RS. Responses on isolated golgi tendon organs of the cat. *J Physiol.* 1977;265:673–689.
14. Tardieu C, Huet de la Teur E, Bret MD, et al. Muscle hypoextensibility in children with cerebral palsy: I.

Clinical and experimental observations. *Arch Phys Med Rehabil.* 1982; 63:97–102.

15. Cooper DL, Fair, J. Developing and testing flexibility. *Phys Sportsmed.* 1978; 6:137–138.

16. Johns RJ, Wright V. Relative importance of various tissues in joint stiffness. *J Appl Physiol.* 1962; 17:824–828.

17. Akeson WH, Woo SLY, Amiel D, et al. The chemical basis of tissue repair: The biology of ligaments. In: Hunter LY, Funk FJ, eds. *Rehabilitation of the Injured Knee.* St. Louis, Mo: C V Mosby Co; 1984:93–148.

18. Fawcett DW. *Textbook of Histology.* 11th ed. Philadelphia, Pa: W B Saunders Co; 1986:136–173.

19. Williams PL, Warwick R. *Grays Anatomy.* 36th ed. Philadelphia, Pa: W B Saunders Co; 1980:411–454.

20. Nimni MC. The molecular organization of collagen and its role in determining the biophysical properties of connective tissue. *Biorheology.* 1980; 17:51–82.

21. Nordin M, Frankel VH. Biomechanics of collagenous tissue. In: Frankel VH, Nordin M, eds. *Mechanics of the Skeletal System.* Philadelphia, Pa: Lea and Febiger; 1980:87–109.

22. Woo SLY. Biomechanics of soft connective tissue. Presented at UCLA Department of Kinesiology; October 26, 1982.

23. Akeson WE, Amiel D, Mechanic GL, et al. Collagen cross linking alterations in joint contracture: Changes in reducible cross links in periarticular connective tissue collagen after nine weeks of immobilization. *Connect Tissue Res.* 1977; 5:15–19.

24. Gay S, Gay RE, Miller EJ. The collagens of the joint. *Arthritis Rheum.* 1980; 23:937–941.

25. Bronstein P. Structurally distinct collagentypes. *Annu Rev Biochem.* 1980; 49:957–1003.

26. Miller EJ. The collagens of the joint. In: Sokolov L, ed. *The Joints and Synovial Fluid.* Orlando, Fla: Academic Press; 1978:205–242.

27. Kleinman HK, Klebe RJ, Martin GR. Role of collagenous matrices in the adhesion and growth of cells. *J Cell Biol.* 1981; 88:473–485.

28. Lane J. Collagen and elastin. In: Owen R, Goodfellow J, Bullough P, eds. *Scientific Foundations of Orthopaedics and Traumatology.* Philadelphia, Pa: W B Saunders Co; 1980:30–35.

29. Rosenberg LC. Proteoglycans. In: Owen R, Goodfellow J, Bullough P, eds. *Scientific Foundations of Orthopaedics and Traumatology.* Philadelphia, Pa: W B Saunders Co; 1980:36–42.

30. Donatelli R, Owens-Burkhardt H. Effects of immobilization on the extensibility of periarticular connective tissue. *J Orthop Sports Phys Ther.* 1981; 3:67–72.

31. Kastelic J, Galeski A, Baer E. The microcomposite structure of tendons. *Connect Tissue Res.* 1978; 6:11–23.

32. Elden HR. Physical properties of collagen fibers. *Int Rev Connect Tissue Res.* 1968; 4:283–348.

33. Akeson WH, Amiel D, Woo SLY. Immobility effects of synovial joints: The pathomechanics of joint contracture. *Biorheology.* 1980; 17:95–110.

34. Stromberg DD, Weiderheilm CA. Viscoelastic description of a collagenous tissue in simple elongation. *J Appl Physiol.* 1969; 26:857–862.

35. Woo SLY, Matthew JV, Akeson WH. Connective tissue response to immobility: Correlative study of the biomechanical and biochemical measurements of normal and immobilized rabbit knees. *Arthritic Rheum.* 1975; 18:257–264.

36. Akeson WH, Amiel D, Mechanic GL, et al. Collagen crosslinking alterations in joint contractures: Changes in the reducible crosslinks in periarticular connective tissue collagen after nine weeks of immobilization. *Connect Tissue Res.* 1977; 5:15–17.

37. Burkhardt S. Tissue Healing and Repair. National Athletic Trainers Association Professional Preparation Conference. Nashville, Tenn; 1979.

38. Dingle JT. The role of lysosomal enzymes in skeletal tissue. *J Bone Joint Surg.* 1973; 55B:87–95.

39. Peacock EE. Collagenolysis: The other side of the equation. *World J Surg.* 1980; 4:297–302.

40. Woessner FJ, Howell DS. The enzymatic degradation of connective tissue matrices. In: Owen R, Goodfellow J, Bullough P, eds. *Scientific Foundation of Orthopaedics and Traumatology.* Philadelphia, Pa: W B Saunders Co; 1980:232–240.

41. Butler DL, Kay MD, Stouffer DC. Comparison of material properties in fasicle-bone units from human patellar tendon and knee ligaments. *J Biomech.* 1986; 19:425–432.

42. Mawghan DW, Godt RE. A quantitative analysis of elastic, entropic, electrostatic and osmotic forces within relaxed skinned muscle fibers. *Biophys Struct Mech.* 1980; 7:17–40.

43. Borg TK, Caufield JB. Morphology of connective tissue in skeletal muscle. *Tissue Cell.* 1980; 12:197–207.

44. Ishikawa H, Sawada H, Yamada E. Surface and internal morphology of skeletal muscle. In: Peachey LD, Adrian RH, Geiger SR, eds. *Skeletal Muscle.* Baltimore, Md: American Physiological Society; 1983:1–22.

45. Kakulas BA, Adams RD. *Diseases of Muscle: Pathological Foundations of Clinical Myology.* 4th ed. Philadelphia, Pa: Harper & Row; 1985:3–60.

46. Podalsky RJ, Schoenberg M. Force generation and shortening in skeletal muscle. In: Peachey LD, Adrian RH, Geiger SR, eds. *Skeletal Muscle.* Baltimore, Md: American Physiological Society; 1983:173–174.

47. Stolov WC, Weilepp TG. Passive length tension relationships of intact muscle, epimysium, and tendon in normal and denervated gastrocmenius of the rat. *Arch Phys Med Rehabil.* 1966; 47:612–620.

48. Schoenberg M, Brenner B, Chalovich JM, et al. Cross bridge attachment in relaxed muscle. *Adv Exp Med Biol.* 1984; 170:269–284.

49. Cecchi G, Griffiths PJ, Taylor S. The kinetics of cross bridge attachment and detachment studied by high frequency stiffness measurements. *Adv Exp Med Biol.* 1984; 170:641–655.

50. Hill DK. Tension due to interaction between the sliding filaments in resting striated muscle: The effect of stimulation. *J Physiol.* 1968; 199:637–684.

51. Stanish WD, Curwin SL, Bryson G. Flexibility in the prevention and recovery from sports injuries. American Academy Orthopaedic Surgeons; 1989. In press.

52. Garrett WE, Califf JC, Bassett HF. Histochemical cor-

relates of hamstring injuries. *Am J Sports Med.* 1984; 12:98–103.

53. Nikolaou PK, MacDonald BL, Bilsson RR, et al. Biomechanical and histological evaluation of muscle after controlled strain. *Am J Sports Med.* 1987; 15:9–14.

54. Garrett WE, Nikolaou BK, Rubbeck BM, et al. The effect of muscle architecture in the biomechanical failure properties of skeletal muscle under passive extension. *Am J Sports Med.* 1988; 16:7–12.

55. Lehto M, Jarvinen M, Nelimarkka O. Scar formation after muscle injury: A histological and artoradiographical study in rats. *Arch Orthop Trauma Scand.* 1986; 104:366–370.

56. Lehto M, Jarvinen M. Collagen and glycosaminoglycan synthesis of injured gastrocnemius muscle in rat. *Eur Surg Res.* 1985; 17:179–185.

57. Lehto M, Sims TJ, Bailey AJ. Skeletal muscle injury: Molecular changes in the collagen during healing. *Res Exp Med.* 1985; 185:95–106.

58. Lehto M, Duance VC, Restall D. Collagen and fibronectin in a healing skeletal muscle injury. *J Bone Joint Surg.* 1985; 65B:820–828.

59. Carlson BM, Faulkner JA. The regeneration of skeletal muscle fibers following injury: A review. *Med Sci Sports Exerc.* 1983; 15:187–198.

60. Snow M. Myogenic cell formation in regenerating rat skeletal muscle injured by mincing. *Anat Rec.* 1977; 188:181–200.

61. Jarvinen M. Healing of a crush injury in rat striated muscle. *Acta Chir Scand.* 1976; 142:47–56.

62. Ippolito E, Natoli PG, Postacchini F. Morphological, immunochemical and biochemical study of rabbit achilles tendon at various ages. *J Bone Joint Surg.* 1980; 62A:583–598.

63. Hana H, Yamauro T, Takeda T. Experimental studies on connective tissue of capsular ligament. *Acta Orthop Scand.* 1976; 47:473–479.

64. Mohan S, Radha E. Age related changes in muscle connective tissue: Acid mucopolysaccharides and structural glycoproteins. *Exp Gerontol.* 1981; 16:385–392.

65. Viidik A. Connective tissues—Possible implications of the temporal changes for the aging process. *Mech Age Dev.* 1979; 9:267–285.

66. Danielson CC. Thermal shrinkage of reconstituted collagen fibrils: Shrinkage characteristics upon in vitro maturation. *Mech Age Dev.* 1981; 15:269–278.

67. Balzas EA. Intracellular matrix of connective tissue. In: Finch C, Hayflick L, eds. *Handbook of the Biology of Aging.* New York, NY: Van Nostrand Reinhold; 1977:222–240.

68. Birari-Varga M, Biro T. Thermoanalytical investigation on the age related changes in articular cartilage, meniscus and tendon. *Gerontology.* 1971; 17:2–15.

69. Kastelic J, Palley I, Baer E. A structural model for tendon crimping. *J Biomech.* 1980; 13:887–893.

70. Boone DC, Azen SP. Normal range of motion of joints in male subjects. *J Bone Joint Surg.* 1979; 61A:756–759.

71. Hunter SC, Etchison WC, Halpern BC. Standards and norms of fitness and flexibility in the high school athlete. *Athlet Training.* 1985; 16:210–212.

72. Kendall HO, Kendall FP. Normal flexibility according to age groups. *J Bone Joint Surg.* 1948; 30A:690–694.

73. Leighton JR. Flexibility characteristics of males ten to eighteen years of age. *Arch Phys Med Rehabil.* 1956; 37:494–499.

74. Tucker JE. *Measurement of Joint Range of Motion of Older Individuals.* Palo Alto, Calif: Stanford University; 1964. Masters thesis.

75. Smith JR, Walder JM. Knee and elbow range of motion in healthy older individuals. *Phys Occup Ther Geriatr.* 1983; 2:31–38.

76. Walker JM, Sue D, Miles-Elkousy N, et al. Active mobility of the extremities in older subjects. *Phys Ther.* 1984; 64:919–923.

77. Boone DC, Azen SP, Lin CM, et al. Reliability of goniometric measurements. *Phys Ther.* 1978; 58:1355–1360.

78. Frekany GA, Leslie DK. Effects of an exercise program on selected flexibility movements of senior citizens. *The Gerontologist.* 1975; 15:182–183.

79. Evans EB, Eggers GWN, Butler JK, et al. Experimental immobilization and remobilization of rat knee joints. *J Bone Joint Surg.* 1960; 42A:737–758.

80. Akeson WH, Woo SLY, Amiel D, et al. The connective tissue response to immobility: Biochemical changes in periarticular connective tissue of the immobilized rabbit knee. *Clin Orthop.* 1973; 93:356–362.

81. Enneking WF, Horowicz M. The intra-articular effects of immobilization on the human knee. *J Bone Joint Surg.* 1972; 54A:973–985.

82. Amiel D, Woo SLY, Harwook FL, et al. The effect of immobilization on collagen turnover in connective tissue: A biochemical–biomechanical correlation. *Acta Orthop Scand.* 1982; 53:325–332.

83. Akeson WH. An experimental study of joint stiffness. *J Bone Joint Surg.* 1961; 43A:1022–1034.

84. Akeson WH, Amiel D, LaViolette D. The connective tissue response to immobility: A study of the chondroitin-4 and chondroitin-6 sulfate and dermatan sulfate changes in periarticular connective tissue of control and immobilized knees of dogs. *Clin Orthop.* 1967; 51:183–197.

85. Akeson WH, Amiel D, LaViolette D, et al. The connective tissue response to immobility: An accelerated aging response? *Exp Geront.* 1968; 3:289–301.

86. Akeson WH, Woo SLY, Amiel D, et al. Rapid recovery from contracture in rabbit hindlimb. *Clin Orthop.* 1977; 122:359–365.

87. Amiel D. Akeson WH, Harwook FL, et al. The effect of immobilization of the types of collagen synthesized in periarticular connective tissue. *Connect Tissue Res.* 1980; 8:27–32.

88. Amiel D, Frey C, Woo SLY, et al. Value of hylauronic acid in the prevention of contracture formation. *Clin Orthop.* 1985; 196:306–311.

89. Peacock EE. Comparison of collagenous tissue surrounding normal and immobilized joints. *Surg Forum.* 1963; 14:440–441.

90. Gossman MR, Sahrmann SA, Rose SJ. Review of length associated changes in muscle: Experimental evidence and clinical implications. *Phys Ther.* 1982; 62:1799–1808.

91. Kelsen SG, Wolanski T. Effect of elastase induced emphysema on diaphragm structure. *Am Rev Resp Dis.* 1982:208.

92. Sunderland S, Ray LJ. Denervation changes in mammilian striated muscle. *J Neurol Neurosurg Psychiatr.* 1956; 13:159–177.

93. Rigby BJ, Hirai N, Spikes JD, et al. The mechanical properties of rat tail tendon. *J Gen Physiol.* 1959; 43:265–283.

94. Mason T, Rigby BJ. Thermal transitions in collagen. *Biochim Biophys Acta.* 1963; 66:448–450.

95. Rigby BJ. The effect of mechanical extension upon the thermal stability of collagen. *Biochim Biophys Acta.* 1964; 79:334–363.

96. Lehmann JF, Masock AJ, Warren CG, et al. Effect of therapeutic temperatures on tendon extensibility. *Arch Phys Med Rehabil.* 1970; 51:481–487.

97. Warren CG, Lehmann JF, Koblanski JN. Elongation of rat tail tendon: Effect of load and temperature. *Arch Phys Med Rehabil.* 1971; 52:465–474.

98. Warren CG, Lehmann JF, Koblanski HN. Heat and stretch procedures: An evaluation using rat tail tendon. *Arch Phys Med Rehabil.* 1976; 57:122–126.

99. Kottke FJ, Pavley DJ, Ptak DA. The rationale for prolonged stretching for correction of shortening of connective tissue. *Arch Phys Med Rehabil.* 1966; 47:345–352.

100. Asmussen E, Boje OVE. Body temperature and capacity for work. *Acta Phys Scand.* 1945; 10:1–22.

101. Saltin B, Hermansen L. Esophageal, rectal and muscle temperature during exercise. *J Appl Physiol.* 1966; 21:1757.

102. Henrickson AS, Fredricksson K, Persson I. The effect of heat and stretching on the range of hip motion. *J Orthop Sports Phys Ther.* 1984; 6:110–115.

103. Lehmann JF, DeLateur BJ. Therapeutic heat. In: Lehmann JF, ed. *Therapeutic Heat and Cold.* 3rd ed. Baltimore Md: Williams & Wilkins Co; 1982:404–563.

104. Olson JE, Stravino VD. A review of cryotherapy. *Phys Ther.* 1972; 52:840–853.

105. Miglietta O. Electromyographic characteristics of clonus and influence of cold. *Arch Phys Med Rehabil.* 1976; 45:508–512.

106. Kelley M. Effectiveness of cryotherapy technique on spasticity. *Phys Ther.* 1969; 49:347–353.

107. Wolf SL, Leibetter MD, Basmajian JV. Effect of a specific cutaneous cold stimulus on single motor unit activity of gastrocnemius muscle in man. *Am J Phys Med.* 1976; 55:177–183.

108. Knight KL. *Cryotherapy: Theory, Technique and Physiology.* Chattanooga, Tenn: Chattanooga Corp; 1986:63–66.

109. Prentice WE. An electromyographic analysis of the effectiveness of heat or cold and stretching for inducing relaxation in an injured muscle. *J Orthop Sports Phys Ther.* 1982; 3:133–140.

110. Halkovich LR, Personius WJ, Clamann HP, et al. Effect of flouri-methane spray on passive hip flexion. *Phys Ther.* 1981; 61:185–189.

111. Newton R. Effects of vapocoolants on passive hip flexion in health subjects. *Phys Ther.* 1985; 65:1034–1036.

112. Koury S, Mamary M, Kagan R, et al. Effect of flourimethane spray on hamstring extensibility during "contract-relax" and active stretching. *Phys Ther.* 1986; 66:806.

113. Leighton JR. A study of the effect of progressive weight training on flexibility. *J Assoc Phys Ment Rehabil.* 1964; 18:101–109.

114. Wilmore JH, Parr RB, Girandola RN, et al. Physiological alterations consequent to circuit weight training. *Med Sci Sports Exerc.* 1978; 10:79–84.

115. Leighton JR, Holmes D, Benson J, et al. A study on the effectiveness of ten different methods of progressive resistive exercise on the development of strength, flexibility, girth and body weight. *J Assoc Phys Ment Rehabil.* 1967; 21:78–81.

116. Tipton CM, Matthes RD, Maynard JA, et al. The influence of physical activity on ligaments and tendons. *Med Sci Sports Exerc.* 1975; 7:165–175.

117. Noyes FR, Trovik PJ, Hyde WB. Biomechanics of ligament failure: An analysis of immobilization, exercise and deconditioning effects in primates. *J Bone Joint Surg.* 1974; 56A:1406–1418.

118. Vailas AC, Tipton CM, Matthes RC, et al. Physical activity and its influence on the repair process of medial collateral ligaments. *Connect Tissue Res.* 1981; 9:25–31.

119. Woo SLY, Ritter MA, Amiel D, et al. The biomechanical and biochemical properties of swine tendons—long term effects of exercise on the digital extensors. *Connect Tissue Res.* 1980; 7:177–183.

120. Kuist M, Jarvinen M. Clinical, histochemical and biomechanical features in repair of muscle and tendon injuries. *Int J Sports Med.* 1982; 3:12–14.

121. Garrick JG, Requa RK. Girls' sports injuries in high school athletics. *JAMA.* 1978; 239:2245–2248.

122. Garrick JG. Characterization of patient population in a sports medicine facility. *Phys Sportsmed.* 1985; 13:73–75.

123. Bass AL. Injuries of the leg in football and ballet. *Proc R Soc Med.* 1967; 60:527–532.

124. Garrett WE, Safran MR, Seaber AV, et al. Biomechanical comparison of stimulated and nonstimulated skeletal muscle pulled to failure. *Am J Sports Med.* 1987; 15:448–454.

125. Agre JC: Hamstring injuries: Proposed etiological factors, prevention and treatment. *Sports Med.* 1985; 2:21–33.

126. Zachazewski JE, Reischl SR. Flexibility for the runner: Specific program considerations. *Top Acute Care Trauma Rehabil.* 1986; 1:9–27.

127. de Vries HA. Evaluation of static stretching procedures for improvement of flexibility. *Res Q.* 1962; 3:222–229.

128. Zebas CJ, Rivera ML. Retention of flexibility in selected joints after cessation of a stretching exercise program. In: Dotson CO, Humphrey JH, eds. *Exercise Physiology: Current Selected Research.* New York, NY: AMS Press Inc; 1985.

129. Schultz P. Flexibility: The day of the static stretch. *Physician Sportsmed.* 1979; 7:109–117.

130. Brukett LN. Causative factors in hamstring strains. *Med Sci Sports Exerc.* 1970; 2:39–42.

131. Voss DE, Ionta MK, Myers GJ. *Proprioceptive Neuromuscular Facilitation Patterns and Techniques.* 3rd ed. Philadelphia, Pa: Harper & Row; 1968:xi–xviii.

132. Wallin D, Ekblom B, Grahn R, et al. Improvement of muscle flexibility, a comparison between two techniques. *Am J Sports Med.* 1985; 13:263–268.

133. Cornelius W, Jackson A. The effects of cryotherapy and PNF on hip extensor flexibility. *Athlet Training.* 1984; 19:183–184.

134. Prentice WE. A comparison of static stretching and PNF stretching for improving hip joint flexibility. *Athlet Training.* 1983; 18:56–59.

135. Louden KL, Bollier CE, Allison KA, et al. Effects of two stretching methods on the flexibility and retention of flexibility at the ankle joint in runners. *Phys Ther.* 1985; 65:698.

136. Markos PD. Ipsilateral and contralateral effects of proprioceptive neuromuscular facilitation techniques on hip motion and electromyographic activity. *Phys Ther.* 1979; 59:1366–1373.

137. Moore M, Hutton R. Electromyographic investigation of muscle stretching techniques. *Med Sci Sports Exerc.* 1980; 12:322–329.

138. Sady SP, Wortman M, Blanke D. Flexibility training: Ballistic, static or proprioceptive neuromuscular facilitation? *Arch Phys Med Rehabil.* 1982; 63:261–263.

139. Tanigawa MC. Comparison of the hold-relax procedure and passive mobilization of increasing muscle length. *Phys Ther.* 1972; 52:725–735.

140. Wiktorsson-Moller M, Oberg B, Ekstrand J, et al. Effects of warming up, massage, and stretching on range of motion and muscle strength in the lower extremity. *Am J Sports Med.* 1983; 11:249–252.

141. Condon SA, Hutton RS. Soleus muscle EMG activity and ankle dorsiflexion range of motion from stretching procedures. *Phys Ther.* 1987; 67:24–30.

142. Entyre BR, Abraham LD. Antagonist muscle activity during stretching: A paradox reassessed. Submitted. *Med Sci Sports Ex.* 1988; 1:285–289.

143. Madding SW, Wong JG, Hallum A, et al. Effects of duration or passive stretching on hip abduction range of motion. *J Orthop Sports Phys Ther.* 1987; 8:409–416.

144. Hubley CL, Kozey JW, Stanish WD. The effects of static stretching exercises and stationary cycling on range of motion at the hip joint. *J Orthop Sports Phys Ther.* 1984; 6:104–109.

145. Garrett WE, Safran MR, Seaber AV, et al. Biomechanical comparison of stimulated and nonstimulated muscle pulled to failure. *Am J Sports Med.* 1987; 15:448–454.

146. Crosman LJ, Chateauvert SR, Weisberg J. The effects of massage to the hamstring muscle group on range of motion. *J Orthop Sports Phys Ther.* 1984; 6:168–172.

147. de Vries HA. Electromyographic observations of the effects of static stretching on muscular distress. *Res Q.* 1961; 32:468–479.

148. de Vries HA. Prevention of muscular distress after exercise. *Res Q.* 1961; 32:177–185.

149. Nelson DL, Hutton RS. Dynamic and static stretch responses in muscle spindle receptors in fatigued muscle. *Med Sci Sports Exerc.* 1985; 17:445–450.

150. Hutton RS, Nelson DL. Stretch sensitivity of Golgi tendon organ in fatigued gastrocoeleus muscle. *Med Sci Sports Exerc.* 1986; 18:69–74.

151. Chavpil M. *Physiology of Connective Tissue.* London: Butterworths Publishers Ltd; 1967.

152. Jarvinen M, Aho AJ, Lehto M, et al. Age dependent repair of muscle rupture: A histological and morphological study in rats. *Acta Orthop Scand.* 1983; 54:64–67.

153. Almekinders LC, Gilbert JA. Healing of experimental muscle strains and the effects of non-steroidal anti-inflammatory medication. *Am J Sports Med.* 1986; 14:303–308.

154. Reed BV. Effect of high voltage pulsed electrical stimulation on microvascular permeability of plasma proteins: A possible mechanism of minimizing edema. *Phys Ther.* 1988; 68:491–495.

14

Weight Training and Conditioning

Michael T. Sanders

INTRODUCTION

Numerous programs of physical exercise have been proposed for improving the physiological capacity of the various systems of the body. To achieve a basic level of performance a scientifically based, systematized program of training is fundamental.[1] Optimizing weight training and conditioning necessitates the systematic application of intensity, the "right exercises," the proper frequency, and appropriate duration of the training program.

A basic background is essential to enable an exercise prescription to reach potential.[2] Comprehension of the dynamics of weight training fundamentals includes understanding specific performance requirements of the individual. All individuals have a specific level of biologic functioning that prevails during various activities.[3] An activity performance profile is used to determine the extent of the certain physiological, neurological, and histological elements to the activity.

Activity Performance Profile

There is a causal relationship between the human body and the environment, with the body adapting to the stimuli to which it is exposed. In training, the work performed is considered to be the cause, while the body's adaptation is the effect.[1]

The three primary factors associated with performance are cardiovascular conditioning, neuromuscular coordination, and skill.[4] In order to achieve an optimal training effect the amount or preparation for activities varies according to the desired outcome of the activity. The specific goals of the training program for each individual must be determined as training progresses. The major thrust in the initial development of the training program is the creation of a performance pyramid model (Fig 14–1).

The model may be pictured as a structure with a base populated by recreational enthusiasts and a peak containing athletes capable of the highest level of physical performance. The first task in analyzing an individual's goals in the training program is to determine what level the individual wishes to attain on the pyramid. Secondly, determination of cardiovascular, neuromuscular, and skill involvement relevant to the pyramid level will lead the program designer to plan training programs that are specific to the event and that are prescribed in appropriate amounts. The quantity of work to be performed in a training session must be set in accordance with

1. Individual abilities
2. The phase of training
3. The correct ratio between the volume and intensity of training

If the training intensity is properly administered, proper athletic development will result, leading to an adequate degree of training (reaching the appropriate level of performance relevant to the person's desired level on the performance pyramid). The next step in the evaluative process is to refer to an Activity Performance Profile (APP) (Fig 14–2), which incorporates a neuromuscular continuum. That is, one end of the continuum is designed to show strength as dominant, while the opposite end stresses muscular endurance. An athletic performance profile is then established for certain activities by subjectively assigning a grade for each primary factor. From these primary factors certain physiological, neurological, and histological elements are ultimately determined as being responsible for physical performance. In assisting an individual to achieve a particular level on the performance pyramid, the sports physical therapist's principal objectives will depend upon the preceding elements. The amount of

239

ELITE ATHLETICS
LEVEL 3[a]

BASIC ATHLETIC PERFORMANCE
LEVEL 2[b]

RECREATIONAL ATHLETIC PERFORMANCE
LEVEL 1[c]

[a]The individuals desiring to achieve this level are only those who have ability to make national, international professional teams or organizations
[b]The individuals desiring to achieve this level are those competing on collegiate levels, high school levels, or involved in organized training or competitions
[c]The individuals desiring to achieve this level are those members who are not part of competing organizations, desiring basic fitness levels or engaging in a training program for rehabilitation of an injury

Figure 14-1. Performance pyramid.

preparation time for activities varies according to the level the individual desires to achieve on the performance pyramid.

The first task in analyzing a performance level is to determine the extent to which cardiovascular conditioning, neuromuscular coordination, and skill contribute to that performance level. The sports physical therapist should understand the physical requirements of that desired performance level and then proceed to develop programs that will meet those requirements.

The first steps in developing a program is to follow preliminary assessment guidelines to determine the parameters of the individual's desired level of fitness and to detect any contraindications to exercise:

1. **To reduce the risks related to any contraindications for exercise individuals should be examined by a physician**
2. **Formal laboratory evaluation if so indicated (e.g., cardiovascular problems, flexibility problems, muscle strength imbalance, orthopedic anomalies)**

	A	B	O	Y	Z	
Anaerobic						Aerobic
Muscular	—|——|——|——|——					Muscular
Strength			Null			Endurance
Power						

Requirements	Distance Running	Football	Golf
Anaerobic	B	B	A
Muscular Strength	B	A	B
Power	B	A	B
Aerobic	Z	Y	O
Muscular Endurance	Z	B	B

Figure 14-2. Activity performance profile.

3. Assessment of current fitness level employing actual strength and cardiovascular testing
4. Determine individuals desired level of performance on the performance pyramid
5. Determine the physiological basis of an individual's activity using the APP
6. Determine specific goals of the program:
   a. Strength development and maintenance
   b. Muscle hypertrophy
   c. Changes in body composition
   d. Improve muscular strength and endurance
   e. Power development

The application of a training program results in several anatomic, physiological, and psychological changes in the body, and a thorough understanding of the physiology of the energy systems will decrease the risk of overtraining and enhance the potential for optimal performance.

Mechanics of the Muscular System

The human body adapts and improves in direct relation to the type of stimuli to which it is exposed. All locomotive muscles are composed of varying proportions of separate and distinct muscle fiber types. The individual involved in training is exposed to a series of stimuli that disturb the muscle fibers and the normal biologic state.[3] Following training there is a period of time during the recovery process when the biochemical sources of energy are not only replaced but may exceed the initial level.[5] If maximal intensity stimuli are overemphasized, however, it has been shown that muscle fibers will be damaged. Microscopic tears to the fibers cause fraying and loss of resilience similar to a rubber band that has been snapped too often. This is a factor in overtraining, although it has not been shown why overtrained muscles lose their ability to contract.[6]

Muscles are composed of varying number of motor units that innervate muscle fibers that contribute to such contractile properties as speed, power, and resistance to fatigue. Some of the more relevant differences between fiber types are outlined below:

1. *Energy source.* Fast fiber types have higher concentrations of glycolytic enzymes but few oxidative enzymes. Energy production is extremely rapid but also terminates rapidly. Slow fibers produce energy more slowly than fast fibers but energy production continues for long periods of time. They contain high concentrations of oxidative enzymes and require a continuous supply of oxygen for optimum function of slow fibers.[7]
2. *Mechanical characteristics.* The contractile apparatus of fast-twitch fibers is extremely developed and suited for major power productive movements. Conversely, the slow-twitch appa-

ratus is suited for long-term submaximal contractions.

3. *Blood supply.* The metabolic apparatus for fast-twitch fibers is not suited for utilization of oxygen; consequently the fibers are not perfused with a large blood supply. The long-term contractile properties of slow-twitch fibers necessitates a greater percentage of capillaries.

4. *Neuromuscular recruitment.* The central nervous system (CNS) controls the specific patterns of contraction and relaxation of the muscular system. The final link between the CNS and the muscular system is the motor unit, which is the nerve plus the muscle fibers it supplies. The CNS dictates which fiber will be recruited for each task, with heavier tasks requiring more fibers.

Relative to the prior information the training program has its effects on the functional state of the neuromuscular system. In this system both the neural (input) component and the muscle function (output) will be affected by training.[8] Because the movement of the muscle is directed by several neural command and feedback systems, it is often difficult to assess in which of the two components the changes caused by training have been most remarkable. Furthermore, it is often impossible to differentiate the pure effects of training from those of learning.[9] Training causes a motor act to be learned. Thus, learning involves training, either physical, mental, or both. Coordination of activity also takes place "inside" the muscle (some researchers refer to this as muscle memory), one of several hundred motor units responsible for the specific activity. Basmajian introduced the concept of motor unit training, which means that human subjects are consciously able to control the firing of the motor unit firing in various skeletal muscle.[9] After a short period of time of training almost all persons are able to isolate one or more motor units from a muscle fiber and turn it on or off in a desired manner. Isolation of several motor units requires a particularly high order of control by the subject, however. The APP illustrates this point by revealing that only elite athletes on the peak of the pyramid would be able to perform these types of neuromuscular activities. Motor unit training can also lead to such skills as the ability to control or deliberately change the firing rate of one spinal motor neuron.[9] It would seem reasonable to suggest that early changes in strength may largely be accounted for by the neural factors with a gradually increasing contribution of the hypertrophic factor as the training increases.[10]

The training program is actually a type of physiological conditioning. Physiological conditioning refers to a planned program of exercise directed toward improving the functional capacity of a particular bodily system. Within the context of these parameters it becomes essential to identify the three types of muscular contractions:

1. *Isometric contraction.* This type of contraction occurs when a muscle attempts to shorten but is unable to overcome the resistance. Considerable muscular force is generated during an isometric contraction, with no noticeable shortening of the muscle.

2. *Concentric contraction.* This type of contraction is the type of muscular contraction that occurs in dynamic rhythmical activities when the muscle endings come together (shortens) as it develops tension.

3. *Eccentric contraction.* This type of contraction occurs when a weight is lowered through a range of motion (ROM) and a muscle lengthens at a controlled rate.

The term muscular contraction may be thought of as the current state of a muscle when tension is generated across contractile proteins (i.e., myosin, actin, tropomyosin, tropinin, C, I, and T). The force of the contraction is dependent upon the external load, the direction of the muscular action, and the magnitude of that action.[9]

Two additional differences between concentric and eccentric contractions should be mentioned. First it is well documented that slopes representing electromyographs and force relationships are different in these two types of contractions.[11] To attain a certain force level requires a much lower level of motor unit activation in eccentric contractions than concentric contractions. Secondly, oxygen consumption is much lower during eccentric exercise than in comparable concentric exercise.[12] These findings indicate that neural input and output relationships of the two exercises are very different and that the mechanical efficiency of eccentric exercises may be several times higher than that of pure concentric exercises. The most important consideration in determining differences between contraction types, however, is the tension that can be produced by a muscle fiber or fiber type. This force of contraction is ultimately dependent upon the following seven variables[4,8]:

1. Number of motor units firing
2. Size of motor units firing
3. Rate of firing of individual motor units
4. Velocity of muscle shortening
5. Length of muscle fiber
6. Condition of muscle fiber
7. Age of the fibers

As mentioned previously, various sports and events make differing demands on the physiological capacities of the body (APP). The principal categories are defined

as anaerobic, aerobic, muscular endurance, muscular strength, and power. Muscular strength is defined as being the greatest force an athlete or an individual is able to exert for a given contraction:

1. The maximum force that can be exerted against an immovable object (isometric contraction)
2. The heaviest weight that can be lifted against gravity where muscle endings come together (concentric contraction)
3. The heaviest weight that can be lowered at a controlled rate and the muscle lengthens (eccentric contraction)

The highest absolute values of strength are necessary for those sports and events in which exceptional external resistance has to be mastered, e.g., weightlifting, football, and throwing events in track and field.

Power is the ability of the individual to overcome resistance by a high-speed contraction. Power (work/time) is dependent upon the individual's level of strength. Time quantification of power has been achieved with the introduction of isokinetic equipment and can be defined as the maximal (or submaximal) torque that can be developed against a preset, prelimiting device at a slow contractile velocity (maximal strength) or a fast contractile velocity (muscular endurance). Thus, although raw strength is an important factor in power output, so too is speed. Individuals may possess great strength, but unless they can exert that strength quickly, they will not be powerful. Experimentally, it has been found that the maximum power output is achieved when lifting a weight that is between one half and two thirds of the maximum that can be moved.[12,13] The two determinants of power output are concerned with the speed of the barbell and the speed of limb movement. When heavy weights are lifted the speed of movement will be low and so will the power output. As the weight is reduced the speed of movement will increase, and provided that the increment in speed exceeds the decrement in weight, the power output will increase.[12,13] This information is of greatest importance to sports physical therapists during the early stages of the program development, when muscular strength is of primary concern.

Muscular endurance is the ability of a muscle to perform repeated contractions against an immovable object (isometric contraction) and against gravity when the muscle endings come together and lengthen (concentric and eccentric).

The effect of conditioning on the physiological system primarily centers on hypertrophy, although strength, endurance, and power gains can be achieved without increases in size.[4,7,8] Table 14–1 compares the biologic changes that result if an individual engages in a conditioning program to enhance muscular strength, endurance, or power.

TABLE 14-1. PHYSIOLOGICAL EFFECTS OF WTC PROGRAMS

Biological Factors	Strength	Endurance	Power
Collagen content	Increase	Increase	Increase
Connective tissue	Increase	Increase	Increase
Tendons and ligaments	Increase	Increase	Increase
Sarcoplasm	Increase	Increase	Increase
Actin			
Myosin			
Tropinin(C,I,T)			
Tropomyosin	Increase	Increase	Increase
Glycogen	Increase	Increase	Increase
Mitochondrion	Decrease	Moderate	Decrease
Fiber type response	FTW	FTW and FTR	FTW

PROGRAM PROCEDURES

The basic principles of training are frequency, volume, and intensity. These must be considered in all training programs, as their proper application will reduce the potential for overtraining and help to maximize performance.

The intensity of training is probably the most important and least understood of all training parameters. In exercise prescription it is sometimes hard to determine the intensity of the exercise that is most suitable for a certain individual. The intensity is the strength of the stimulus, or the concentration of the work executed per unit of time within a series of stimuli. Intensity may also be thought of as the quality of the training unit.[1,3] For cardiovascular endurance, the units of measurement of intensity consist of heart rate, stride rate, and so on. For conditioning programs, "spheres of intensity" are used and include parameters such as the weight lifted and the height, distance, or speed at which the training modality is performed. Thus the more work that is performed per time unit, the higher the intensity. Intensity is a function of the following parameters:[1,3,8,9]

1. Strength of the nervous system stimuli employed in training
2. The load and speed of performing a movement, which determines the strength of the stimulus
3. The variation of the exercise bouts
4. The rest between repetitions
5. The psychological strain that results from the exercise bout

Obviously the intensity of an exercise varies in accordance with different activities. Intensity in condi-

tioning programs is fairly easy to quantify. For exercise performed against resistance, or exercises developing high velocity, a percentage of maximal intensity is employed. Repetition maximum (RM) is defined as the maximum amount of weight that can be lifted for a specific number of repetitions. The "sphere of intensity"[1,3] shown in Table 14–2 illustrates the percentage differences between maximum intensity, medium intensity, light intensity, and easy intensity.

The volume of training, which is sometimes referred to as duration of training incorporates three parts:

1. The time or duration of training
2. The distance or total weight lifted per time unit
3. The number of repetitions of an exercise

The term volume indicates the total quantity of work completed during a session of exercise. The unit of measurement most often employed is kilograms. The volume of each work bout should be carried to the fatigue point or to the required percentage of the fatigue point (repetition maximum). The fatigue point results when the exercise cannot be performed or sustained. It is not known what causes the fatigue point at a maximal level of intensity but phosphagen depletion appears to be primarily involved.[3,5,7,8,10,13-16] The mechanisms involved in controlling adaptations to higher levels of exercise intensity are poorly understood at this time. Some of the more widely accepted effects of exercise on the bodies functional capacities appear to be[3,5,7,8,10,13-16]:

1. Glycogen depletion in the muscle
2. Inactivation of the mitochondria
3. Low blood sugar
4. Fluid and mineral imbalances
5. A compromise of the ability of the contractile proteins to transduce energy into movement
6. Depressed blood circulation
7. Redistribution of the blood flow

The dynamics of volume of training are directly related to the performance level desired by the individual, the performance requirements of the activity, and the training objectives for that particular cycle of training.

The time unit at which an individual is exposed to a series of stimuli is called the frequency of training. The term frequency refers to the relation expressed in time between working and recovery phases of train-

ing.[17] The specific rest interval between sets of exercise or days of exercise depends directly on the specified volume and intensity of training. Frequent bouts of maximal intensity and high volumes of training will lead to critical fatigue, high exhaustion, or even injury. A positive training process is the result of correctly timed alternation between stimulation and regeneration, between work and rest. The adaptability processes occur only when the stimuli reach an intensity proportional to an individual's threshold capacity.[18] A high volume of work below a minimal intensity level (below 30% of one's RM) does not result in adaptation because a higher level of intensity is required to initiate such adaptation.[2] It is possible to exceed the optimal level of stimulation by demanding too much work from the individual or by miscalculating the training ratio for volume and intensity.

Periodization

The concept of periodization was originally proposed by Matveyev in 1961 to increase training efficiency by employing a variety of plans.[1,3,17] These plans extend from short-term to long-term elite athlete training programs. If scientific training guidelines are used, planning can become a primary tool by which the sports physical therapist can maximize stated training objectives. The typical cycles of training are called macro, meso, and micro, depending on their duration[1,3,17,18]:

1. Macro-cycles. Half-yearly cycles, yearly cycles, or even 4-year Olympic cycles for elite athletes
2. Meso-cycles. Cycles with a duration of 3 to 6 weeks
3. Micro-cycles. The cyclical structure of a training session up to weekly cycles

Periodization is the continuous sequence of cycles in the process of achieving the training objectives.[18] There are limits to the capacity of the individual to keep improving. Research has shown that this developmental process cannot continue steadily in a linear fashion.[1,2,3,5,13,14,16] This would seem to indicate that in designing a program regardless of the duration it becomes a matter of demarcating more clearly the relationship between the basic categories of training:

Aim of performance	Level on the performance pyramid
Structure of performance	Activity performance profile
Training load	Frequency, volume, and intensity

Consequently considerations for increasing demands on the individual should only proceed from the assumption that all of the above factors are interrelated and jointly affected.

TABLE 14-2. "SPHERES" OF INTENSITY

Heavy intensity—90%–100% of maximal effort
Medium intensity—80%–89% of maximal effort
Light intensity—70%–79% of maximal effort
Low intensity—below 70% of maximal effort

Specific Training Programs

For over 30 years the active investigation of the optimal weight training program has been examined. From various training modalities to the optimum number of repetitions and sets, this optimal program has been thoroughly researched and absorbed into the practitioner's program development. There remain many questions regarding the integration and regulation of intensity, however.

In 1948, Delorme and Watkins were primarily concerned with rehabilitation of patients with knee injuries.[19] Their exercise regimens allowed the practitioner to quantify and objectify the loading. Identifying the terms RM, and the number of complete and continuous executions of an exercise (set) were major contributions. The Delorme technique of training is to start with a light weight for a given number of repetitions and progressively increase the resistance until 10 RM is achieved.

Zinovieff believed that the Delorme technique was too fatiguing and placed too great a strain on the muscular system.[20] Employing the "Oxford Technique" the researcher merely reversed Delorme's procedure, beginning with 10 RM and decreasing until 50% of 10 RM was achieved.

Studies conducted by Macqueen,[21] Berger,[22,23] Stull and Clarke,[24] Dons and Bollerup,[25] Sanders,[26] and Atha[27] examined the following parameters of weight training programs:

1. The optimal amount of resistance for achieving gains in muscular strength and endurance
2. The optimal number of repetitions and sets for training programs
3. The effects of different modalities of training on muscular strength, endurance, and power
4. The effects of concentric, eccentric, and isometric contractions on muscular strength, endurance, and power

It is known that the intensity of the loading on the muscular system is the main determinant of whether or not increments in strength, power, and size will occur. Training at low resistance (30% RM) is ineffective for increasing strength, even though the individual may perform hundreds of contractions in a training session. On the other hand five to six contractions at 90% RM will prove effective in increasing both the size and strength of the muscle groups.[27]

Table 14–3 presents a compilation of various weight training programs that are currently employed by sports physical therapists.

As mentioned previously, differences in training program objectives change the configuration of the exercise stimulus. Adaptive changes that take place are a result of the frequency, volume, and intensity incorporated. The greater the need for transfer of training ef-

TABLE 14-3. TRAINING PROGRAMS

Programs	Set	Repetition (%RM)
Delorme and Watkins[19]	1st	10 (50% of 10 RM)
	2nd	10 (75% of 10 RM)
	3rd	10 (100% of 10 RM)
Oxford technique[20]	1st	10 (100% of 10 RM)
	2nd	10 (75% of 10 RM)
	3rd	10 (50% of 10 RM)
Macqueen[21]	3 sets	10 (100% of 10 RM)
	4–5 sets	2–3 (100% of 2–3 RM)
Berger[22]	3 sets	6 (100% of 6 RM)
Stone and Kroll[28]	1st	8 (50% of 4 RM)
	2nd	8 (80% of 4 RM)
	3rd	6 (90% of 4 RM)
	4th	4 (95% of 4 RM)
	5th	4 (100% of 4 RM)

fects to a specific skill movement the more important it is that the exercises selected mimic the angles, speed, and type of contraction desired.[1,3,5,28] Individuals requiring basic fitness will train much differently after the initial phases of training than an athlete requiring a high level of performance. Although the same is true for rehabilitation of an injury. The mechanics of the program are the same, the frequency, volume, and intensity are far different.

PLANNING THE PROGRAM

When the sports physical therapist develops a training plan one must follow certain requirements. Because the major objective of any training program is improvement of performance the typical goals associated with participation in the training program include

1. Muscular strength improvement
2. Muscular endurance improvement
3. Power development
4. Muscle hypertrophy or density
5. Changes in body composition

Consequently the development of the overall plan to achieve stated objectives will increase efficiency of the training program. The incorporation of a scientific basis in the methodology of planning is a necessity if the sports physical therapist and the client expects high efficiency. The following sections provide a detailed outline of the operational plan for a sports physical therapist (Table 14–4).

Medical Evaluation

Of major importance is determining whether the individual has any contraindication for specific exercises and the movements required for their performance. For postsurgical patients the restrictions are somewhat

TABLE 14-4. PLANNING THE TRAINING PROGRAM

1. Medical evaluation
2. Determine individuals major performance goals.
3. Determine physiological requirements of the activity.
4. Determine frequency of training program.
   a. Length of the training cycle(s)
      (1) macro-cycle—6 months to multiple years
      (2) meso-cycle—3 weeks to 6 months
      (3) micro-cycle—1 to 3 weeks
   b. Number of workouts per week
5. Determine repetition and set system to be used.
6. Select training modalities.
7. Select actual exercises to be used.
8. Select the order of the exercises.
9. Determine the volume of training to be done per session.
10. Determine integration and regulation of the intensity.
11. Determine starting load for training program.
12. Overtraining principles

higher. The selection of a training program or modality becomes a problem of time, money, space, availability, and the current status of the individual.

Performance Goals

Determination of the performance goals of the training program can be done by referring to the performance pyramid. The individual can express goals by identifying what level of the pyramid he or she would like to attain. This will directly affect the levels of volume and training that will be incorporated. Specific goals relative to rehabilitation, strength endurance, and power development will also determine volume and training parameters.

Physiological Requirements

This area can be directed to the APP, which will elicit the specific energy demands of the activity. As far as the physiological profile of activities are concerned, in the first 15 to 20 seconds the energy demands are supplied by the phosphate system [adensonine triphosphate–creatine phosphate (ATP/CP)] followed by the lactic acid (LA) system up to 2 minutes. If the event continues for longer periods of time, then the energy demands are supplied by the Krebs cycle and electron transport system.[1,3]

Frequency of Program

It is important in all training programs to determine the desired length of the training. To enhance the individual's adaptation to training as well as regeneration following demanding training sessions the specific cycle length must be determined. In order to avoid overtraining and stagnation the specific cyclical alternations of high- and low-intensity stimuli must be followed so that fatigue and rest are partners. There exists a wide variation in frequency patterns of workouts, from as many as five per week to as few as two per week.[4] Those physiological properties associated with protein turnover and the glycogen restoration appears to be the most important factors in returning muscle glycogen to the preexercise levels and restoring functional ability.[5,7,8,13,15,16] This suggests that the ideal pattern would be alternate days of training and rest.

Repetition and Set System

Many enigmas still surround the employment of specific rep and set systems. The major factor that determines the system to be employed is the goal of the training program. A javelin thrower will not utilize Delorme's repetition and set system for an entire macro-cycle, nor will a patient recently undergoing knee surgery employ four sets of 5 RM on terminal knee extension. Regardless of the goals of the training program the most often employed repetition and set regimen for the initial micro-cycle is Delorme's. During this initial cycle the following is, hopefully, achieved[18]:

1. Improved general physical preparation
2. Improved motor capabilities for specific activities
3. Improved exercise technique
4. Stimulated organism adaptation to increasing levels of high volume and intensity

After the initial base phase of conditioning the specific goals of the training program will necessitate the inclusion of different repetition and set regimens. A progressive increase in volume and intensity with a decrease in the number of repetitions would be the most efficient approach for optimal strength, endurance, and power gains. The training program for any elite sporting activity should replicate the demands of that activity (specificity training). There are numerous combinations of loading, repetition, and set regimens that may be used. The fact that many physiological factors play a role in athletic as well as normal activities dictates that many combinations of loading systems can be employed. The research relative to repetition and set systems can be summarized as follows:

1. Resistances of five to six repetitions seem to result in the greatest strength and power gains.
2. The effective range for muscular strength and endurance gains appear to be in the 2- to 10-RM range.
3. Beyond 20 RM strength gains are more related to biomotor and muscular endurance enhancement with very small gains (<5% in the 1 RM) in muscular strength.
4. Mere repetition of contractions (<30% RM) places little stress on the neuromuscular system and has little effect on the functional capacity of the muscular system.[19-27]

Training Modalities

The modality of training resulting in the most rapid muscular strength, endurance, and power development gains has not been clearly established. Several investigators have compared the effects of isometric, isotonic, and isokinetic forms of training for improving various physiological parameters.[19-26] Results indicate that the muscular adaptations that occur as a result of overloading appear to be specific to the modality used. Almost any modality used will result in some strength gains. The problem in training for a specific goal is to identify the specific adaptations that are required for specific muscle groups and then to adopt those methods of exercise that will produce them most efficiently. Pathological conditions require a more moderate approach, as a straight leg raise might be 1 RM for a knee patient. The selection of various training modalities—isotonic, isometric, or isokinetic—is determined by their availability, the current status of the individual, and the desire of the individual.

Order and Selection of Exercises

The selection and order of specific exercises are based on the analysis of the muscles and joint angles to be trained. Adaptations in the structure and function of the organism occur in such a fashion that the organism is better able to handle the stress that has or will be placed upon it. This is known as the SAID principle—specific adaptations to imposed demands.[28] A specific movement, speed of movement, or angle of movement necessitates the proper selection and subsequent arrangement of those exercises for performance. For elite athletic performance high-skill movements such as the power clean and snatch have a high degree of transferability for training in many sport skills. These exercises would not be appropriate, however, for individuals desiring basic fitness. The sequencing of exercises usually begins with those movements requiring large muscle groups and then proceeds to small muscle groups. Circuit weight training involves the sequential arrangement of exercises resulting in continuous activity.[2,4,28] Circuit weight training exercises are arranged in a circuit so that there is an alternation of leg, chest, back, and arm movements to prevent fatigue in any single area before the circuit is completed. Circuit training is used for basic fitness development and for those individuals who have not participated in training programs before. Regardless of the selection and order of the exercises, progressively overcoming increased loading is necessary for the development of strength, power, and endurance.

Volume and Intensity

In order to maximize the training program the individual has to plan programs specific to the desired outcome and that properly integrate the volume and intensity.[3] The appropriate stimulus administered at the correct time will result in maximum training efficiency. A positive adaptation process to increased training loads is the result of correctly timed alternation between stimulation and regeneration and between work and rest. As was mentioned previously the initial micro-cycle of base training has a general training effect regardless of the current state of the individual; beginners will show a dramatic change during the initial 3 weeks, but will eventually reach a plateau. Constant high volume and high intensity will eventually lead to overtraining and injury.[6] Volume is determined by multiplying the resistance by the repetitions performed, for example, 100 lb × 10 repetitions = 1000 lb of volume. Intensity is determined by the percentage of the repetition maximum for that specific number of repetitions. According to Harre, the adaptability process occurs only when the stimuli reach an intensity proportional to the individual's threshold capacity (RM).[18] Despite a high volume of work, if the intensity is below a minimal level (30% RM), adaptation will not result.[1]

The particular phases of training that an individual will perform include a base phase, a strength phase, and a conversion phase. The base phase is to develop a general foundation for the more difficult program to follow. Regardless of the current state of the individual all participants will employ Delorme's repetition and set scheme during the time period.[19]

During the next phase (the strength phase), the major purpose is to develop the highest level of strength possible. Because most sport activities require power development, and as the primary goal of rehabilitation is strength enhancement and then power, strength acquisition is essential during the initial micro- and mesocycles. Power as we know it is a by-product of strength and speed (force × distance/time). Consequently, it is logical to develop the highest level of strength before converting it to power. The conversion phase entails the inclusion of more power type of movements in the actual training program. The power movements consist of actual sport activities (plyometrics, sprinting, jumping etc.) or the inclusion of Olympic style movements with the barbell. These movements include derivatives of the clean and jerk as well as the snatch. Training modalities that are included as power movements are those movements whose muscular contractions (or barbell velocity) approximates 180 degrees of limb speed velocity per second.[29] During the conversion phase, the specific goals of the individual's training program will be attained. The strength levels that have been developed in the prior two phases can now be converted into power or endurance. The training ratio will now shift so that strength will still be maintained but the major thrust of the training program will be specific goal attainment. According to the APP, a shotputter whose event performance lasts about 3 seconds will be per-

forming athletic movements and weight lifting movements geared toward these energy release mechanisms, whereas a distance runner (10,000 m) will be conserving strength in the weight room but engaging in heavy interval work on the track. The length of the conversion phase (macro-cycle) depends upon the ultimate goal of the training program. Table 14–5 illustrates a sample training program for a specific lift (barbell squat), which includes a base strength and conversion phase as well as samples of a base phase intensity regimen. The intensity regimen is an adaptation of Bompa's 2-week micro-cycle that includes 6 days of training in the 2-week period.[3,17] The regulation of intensity proceeds in a wavelike pattern with alternate days of varying intensities. The key to success in the training programs is always striving to increase resistance without sacrificing good mechanics. Regardless of the intensity regulation that is followed, progressively increasing the resistance is essential for maximizing strength, endurance, and power development. During the two heavy-intensity days in the sample program the amount of resistance added should be the minimum possible increment with respect to the training modality. For various machine modalities 10 lb is often the smallest increment, whereas in free weight 1½ lb may be the smallest increment. The combination of training modalities and intensity regulations are endless. This presents a unique situation for the sports physical therapist, as awareness of the demands of the activity, current status of the individual, and the training modalities available all must be taken into consideration in the program development.

Starting Load

The last major obstacle to overcome in the development of the training program is the determination of starting weights for each specific exercise in the regimen. Sanders implemented a formula for using one's body weight for baseline exercise loading.[30] These percentages are merely median points for various body parts and include a very small number of the exercises that are possible. Some machine modalities are restricted to starting resistances and include very large increments between levels. Rehabilitation situations as well as some beginning participants would preclude the use of these modalities, as some loading increments would only lead to poor performance and possibly injury. Determination of the RM is not an easy task. Under no situation should a 1 RM be determined the very first day of training, as this will result in poor technique performance, high risk of injury, and prolonged residual muscular soreness. The percentages shown in Table 14–6 should only serve as a guideline for the base phase of training.

Overtraining

Although poorly understood at times, overtraining is a real problem to the elite athlete as well as the beginner. Highly motivated and compulsive individuals are most at risk. Sixty-four percent of the women, and 60% of the men at the 1988 Olympics have suffered from overtraining at some point in their competitive lives.[6] The telltale signs of overtraining resemble those of depression: lack of motivation, loss of appetite, inability to sleep, and quite possible the presence of "nagging injuries." The only way to successfully overcome the effects of overtraining is to stop training. This is the time to determine the causes of overtraining by review of the individual's training, dietary habits, and social demands. Regardless of the causes, if overtraining is not identified early recovery can be a lengthy process.

Sample Programs

Physical conditioning for any sport activity should replicate the physiological demands of the activity. Not

TABLE 14–5. PHASES OF TRAINING

	Base	Strength	Conversion
Duration	2–3 weeks	3–6 weeks	6 weeks–?
Repetitions	10	5–6 wk	2–6
Sets	3	4–6 wk	4–6 wk
Intensity	50%–100% RM	30%–100% RM	30%–100% RM

Sample 2-wk micro-cycle—Base Phase (Barbell Squat 10 RM = 100 lb)
Day 1—medium intensity (up to 89% RM)
Day 2—heavy intensity (>90% RM)
Day 3—medium intensity (up to 89% RM)
Day 4—medium intensity (up to 89% RM)
Day 5—heavy intensity (>90% RM)
Day 6—light intensity (30% and 79% RM)
The individual will be doing three sets of ten repetitions, with the last set being the intensity level for that day, for example, for the first day the progression will be
- 1 set of 10 repetitions at 50% of 10 RM = 50 lb
- 1 set of 10 repetitions at 75% of 10 RM = 75 lb
- 1 set of 10 repetitions at 89% of 10 RM = 89 lb

TABLE 14-6. BODYWEIGHT PERCENTAGES

Lift	Percentage of Body Weight	Repetitions
Barbell squat	45%	10
Universal leg press	50%	10
Barbell bench press	30%	10
Universal bench press	30%	10
Universal leg extension	15%	10
Weight boot leg extension	15%	10
Universal leg curl	10%	10
Weight boot extension	10%	10

only is the intensity system important but so too are the selection and order of exercises. A female distance runner would not have much transfer of training doing a barbell squat of 300 lb. For the person concerned with a basic fitness program, doing single repetitions of the snatch would not be as important as the high jumper performing the same lift. Sample training programs are shown in Table 14–7 and represent a cross section of individuals who have different goals and training backgrounds:

- Subject 1: 35-year-old female distance runner (5,000 to 10,000 m)
- Goals: Upper body strength, hamstring strength
- Contraindications: None
- Prior training: None
- Length of program:?

- Subject 2: 50-year-old man
- Goals: General fitness, achieve 17% body fat
- Contraindications: No squatting or heavy power movements
- Prior training: None
- Length of training: Achieve body fat goals

- Subject 3: 24-year-old male javelin thrower
- Goals: Increased power development
- Contraindications: None
- Prior training: 5 years
- Length of training: 6 months to national competition

- Subject 4: 17-year-old woman
- Goals: Lose weight and increase muscle tone, 15% body fat

TABLE 14–7. SAMPLE PROGRAMS

Subject 1

Program: Goals—Upper body strength, hamstring strength
       Cycle—Three-week micro-cycle followed by evaluation of hamstring
WTC program—Delorme's three sets of ten repetitions, three times weekly
Modality—Barbell, dumbells, leg extension, and leg curling machine
Exercises—Upper body: bench press, upright rowing, dumbell press, tricep extension, barbell curl
    Lower body: leg extension, leg curl, and calf raises
Intensity—Bompa's 2-week, 6-day program: day 1 (M), day 2 (H), day 3 (M), day 4 (M), day 5 (H), day 6 (E), day 7
    retest hamstrings (H,M,L,E refers to the level of intensity that will be followed)
Starting weight—Employ % of bodyweight for all exercises

Subject 2

Program: Goals—General fitness and 17% body fat
       Cycle—Six-week meso-cycle, with periodic body fat evaluations
WTC program—Two weeks of Delorme's three sets of ten repetitions, three times weekly, 4 weeks of Berger's
    three sets of six, three times weekly
Modality—Barbells, dumbells, and various machines
Exercises—Total body workout, with the elimination of heavy Olympic movements and squatting
Intensity—Follow repeated micro-cycles of H,H,E,M,H,L intensity levels
Starting weight—Employ percentage of body weight for all exercises
Special notes—To achieve body fat goals begin an aerobic running program on alternate days, dietary con-
    sulting, and periodic assessment of body fat

Subject 3

Program: Goals—Increase power development
       Cycle—Six-month macro-cycle
WTC program—Two micro-cycles of Delorme's three sets of ten repetitions, followed by two micro-cycles of
    Berger's three sets of six, followed by Macqueen's Pyramid of four to five sets of two to three repetitions
Exercises—Heavy assortment of Olympic-style movements (snatch and power clean), heavy squatting and
    pressing exercises, with additional supplemental exercises
Intensity—Follow Delorme's, Berger's and Macqueen's progressions
Starting weight—Since individual has been training, determine 10 RM the first week on all exercises. Subse-
    quent increments can be derived from this

Subject 4

Program: Goals—General fitness and maintain body fat percentage
       Cycle—Eight-month macro-cycle with periodic body fat and fitness evaluations
WTC program—Begin with Delorme's scheme, and alternate Berger's regimen during the length of the 8-
    month cycle
Modality—Assortment of machines and free weight apparatus
Exercises—Total body workout with upper and lower body exercises included
Intensity—Alternate Bompa's 2-week micro-cycle for the 8-month period
Starting weight—Employ % of body weight
Special notes—Begin an aerobic running program 3 times/weekly and dietary consulting

- Contraindications: None
- Prior training: None
- Length of training: Achieve goals and maintain those levels.

Obviously, the sports physical therapist has to be concerned with other components of the individual's life. Dietary habits, anaerobic and aerobic running programs, social demands, and motivation all contribute to the achievement of the goals of the training program.

Conclusion

The principles involved in planning the training program should be seen as a reference structure. The complexity of the individual and situations that arise suggest an immense permutation of variables of which the sports physical therapist must be aware. Interpretation of these values will be represented by a modification in the total program. Training is a complex concept; improvement will result from an organized and well-planned training program based on sound principles of frequency, volume, and intensity. Training is the systematic athletic ability, progressively and individually graded, aimed at manifesting the organism's physiological as well as psychological functions to meet demanding tasks.

REFERENCES

1. Dick F. *Training Theory.* 2nd ed. London: British Amateur Athletic Board; 1984:7–76.
2. Kraemer WJ, Fleck SJ. Resistance training: Exercise prescription. *Phys Sportsmed.* 1988; 16(6):69–81.
3. Bompa TO. Physiological intensity values employed to plan endurance training. *Athlet Training.* 1988; 3(4):37–52.
4. Sanders MT, Sanders BR. Mobility: Active resistive training. In: Gould JA, Davies GJ, eds. *Orthopaedic and Sports Physical Therapy.* St. Louis, Mo: C V Mosby Co; 1985; 2:228–241.
5. DeVries HA. *Physiology of Exercise for Physical Education and Athletics.* Dubuque, Iowa: William C Brown Co; 1980:25–78.
6. Jackson DL. *Overtraining. Bulletin Section of Sports Medicine,* Lexington, Ky: University of Kentucky Press; 1988.
7. McKain H, Peterson RA. The University of Northern Colorado physiologically based swimming and conditioning program. *Swim Techn.* 1976; 12(4):110–114.
8. Edgerton VR, Roy RR, Gregor RJ, et al. Morphological basis of skeletal muscle power output. In: Jones NL, et al, eds. *Human Muscle Power.* Champaign, Ill: Human Kinetic Publishers; 1986:43–59.
9. Basmajian JV. *Muscles Alive; Their Functions Revealed by Electromyography.* 4th ed. Baltimore, Md: Williams & Wilkins Co; 1979:115–130.
10. Moritani T, DeVries HA. Neural factors versus hypertrophy in the time course of muscle strength gains. *Am J Phys Med.* 1979; 58(3):115–130.
11. Komi PV. The stretch-shortening cycle and human power output. In: Jones NL, McCartney N, McComas et al, AJ, eds. *Human Muscle Power.* Champaign, Ill: Human Kinetic Publishers; 1986:27–39.
12. Asmussen E. Some physiological aspects of fitness for sport and work. *Proc Soc Exp Biol Med.* 1969; 62:1160–1164.
13. Macdougall JD. Morphological changes in human skeletal muscle following strength training and immobilization. In: Jones NL, McCartney N, McComas AJ, eds. *Human Muscle Power.* Champaign, Ill: Human Kinetics Publishers; 1986:269–288.
14. Kraemer WJ, Noble BJ, Clark MJ, et al. Physiologic responses to heavy-resistance exercise with very short rest periods. *Int J Sports Med.* 1987; 8:247–252.
15. Macdougall JD, Ward GR, Sale DG, et al. Biochemical adaptation of human skeletal muscle to heavy resistance training and immobilization. *J Appl Phys.* 1977; 43:700–703.
16. Wolf SL. The morphological and functional basis of therapeutic exercise. In: Basmajian JV, ed. *Therapeutic Exercise: Student Edition.* Baltimore, Md: Williams & Wilkins Co; 1980:1–32.
17. Bompa TO. *Theory and Methodology of Training: The Key to Athletic Performance.* Dubuque, Iowa: Kendall Hunt; 1985:1–180.
18. Harre D. *Principles of Sport Training.* Berlin: Sportverlag; 1981:6–175.
19. Delorme TL, Watkins AL. Techniques of progressive resistance exercise. *Arch Phys Med Rehabil.* 1948; 29:263.
20. Zinovieff AN. Heavy resistance exercise, the Oxford technique. *Bri J Phys Med.* 1951; 14:129.
21. Macqueen IF. Recent advances in the technique of progressive resistance. *Br Med J.* 1954; 11:1193.
22. Berger RA. Optimum repetition for the development of strength. *Res Q Exerc Sport.* 1962; 33:334–338.
23. Berger RA. Comparison between resistance load and strength improvement. *Res Q Exerc Sport.* 1967; 33:637.
24. Stull GA, Clarke DH. High-resistance, low repetition training as a determiner of strength and fatigability. *Res Q Exerc Sport.* 1970; 41:189–193.
25. Dons B, Bollerup K. The effect of weightlifting exercise related to muscle fiber-type composition and muscle cross-sectional area in humans. *Eur J Appl Physiol.* 1979; 40:94.
26. Sanders MT. A comparison of two methods of training on the development of muscular strength and endurance. *J Orthop Sports Phys Ther.* 1980; 1:210–213.
27. Atha J. Strengthening muscle. In: Miller DI, ed. *Exercise and Sport Science Reviews.* American College of Sports Medicine Series; 1981; 9:1–73.
28. Stone WJ, Kroll WA. *Sports Conditioning and Weight Training: Programs for Athletic Conditioning.* Boston, Mass: Allyn & Bacon Inc; 1982:1–15.
29. Wyatt MP, Edwards AM. Comparison of quadriceps and hamstring torque values during isokinetic exercise. *J Orthop Sports Phys Ther.* 1981; 3:48–56.
30. Sanders MT. Unpublished study on resistive training. Collegeville, Minn: St. John's University; 1978.

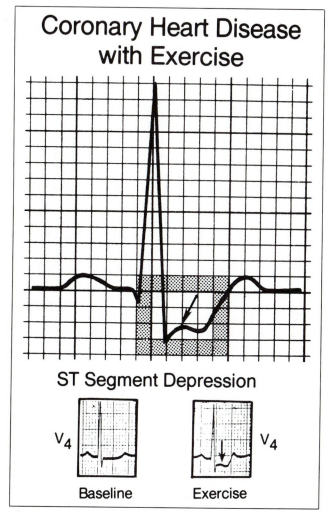

Figure 15-7. Ischemic ECG response during exercise testing. *(From Stein E.* Clinical Electrocardiography: A Self-Study Course. *Philadelphia, Pa: Lea & Febiger; 1987, with permission.)*

RPE	
6	
7	Very, very light
8	
9	Very light
10	
11	Fairly light
12	
13	Somewhat hard
14	
15	Hard
16	
17	Very hard
18	
19	Very, very hard
20	

Figure 15-8. Borg perceived exertion scale. *(From Borg G. Psychophysical bases of perceived exertion.* Med Sci Sports Exerc. *1982; 14:5, with permission.)*

quire very detailed measures, including a multiple-lead electrocardiogram (ECG) to help determine ischemic responses to exercise stress (Fig 15–7).[34] Exercise testing of athletic populations might include the actual measurement of VO_2 max using commercially available metabolic cart equipment, for example.

An easy variable to obtain during all forms of exercise testing is "perception of effort." This variable can be measured by using Borg's scale of perceived exertion (Fig 15–8).[35] Perceived exertion is very useful in exercise prescription (see the case studies below).

Finally, several variables can complicate the actual exercise testing session, for example, use of medications, determination of end points for the test, test interpretation, follow-up of abnormal results, and briefing of the individual about the test results. All of these situations present unique challenges to the sports physical therapist and therefore require special train-

ing, preparation, and practical experience in the exercise sciences.

EXERCISE PRESCRIPTION

Exercise must be prescribed in the appropriate amount to be effective in improving CR fitness. When coupled with the principles of CR training, the principles of exercise prescription provide the sports physical therapist with the base to design sound preventive/rehabilitative sports medicine programs.

The ACSM, in a position statement, has made recommendations regarding the quality and quantity of exercise necessary for developing and maintaining CR fitness in healthy adults.[36] These recommendations are discussed in more detail elsewhere.[24]

The primary components of sound CR exercise prescription include the mode (type of activity), the intensity, the duration, the frequency, the rate of progression, and special situations (Table 15–5). All these factors must be determined based upon each individual's needs and each component must be addressed, whether

TABLE 15-5. RECOMMENDATIONS FOR EXERCISE PRESCRIPTION

1. Frequency	3–5 days per week
2. Intensity	60%–90% of maximum heart rate (HR max) reserve, 50%–80% of maximum oxygen uptake
3. Duration	15–60 min (continuous)
4. Mode–activity	Run, jog, walk, bicycle, swim, or endurance sport and dance activities
5. Initial level of fitness	High = higher work load / Low = lower work load

From American College of Sports Medicine. Position statement on the recommended quantity and quality of exercise for developing and maintaining fitness in healthy adults. Med Sci Sports Exerc. 1979; 10:3, and Pollock ML, Wilmore JH, Fox SM. Exercise in Health and Disease. Philadelphia, Pa: W B Saunders Co; 1984, with permission.

the individual is an elite athlete or a cardiac patient who develops symptoms upon physical exertion.

The mode or type of activity should be based on the CR training needs of the individual. Aerobic as well as anaerobic work may be prescribed following an evaluation of the strengths and weaknesses of the person's health–fitness profile. Table 15–6 provides some examples of various modes of training.

Aerobic activities include large muscle groups and are rhythmic and continuous in nature. The principal difference between primary and secondary aerobic activities involves whether or not there are short, low-intensity breaks in the activity.

Anaerobic activities can complement the CR training of individuals for general health and daily living and help improve peak athletic training. Resistance training refers to exercise done with free weights, isokinetics, variable resistance, or isometrics. Plyometrics exercises involve an eccentric muscle contraction followed immediately by a concentric muscle contraction of the same muscle. Further information about anaerobic training is available elsewhere.[37,38]

Circuit (resistance) training has been used as an alternative mode to primary or secondary aerobic ac-

TABLE 15-6. MODES OF EXERCISE

Aerobic		Anaerobic
Primary	**Secondary**	
Running/jogging	Handball	Sprints
Swimming	Basketball	Plyometrics
Cycling	Racquetball	Resistance training
Ice skating	Rope skipping	
Cross-country skiing	Aerobic dance	

From Pate RR, McClenaghan B, Rotella R, eds. Scientific Foundations of Coaching. Philadelphia, Pa: Saunders College Publishing; 1984, with permission.

tivities to increase CR fitness. It usually includes several stations typically involving weight lifting or other resistance training. The individual moves through the stations, performing 30 seconds worth of work (for example) at each station until a complete circuit of the stations has been made. This type of exercise training is used extensively in commercial health clubs and many public school programs. There is some evidence that this type of resistance training can have some positive effects on resting blood pressure, total blood cholesterol, HDL cholesterol, and VO_2 max. These changes are smaller in magnitude than those resulting from primary or secondary aerobic CR training, however.[37]

Establishing exercise intensity for CR training and conditioning is probably the most difficult component of exercise prescription to determine. Exercise is essentially like medication, with the proper dosage needed for the desired result and an overdosage capable of causing serious injury. Table 15–7 illustrates three methods commonly used to establish the proper exercise intensity or training zone for healthy adults.[39] These methods include criteria based on VO_2 max, HR, and ratings of perceived exertion (RPE).

Exercise intensity can be based upon a percentage of the individual's VO_2 max, as determined from a laboratory or field test assessment. For example, if a 30-year-old healthy woman had a VO_2 max of 43.02 mL/kg/min (or about 12 mets), her CR intensity training zone should be between 6 and 10 mets (Fig 15–1).

The most consistent HR method for determining exercise intensity is based upon the Karvonen formula or HR max reserve methods.[39,40] For example, our 30-year-old healthy woman's HR exercise intensity (training zone) can be calculated as follows:

$$(MHR - RHR) \times 0.6 + RHR,$$

where

1. MHR is the maximum HR; MHR = 220 − age, if the individual is not taking HR-reducing medication;
2. RHR is the resting HR; and
3. 0.6 represents the minimum HR intensity from Table 15–5.

TABLE 15-7. RECOMMENDED TRAINING ZONE FOR EXERCISE PRESCRIPTION

Oxygen uptake	50% — — — → 85%	
Heart rate	60% — — — → 90%	
RPE	12 — — — — → 16	
	Somewhat hard	Hard

From Pollock ML, Wilmore JH, Fox SM. Exercise in Health and Disease. Philadelphia, Pa: W B Saunders Co; 1984, with permission.

If our young woman's resting heart rate is 70 bpm, her HR exercise intensity by substitution would be

$$MHR = 220 - 30 = 190,$$
$$RHR = 70,$$
$$(190 - 70) \times 0.6 + 70 = 142 \text{ bpm}.$$

This value would represent the minimal exercise intensity for CR training. For maximal exercise intensity we would do the same calculation except that the percentage of HR intensity would be 90%. Thus, again by substitution:

$$(190 - 70) \times 0.85 + 70 = 172 \text{ bpm}$$

Therefore, our young woman should engage in CR exercise at a HR intensity between 142 and 172 bpm.

A third method of determining exercise intensity is RPE, in which the individual is taught to use the Borg Scale (Fig 15–8). Thus, our 30-year-old woman should exercise at an RPE of between 12 and 16. The RPE method of prescribing intensity is simple, but requires that the individuals gain experience over time in CR training to accurately predict how hard they are working.

The duration of CR training and conditioning should be based upon its interaction with the intensity of work. Exercise for longer durations at low intensity requires a similar total expenditure of kilocalories as exercise for shorter durations at high intensity. For example, if an individual ran a mile in 6 minutes he or she would expend approximately the same amount of kilocalories as an individual who walks a mile in 20 minutes. Obviously, a person who has a high capacity for tolerating greater intensities and durations will expend more kilocalories per unit of time than a person with a lower capacity to do so. The key, once again, is to tailor the duration of work to the individual's needs and abilities.

An initially low-fit, overweight person should strive to exercise at minimal intensity for a longer period of time, whereas a high fit person might obtain similar CR results by exercising for fewer minutes at a high intensity. The general guidelines for CR exercise duration are 15 to 60 minutes of primary or secondary aerobic exercise.[12,24]

The frequency of CR training and conditioning is also best determined by considering the interaction between intensity and duration. The normal recommendation for frequency is 3-7 days/wk.[12,24] The minimal threshold for frequency should be 3 days/wk, based on an alternate-day schedule. An individual may need to exercise more times per week, particularly if he or she can work only at low intensities or for short durations. Individuals may wish to work more often if they desire to exceed minimal CR adaptations, such as improving their personal 10-kilometer running time, for example.

Certainly many sports require that an individual train 6 to 7 days/wk for optimal performance.

It is important to emphasize that increasing the frequency, intensity, or duration of training can expose individuals to an increased risk of injury. Therefore caution should be used when manipulating the frequency of CR training. In addition, the sports physical therapist should reassure overly enthusiastic individuals that missing training for 1 or 2 days will not result in any significant loss of CR conditioning. In fact, a 1- or 2-day layoff may allow the body to adapt to training more effectively.

The rate of progression of CR training and conditioning should be based on the individual's age, sex, body weight, heredity, and initial fitness level.[12,24,39] This aspect of the exercise prescription involves application of the exercise training principles discussed in the following section.

According to the ACSM the rate of progression can be determined by designing an initial conditioning stage, an improvement conditioning stage, and a maintenance conditioning stage for each individual.[24] Table 15–8 illustrates an example of the rate of progression for a symptomatic cardiac patient. It is rare that the intensity, frequency, and duration of exercise are all changed at the same time. It is best to change only one of these factors at a time to allow the body to adapt. Other examples of rates of progression are discussed in the case studies.

The final component of exercise prescription involves adaptation to special situations or special populations that every sports physical therapist will face at one time or another. Among the unique challenges faced by the sports physical therapist are (1) cardiac patients, (2) children, and (3) elite athletes.

Table 15–9 contains guidelines for exercise prescription for post–myocardial infarction (MI) and post–coronary artery bypass graft (CABG) patients.[41] Note that these guidelines represent adjustments to the general recommendations already discussed in this section.

The exercise prescription for a child must take into account the unique responses of children to exercise compared to adults. Table 15–10 contains selected CR responses of children to exercise. Again, the exercise prescription framework would remain the same except for adjustments based on this special population.[42]

The elite athlete poses another special situation or problem when one tries to determine an appropriate exercise prescription. Elite athletes can usually work at higher intensities, more frequently and for longer durations than other groups of individuals. They also need more specific and diverse types of CR training and conditioning to achieve maximal performance. Unfortunately, this group is also at higher risk for the negative mental and physical effects of overtraining than other groups.[42]

TABLE 15-8. EXAMPLE: PROGRESSION OF THE SYMPTOMATIC PARTICIPANT USING A DISCONTINUOUS AEROBIC CONDITIONING PHASE[a]

Endurance Aerobic Phase	Weeks	Total Minutes at % FC[b]	% FC	Minutes at Exercise Intensity (60%-80% FC)	Minutes at Rest Phase Lower Than Exercise Intensity	Repetition
Initial Stage	1	12	60	2	1	6
	2	14	60	2	1	7
	3	16	60	2	1	8
	4	18	60-70	2	1	9
	5	20	60-70	2	1	10
Improvement Stage	6-9	21	70-80	3	1	7
	10-13	24	70-80	3	1	8
	14-16	24	70-80	4	1	6
	17-19	28	70-80	4	1	7
	20-23	30	70-80	5	1	6
	24-27	30	70-80	Continuous		
Maintenance Stage	28+	45-60	70-80	Continuous		

[a]Clinical status must be considered before advancing to the next level.
[b]Functional capacity.
From American College of Sports Medicine. Guidelines for Exercise Testing and Prescription. 3rd ed. Philadelphia, Pa: Lea & Febiger; 1986, with permission.

When properly applied, the principles of exercise prescription allow for the safe, scientific development of CR fitness. When the sports physical therapist must adapt the exercise prescription for special situations, he or she should review the available professional literature for guidance.

EXERCISE TRAINING PRINCIPLES

Once the sports physical therapist has successfully developed the skills to write accurate exercise prescrip-

tions, he or she should construct their CR training and conditioning programs based upon scientific exercise principles. Some of the more important CR training principles include: overload, consistency, specificity, state of training, progression/periodization, individuality/reversibility/detraining, and overtraining/psychological stress.[24,26,43,44] The application of these scientific principles to CR training represent an art that must be developed through professional preparation and experience.

The overload principle refers to the fact that CR development is systematic in nature. That is, the physio-

TABLE 15-9. GUIDELINES FOR EXERCISE PRESCRIPTION FOR CARDIAC PATIENTS AS RECOMMENDED AND PRACTICED AT MOUNT SINAI MEDICAL CENTER, MILWAUKEE, WISCONSIN[a]

Prescription	Phase I (inpatient program)	Phase II (discharge → 3 mo)	Phase III (30 mo →)	Healthy Adults
Frequency	2-3 times/day	1-2 times/day	3-5 times/wk	3-5 times/wk
Intensity	MI: RHR + 20 CABG: RHR + 20	MI: RHR + 20[b], RPE 13 CABG: RHR + 20[b], RPE 13	70%-85% HR max reserve	60%-90% HR max reserve
Duration	MI: 5-20 min CABG: 10-30 min	MI: 20-60 min CABG: 30-60 min	30-60 min	30-60 min
Mode-activity	ROM, TDM, bike, 1 flight of stairs	ROM, TDM (walk, walk-jog), bike, arm erg, Wgt Trg	Walk, bike, jog, swim, cal, Wgt Trg, endurance sports	Walk, jog, run, bike, swim, endurance sports, Wgt Trg, cal

[a]Symbols and abbreviations: MI, myocardial infarction patient; CABG, coronary artery bypass graft surgery patient; HR, heart rate, beats/min; RHR, standing resting HR; ROM, range of motion exercise; TDM, treadmill; arm erg, arm ergometer; cal, calisthenics; Wgt Trg, weight training; RPE, rating of perceived exertion.
[b]Within 6-8 wk after surgery or event, a symptom-limited exercise test is performed. Heart rate intensity is then based on 70% maximum HR reserve.
From Pollock ML, Foster C, Knapp D, Schmidt DH. Cardiac rehabilitation program at Mount Sinai Medical Center, Milwaukee, Wis: J Cardiac Rehabil. 1982; 2:458-463, with permission.

TABLE 15–10. HEMODYNAMIC AND RESPIRATORY CHARACTERISTICS OF CHILDREN'S RESPONSES TO EXERCISE

Function	Typical for Children (Compared With Adults)
Hemodynamic	
HR at submaximal power load	Higher, especially at first decade
HR_{max}	Higher
$SV_{submax\ and\ max}$	Lower
Q at given V_{O2}	Somewhat lower
AVD-O_2 at given V_{O2}	Somewhat higher
Blood flow to active muscle	Higher
SBP,$DBP_{submax\ and\ max}$	Lower
Respiratory	
V_E at given V_{O2}	Higher
V_E "breaking point"	Similar
Respiration rate	Higher

From Bar-Or O. *Importance of differences between children and adults for exercise testing and exercise prescription.* In: Skinner JS, ed. *Exercise Testing and Exercise Prescription for Special Cases. Philadelphia, Pa: Lea & Febiger; 1987,* with permission.

logical systems of the body adapt to specific demands presented. Overload is primarily controlled by adjusting the intensity, duration, frequency, and rate of progression.

Adaptations in the CR system of the body occur over time. These CR adaptations occur at different rates when compared to those changes in tendons, ligaments, and connective tissue. Thus, although the body might be ready for increased CR overload, the increase may overstress the tendons, ligaments, or connective tissue. This points out the importance of designing CR programs that allow for gradual adaptations which avoid high risks of injury. Therefore, the adjustments made with intensity, duration, frequency, and rate of progression during training must be systematic for CR improvement, but not so rapid and diverse that injuries result.

Consistency in CR training and conditioning ensures that the individual will make gradual improvements in health and performance. Long-term commitment to training is required to develop and maintain CR health. It is important to discourage individuals from taking long layoff periods (detraining) from CR training because it is much easier to maintain a desirable level of CR fitness than it is to develop it.[39]

The specificity principle involves several different elements when applied to CR training and conditioning. The effects of training are always highly specific. The aerobic energy system is specifically challenged by CR training. The specific adaptations to CR training will also depend upon the mode used. If a person is trying to improve his or her running time in a 10-km race, for example, he or she should spend most of their training time running. Also, the muscle groups that are overloaded specifically in training will be the ones that adapt and allow for improvements in economy of movement.

The specificity principle even more dramatically applies to athletic individuals in terms of the development of their optimal CR performance. For example, a male collegiate distance runner should include several different kinds of CR training. He should incorporate long–steady running, intervals, repetition runs, tempo runs, and strides.[45] Such a pattern of diverse training will ensure the specific CR adaptations necessary for success in his sport. The sports physical therapist may need to consult the available literature to develop the "best" CR program for individuals or groups who need comprehensive CR development.

The individual's initial level of fitness or state of training will help determine the rate of progression. Generally, the individual that is inexperienced with CR training should start slower but will see greater initial improvements. The experienced individual (high fit) can work harder initially but will demonstrate smaller CR improvements.[47,48] The state of training should be assessed in the initial health/fitness evaluation of the individual by the sports physical therapist.

The progression principle has already been addressed in the exercise prescription section of this chapter. Periodization refers to the staging of exercise training in cycles of development and is directly related to progression. Figure 15–9 illustrates an example of progression/periodization in aerobic training for the average healthy adult.[46] The figure indicates that it may take several weeks to months to achieve the maintenance stage that is consistent with CR health (300 to 400 kcal per workout).

Progression/periodization may differ substantially for athletic individuals or groups (as opposed to patients). There should be periods of CR training that might be more intense and demanding for the athletes than others. There should also be a recovery phase designed into training that allows for adequate rest or peaking for maximal performance.

Each individual responds differently to CR training and conditioning. Factors such as age, sex, heredity, maturity, diet, current fitness level, and other physiological and psychological characteristics need to be considered in the design of the training program. The individuality principle points out the importance of conducting in-depth accurate initial evaluation of individuals. It is unrealistic to expect individuals or groups to all adapt or respond to the CR training stimulus in the same way.

The reversibility/detraining principle states that the associated positive physiological adaptations of a regular CR training and conditioning program are gradually lost as the program is discontinued. The major studies that have addressed this topic have either

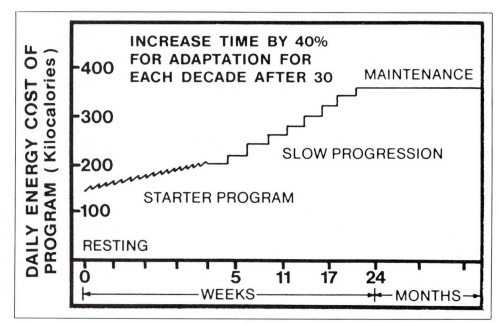

Figure 15-9. Schematic illustration for average in regard to progression in an aerobic training program. *(From Pollock ML, Wilmore JH, Fox SM. Exercise in Health and Disease. Philadelphia, Pa: W B Saunders Co; 1984, with permission.)*

been studies of patients confined to bed or formerly high-fit individuals who have stopped training for various periods of time. In 1968 Saltin and coworkers evaluated the effects of 3 weeks of bed rest followed by 8 weeks of aerobic training on 5 men.[49] They found that VO_2 max was 3.3 L/min before bed rest, 2.4 L/min after bed rest, and 3.92 L/min after training. Bed rest represented a 27% loss in CR fitness (primarily due to stroke volume decreases) for the subjects.

In a series of studies, Coyle and coworkers evaluated the effects of detraining on formerly active high-fit men.[50-52] Following 84 days of detraining Coyle et al found that the subjects had significant decreases in SV, VO_2 max, a-vO_2 difference, and mitochondrial enzyme activity. These changes occurred as early as 12 days after detraining. The subjects in these studies did not, however, regress to typical CR levels seen in inactive individuals who have never experienced intensive CR training.

The results of the studies conducted by Saltin et al and Coyle et al indicate that the reversibility/detraining principle is very important to consider during the development of CR training programs. The sports physical therapist must be able to minimize the deconditioning effects of bed rest and educate individuals about the negative effects of detraining on CR fitness.

Overtraining is a term that has been used in recent years to describe the negative effects of lack of adaptation to increased intensity of physical training. Overtraining may result in negative physical as well as psychological symptoms. Physical symptoms of overtraining include weight loss, increased training HR, increased muscle soreness, and insomnia.[55,56] Psychological symptoms of overtraining include increases in tension, de-

pression, anger, fatigue, confusion, and decreased vigor.[56] Because of these risks associated with overtraining, individuals should have their physiological and psychological responses to CR training closely monitored.

Overtraining and psychological stress can lead to staleness during CR training.[53] For example, the yearly incidence of staleness in collegiate swimmers who train up to 14,000 m/day is about 10%, whereas the career prevalence of staleness in elite runners has been reported to be 60%.[56] Little data are available about the incidence of overtraining in average healthy adults or physically compromised populations.

It does appear that staleness can be prevented by monitoring changes in psychological mood states.[54,56] The profile of mood states instrument has been used to assess change in tension, depression, anger, vigor, fatigue, and confusion.[57]

The exercise training principles mentioned in this chapter can help one develop CR fitness programs. Currently there is an explosion in the available literature related to new techniques for the application of exercise training principles. It is extremely important that sports physical therapists remain up-to-date so that they can apply these new techniques to their CR training and conditioning programs.

CHRONIC ADAPTATIONS TO CARDIORESPIRATORY TRAINING

The major goals of CR training and conditioning should be (1) to reduce the energy demands for individuals at submaximal work loads and (2) to increase the

total energy output capability at maximal exercise following training. The CR adaptations that occur within the body, following endurance training, allow increases in the supply of oxygen and other nutrients that more effectively meet the demands of exercise.

Some of the general changes (for healthy adults) with CR training and conditioning are listed in Table 15–11 and are highlighted here.[58] These may differ in patients with pulmonary or cardiovascular disease.[2,39,58]

Improvements in CR function require a mini-

TABLE 15–11. CHANGES IN CARDIOVASCULAR AND PULMONARY FUNCTION AS A RESULT OF ENDURANCE-TYPE PHYSICAL TRAINING[a]

Measurement	Resting Pre		Post	Upright Submaximal "Steady-State" Exercise Pre		Post	Upright Maximal Exercise Pre		Post
Heart rate (bpm)	70	0,−	63	150	−	130	185	0,−	182
Stroke volume (mL/beat)	72	+,−	80	90	+,−	102	90	+	105
Cardiac output (L/min)	5.0	0,+	5.0	13.5	0	13.2	16.6	+	19.1
(a-v)O_2 difference (Vol %)	5.6	0	5.6	11.0	+	11.3	16.2	0,+	16.5
O_2 uptake (L/min)	0.280	0	0.280	1.485	0,−	1.485	2.685	+	3.150
(mL/kg/min)	3.7	0	3.7	19.8	0,−	19.8	35.8	+	42.0
(Mets)[b]	1.0	0	1.0	5.7	0	5.7	10.2	+	12.0
Work load (mL/kg/min)	—		—	600	0	600	1050	+	1500
Blood pressure (mm Hg)									
Systemic arterial systolic BP	120	0,−	114	156	0,−	140	200	0,−	200
Systemic arterial diastolic BP	75	0,−	70	80	0,−	75	85	0,−	75
Systemic arterial mean	90	0,−	88	126	0,−	118	155	0,−	152
Total peripheral resistance (dyn/sec/cm⁵)	1250	0	1250	750	0,−	750	450	0,−	390
Blood flow (mL/min)									
Coronary	260	−	250	600	−	560	900	0,+	940
Brain	740	0	740	740	0	740	740	0	740
Viscera	2400	0	2500	900	0,+	1000	500	0,−	500
Inactive muscle	600	+,−	555	500	0,−	500	300	0	300
Active muscle	600	−	555	10,360	0	10,000	13,760	+	16,220
Skin	400	0	400	400	0	400	400	0	400
TOTAL	5000		5000	13,500		13,200	16,600		19,100
Blood volume (L)	5.1	0,+	5.3						
Plasma volume (L)	2.8	0,+	3.0						
Red cell mass (L)	2.3	0,+	2.3						
Heart volume (mL)	730	0,+	785						
Pulmonary ventilation (L/min)	10.2	0	10.3	44.8	0,−	38.2	129	+	145
Respiratory rate (breaths/min)	12	0	12	30	−	24	43	+	52
Tidal volume	850	0,+	855	1.5	0,+	1.6	3.0	0,−	2.8
Lung diffusing capacity (D_L) (mL at STPD)[c]	34.1	0,+	35.2	40.6	0,+	42.8	48.2	+	50.6
Pulmonary capillary blood volume (mL)	90.1	0,+	97.2	129.3	+	141.2	124.5	+	220.0
Vital capacity (L)	5.1	0,+	5.2						
Blood lactic acid (mmol/L)	0.7	0	0.7	3.9	−	3.0	11.0	0,+	12.4
Blood pH	7.43	0	7.43	7.41	0,+	7.43	7.33	0,−	7.29
Recovery rate					+			+	

[a]Estimated for a healthy man, age 45, weighing 75 kg. Pre, pretraining; Post, posttraining. Minus (−) sign means usually decrease in value with training. Plus (+) sign means usually increase in value with training. Zero (0) sign means usually no change in value with training.

[b]A MET is equal to the O_2 cost at rest. One MET is generally equal to 3.5 mL/kg of body weight per minute of O_2 uptake or 1.2 kcal/min.

[c]STPD, standard temperature (0°C), pressure 760 mm Hg.

From Brooks GA, Fahey TD. Exercise Physiology Human Bioenergetics and Its Applications. *New York, NY: John Wiley and Sons; 1984, with permission.*

mum of 6 to 8 weeks of training. Months to years of training and conditioning may be necessary, however, to maximize CR improvements.

An increase in VO$_2$ max during maximal exercise following CR training is primarily due to increases in SV and a-vO$_2$. During submaximal exercise, VO$_2$ max is unchanged or reduced although there are slight changes in HR, SV, and a-vO$_2$. Resting HR generally decreases after CR training whereas SV increases. As Table 15–11 illustrates, the energy demand at submaximal work loads is reduced while more work can be performed at maximal exercise.

After CR training, resting BP is unchanged or slightly reduced, usually due to decreases in SBP. The SBP and DBP are reduced at submaximal work loads. At maximal exercise SBP remains fairly constant whereas DBP may decrease slightly. The TPR is unchanged at submaximal work loads after training but does decrease slightly at maximal exercise. The changes with BP following CR training reduce the stress on the heart and blood vessels of the body.

Blood flow redistribution in the body with exercise is critical for meeting the demands of physical activity. Following CR training, blood flow at rest and submaximal exercise is unchanged, but it increases at maximal exercise. The improved redistribution of blood flow is primarily due to increases in a-vO$_2$.

Increases in blood volume (due to plasma volume increases) and heart volume are often observed following CR training. These adaptations allow for improvements in the supply capacity of the CR system.

The resting pulmonary function values, following CR training, remain approximately the same. At submaximal work loads and maximal exercise, however, there are significant changes in MV, f, and TV. The changes in Table 15–11 represent the major pulmonary adaptations expected with CR training.

Following CR training, blood lactate levels and blood pH levels are unchanged at rest. At submaximal work loads, the blood lactate breakpoint or AT is slightly shifted to the right. This allows more work to be performed before significant amounts of lactate accumulation. The blood lactate clearance capability (blood pH) is also slightly improved at submaximal work loads. At maximal work loads the blood lactate levels increase and blood pH decreases. The changes at maximal work loads are probably due to improvements in lactate turnover, anaerobic mechanisms affected by higher intensity CR training, and increased psychological tolerance to work.

In summary, the chronic adaptation to CR training and conditioning allow the individual to do more work in a more economical manner. By supplying the right CR training ingredients, the sports physical therapist can successfully reduce the practical CR demands of daily life for their patients.

CASE STUDIES

The final section of this chapter is devoted to providing the reader with realistic CR training and conditioning case study examples. The case studies are designed to demonstrate the development and implementation of successful CR training and conditioning programs. The cases that follow include examples of CR programs for a teenager, a healthy adult, a cardiac patient, and an elite athlete.

Case Study One

Tina is a 15-year-old healthy high school student who is very interested in her current personal fitness level because over the last year she has gained 15 pounds and noticed that she fatigues easily. She has been told that her weight gain is related to growth and development. She has participated in little physical activity during the last year, however, and has depended on fast foods as a primary dietary source.

Tina's mother has encouraged her to visit a local Sports Medicine Clinic that has advertised individualized programs for personal health/fitness. Tina has decided to give the program a try because her physical education class at school emphasizes athletic games and dodgeball, but not fitness. She has mentioned to her mother that this is why she hates to exercise.

Based upon her initial visit to the Sports Medicine Clinic, Tina's sports physical therapist made the following assessments and recommendations based on her individual needs and health/fitness evaluation:

Assessment	*Goal/Plan*
1. Healthy teenage female who is 30% body fat (based on skinfold evaluation) who needs to reduce body fat levels to 20% to 25%.	Lose 10 to 15 lb based on body composition analysis. Participate in a nutrition/weight control program (one that combines caloric intake control and increased caloric expenditure) conducted at the clinic.
2. Low health-related fitness based on the results of the Fit Youth Today (FYT) Fitness Test.[59] The FYT test consists of four criterion referenced activities (curlups, sit and reach, body composition, and a 20-minute steady-state jog). Tina scored as follows: curlups—30 in 2 minutes; sit and reach—2 inches before toes; body composition—30% fat, steady-state jog—1 mile.	Improve abdominal tone, body composition, and CR endurance. Follow the FYT 8-week conditioning protocol to achieve the above goals and to increase caloric expenditure (Table 15–12).[60] Specific FYT goals: curlups—40 in 2 minutes; sit and reach—touch toes; body composition—25% fat;[61] steady-state jog—2 miles.

TABLE 15–12. FYT CONDITIONING PROTOCOL

Day	Jog (min)	Rcvry[a] (mins)	Jog (min)	Rcvry (min)	Jog (min)	Rcvry (min)	Ttl Time (min)	Curlups
1	2	1	2	1	2	1	9	10
2	2	1	2	1	2	1	9	10
3	3	1	2	1	2	1	10	12–14
4	3	1	2	1	2	1	10	12–14
5	3	1	3	1	3	1	12	15
6	4	1	3	1	2	1	12	15
7	4	1	3	1	2	1	12	15–18
8	5	1	4	1	3	1	15	18
9	5	1	4	1	3	1	15	18
10	5	1	4	1	3	1	15	18–20
11	6	1	4	1	4	1	17	18–20
12	12-min steady state jog						12	20
13	7	1	4	1	3	1	17	20–22
14	8	2	7	2			19	20–22
15	8	2	7	2			19	22–24
16	10	2	7	2			21	25
17	10	2	7	2			21	25
18	12	2	8	2			24	25
19	12	2	8	2			24	25–27
20	15	2	8	2			27	27–30
21	15	2	8	2			27	30–34
22	18	2	6	2			28	34–36
23	18	2	6	2			28	36–40
24	20	2					22	40

[a]Rcvry, recovery time.

From American Health and Fitness Foundation. FYT Program Manual. 2nd ed. Austin, Tex: American Health and Fitness Foundation; 1988, with permission.

The sports physical therapist designed the following exercise prescription for Tina based on his evaluations and conversations with her concerning her individual goals (weight maintenance and improved CR endurance):

Mode: walk/jog, cycle, swim
Intensity: Heart rate range, 145 to 185 bpm RPE, 13 to 15 "somewhat hard to hard"
"Talk Test," be able to carry on a conversation
Duration: Minimum of 20 minutes, work up to 30 to 45 minutes.
Frequency: 3 days per week
Progression: Follow the FYT Conditioning Protocol
Special Situation: Follow-up FYT evaluation in 8 to 10 weeks, check in at the clinic as needed for excessive muscle soreness or injury.

Although Tina's success in her personal fitness program will depend on several other factors (e.g., motivation, consistency, inherent ability, etc.), a sound assessment combined with realistic goals and plans can provide the framework to her enhanced future CR fitness.

Case Study Two

Robert is a 50-year-old man who was referred to the Sports Medicine Clinic by his personal physician following his recent physical examination. His health history includes a 30-pack-year smoking habit (currently 2 packs per day). He has had no previous operations. He is 5 feet 8 inches tall and weights 210 pounds. He has low back pain occasionally while sitting at his desk at work. He reports some moderate job-related stress. He drinks in moderation (6 glasses of wine per week). His father died of a myocardial infarction (MI) at the age of 62.

The analysis of his blood chemistry from his physical examination indicates that his total serum cholesterol value is 270 mg/dL, HDL is 40 mg/dL, and triglyceride level is 150 mg/dL. His fasting blood glucose is 95 mg/dL. He has not been physically active (less than 500 kcal/wk) for the past 25 years. His physician has suggested that he stop smoking, lower his cholesterol, lose weight, and start a regular exercise program.

Based upon his initial visit to the Sports Medicine Clinic, Robert's sports physical therapist suggested the following treatments to fulfill the physician's recommendations:

1. Participate in a smoking cessation class taught by a behavioral psychologist for 8 weeks in the clinic teaching classroom
2. Attend a nutrition/weight-control (low-cholesterol, low-sodium) class held weekly (for 8 weeks) in the clinic meal preparation classroom
3. Take a treadmill CR exercise evaluation with physician interpretation

Robert's exercise evaluation was performed with the following results:

Protocol: Bruce treadmill test
Resting Data: HR, 80 bpm; BP, 130/80 mm Hg; 24% body fat assessed with three-site skinfold.
Maximal Data: Stage 3 (3.4 mph, 14% grade)
        Total time, 8 minutes
        HR, 170 bpm
        BP, 190/84 mm Hg
        RPE, 19
        Predicted VO_2 max, 30 mL/kg/min
        Test terminated due to fatigue and extreme shortness of breath.

The sports physical therapist designed the following initial exercise prescription for Robert based upon his health history, treadmill evaluation, and conversations with him concerning his individual goals (smoking cessation, weight loss, lowered cholesterol, and improved CR endurance):

Mode: Stationary cycle (primarily to avoid weight-bearing injuries), light weightlifting for muscle toning
Intensity: Heart rate range (by the Karvonen formula), 134 to 152 bpm; RPE, 13
Duration: Work up to 20 to 30 minutes
Frequency: Initially three times weekly with a goal of 5 times weekly after 12 weeks
Progression: Follow minimum guidelines for CR work load until follow-up at 12 weeks
Special situations: Strive to lower CHD risk. Take whatever possible measures to stop smoking, once Robert is motivated to do so. Weight loss should not exceed 1 to 2 lb/wk. Encourage Robert to purchase a quality stationary cycle with an adjustable seat and handlebars (or workout regularly on the clinic cycle). The cycle should have variable resistance to allow increases in work load to reflect the training heart rate range. Advise Robert to work his CR exercise program into his daily routine, which will ensure consistency.

Robert's success in achieving all his goals (i.e., stopping smoking, losing weight, lowering cholesterol, and improving his CR fitness) is unlikely during the initial 3 months of training. With regular clinic follow-up and peer encouragement, however (assuming he maintains his intrinsic motivation), Robert should see some beneficial changes in his CHD risk profile as soon as 3 months. These early potential improvements in CR health/fitness can have a dramatic impact on Robert's future risk for chronic disease (mainly CHD) and will improve his physical work capacity.

Case Study Three

Patient Profile: Mary is a 60-year-old white female.

Problem: Patient is post-MI having increasing angina and marked decrease in exercise tolerance.

Diagnosis: CHD manifested by prior anteroseptal and subendocardial MI, with current angina and marked dyspnea on exertion and decreased exercise tolerance, with documented left ventricular dysfunction at rest. No congestive heart failure. Normal sinus rhythm, Functional Therapeutic Class III-C.

Subjective: Patient is a 60-year-old white female who was hospitalized in January 1983 for hysterectomy. The surgery was not complicated, however; after her surgery during her recovery in the hospital, the patient suffered severe chest pain, which was later found to be an anteroseptual MI. The patient recovered from her MI without incident and was discharged from the hospital to begin post-MI rehabilitation program. The patient remained asymptomatic until about June 1987 when she noted a marked decrease in her exercise tolerance. She had no chest pain at that time. The patient suffered another MI, diagnosed as subendocardial MI in July 1987 with peak CPK being 1554. When the patient was discharged, tolerance was greatly decreased and she had stable angina until approximately the end of November and the middle of December 1987, at which time her angina increased to almost a daily basis. She states that she could only walk about half a block before she would get short of breath and a pressure sensation in her chest requiring her to stop. The patient has markedly curtailed her daily activities. The patient was unable to tolerate Isordil and she was treated with Inderal and Procardia, in increased dosages during the past 2 months. The patient states that now she has less angina mainly because she has markedly decreased her activity level but she still notes the significant degree of fatigue and limited exercise tolerance.

Past Medical History: Patient has had hypertension for 10 years; otherwise unremarkable.

Family History: Noncontributory

Risk Factors: Positive for hypertension and cigarette smoking, otherwise negative

Allergies: No known medical allergies

Current Medications: Inderal 40 qid, Procardia 20 mg qid, and sublingual nitroglycerin prn.

Physical Examination: Height 5'4", weight 165 lb, BSA 1.8 m², BP 110/72, P 60 and regular. Carotid pulses and neck veins are within normal limits. The PMI is laterally displaced but no palpable gallops can be appreciated. On auscultation there is a regular rate and rhythm with a normal S1 and S2. There is a positive S3 at the apex. No fourth heart sounds or murmurs. Patient has good pulses in extremities. There is no peripheral edema noted. She has an abdominal surgical scar which is well healed and otherwise physical examination is remarkable.

Exercise Stress test:

Protocol: Bruce
Resting data: HR = 65 bpm, BP = 110/72 mm Hg
Maximal data: Stage 2 (2.5 mph, 12% grade)
Total time: = 5 minutes
HR = 105 bpm
BP = 120/70 mm Hg
RPE = 20

Test terminated due to marked dyspnea and exhaustion. ECG had minor ST flattening laterally.
Resting multigated acquisition nuclear study:

LVEF = 29%
Dilated LV anteroapical hypokinesis, inferior dyskinesis

Mary was referred by her physician to the Sports Medicine Clinic in order to help her develop an appropriate CR program to achieve three goals: (1) interaction with peers in a supervised cardiac rehabilitation program to prevent and control depression over her current physical health status, (2) teach the patient her exercise tolerance level for exertional angina, and (3) to maintain or improve her current physical work capacity and control her CHD risk factors. The physician has determined that Mary is not a good candidate for coronary artery bypass graft surgery or angioplasty.

Obviously, the sports physical therapist who would have to develop the CR program for Mary has a complex task. Her exercise prescription should be designed to achieve the desired physician goals and based on her treadmill stress test. It will also have to be a conservative exercise prescription due to the symptomatic CHD.

A working updated knowledge of cardiac medications is essential to the development of Mary's exercise prescription. Inderal is a β-blocker medication that lowers resting and exercise HR as well as resting and exercise BP. It also improves exercise performance when the patient has angina. Procardia is a calcium-channel blocker that increases exercise HR but lowers exercise BP response. It may delay the ischemic response in cardiac patients.[24]

A typical exercise prescription for Mary might be written as follows:

Mode: walking, stationary cycling in the sports medicine clinic during supervised cardiac rehabilitation sessions.
Intensity: HR range should be based on her most recent treadmill stress test while on her medications. Her HR range would be 87 to 98 bpm or below whatever HR is associated with ischemic ECG changes.
Duration: 5 to 10 minutes at first, working up to 20 to 30 minutes. Patient may have to work in several short intervals in her training HR zone to avoid exertional angina.
Frequency: 3 times weekly, gradually increasing to 5 times weekly if possible.

Progression: Maintain 20 to 30 minutes 3 to 5 times weekly, follow-up with physician as needed.
Special situations: Teach patient the Borg scale and how to recognize anginal threshold. Be conservative as she will not be able to improve pump (SV) function. Have emergency equipment available.

Mary's success at achieving her physician's goals will be very difficult to accomplish. Coronary heart disease is a progressive disease and therefore limits currently available treatments. Mary may be able to carry out her daily living tasks more effectively if she maintains her medication schedule and is physically active. Both medication and physical activity can help in the control of ischemic CHD. There are currently no treatments available that eliminate this disease, however. A CR program for Mary may also help her control some of her anxiety and depression associated with her health status.

Case Study Four

Larry is a 23-year-old long distance runner (he competed in collegiate cross-country and track) who is interested in competing in road racing (5 km to marathon distance). He dropped in at the Sports Medicine Clinic to inquire about getting a treadmill test evaluation and CR training advice.

Larry is in good health and eats a normal healthy diet. He has never run a marathon but has run 5 km in 16:00, and 10 km in 32:00. He is currently at 7% body fat, which is consistent with peak endurance running performance. Larry usually trains by running 6 to 10 miles daily.

Based upon Larry's baseline data the sports physical therapist decided to have Larry perform a 2-mile time trial for the prediction of his VO_2 max. Larry ran 9:30 for the 2-mile distance. Based on the equation given earlier, Larry's predicted VO_2 max is 68 mL/kg/min. This value is high for his age and sex (Table 15–4) and consistent with road racing success.

From interacting with Larry and by referring to the training literature, the sports physical therapist designed the following CR program[32]:

Mode: Running, light weightlifting to enhance strength and flexibility. Include easy steady runs, moderately hard steady (tempo) runs, interval running, and repetition running.
Intensity:

1. Easy steady runs—60% to 75% of VO_2 max. These help in injury prevention, CR development, metabolic enhancement, and confidence.
2. Moderately hard steady (tempo) runs—85% of VO_2 max or between 10-km and marathon pace. These develop anaerobic threshold.
3. Interval runs—95% to 100% of VO_2 max. These help improve VO_2 max.
4. Repetition runs—a little faster than 5-km race pace. These develop running economy (decreased O_2 consumption at a given speed).

Frequency: 6 to 7 days/wk

Progression: Incorporate the four types of runs such that you cover 70 miles per week with: one long run 10 to 15 miles, one tempo run (20 minutes long) every 10 days, 1 interval or repetition session every 10 days, and race no more than every other week.

Special situations: Focus on specific training for the distance desired during different parts of the year. For example, longer runs for a marathon during late fall, and short, faster training for a 5-km raced in summer. Be consistent in training but beware of overtraining symptoms. Do not neglect aches and pains—treat them and rest.

Larry's success in his CR training program will be based on his ability to adapt to the new training format. With proper guidance from the sports physical therapist he should expect improvements on his personal bests and be able to complete a marathon race in the future.

CONCLUSION

Physical activity and regular exercise are the backbone of the physical therapy profession. Therefore, it is very important that sports physical therapists understand the concepts required to implement CR training and conditioning programs successfully. By studying and applying exercise science principles, professionals can narrow the current knowledge gap concerning exercise and its health benefits. The topics highlighted in this chapter were designed to generate interest and raise questions concerning the CR training and conditioning literature. I feel that by pursuing a consistent program involving excellence in teaching, service, and research that future sports physical therapists can meet the diverse CR training and conditioning needs of their patients.

REFERENCES

1. Cooper K. Forewood. In: Blair SN, Painter P, Pate RR, et al, eds. *Resource Manual for Guidelines for Exercise Training and Prescription* Philadelphia, Pa: Lea & Febiger; 1988.
2. Astrand PO, Rodahl K. *Textbook of Work Physiology.* 3rd ed. New York, NY: McGraw-Hill Book Co; 1986.
3. American Heart Association. *Heart Facts.* Dallas, Tex: American Heart Association; 1989.
4. Stamler J. Major coronary risk factors before and after myocardial infarction. *Postgrad. Med.* 1981; 57:34.
5. Paffenbarger RS. Contributions of epidemiology to exercise science and cardiovascular health. *Med Sci Sports Exerc.* 1988; 20:5.
6. Paffenbarger RS, Hyde RT, Wing AL, Hsieh CC. Physical activity, all-cause mortality, and longevity of college alumni. *N Engl J Med.* 1986; 314:605.
7. Paffenbarger RS, Hyde RT, Wing AL, Steinmetz CH. A natural history of athleticism and cardiovascular health. *JAMA.* 1984; 252:491.
8. Ross JG, Gilbert GG. The national children and youth fitness study. A study of findings. *JOPERD.* 1985; 56:45.
9. Updyke WF. *Planters–AAU Physical Fitness Program: Annual Report of Results.* Bloomington, IN: Indiana University, School of HPER. 1986.
10. Texas Association of HPERD, Governor's Commission on Physical Fitness, American Heart Association. *Texas Youth Fitness Study.* Austin, Texas; 1986.
11. US Department of Human Services. *Promoting Health/Preventing Disease.* Washington, DC: US Government Printing Office; 1980.
12. American College of Sports Medicine. Opinion statement on physical fitness in children and youth. *Med Sci Sports Exerc.* 1988; 20:4.
13. Zinkgraf S, Johnson C, Murthy L. The FYT program: The results of a large-scale pilot study. *Tex Assoc HPERD J.* 1988; 56:2.
14. Gollnick P. Metabolism of substrates: Energy substrate metabolism during exercise and as modified by training. *Fed Proc.* 1985; 44:353.
15. Sherman WM, Costill DL. The marathon: Dietary manipulation to optimize performance. *Am J Sports Med.* 1984; 12:44.
16. Holloszy J. Muscle metabolism during exercise. *Arch Phys Med Rehabil.* 1982; 63:231.
17. Holloszy J, Coyle E. Adaptations of skeletal muscle to endurance exercise and their metabolic consequences. *J Appl Physiol.* 1984; 56:831.
18. Durstin JL, Pate RR. Cardiorespiratory responses to acute exercise. In: Blair SN, Painter P, Pate RR, et al, eds. *Resource Manual for Guidelines for Exercise Training and Prescription (American College of Sports Medicine).* Philadelphia, Pa: Lea & Febiger; 1988.
19. Clausen JP. Effect of physical training on cardiovascular adjustments to exercise in man. *Physiol Rev.* 1977; 57:779.
20. Rowell LB. What signals govern the cardiovascular responses to exercises? *Med Sci Sports Exerc.* 1980; 12:307.
21. Blomquist CG, Saltin B. Cardiovascular adaptations to physical training. *Annu Rev Physiol.* 1983; 45:169.
22. American Heart Association. *Exercise Testing and Training of Apparently Healthy Individuals: A Handbook for Physicians.* Dallas, Tex: American Heart Association; 1972.
23. American Heart Association. *Exercise Testing and Training of Individuals With Heart Disease or at High Risk for Its Development: A Handbook for Physicians.* Dallas, Tex: American Heart Association; 1975.
24. American College of Sports Medicine. *Guidelines for Exercise Testing and Prescription.* 3rd ed. Philadelphia, Pa: Lea & Febiger; 1986.
25. Smith KW, McKinlay SM, Thorinton BD. The validity of health risk appraisal instruments for assessing coronary heart disease risk. *Am J Public Health.* 1987; 74:419.
26. Blair SN, Painter P, Pate RR, et al, eds. *Resource Manual for Guidelines for Exercise Testing and Prescription (American College of Sports Medicine).* Philadelphia, Pa: Lea & Febiger; 1988.

27. Cooper KH. *The Aerobics Way.* New York, NY: Bantam Books; 1978.
28. Kline GM, Porcari JP, Hintermeister R, et al. Estimation of VO₂ max from a one-mile track walk, gender, age, and body weight. *Med Sci Sports Exerc.* 1987; 19:3.
29. Fardy PS, Yanowitz FG, Wilson PK. *Cardiac Rehabilitation, Adult Fitness, and Exercise Testing.* 2nd ed. Philadelphia, Pa: Lea & Febiger; 1988.
30. Daniels J, Scardira N, Hayes J, Foley P. Elite and subelite female middle- and long-distance runners. In: Landers DM, ed. *Sport and Elite Performers.* Champaign, Ill: Human Kinetics. 1986.
31. MacDougall JD, Wenger HA, Green HJ, eds. *Physiological Testing of the Elite Athlete.* Mutual Press, Canadian Association of Sports Sciences; 1982.
32. Daniels J. A physiologist's view of running economy. *Med Sci Sports Exerc.* 1985; 17:3.
33. Jackson AS, Squires WG, Crimes G, Beard EF. Prediction of future resting hypertension from exercise blood pressure. *J Cardiac Rehabil.* 1983; 3:4.
34. Stein E. *Clinical Electrocardiography: A Self-Study Course.* Philadelphia, Pa: Lea & Febiger; 1987.
35. Borg G. Psychophysical bases of perceived exertion. *Med Sci Sports Exerc.* 1982; 14:5.
36. American College of Sports Medicine. Position statement on the recommended quantity and quality of exercise for developing and maintaining fitness in healthy adults. *Med Sci Sports Exerc.* 1979; 10:3.
37. Fleck SJ, Kraemer WJ. *Designing Resistance Training Programs.* Champaign, Ill: Human Kinetics Books; 1987.
38. Vogel JA (Chairperson). Physiological responses to resistance exercise. *Med Sci Sports Exerc.* 1988; 20 (suppl):5.
39. Pollock ML, Wilmore JH, Fox SM. *Exercise in Health and Disease.* Philadelphia, Pa: W B Saunders Co; 1984.
40. Karvonen M, Kentala K, Musta O. The effects of training heart rate: A longitudinal study. *Ann Med Exp Biol. Fenn.* 1957; 35.
41. Pollock ML, Foster C, Knapp D, Schmidt DH. Cardiac rehabilitation program at Mount Sinai Medical Center, Milwaukee, Wis: *J Cardiac Rehabil.* 1982; 2:458–463.
42. Bar-Or O. Importance of differences between children and adults for exercise testing and exercise prescription. In: Skinner JS ed. *Exercise Testing and Exercise Prescription for Special Cases.* Philadelphia, Pa: Lea & Febiger; 1987.
43. Pate RR, McClenaghan B, Rotella R, eds. *Scientific Foundations of Coaching.* Philadelphia, Pa: Saunders College Publishing; 1984.
44. Sharkey BJ. *Coaches Guide to Sport Physiology.* Champaign, Ill: Human Kinetics Publishers; 1986.
45. Daniels JT. Over and out. *Runner's World.* 1986; 21:7.
46. Pollock ML, Wilmore JH, Fox SM. *Health and Fitness Through Physical Activity.* New York, NY: John Wiley and Sons; 1978.
47. Sharkey BJ, Jackson JH, Johnston LP. Cardiorespiratory adaptations to training at specified intensities. *Res Q.* 1968; 39:2.
48. Saltin B, Hartley L, Kilbom A, Astrand I. Physical training in sedentary middle-aged men. II. *Scand J Clin Lab Invest.* 1969; 24:4.
49. Saltin B, Bloomquist G, Mitchell JH, et al. Response to exercise after bedrest and after training. *Circulation.* 1968; 38:5.
50. Coyle EF, Martin WH, Sinacore DR, et al. Time course of loss of adaptations after stopping intense endurance training. *J Appl Physiol.* 1985; 57:6.
51. Coyle EF, Martin WH, Bloomfield SA, et al. Effects of detraining on responses to submaximal exercise. *J Appl Physiol.* 1985; 59:3.
52. Coyle EF, Hemmert MK, Coggan AR. Effects of detraining on cardiovascular responses to exercise. *J Appl Physiol.* 1986; 60:1.
53. Morgan W. Affective beneficience of vigorous physical activity. *Med Sci Sports Exerc.* 1985; 17:1.
54. Costill DL, Flynn MG, Kirwan JP. Effects of repeated days of intensified training on muscle glycogen and performance. *Med Sci Sports Exerc.* 1988; 20:3.
55. Kirwan JP, Costill DL, Flynn MG. Physiological responses to successive days of intense training in competitive swimmers. *Med Sci Sports Exerc.* 1988; 20:3.
56. Morgan WP, Costill DL, Flynn MG, et al. Mood disturbance following increased training in swimmers. *Med Sci Sports Exerc.* 1988; 20:4.
57. McNair DM, Lorr M, Droppleman LF. *Profile of Mood States Manual.* San Diego, Calif: Educational and Individual Testing Service; 1971.
58. Brooks GA, Fahey TD. *Exercise Physiology Human Bioenergetics and Its Applications.* New York, NY: John Wiley and Sons; 1984.
59. American Health and Fitness Foundation. *FYT Program Manual.* 2nd ed. Austin, Tex: American Health and Fitness Foundation; 1988.
60. Murray TD. Description and rationale for the FYT conditioning protocol. *Tex Assoc HPERDJ.* 1988; 56:2.
61. Jackson AS, Pollock ML. Practical assessment of body composition. *Physician Sports Med.* 1985; 13:5.

Nonorthopaedic Problems

Michael J. Dreibelbeis

INTRODUCTION

This chapter's intention is to provide an overview of the more common nonorthopedic problems faced by the sports physical therapist on a daily basis. I have tried to include simple remedies that may be helpful as well as suggestions for when a referral is needed.

LACERATIONS

Lacerations are the result of a tearing force of sufficient magnitude to open the skin.[1] They are otherwise known as cuts, gashes, tears, or rips. The laceration thus allows an opening for infection into the body as well as causing the destruction of skin and underlying tissue. Treatment of the wound will vary, but, in general, the laceration should be cleansed with soap and water or hydrogen peroxide to decontaminate the area. It is then covered with a sterile dressing. It should be evaluated by a physician within 2 hours after the injury occurs. The wound may be closed with a butterfly bandage, a steri strip, or sutures, depending on the site of the injury, the depth of the damage, and the physician's preference.

PUNCTURES

Puncture wounds are very difficult to cleanse and thus frequently become infected. Every attempt should be made to find the object that caused the puncture and remove it from the playing environment to prevent injury to another athlete. If the athlete has a tiny sliver-type of puncture, the sports physical therapist should cleanse the wound with soap and water or hydrogen peroxide and remove the object using good clean technique. The wound is cleansed again and dressed with an antibiotic ointment and then appropriately bandaged. In the case of a deep puncture the object is left

in place and the athlete is evaluated by a physician. There is potential for damage to deep structures. The athlete's record should be checked to see that he or she is currently immunized for tetanus. In general, the athlete should have been vaccinated in the last 5 to 10 years, but the team physician should make the decision on a case by case basis.

ABRASIONS

Floor burns, turf burns, grass burns, strawberries, and sliding burns are all common terms for abrasions.[2] The cause of an abrasion is friction or scraping of the skin that leaves an open wound that is tender, oozing, and red. There is loss of the epidermal layer and the athlete has moderate local pain and stiffness. If, as is often the case, the abrasion is on the lateral thigh, there may be a marked limp when the athlete walks.

It is important that the wound be cleansed with soap and water or hydrogen peroxide and debrided with a gauze pad or soft brush to remove all foreign particles to reduce the risk of infection and scarring. This must be done despite the athlete's protest about the associated pain. A wet towel filled with ice may be placed over the wound prior to debridement to achieve local anesthesia.

INCISIONS

The most common cause of incisions in athletes is the surgeon's scalpel. These are most often closed with material such as staples, silk (a black, single-strand material), a monofilament product (which is typically light blue in color), or a tape closure, like steri strips. Incisions should be kept dry for 5 to 7 days. This means no showers without covering the wound with plastic and no soaking in the tub or whirlpools during that time. These rules are to prevent the infectious agents in water

from following the suture material into the wound, thus causing an infection. These are, however, only guidelines. Because opinions differ widely, the team physician or surgeon should be consulted for his or her guidelines.

BLISTERS

Blisters are caused by friction. Eliminate the friction and you eliminate the problem. Blisters are most common early in the season when the feet or hands have not become accustomed to the friction and shearing stresses that are applied to them.[3] Blisters are frequently caused by poorly fitting shoes, new shoes, old or dirty socks, and excessive callus buildup.

The first treatment for blisters is prevention by education of the athlete. The athlete should wear a thick, double knit sock or a thin cotton sock with a heavy wool sock or cotton sock over it. The wool actually has a greater cushion effect and is preferable. The socks should be clean and dry before each practice. If the practice area is wet and the athlete is particularly susceptible to blisters, he or she may wish to change to dry socks during practice. The athlete should be taught how to buy good shoe gear. All too often in junior and senior high school an athlete will try to stretch two or three seasons out of one pair of shoes. This practice should be discouraged due to the increased chance of blisters and the potential of problems in the lower kinetic chain from worn-out shoes.

Athletes must also be taught that, if they feel a hot spot, a friction area, or a blister forming, they should:

1. Cease activity immediately.
2. Remove their shoes and socks.
3. Apply ice, if available, for about 10 minutes.
4. Dry their feet and apply a lubricant such as petroleum jelly or Skin Lube. An ointment such as Neosporin could also be used because the base is petroleum jelly. New skin could also be used.
5. Cover the hot spot with a Band-Aid.
6. Replace their socks and shoes to see if the friction area is gone. If it is, they can return to play. If it is not, it must be reevaluated.

Athletes must understand that by taking these six steps immediately they will reduce the chance of missing practice due to a preventable blister.

The treatment of a blister in an athlete is generally more aggressive than that of a blister in the general public because the blister is more likely to be opened during the sport activity. The primary concept of blister care is to prevent or minimize the chances of infection. If the athlete has a 2- or 3-day break without practice, such as a weekend, and the blister is in a location that is likely to be torn open during activity, then it may be drained. This can be done by two methods. The blister area must first be thoroughly cleaned with soap and water. Betadine or alcohol may also be used.

The first method involves cutting a small, triangular piece out of the top of the blister. This will allow the serous fluid to drain out of the blister and Betadine can be poured into the wound to clean under the skin flap. The skin flap can be left on over the next 24 to 48 hours to make the athlete more comfortable. A blister doughnut, cut out of 0.25-in adhesive foam and placed around the blister, will protect the area. A tape adherent, such as Tuf-skin or tincture of Benzoin compound will enable the foam to adhere better. The blister should then be covered with an antibiotic ointment and a Band-Aid. The athlete should be instructed to wash the foot daily, and reapply the doughnut, ointment, and Band-Aid as well as watch for signs of infection around the blister.

A second method of draining the blister is to use a sterile 21-gauge or smaller hypodermic needle. The blister and surrounding area are thoroughly cleaned. The needle is introduced into the epidermis about 0.25 in away from the blister and then directed into the cavity of the blister itself. The fluid is expressed by applying pressure to the blister or a syringe is used to draw the fluid out of the area. After all of the fluid is removed, a nonadhesive pad should be placed on the blister to apply pressure to the area so that the blister will not refill with fluid. The needle (and syringe, if used) should be disposed of in a contaminated waste container. In 3 to 5 days, when the tenderness of the blister has subsided, the loose skin may be cut away using sterile scissors and forceps. The skin should be cut on a bevel as close to the outside margin of the blister as possible.

When there is little chance of the blister tearing, it is preferable to treat it with a more conservative approach. A doughnut pad is placed around the blister, if it is needed for pain relief, and a Band-Aid is put over that to keep it clean if it should tear.

When a blister is torn it should be treated in the following manner:

1. Clean the wound with soap and water.
2. Apply an antiseptic (such as Betadine).
3. Cut the skin flap on a bevel as close to the outside margin as possible.
4. Apply an antiseptic or antibiotic ointment to the blister.
5. Cover with a Band-Aid to keep the wound clean. A doughnut pad may be used to reduce pain.
6. The athlete may return to full activity as pain allows, but the wound should be protected for

3 to 7 days or until the underlying skin hardens sufficiently.

CALLUSES

A callus is the body's natural reaction to excessive friction on the skin. Callus formations on the foot in running athletes and the hands of gymnasts are common findings. If the callus becomes thick and hard, it may lose its elasticity and tends to tear or crack open.[4] This provides a site for infectious agents to enter the body. The athlete who has hard callus formation should be encouraged to use a callus file or 150-grit sandpaper on the callus two or three times each week to decrease its thickness. Lanolin massaged into the callus twice a week helps to keep the area more elastic.

Excessive callus formation is often preventable. This is accomplished by assuring that shoes fit well. Socks should be clean and provide adequate cushioning.

SUNBURN

Sunburn is a photodermatitis known as erythema solare or actinic dermatitis. It is caused by the ultraviolet radiation from the sun. There are two categories of sunburn, generally known as first and second degree.

First-degree sunburn is characterized by a mild to moderate pink or red color of the exposed skin. There is no open lesion, or blister formation. A mild amount of pain is present.

Second-degree sunburn is characterized by its red color and the formation of blisters. It is more painful than the first degree and there is usually associated swelling and itching. If a large area of the body (more than 10%) suffers second-degree burn, the athlete should be seen by a physician. Usually the burns are small and simple first aid and home remedies may be sufficient. Many physicians suggest two 5-grain tablets of aspirin three times daily[5] as well as 4 mg of chlorphenramine maleate (Chlor Trimeton) for an antihistamine. If the athlete is itching, Benadryl may be helpful. This is available by prescription or is present in Benalyn cough syrup.

Athletes tend to report sunburn more often when on the road. This is due to ready access to a clinician, absence of usual home remedies, and increased time spent in the sun. The athletes should be educated about using a sunscreen that is appropriate for their location. It is important the athletes know that the sun's rays are more direct the closer their location is to the equator and that there is a greater chance of getting a sunburn.

Sunburn should be prevented not only because it is painful and may affect the player's performance but also because sun exposure has been linked to the increased chance of skin cancer.

INFECTIONS

Infections are the result of the body's inability to initially defend itself against foreign agents. The most common infections seen in sports activities are caused by bacteria and fungal and viral microorganisms.

Viral Infections

A virus is a small microbe that is incapable of reproduction and growth outside of living cells. The particles vary in size from 15 to 300 μm.[6] Handwashing is a highly effective method of preventing the spread of common virus infections such as influenza and the common cold. Handwashing should be encouraged whenever possible in the training room. When on the field, a rinse of the hands with rubbing alcohol will help deter the spread of a virus. As a general rule, serious viral infections, such as measles, rubella, and polio are prevented with vaccinations.

Herpes Simplex. Commonly known as cold sores or fever blisters, there are two types of herpes simplex infections found in humans. Although historically type I was thought to occur above the waist and type II to occur in the genital area, this distribution has become less clear-cut as we have learned more about this viral infection.

Herpes simplex presents as a cluster of small (1 to 2 mm) blisters that progress to ulcers and then crust over before healing.[7] Herpes simplex is contagious and the infected athlete should avoid contact with other athletes until the lesions have dried and are no longer contagious. The nontreated lesion will heal in 10 to 21 days. The lesion can be treated with drying agents and astringents used for the treatment of acne.[8]

Warts. Warts are benign epithelial tumors due to a local viral infection. Warts commonly involve many sites on the skin and mucous membranes. Warts are contagious to susceptible individuals through direct or indirect contact. Warts may or may not grow in size and may or may not be painful.[9]

If an athlete has warts and they are not causing problems or are not painful, they should be left alone.

Warts on the plantar aspect of the foot are called plantar warts. They are commonly mistaken for calluses. Upon closer examination, however, the plantar wart is found to have a central core of tiny dark spots that are tiny blood vessels and nerve endings. Plantar warts frequently become painful. They can be treated

with low-intensity ultrasound. The ultrasound seems to be most effective if the wart has not been previously treated with chemicals or cauterization. The procedure we use in the clinic is as follows:

1. Identify the wart and measure its diameter
2. Apply ultrasound for 10 minutes at 0.5 W/cm using mineral oil as the couplant
3. Frequency: Once each week
4. Duration: two to four treatments

Physicians more commonly employ electrosurgical removal, liquid nitrogen treatment, or trichloracetic acid application to remove warts. Each of these methods have their own advantages and disadvantages.

Mononucleosis. Infectious mononucleosis is an acute proliferation of the white blood cells called monocytes. It is caused by the Epstein–Barr virus. The disease is essentially self-limiting but in severe cases produces high fever and swelling of the tonsilar tissue, sometimes causing partial airway obstruction and occasionally encephalitis. The signs of "mono" include sore throat, fatigue, headache, fever, and occasionally jaundice. Examination of the throat frequently reveals small white spots on the tonsilar pillars.[34] Palpation of the abdomen often reveals an enlarged spleen. The spleen must be two to three times normal size to be palpated below the ribs.

Treatment is essentially supportive. Once the fever and fatigue phase of the disease has passed the athlete may wish to return to activity. There is no evidence that activity will retard the recovery process. The enlarged spleen poses a potential hazard particularly in contact sports if it extends below the protection of the ribs. The enlarged spleen may be present for up to 6 months. Authorities are somewhat divided on when an athlete can return to contact participation if the spleen is enlarged. Some say as long as 6 months after the acute phase. Many others feel that once the athlete is tolerating activity without fatigue or fever for 10 to 14 days and understands the risk of splenic rupture, he or she may be allowed to return to competition, wearing additional rib or abdominal pads to provide protection to the area.

Bacteria

Bacteria are plantlike organisms that lack chlorophyll and may destroy blood cells.[10] Bacterial infections are common complications of skin injury. The most common infectious bacteria are staphylococci and streptococci.

Impetigo. Impetigo is an acute, contagious skin infection commonly caused by either staphylococci or streptococci. The infection is characterized by an eruption of small blisterlike vesicles that after 3 to 5 days de-

velop a yellow crustation. Impetigo is highly contagious and the athlete should be isolated from teammates immediately. The athlete's equipment should be disinfected according to the manufacturer's recommendation.

The athlete must pay particular attention to personal hygiene and wash the area 3 to 5 times daily with soap and hot water. The area should then be thoroughly dried. Although there is much controversy regarding the utility of topical antibiotics, many clinicians routinely use an antibiotic ointment (Bacitracin) over the lesion.[11]

Acne. This common skin problem occurs most often during adolescence but may be seen due to an athlete's use of anabolic steroids. Acne is a chronic inflammatory disease of the sebaceous glands. Acne presents with blackheads, cysts, and pustules. Acne is common in adolescents and many young athletes need to be reassured that the disease rarely results in scarring or permanent disfigurement. The athlete with acne should seek the advise of a physician concerning treatment of the disease. The treatment, usually symptomatic, consists of frequent washing with soap, hot water, and a washcloth followed by the use of an astringent agent to dry the skin. The athlete should be educated not to pick at the lesions or try to pop the blackheads.

Folliculitis. This infection of the hair follicles is common in wrestlers and athletes who use community whirlpools. The infection occurs most often in areas where the skin is frequently rubbed or shaved (face, neck, groin, and thighs). The athlete with folliculitis should not participate in contact sports until the infection has cleared and he has been seen by the team physician for evaluation.[12]

Fungal Infections

In most cases fungi are a part of the normal flora found on the skin and in the mouth, abdominal tract, and rectal and vaginal areas. Fungi are not generally pathogenic unless the host's defenses are decreased by disease or other stress or the host provides the right conditions for the fungi to thrive. The fungi thrive in dark, warm, moist areas such as the feet and the groin.

When a fungus attacks the body, it attacks the keratin layer of the skin. The common fungal genera seen in athletes are microsporum, trichophyton, and epidermophyton. These are given the common name of ringworm and tinea. They are then further classified according to where the infection occurs.

Tinea Pedis. Tinea pedis is commonly called "athlete's foot." Symptoms are itching or burning between the toes and on the sole of the foot. Signs include a rash with small blisters that may break and exude a yellow

serum. Scaling is frequently seen, with the color ranging from red to grey. The area is often scratched due to the persistent itching. This can lead to a secondary bacterial infection in the area. Treatment is usually with antifungal ointment and liquids that are available as over-the-counter products at the local drug store. Common over-the-counter antifungal products are Tinactin, Mycitracin, and Desenex. There are also prescription products available if the over-the-counter product does not clear up the situation in 7 to 10 days.[13] Prevention is the mainstay in the sports medicine arena when dealing with the fungal skin disorders. The athlete should:

1. Keep the feet dry
2. Wear clean, dry socks for each practice session
3. Allow shoes to dry between practices. They should not be buried in the bottom of the locker. If possible, two pairs of shoes should be alternated
4. Dust shoes lightly with antifungal powder on a daily basis
5. Thoroughly dry feet after showering paying special attention to the area between the toes
6. Maintain a clean, well-ventilated, locker room area that is disinfected on a daily basis
7. Not share towels

Tinea Cruris. Tinea cruris is commonly known as "jock itch." The symptoms are itching or burning in groin area. Signs include bilateral, commonly symmetrical, brownish red elevated lesions that usually spare the scrotum. This is frequently butterfly shaped. The treatment is to thoroughly clean the area with soap and water and have the athlete change into a clean supporter or underwear twice daily. An antifungal powder should be used two or three times daily. The area should be allowed to dry daily. A portable hair dryer on the cool setting may be used to speed up the process.

Tinea cruris is sometimes mistaken for the yeast infection *Candida albicans*. If the "jock itch" does not respond to antifungal powder in 3 to 5 days, and the itching is severe or if the scrotum is red and well involved, it may be a yeast infection. This is more common in diabetic athletes.

EYES, EARS, AND NOSE

Prevention of Eye Injuries

Prevention of ocular injuries is preferable to treatment. This involves education of all concerned about the risk of eye injury in sports, especially those played with projectiles such as racquetball, golf, and hockey. Proper inflation of air-filled balls may help prevent eye injury. An underinflated ball will conform more easily to the eye anatomy, causing direct ocular trauma. Eye protection is very important.[14]

Polycarbonate lenses and eye guards approved by the American Society for Testing and Materials (ASTM) should be used. The use of open eye guards without lenses is not recommended due to the fact that a ball may push through the opening and cause injury.[15]

Corrective Lenses. The current feeling among medical experts regarding vision correction for sports is shifting slightly from support for soft contact lenses back to the wearing of glasses with lenses made of polycarbonate. As enumerated below, there are advantages and disadvantages to both types of vision correction.

Generally the decision should be made according to the athlete's preference in consultation with the physician.

SOFT LENSES

PRO	CON
Seldom dislodged	Easily damaged
Can't fog	Must be disinfected daily
	Dirt under lens causes irritation

GLASSES

PRO	CON
Protects eye from projectiles	May slip off
	May fog
Easy to clean	Will not fit in some head gear
Sturdy, seldom broken	Can't be worn in wrestling

Conjunctivitis (Red Eye). Conjunctivitis is an inflammation of the mucous membrane covering the anterior surface of the eyeball and the under surface of the eyelid. It is the most common eye disease seen in sports. The causes may be viral infection, bacterial infection, allergy, or chemical contamination. A condition that has a similar presentation is iritis. This should be considered as a differential diagnosis.

Conjunctivitis is highly contagious. Special attention should be paid to handwashing by the athlete and the practitioners who treat them. The athlete should be instructed to dry each eye with different parts of the towel so that the infection does not spread from one eye to the other.

Examination of the eye will reveal red eyelid margins and conjunctiva. The eye may be slightly swollen and a small amount of mucopurulent (pus) drainage may be noted. There is frequently increased tearing and nighttime matting of the eyelashes.

Viral conjunctivitis is the most common type and is frequently associated with cold and flu symptoms.

The virus will run its course in 5 to 7 days with or without treatment. There is rarely puslike drainage or pain with viral conjunctivitis. Viral and allergic conjunctivitis are similar to their clinical presentation.

Allergic conjunctivitis most commonly occurs in the spring, summer, or fall in individuals who have allergies or hay fever. Frequently both eyes are involved. Treatment involves the use of oral antihistamine medications and treatment of the underlying allergy.

Chemical conjunctivitis is commonly seen in contact lens wearers. A thorough history should be taken to determine if the athlete has changed solutions, opened a new bottle of solution, or is cleaning his or her contacts properly. Once the offending chemical is found its use is discontinued. The use of artificial tears may help to make the athlete more comfortable.

Bacterial conjunctivitis may be associated with mild sensitivity to light, mild discomfort, itching, burning, and matting of the eyelashes especially at night. *Streptococcus* and *Staphylococcus* are the most commonly involved organisms.[16] The treatment is generally with antibiotic ointments or eyedrops. Care must be taken to avoid touching the eye with the medication as the container may recontaminate the eye during the next application of the medicine. If the athlete continues to compete the drops may be preferable during the time of competition as it does not blur the vision of the athlete.

Corneal Abrasion.

Corneal abrasion is a serious traumatic condition that is caused by the physical rubbing or denuding of the cornea. This may be caused by contact lens abuse, a foreign body in the eye or chemical irritants.

The athlete will complain of something in the eye and moderate to severe pain with eye opening as well as photophobia. First aid measures include irrigation of the eye. The eyelid should be inverted with the irrigation. The eye should then be patched and the athlete examined by a physician for a more thorough evaluation. This includes fluorescein staining of the eye and examination under blue light, which will highlight the abraded area. The athlete is then given antibiotic ointment for the eye and it is patched for 24 to 48 hours.[17] Analgesics are needed, as this is a very painful condition; codeine is frequently ordered for the first 24 hours. The athlete should be confined to bed or quiet rest during this time and should be reexamined the following day to ensure that proper healing is taking place.

Penetrating Eye Injuries.

Although penetrating eye injuries are uncommon in sports, they do occur. The outcome of such injuries is commonly the loss of vision in the eye or the eye itself. One series of 2089 sport-related eye injuries reported 70 penetrating injuries.[18]

The most common penetrating objects are hockey sticks, ski tips, golf balls, racquetballs, and tennis balls.

On the field the examination will reveal a spasm of the obicularis oculi muscle, which makes it difficult to open the eyelid. If the lid can be gently opened, the eye will appear soft and sunken back in the orbit. There is generally no vision except perception of movement or light. Both eyes should be lightly patched to prevent movement of the involved eye. Care should be taken so that no pressure is placed on the involved eye. The athlete is then transported to the emergency department with the head slightly elevated.

Hyphemia.

Hyphemia is bleeding or a collection of blood in the anterior chamber of the eye. This is a traumatic condition seen most commonly in sports that use an air-filled ball such as soccer, basketball, or racquetball. Examination of the eye reveals a haze in front of the iris and an irregularly shaped iris. This is a serious condition and must be recognized. An athlete should be examined immediately after any impact to the eye and then reexamined a few minutes later. If there is blood in the anterior chamber of the eye, the eye should be patched and the athlete sent to the emergency department for evaluation by an ophthalmologist. Typical treatment for this condition includes measurement of intraocular pressure to watch for acute glaucoma, and bed rest with one or both eyes patched for 2 to 5 days. The major cause of concern is a secondary hemorrhage which increases the chances of glaucoma.

Ear Injuries

Swimmer's Ear.

Swimmer's ear is an external otitis infection that is common in swimmers because their ears are so frequently exposed to water. The presentation of swimmer's ear is that of pain on movement of the external ear, itching, and dry scaly external ear canal. Swimmer's ear is a totally preventable condition. A frequent mechanism is from water becoming trapped in the ear canal behind a wax plug. The wax plug can act as a one-way valve in the ear, allowing water into the ear canal but not out. The treatment is first to remove the wax plug by using a product such as Debrox, which softens the wax and helps to remove it. After the wax buildup has been removed, the swimmer should be instructed to dry the ears carefully after each exposure to water. A towel should be used on the external portion of the ear and a cool blow dryer pointed at the ear to dry the canal. The athlete should never put cotton swabs into the ear canal, as the swab will leave cotton lint in the ear canal, which makes the wax much harder to remove. After thoroughly drying the ear, the athlete should also instill a solution of 5% acetic acid in isopropyl alcohol, commonly called swimmer's drops. A

home-made solution of isopropyl alcohol and white vinegar mixed in a 1:1 ratio can also be used.[19] The drops help to create an environment in which fungus will not grow. Particularly susceptible swimmers may also use silicone ear plugs to keep the water out of the ear.

Cauliflower Ear or Wrestler's Ear. The external ear is prone to blunt trauma, which can frequently develop into cauliflower ear or wrestler's ear. This is preventable if the wrestler will simply wear his headgear at all times. This includes practice as well as meets.

The problem is that the cartilage of the ear has no direct blood supply and must depend on the perichondrium for nourishment. When significant trauma occurs to the external ear, it tears the overlying tissue away from the cartilage and causes fluid accumulation and hematoma between the cartilage and the skin. If the fluid is not evacuated from the ear promptly, fibrosis ensues, resulting in an elevated, white, rounded keloid formation that resembles a cauliflower.

Evacuation of the hematoma by the physician is a relatively simple procedure. First the ear must be scrubbed for 10 minutes using a Betadine-type scrub. One milliliter of lidocaine with epinephrine is injected into the hematoma using a 21-gauge needle and a 5-mL syringe. The area is gently massaged. The needle is reinserted and the lidocaine and hematoma are then removed. After the fluid is removed, direct digital pressure must be placed over the ear; a form-fitted compression dressing is then applied. The compression dressing can be fashioned out of plaster or cotton and flexible collodion. The dressing should be left in place for 48 hours and then inspected for signs of infection.

Nosebleeds

Most nosebleeds (epistaxis) seen in sports are associated with direct, blunt trauma. Sometimes they are associated with a fracture of the nasal bone and cartilage. Recognition of a fracture of the nose is generally not difficult because of obvious deformity.

Treatment of epistaxis is relatively easy. The athlete is instructed to sit up with the head slightly forward and gently blow each nostril.[20] This will remove any old clots and allow the vessels to contract and retract, thus stopping the bleed. The nose is then gently packed with cotton dental rolls that have been moistened with $\frac{1}{8}$% Neo-Synephrine. For athletes involved in a sport where they need to return immediately, such as wrestling, they may if they feel ready. It is preferable that the athlete remain quiet for 10 to 15 minutes. The packs can be removed after 30 minutes. There may be a small amount of bleeding just after the packs are removed. If the bleeding persists for more than a half an hour, the athlete is referred to the physician for an evaluation. If an athlete has frequent nosebleeds and is in

a sport where the nose cannot be well protected, the physician may choose to cauterize the superficial bleeding site. This should decrease the frequency of the nosebleeds.

Dental Injury

Although the number of dental injuries seen in sports has decreased over the past three decades, they are still quite common. Authorities agree that most dental injuries are preventable through the use of a well-fitting mouth guard and effective facial protectors. At this time only football and youth ice hockey require mouth guards and face guards. Athletes in other sports such as wrestling, basketball, baseball, and field hockey should be encouraged to wear well-fitted mouth guards. These serve to decrease the potential for dental and oral injury, and are felt to decrease the incidence of cerebral concussion as well.

When dental injury occurs, the management of the injury on the field will make a difference as to whether or not the tooth can be reimplanted.[21] Most authorities agree that if a tooth has been avulsed or knocked out of the mouth, there is approximately 1 hour to reimplant the tooth and have it splinted by the dentist or oral surgeon. This time pressure necessitates a dental emergency plan so that the athlete will know where to go for treatment.

In the case of the avulsed tooth, every attempt should be made to find the tooth on the ground or in the grass. When the tooth is found, it should be left intact. Dirt or tissue should not be removed. The front and back of the tooth should be identified. The tooth is then replaced in the socket in the appropriate position. The bottom surface of the replaced tooth should set at approximately the same level as that of the surrounding teeth. If it protrudes, then firm pressure should be used to reseat it in its socket. The athlete should stabilize the replaced tooth with his or her finger if it is so unstable that it will not stay in place.

If it is not possible to reseat the tooth, it should be stressed that immediate action to replace the tooth will play a key roll in its survival. Two alternative methods of transporting the tooth are available if you cannot reseat the tooth.

1. If the athlete is alert, cooperative and reliable, the tooth may be placed under the tongue (where an oral thermometer would go). The athlete is cautioned not to swallow the tooth during the transport process.
2. If milk is immediately available, it may be poured into a cup and the tooth placed in the milk. The patient's saliva works as well as milk. The tooth is placed in a cup and the athlete is asked to spit into it until the tooth is covered with fluid.

In the case of a nonavulsed tooth injury, typically the athlete will have a cut lip or will notice a "loose tooth." The extent of dental trauma is difficult to assess because the damage may be below the gum line.

To evaluate the loose tooth, one must first identify the source of the bleeding in the mouth. Gauze is used to wipe the blood from the area. Bleeding from a lip laceration can be controlled with direct pressure. If the primary source of blood is seepage around the base of the tooth, the tooth should be considered injured. To evaluate the degree of looseness, the examiner stabilizes the athlete's head with one hand. The tip of the index finger of the examiner is placed on the biting surface of an apparently noninjured tooth. Mild pressure is put on the tooth, first toward the tongue and then toward the lips. The easy motion and amount of motion in the noninjured teeth is noted. The test is repeated on the injured tooth, and the ease and amount of motion of both are compared. The normal tooth will move very slightly but will not be painful. If the suspected tooth movement is similar to the noninjured tooth and the tooth is not obviously fractured, painful, or numb, the source of the bleeding is probably the gum tissue and the athlete may return to play.

If there is a marked increase in motion, pain, or numbness in the tooth compared to the surrounding teeth, the athlete should be seen by the dentist on an emergency basis.[22]

Tooth Fractures. There are three common types of tooth fractures: enamel fractures, where the enamel is slightly chipped off the tooth; dentin fractures, a slightly deeper fracture where the tooth is sensitive to inhaled air; and pulp fractures, where the pink pulp of the tooth is exposed.

The tooth is first examined for looseness, as described in Table 16-1. The sports physical therapist should then have the athlete perform an inhaled air test. The athlete is asked to inhale vigorously two or three times. If the tooth is sensitive to the inhaled air test, then the athlete is asked to tip the head back and the injured tooth is visually examined to see if the pink pulp is visible in the fracture or if there is a small drop of blood in the center of the fracture. Either sign indicates a fracture that extends into the dental pulp. The athlete with a pulp fracture should receive emergency dental treatment for the fracture.[23] Generally the athlete with this type of fracture will stop playing due to the intense pain of air passing over the fractured tooth.

Mouth Guards. Most dental trauma is preventable if an athlete wears a properly fitted intraoral mouth guard. The mouth guard is designed to fit tight and comfortably over the upper teeth. If correctly fit, it allows speech and no obstruction of the air passages. The mouth guard should extend back as far as the last molar. If it is longer, it will possibly impede the airway and become uncomfortable.

The mouth guard should be constructed of a flexible resilient material that can be easily fit to the teeth in the upper jaw. The combination of proper fit and good construction not only protects the teeth but also absorbs shock from a blow to the chin, which may prevent a concussion. In fact, the United States Public Health Services feels mouth guards are so important that it recommends all junior high, high school, college, and university students who play collision and contact sports wear an intraoral mouth guard.

Selection of mouth guards is relatively simple, as most of the commercially available intraoral mouth guards are well constructed. Generally, the guard is dipped in hot or boiling water for 10 to 30 seconds, removed from the water, quickly rinsed in cool water for 2 to 3 seconds, and then fit to the athlete's upper teeth. The fitting is done by putting the guard on the athlete's upper teeth and pressing the bottom of the guard onto the teeth. The athlete is now allowed to bite gently with even pressure on all teeth. The athlete should not bite hard on the mouthpiece at this point, as this may decrease the shock absorption properties of the mouth guard. The guard is held in the mouth until cool. It is then removed and rinsed in cool water. The

TABLE 16-1. COMMON TOOTH FRACTURES

Type	Observation	Loose Tooth Test	Inhaled Air Sensitivity	Treatment
Enamel fracture	Small chip off the tooth	Negative	No	Continue play. See dentist in 48 hours
Dentin fracture	Slightly larger chip or fracture	Negative	Yes	Evaluate for pulp fracture. Continue play if tolerated. See dentist in 24 hours or less.
Pulp fracture	Similar to dentin fracture. Pink pulp visible or drop of blood from center of fracture	Negative	Yes, unless tooth is numb	Emergency dental referral and treatment

fit should then be rechecked. These are general guidelines for fitting of the mouth guards, but the directions specified by the manufacturer will yield the best results.

An alternative to the dip-and-fit mouth guard is the custom-made guard fit by a dentist. These are more expensive but will fit better and are preferred by most athletes. Any athlete with braces should have this type of guard.[24] The custom-fit guard is also preferable for those athletes who need to talk with the guard in place, such as quarterbacks and basketball players.

RESPIRATORY CONDITIONS

The respiratory system is intricately involved in the delivery of oxygen to exercising muscles and in the elimination of CO_2, a by-product of exercise. The respiratory system comprises the nose, nasal pharynx, oropharynx, larynx, trachea, bronchi, and other associated lung structures. When the system is congested or compromised, it may well lead to submaximal athletic performance.

Cold and Flu

The common cold and flu are regular visitors to the locker room in the fall and winter. Both are viral infections of the upper respiratory tract. The infection is spread via respiratory droplets and is best controlled by the use of disposable tissues for nasal drainage and good handwashing habits.

What generally differentiates the common cold from influenza is that influenza occurs in epidemics. Influenza also lowers the white blood cell (WBC) count and generally results in more severe symptoms.

Fatigue and sluggishness are the principal symptoms of colds and the flu. The athlete may complain of chills or headache. There is general sneezing and watery to mucopurulent discharge from the nose. The throat is dry, scratchy, and sore but seldom painful. The cervical lymph nodes are sometimes enlarged. A low-grade fever may be present, and often there are increased complaints of aching muscles.[25]

No specific treatment is needed, but the athlete should be isolated from his or her teammates to prevent spread of the disease. Symptomatic treatment for aches and pains is acetaminophen 650 mg as needed, and rest in bed when possible for 24 to 72 hours. Antibiotics are of no value in the treatment of a viral cold or influenza. Over-the-counter decongestants such as pseudoephedrine (Sudafed) 60 mg three times a day may help ease breathing and decrease the runny nose.

The cough may be treated with a cough syrup such as Robitussin DM. If this does not stop the cough and the athlete is *not* allergic to codeine, pharmacies sell nonprescription cough mixtures with codeine, but the

nonnarcotic medication should be tried first. If the athlete is having trouble sleeping, he might try Benylin Cough Syrup, as this mixture makes many people a little drowsy due to the drug diphenhydramine.[26]

Of course, the athlete should not be allowed to play until the fever is gone and the symptoms are well controlled. This generally takes 2 to 5 days.

The nasal congestion that accompanies colds and flu is often the limiting factor in the decision to determine to play. Nasal congestion markedly decreases the amount of normal breathing done through the nasopharynx. This limits the amount of heat and humidity supplied by the pharynx to the air before passing into the lungs, which must now take on that task. If, as is often the case, the tracheobronchial mucosa has been damaged by the viral infection, the poorly humidified air dehydrates it further, providing an excellent medium for a bacterial infection to develop on top of the viral infection. If the athlete has symptoms of fever, productive cough, or fatigue lasting more than 5 days, then it is likely that there is a superimposed bacterial infection. This athlete needs to be seen by the physician and may well be placed on antibiotics for the superimposed bacterial infection.

To prevent the cold or flu, the athlete should:

1. Avoid overfatigue especially with travel.
2. Establish regular eating habits and proper nutrition.
3. Maintain high standards of cleanliness.
4. Be educated on prevention.

The most common time for the flu epidemic to hit a team is after Thanksgiving, Christmas, and New Years holidays, when everyone has visited friends and family and brought new viruses back to "share" with their teammates. The athletes should be taught to stay away until their symptoms are gone to decrease the chance of a teamwide outbreak.

Despite widespread claims and many believers, vitamin C has not been shown to be helpful prophylactically or therapeutically in the treatment of these diseases.[27]

Asthma

Asthma is a respiratory ailment found often in young athletes but occurs in all ages. Asthma is characterized by a prolonged expiratory phase of breathing with audible wheezing. There are also recurrent attacks of dyspnea and coughing. The cough is frequently productive of thick, mucoid sputum. The wheezing component is a result of reduced diameter of the bronchioles, which occurs in response to provocation by an external allergen or other internal provocation. This bronchiole constriction is reversible, but the degree of its reversibility varies from athlete to athlete. This variability in airway obstruction will allow some athletes to compete with

almost no measurable airway obstruction whereas other athletes, despite treatment, will compete with a considerable amount of airway obstruction.

There are two basic types of asthma, extrinsic and intrinsic. Extrinsic asthma is also referred to as allergic or atopic asthma. It usually begins in childhood and often there is a familial history of asthma. Many of these people can identify and avoid the allergens, such as foods, pollens, and many types of dust, that trigger the asthma attacks.

People with intrinsic asthma do not have identifiable allergens or a family history of asthma. Intrinsic asthma is also most likely to occur initially during adulthood.

There are a number of bronchial irritants that commonly trigger asthma attacks in all asthmatics. The most common are bronchitis and pneumonia. Other irritants include solvent fumes, cold air and exercise.

Exercise-Induced Asthma. The fact that exercise can cause an asthmatic attack was first documented in the second century A.D.[28] In 1869, H. H. Satter observed exposure to cold triggered exercise-induced asthma (EIA). He speculated that the passage of cold air over the bronchial mucosal membranes might trigger the attack directly or by irritating nervous tissue. EIA may be the first and only symptom of asthma in an athlete. Exercised-induced asthma may present with a mild coughing attack or an unusually dyspneic appearance of the athlete if the attack is mild. In a severe attack of EIA, the athlete will present with wheezing and severe shortness of breath. The athlete will be quite anxious and will appear fatigued. This will affect his or her athletic performance.

Exercise-induced asthma is preferred over the older term, exercise-induced bronchospasm. Recent information shows bronchospasm, edema, and inflammation can occur individually or in any combination in the respiratory tract of an individual with EIA.

The diagnosis of EIA is relatively easy if the athlete presents with wheezing after each workout session. Often this is not the case. The athlete will present with mild shortness of breath and a persistent hacky cough. Pulmonary function tests postexercise may be decreased by 20% to 30% without any wheezing noted audibly or by auscultation.

Exercise-induced asthma can be diagnosed by means of an exercise challenge test that includes pulmonary function tests given before and after the athlete exercises and that are supervised by a pulmonary specialist. The test can be repeated with the athlete taking medication to see how effective the treatment is for that athlete. The medication can be titrated to that particular athlete using this method.

When an athlete is placed on an asthma medication, consideration must be given to whether he or she will be competing in an international or national event where drug testing will take place. Some common asthma medications are on the list of banned substances and use of these would cause the athlete to be disqualified. Most asthma can be controlled with approved drugs. The list of banned substances can be obtained from the Olympic Training Center in Colorado Springs, Colorado.

Once the diagnosis of EIA is made, the athlete must be educated about asthma and ways to reduce the chances of triggering an attack. This is done by learning to breathe through the nose, which will warm and humidify the air before it goes into the lungs. In cool weather, he or she should wear a mask that will aid in warming the air. An asthmatic athlete who is suffering from a cold or the flu or is just recovering from these ailments must be careful about returning to sports too soon because of the chance that the airways may be more sensitive to irritants. The athlete should also be educated about "working through" an attack so that he or she can continue participating. Although the mechanism is not well understood, asthmatic symptoms tend to peak at about 6 minutes into the exercise and plateau until 12 to 16 minutes, when the symptoms tend to decrease.[29]

Asthmatic athletes often perform best if they warm up for 15 to 20 minutes 1 to 1½ hours before competition. This is because the second exercise session in less than 90 minutes will often cause less severe symptoms than those experienced during the first exercise session.[30]

The most effective way to deal with both asthma and EIA is through pharmacological agents administered following exercise. Almost every asthmatic can be managed by the proper administration of prescription bronchodilators. These are most commonly administered by inhalation. They are rapid acting, sustained-action medications that are generally used every 4 to 8 hours. The athlete must adhere closely to the schedule of administration designed by the physician to achieve maximum benefits.

Asthmatic athletes may also be on oral bronchodilators. These drugs are considered by many to be the mainstay treatment for chronic asthmatics, unlike the bronchodilators, which are helpful once an asthma attack has started. When inhaled prior to the start of exercise, cromolyn sodium (Intal) works to reduce the chance of an extrinsic allergen causing an attack.

Asthmatic athletes often do the best in skill- and coordination-type activities as opposed to endurance sports.[6] Swimming is a good choice, however. This is probably due to the fact that the swimming environment is warm and humid, thus decreasing the dehydration of the bronchial tree. Swimming also necessitates rhythmic, deep, forced breathing, which promotes maximum emptying of the lungs. This breathing pattern reduces the chances of an asthma attack.

Few children can truly use asthma as a reason for

not participating in sport activities. Most athletes with asthma can be helped through education and medications to participate and excel in the athletic event of their choice.

CARDIOVASCULAR CONDITIONS

Excluding trauma, sudden death in young athletes is almost always due to a cardiovascular abnormality. Although most authorities agree that all athletic heart deaths are not foreseeable, our emphasis is in prevention via the preparticipation screening examination.

The examining physician should perform a simple yet thorough cardiovascular exam that generally rules out significant pathology. The physician should be alert to systolic heart murmurs $\frac{3}{6}$ or greater as well as murmurs that last through both systole and diastole.[31] Also important are resting blood pressures higher than 130/80 mm Hg in children ages 6 to 11 and 140/90 mm Hg in children 12 years and older, as well as any heart arrhythmias or discrepancies between simultaneous monitoring of brachial and femoral pulses. These are signs of possible cardiac problems and deserve further investigation before participation is allowed.

Heart Murmur

Many athletes have functional heart murmurs. These are abnormal sounds produced during the filling of the chambers or ejection of blood from the heart that are not associated with disease. The most common functional murmur is the systolic ejection type.

A click murmur is indicative of mitral valve prolapse, which is the most common cardiac abnormality found in athletes. Healthy young women have a reported incidence of 16%. The syndrome of mitral valve prolapse includes the click murmur, pectus excavatum, and (mild) scoliosis. Mitral valve prolapse may be the initial manifestation of a cardiomyopathy and should be investigated further.

Marfan's Syndrome

Marfan's syndrome is occasionally associated with mitral valve prolapse. Marfan's syndrome is a genetic disorder with variable autosomal dominant characteristics. The diagnosis of Marfan's syndrome is difficult, as the physical examination, ECG, and chest x-ray are often within normal limits. Keys to the diagnosis is a family history of unexplained sudden death and other family members with physical signs such as unusually long arms or recurrent dislocations of the patella as well as chest wall deformities.[32] The common hallmark of Marfan's syndrome is disproportionate height and long arms. These findings are not diagnostic, however. Diagnosis includes positive findings in two of these four categories: family history, ocular lens displacement, echocardiographic findings of aortic root dilatation or mitral valve prolapse, and height or arm length greater than the 95th percentile. An athlete with confirmed Marfan's syndrome should not be allowed to participate in vigorous competitive sports[33] and should receive regular medical reassessments.

Hypertension

Hypertension or high blood pressure is a common finding at preseason screenings. The findings of an athlete with elevated blood pressure (130/80 mm Hg, 6 to 11 years, and 140/90 mm Hg, 12 years and older) requires serial measurement in a more relaxed setting during the subsequent 7 to 10 days to determine whether or not the blood pressure is chronically elevated. The measurement of blood pressure seems like an easy enough task but one must use an appropriately sized cuff to ensure accurate readings. The bladder of the blood pressure cuff should cover at least two thirds of the upper arm and circle more than half of the circumference of the arm. The total length of the cuff should easily wrap around the arm one and one-half to two times.

If the athlete is found to be hypertensive, examination of blood pressure during exercise should be carried out along with a thorough workup to find the cause of the hypertension. Care should be taken to examine the blood pressure during both dynamic and isometric activities. Generally if systolic measurements do not exceed 220 systolic or 100 diastolic, the athlete can safely participate with blood pressure medication. The hypertensive athlete's blood pressure should be routinely monitored throughout the season to detect any changes that might occur.

BLOOD DISORDERS

Anemia

Anemia is a common clinical finding in both athletic and nonathletic populations. When an athlete develops anemia, it is important to determine the cause of the anemia. It is not good medicine to assume that the anemia is due to sport participation or low iron intake and simply treat the athlete with iron supplements. The athlete deserves a thorough history and physical examination by a physician as well as a comprehensive set of diagnostic laboratory studies to determine the cause of the anemia.

The causes of anemia range from severe infection, cancer, or depressed bone marrow function to recent severe loss of blood volume, increased menstrual flow, low dietary intake of iron, and chronic exercise. Several authors have found that trained athletes have hemoglobin and hematocrit levels that are in the low range of normal or slightly below normal. This is often referred to as "sports anemia."[35] There is evidence that chronic exercise increases the plasma volume, which will alter the standard hemoglobin and hematocrit tests. It has

been shown that a hematocrit level of about 40% yields an increase in oxygen delivery compared with higher hematocrit values. The higher hematocrit value will cause an increase in blood viscosity, forcing the heart to work harder to move the same volume of blood. The increased work load decreases the athlete's efficiency, and the body works to increase the plasma volume, thus decreasing the viscosity of the blood.

Iron deficiency may result from lack of iron intake in the diet and loss from exercise. Most athletic diets are relatively high in calories and should be well balanced from a nutritional standpoint. Studies show, however, that 10% to 15% of female athletes do not receive adequate iron in their diets. Although some authors suggest iron supplementation prophylactically in menstruating athletes, studies have not demonstrated this practice to be helpful in increasing iron storage.[36] Iron deficiency can develop from exercise as a result of hemoglobinuria and as a result of excessive sweating. As much as 0.25 to 1 mg of iron may be lost per day through sweat. Iron deficiency in the absence of anemia can cause diminished exercise performance that is unrelated to the oxygen carrying capabilities of the hemoglobin. Compounds in the muscles such as myoglobin use iron compounds. Lack of iron may limit the ability of the myoglobin to store oxygen in the muscle tissue.

If the iron deficiency or anemia is due to low iron intake from the diet, the athlete should receive dietary counseling. Iron is found in high concentration in foods such as liver, beef, pork, nuts, beans, peas, and spinach. Iron absorption is facilitated by ascorbic acid or vitamin C and is impaired by the intake of tea.

Sickle Cell Disease

Sickle cell disease is a genetic disorder confined essentially to blacks. Both parents transmit the abnormal sickle cell gene to the offspring. This hemolytic disorder causes accelerated red blood cell (RBC) destruction due to a structural defect in the hemoglobin molecule. Most of the hemoglobin in these patients is of the sickle cell type. Sickle cell disease is generally diagnosed in childhood via routine laboratory screening tests. Patients with sickle cell anemia seldom have a hemoglobin higher than 7 g/dL. (Normal hemoglobin is 11 to 16 g/dL.) Most people with sickle cell disease do not participate in sports.[37] This is due to moderate to severe anemia, painful attacks of bone and joint pain, and occasional acute abdominal crises that resemble the surgical abdomen.

Sickle cell trait carrier is a common disorder with an incidence of 6% to 9% of the black population. This individual has received only one recessive sickle cell gene. Less than 50% of his or her hemoglobin is of the sickle cell type. There is usually no anemia and RBC life-span is normal. The sickle cell trait athlete may experience a sickle cell crisis when performing at an altitude greater than 4000 ft above sea level. The relative scarcity of oxygen causes the RBC to deform and decreases its oxygen carrying capacity. The athlete in crisis will have moderate pain somewhere in the abdomen and should be sent to the emergency department for evaluation.

Exercise-Related Hematuria

Exercise-related hematuria or blood in the urine is not uncommon in sports. It is usually seen with endurance activities such as marathons. One possible cause for the hematuria is rupture of the renal capillaries as a result of increased renal vascular resistance. A second possible mechanism is traumatic injury to the lower urinary tract from the continuous up and down movement of the sport activity. If hematuria is excessive, it can be a cause of anemia through blood loss, although this is not common.

GASTROINTESTINAL DISORDERS

The gastrointestinal (GI) tract's basic function is the digestion of food and provision of energy for the work that the body must perform. The balance of intake of food and water and output of work is a delicate one. If this balance is not maintained, the athlete will not be able to perform optimally. Gastrointestinal upset is characterized by loss of appetite, nausea, abdominal pain, diarrhea, constipation, and vomiting.

Indigestion

Indigestion is the failure of the digestive tract to digest and absorb foodstuffs. Indigestion is common in athletes because many athletes have food superstitions or habits and any variation from these habits can cause the athlete to become distressed. This emotional stress causes increased secretion of hydrochloric acid and may cause nausea, flatulence, or diarrhea. All of these can take the athlete's mind off of the competition. The easiest way to avoid this type of emotional development of symptoms is to establish a preevent routine and stick to it. If an athlete has frequent GI upset, the athlete should be evaluated by a physician for other GI problems.[38]

Diarrhea

Diarrhea is another common problem for athletes when they are nervous or have problems with the travel schedule they must keep. Diarrhea is simply abnormal passage of fluid, unformed stools. Elimination of stools may occur 3 to 20 times daily, quickly leading to dehydration. Strict monitoring of the athlete's weight should assist in the assessment of dehydration. Because diarrhea is a sign of many disease processes, its cause must be determined. Less severe causes of diarrhea are treated symptomatically, generally by a kaolin-pectin mixture such as Kaopectate after each loose stool and

the ingestion of a bland diet until the symptoms subside. Recently approved for over-the-counter use, immodium is quite effective in relieving the diarrhea. If the diarrhea persists for more than 3 days, a physician should be consulted.

Strenuous training or severe increases in aerobic training will sometimes cause "runner's trots." The common complaints are lower abdominal cramping and bloating. The symptoms generally subside if the intensity of training is decreased or held constant until the athlete's symptoms subside. The athlete should be watched for dehydration.

Constipation

Athletes will occasionally complain of constipation with the stress of competition. The complaint is often an observation of decreased stool frequency or change in bowel function. The athlete should be considered constipated if defecation is delayed by several days or if the stools are unusually dry and hard. Lack of bowel movements is often a sign of poor eating habits. If food is not taken in, it cannot be evacuated. Simple constipation often can be treated by a change in diet.

Constipation may be relieved by eating foods with high fiber content such as fruits, vegetables, and bran. The constipation may also be relieved by adequate hydration of the athlete. He or she should be consuming at least 80 oz of water daily. Medications are seldom needed in the treatment of constipation in the athletic population. If a laxative is needed to relieve the symptoms, the athlete should be seen by the team physician.

Hemorrhoids

The constipated athlete is susceptible to hemorrhoids due to increased straining with defecation. The same mechanism occurs when an athlete holds his or her breath during weightlifting. The hemorrhoid is a varicosity of the venous plexus of the anus. It may be internal or external to the anus. Most often hemorrhoids are painful, nodular swellings near the sphincter of the anus. They often bleed slightly and cause itching. Treatment of hemorrhoids are mostly palliative:

1. Avoidance of straining
2. Proper diet and hydration
3. Use of an anorectal cream such as Anusol or Preparation H to decrease the pain and itching

As with any rectal bleeding, if it persists for more than 5 days, the physician should be consulted, as rectal bleeding may be an early sign of colorectal cancer.

EATING DISORDERS

Anorexia Nervosa

Anorexia nervosa is a personality disorder in which the person develops an extreme aversion to food. This results in a life-threatening weight loss and electrolyte imbalance. Anorexia is seven times more common in women than in men. The exact etiology of the disease is not known but multiple psychological factors play a role.

Athletes who are overly concerned about weight control are the most likely to develop eating disorders. Typically the anorectic athlete is female, 15 to 30 years of age, and believes she is overweight despite being too thin. She will deny hunger and typically exercise excessively. This behavior is thought to stem from a desire to conform to an impossible goal. It is important that athletes who exhibit these behaviors be evaluated by a team of professionals experienced in dealing with eating disorders.

Bulemia

Bulemia is a condition most common to women 15 to 30 years of age who are concerned about being overweight. The bulemic athlete will go through binge–purge cycles, consuming thousands of calories one day and then going days without a meal before entering into another binge of eating. Typically the athlete eliminates the food eaten during binges by inducing vomiting either by sticking a finger in the throat or the use of Ipecac syrup. The athlete is often obsessed with diets and recipes and often prepares large meals for others. The hazards of bulemia include stomach rupture, liver damage, heart dysarrhythmias, and dental caries from the stomach acid on the tooth enamel. It is not uncommon for bulemic athletes to have calluses on the dorsal surface of the index and long fingers in the area of the metacarpophalangeal joint. This is secondary to the teeth scraping on the finger when vomiting is induced.

As is true of all athletes suspected of having an eating disorder, the suspected bulemic should be evaluated by experts in the field. Both bulemia and anorexia nervosa are quite difficult to treat and are potentially lethal. Some estimates say that 15% to 20% of people with these disorders will die from them.[39]

DIABETES MELLITUS

More than 10 million people in the United States today have diabetes mellitus. There are two forms of diabetes: type I (insulin-dependent or juvenile-onset) diabetes, which is usually characterized by total endogenous deficiency of insulin; and type II (non-insulin-dependent or adult-onset) diabetes, which usually occurs in middle-aged individuals who are overweight. In type II diabetes there is a relative deficiency of insulin.

The key to control of both types of diabetes is the control of blood sugar levels. Diet, insulin, blood sugar monitoring, and exercise are important factors that the diabetic athlete must manage to achieve optimal blood sugar control. Diabetics who engage in sports are usu-

ally in better control of their disease than their nonathletic counterparts, due in part to their regimented activity and their desire to participate. This motivates the athlete to take good care of himself or herself.[40]

Experienced athletes will not alter their insulin usage in season but will alter their eating pattern to compensate for changes in exercise. Athletes who are just starting a new sport or exercise program may need to have their insulin dose adjusted. Athletes are encouraged to use abdominal injection sites, as these sites provide a more controlled release of the injected insulin than leg sites, which are more actively involved in exercise.

Diabetic athletes should take responsibility for their own care. Sometimes, however, school rules make this difficult if athletes have to check their blood sugar or self-administer their insulin.[41] The logistics of this should be thought out before it presents as a problem.

Often the athlete will need a prepractice or competition snack. A sandwich, milk, peanuts, or cheese work well, but each athlete will decide what works best. If a practice runs long or is more vigorous than the athlete had planned, he or she may need a snack during the activity.

Monitoring is the key to prevention of problems associated with too much or too little blood sugar, but occasionally an athlete will suffer from insulin shock (too much insulin or exercise) or diabetic coma (too little insulin or too much blood sugar).

The signs and symptoms of both conditions are detailed in Table 16–2.[42] If the athlete is conscious and has been feeling poorly for the last few days and *not* taken insulin, the problem is most likely diabetic coma. If the athlete has taken insulin but not eaten or has exercised excessively, the problem is probably insulin shock or hypoglycemia. A high-sugar snack should be kept nearby in case of hypoglycemia.

EPILEPSY

Epilepsy is a chronic disorder characterized by paroxysmal attacks of brain dysfunction. Epilepsy is a symptom and not a disease process. The cause of epileptic attacks is not always known but hypoglycemia, adrenalin release, closed head injury, and hyperventilation are conditions that may induce seizures. There is no evidence that vigorous physical activity, even repeated tackling with the head in football, can cause more seizure activity in the epileptic athlete than when the same athlete is asleep at home. Injury rates are identical in epileptics and in nonepileptic athletes participating in all sports, including boxing and football.[43]

Each athlete should be individually evaluated to determine whether any sport restrictions are needed. If an individual has major seizures weekly, most authorities recommend avoidance of all collision sport participation. A seizure during a collision sport would place the athlete at risk of injury because of the contact caused by the injury rather than the seizure. If seizure activity is controlled, the athlete is allowed to participate in all sports, with the possible exceptions of scuba diving and participation at great heights such as mountain climbing.

Management of an epileptic seizure is not difficult. The athlete may experience an aura. This is a signal of an impending seizure. The athlete can then lie down to protect himself or herself from a potential fall. If a seizure occurs without warning, care should be taken to:

- Cushion the athlete's fall if possible
- Clear the area of potential injury-producing objects
- Protect the athlete from any hazards
- Avoid restraining the athlete

TABLE 16–2. DIABETIC EMERGENCIES

Signs	Diabetic Coma	Insulin Shock
Insulin intake	Insufficient insulin	Too much insulin
Period of onset	Gradual—days	Sudden—minutes
Skin appearance	Red, dry	Pale, clammy
Thirst	Intense	Absent
Breathing	Deep and rapid Sweet fruity odor	Normal
Blood pressure	Low	Normal
Pulse	Rapid	Normal
Headache	Present	Absent
Mental state	Restless	Apathy, fatigue
Vomiting	Common	Uncommon
Seizures	None	In more severe cases
Treatment	Transport to hospital	Rest 15 to 30 minutes Ingestion of sugar, e.g., soda, orange juice If no improvement in 30 minutes, transport to hospital

- Loosen tight clothing
- Allow the athlete to awaken normally after the seizure with a minimum of onlookers to decrease the embarrassment that commonly occurs
- Monitor the *Airway*, *Breathing*, and *Circulation* once the seizure has stopped
- Transport the athlete to a medical facility

REFERENCES

1. Klafs CE, Arnheim DD. *Modern Principles of Athletic Training*. 4th ed. St. Louis, Mo: C V Mosby; 1977: 259.
2. American Medical Association. *Standard Nomenclature for Athletic Injuries*. Chicago, Ill: American Medical Association; 1968.
3. Klafs CE, Arnheim DD. *Modern Principles of Athletic Training*, 4th ed. St. Louis, Mo: C V Mosby; 1977: 292.
4. Klafs CE, Arnheim DD. *Modern Principles of Athletic Training*. 4th ed. St. Louis, Mo: C V Mosby; 1977: 291.
5. Strauss RH. *Sports Medicine*. Philadelphia, Pa: W B Saunders; 1984: 101.
6. Kulund DN. *The Injured Athlete*. 2nd ed. Philadelphia, Pa: J B Lippincott; 1988: 64.
7. Krupp MA, Chatton MJ. *Current Medical Diagnosis and Treatment*. Los Altos, Calif: Lange Medical Publications; 1980: 57.
8. Strauss RH. *Sports Medicine*. Philadelphia, Pa: W B Saunders; 1984: 95.
9. Sauer GC. *Manual of Skin Disease*. 3nd ed. Philadelphia, Pa: J B Lippincott; 1973: 145–155.
10. *Steadman's Medical Dictionary*. 23rd ed. Baltimore, Md: Williams & Wilkens Co; 1976.
11. Strauss RH. *Sports Medicine*. Philadelphia, Pa: W B Saunders; 1984: 93–94.
12. Klafs CE, Arnheim DD. *Modern Principals of Athletic Training*. 4th ed. St. Louis, Mo: C V Mosby; 1977: 301.
13. Stauffer LW. How I manage athlete's foot. *Physician Sportsmed*. 1986; 14(7): 102–108.
14. International Federation of Sports Medicine Position Statement. Eye injuries and eye protection in sports. *J Osteopath Sports Med*. Dec 1988: 18–20.
15. Easterbrook M. Eye protection in racket sports: An update. *Physician Sportsmed*. 1987; 15(10): 180–192.
16. Kulund DN. *The Injured Athlete*. 2nd ed. Philadelphia, Pa: J B Lippincott; 1988: 187.
17. Pashby R, Pasby T. Occular injuries in sport. *Current Therapy in Sports Medicine*. St. Louis, Mo: C V Mosby; 1985–1986: 142–147.
18. Orlando RG. Soccer related eye injuries in children and adolescents. *Physician Sportsmed*. 1988; 16(11): 103–106.
19. Marcy SM. Swimmer's ear: Timely management tips. *Patient Care*. May 1987; 28–43.
20. Stevens H. Epistaxis in the athlete. *Physician Sportsmed*. 1988; 16(12): 31–40.
21. Comer RW. Oral trauma emergency care of lacerations, fractures and burns. *Postgrad Med*. 1989; 85(2): 34–41.
22. Castaldi CR. First aid for sports related dental injuries. *Physician Sportsmed*. 1987; 15(9): 81–89.
23. Hale ML. Traumatic injuries of the teeth and alveolar process. In: *Textbook of Oral and Maxillofacial Surgery*. 5th ed. St. Louis, Mo: C V Mosby; 1979.
24. Personal communication: Thomas Strub, D.D.S., Albert Lea, Minn.
25. Krupp MA, Chatton MJ. *Current Medical Diagnosis and Treatment*. Los Altos, Calif: Lange Medical Publications; 1980: 827.
26. Personal Communication: James E. Dreibelbeis, R.Ph., West Liberty, Iowa.
27. Strauss RH. *Sports Medicine*. Philadelphia, Pa: W B Saunders; 1984: 111.
28. Katz RM. Coping with exercise induced asthma in sports. *Physician Sportsmed*. 1987; 15(7): 100–111.
29. Godfrey S, Silverman M, Anderson SM. Problems of interpreting exercise induced asthma. *J Allergy Clin Immunol*. 1973; 52: 199–203.
30. Kulund DN. *The Injured Athlete*. 2nd ed. Philadelphia, Pa: J B Lippincott, 1988: 59.
31. Braden DS, Strong WB. Preparticipation screening for sudden cardiac death in young athletes. *Physician Sportsmed*. 1988; 16(10): 128–142.
32. Bracker MD. Suspected Marfan's syndrome in a female athlete. *Physician Sportsmed*. 1988; 16(2): 69–77.
33. Cantell JD. Marfan's syndrome: Detection and management. *Physician Sportsmed*. 1986; 14(7): 51–55.
34. Strauss RH. *Sports Medicine*. Philadelphia, Pa: W B Saunders; 1984: 120.
35. Kulund DN. *The Injured Athlete*. 2nd ed. Philadelphia, Pa: J B Lippincott; 1988: 101.
36. Strauss RH. *Sports Medicine*. Philadelphia, Pa: W B Saunders; 1984: 124.
37. Klafs CE, Arnheim DD. *Modern Principles of Athletic Training*. 4th ed. St. Louis, Mo: C V Mosby; 1977: 462.
38. *Current Therapy in Sports Medicine*. St. Louis, Mo: C V Mosby; 1985–1986: 42–47.
39. Blacket PR. Children and adolescents with diabetes. *Physician Sportsmed*. 1988; 16(3): 133–149.
40. American Medical Association. *Diabetic Athlete*. Chicago, Ill: American Medical Association; 1980.
41. American Academy of Orthopaedic Surgeons. *Emergency Care and Transportation of the Sick and Injured*. Chicago; 1977: 243.
42. Corbitt RW. Epilepsy and contact sports. *JAMA*. 1974; 229: 820–821.

17

Protective Equipment

Tyrone McSorley

THE INJURY FACTOR

Based on data from 1986–1987 projections by the NATA, of the estimated 5.8 million interscholastic athletes in the United States, there will be 1 million injuries.[1] This does not consider amateur, college, semiprofessional, or professional levels of competition. Football is widely considered to be a high-risk sport,[2,3] but wrestling and gymnastics are also potentially dangerous, and only minimal protective equipment is used in these two sports.[4] One study showed a high school hockey injury rate of 75%![5] The sports injury rates among male and female basketball players were roughly equivalent, with approximately 23% of the high school participants being sidelined at least once during the 1987–1988 season. More than half of the injuries occurred during practice; of those injuries sustained in games, 65% to 67% occurred in the second half.[6]

Thus, one can see that injury rates may be linked to fatigue, as well as longer playing times for the more talented athletes, elements that can be perplexing when attempting to draw cause and effect relationships to protective equipment. What this may imply is that sports now utilizing minimal equipment may need more, or that events involving a tremendous amount of protection may need further changes in rules, stricter enforcement, or simply different utilization of players relative to fatigue/conditioning factors.

Quite simply, equipment is not the final answer to the problem; it can be part of the solution, or a catalyst to the injury. We must understand as many of the principles involved as possible to best protect the athlete and ourselves.

CEREBRAL, SKULL, AND FACIAL PROTECTION

Helmets

Protecting the floating brain from impact forces is extremely important and equally difficult. It was once

reported that a famous professional football running back suffered two concussions during his years of repeated blows, but neither was from contact. Both were from going up for a pass, having his feet knocked out from under him, and striking the ground on his gluteal region. The helmet did not strike the ground, and yet the "contre-coup" whiplash forces caused severe cerebral bleeding. One can extrapolate from auto accidents involving a well-stabilized victim that upper motor neuron injuries do not require contact with anything except the inside of the cranium.

The line of thought "football helmets–brain or spinal cord injuries–legal liability," has led to the demise of helmet manufacturers. During the 1960s, there were at least 20 helmet manufacturers; now only two remain—Riddell, Inc, and Athletic Helmets Inc.[7] In the last 15 years, 25 helmet liability cases have gone to court, awarding $46,000,000 in verdicts (50 more cases are pending).[7]

The 1987 survey of football deaths showed three deaths directly related to head injuries, with two of these resulting from neck injuries that occurred while tackling.[8] Interestingly, only 14% of spinal cord injuries are due to sports, and, of that amount, only 6.1% is due to football. Diving is the leading "sports" cause. The other principal areas are motor vehicle accidents (47.7%), falls (20.8%), and violence (14.6%).[9]

Football Helmet Design. Prior to the institution of a leather cranial covering in 1918, there was no protection for the head. In 1932, suspension webbing was introduced, and in 1950, the plastic shell appeared. Today, three main styles are used—padded, suspension, and, most recently, air–fluid, which allows a more custom fit, as the cell can be pumped tight against the head. The National Operating Committee on Standards for Athletic Equipment (NOCSAE) certifies helmet manufacturers. They test for simultaneous three-site forces, and repeated falls onto a force meter.[10] A study done by Houston in 1982 showed 75% of 3-year-old high school helmets failed to pass the NOCSAE

tests.[11] Coaches and equipment purchasing administrators need this type of information.

Fitting a Helmet. Circumferential head measurements will provide an initial size, but custom sizes may be needed. The initial guidelines are as follows:

1. Approximately three-fourths inches above eyebrows
2. Ear holes match up
3. Cheek pads snug
4. Covers base of skull

The fit is tested by

1. Compressing from above (there should be no recoil)
2. Applying manual pressure from front/back/oblique angles (there should be no shifting or rotation)
3. Checking to see that the face mask and chin straps are secure
4. Confirming that a tongue depressor will not slide easily between the head and liner

Air–fluid helmets should be fitted with the cells partially drained and then inflated in the following order: (1) top of head, (2) front, (3) back, (4) neck, and (5) sides (Fig 17–1).[10]

Proper fit should be checked often, especially during the first few days of contact.

Chin Strap. A new device called the "Heads up! Chin Strap" helps absorb compression forces on the neck when it goes into forced flexion. It was tested by Voigt R. Hodgson, the principal investigator of NOCSAE since 1970. His evaluation showed effectiveness in the neck by reducing forces to the neck from 1460 down to 520 lb using a 2 in roll[12]; following 5 years of testing in

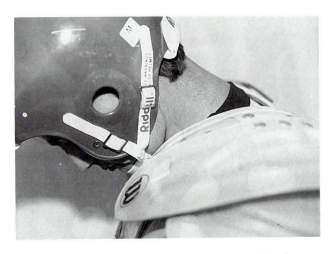

Figure 17–2. Hyperflexion is a very dangerous position for contact sports.

Texas high schools, it was used by schools in Las Vegas with excellent subjective responses.[12] It would appear that these straps can potentially diminish head down hitting, which is the most common cause of quadriplegia in high school football players.[13] Constant reminders to the coaching staff and players of proper technique and further research in this area are also vital (Figs 17–2 through 17–4).

Baseball Helmets. Baseball/softball batting helmets now offer ear protection, as well as a mandibular protection bar, thus reducing the possibility of a ball reaching the face at all.[14] Batting helmets must be able to absorb high-velocity impact. It would appear that a simple chin strap to hold the helmet in place would improve its function tremendously, as sliding or contact with the ground or another player can cause these helmets to come off, possibly at the same time a throw is being received.

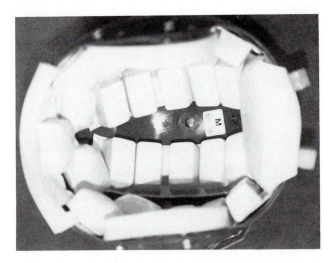

Figure 17–1. The interior of a fluid–air helmet.

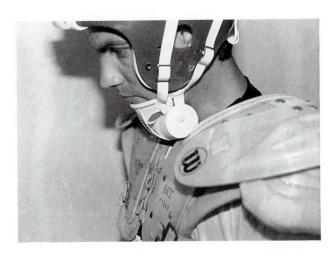

Figure 17–3. This chin strap is designed to help control hyperflexion.

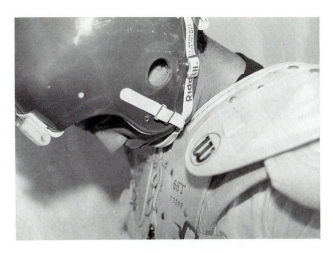

Figure 17-4. Coaches and athletes should be constantly reminded that no helmet or padding can protect against compression.

Ice Hockey and Lacrosse Helmets.

Hockey helmet standards are set by the Canadian Standards Association. Bishop et al[10] and Hayes[10] examined the effectiveness of the equipment, demonstrating the need for more research in the late 1970s. A recent evaluation of hockey injuries showed that mandatory usage of face masks has drastically reduced the number of injuries to the head/face/scalp, accounting for 50% of all injuries.[15] Most notably, the serious eye injuries have been "dramatically decreased." Professional players do not have to wear face masks, but some clear shields are seen on a few players. Sim and Simonet stated that little research has been done to date showing the impact absorption capabilities of the newer equipment. Players over 12 years old must now wear a full face mask with an internal mouthpiece, or half mask with an internal/external mouth guard. The full face shield used in lacrosse is a design many other sports should have copied years ago.

Helmets in Other Sports.

Taekwondo, boxing, and many other sports use a soft, shock absorbency type of protection.

Head injuries in biking are the leading cause of death—more than 1000 per year on US roads, 75% of which are due to head trauma.[15] Burkes states that two standards are now being used to rate bike helmets.[15] His article also quotes guidelines regarding impact forces[16]:

1. below 150g—little or no injury
2. 151 to 250g—light concussion, amnesia
3. 251 to 400g—extended loss of consciousness, traumatic amnesia
4. over 401g—definite brain bleeding
5. over 200g—likely permanent brain damage, possible death

The American National Standards Institute (ANSI) and the Snell Memorial Foundation rate helmets as well, with 36 helmets currently "approved."[16] A California law now requires that children under the age of 4 must wear an approved helmet if either a passenger or an operator.

Other sports participants, such as equestrian riders, wear head protection specific to the appearance/protection needed. Often the athletes themselves can help you understand potential dangers. A world-class speed skier (over 100 mph) taught me that his helmet has to be skin tight to protect from "bucketing," (quickly filling with water) when he falls, which could cause a severe distraction force in contrast to the normal compression.

Legal/Liability Issues.

The July 1988 issue of *Sports Illustrated* presented an article on a youth who suffered a bilateral facet dislocation of C3–C4 due to a football injury.

Apparently, the helmet he was wearing had a strap attached to the face mask to keep it from going into extension. The article brings up important ethical questions about allowing the player to play if he or she is unable to practice or if there has been any alteration of equipment.

A written and verbal explanation of all potential injuries from a given sport should be provided for the entire team, with all coaches and staff present, and it should be dated and signed. Helmet manufacturers now have warnings on the back of football headgear.

Face Guards

As noted in the previous section, there are now face shields for baseball players (catchers, of course) and lacrosse players. These are mandatory for all but professional hockey players. Goalies are especially well protected, but their equipment should be checked often. Specific soft face guards are also available for wrestling (Fig 17–5).

Football Face Masks.

The following guidelines should be kept in mind:

1. There should be no less than two bars (kickers often wear one, perhaps unwisely).
2. They should be mounted 3 in above edge of helmet.
3. No helmet should be drilled more than one time per side.
4. There should be clearance of 1 to 1.5 in between the nose and face guard
5. Stop use and replace if cracked (watch for stress lines) (Fig 17–6).

One of the most important safety factors regarding a face mask is the capacity for "safe removal" if the

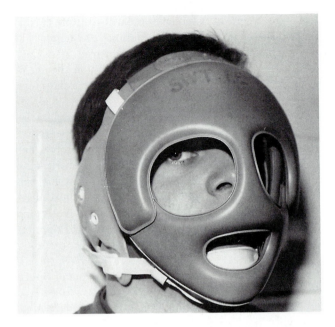

Figure 17-5. Facial protection, used with wrestling headgear, is often used postinjury.

player is unconscious or suspected of a cervical injury (that is, removal of the mask without releasing the chinstrap or helmet!). Thus, one would be able to safely monitor or apply cardiopulmonary resuscitation (CPR) without risking further injury. The sports physical therapist should carry the razor or screwdriver necessary for facemask removal. The time between needing it and finding it could be neurologically damaging or life-threatening.

Mouth Guards

Mouthpieces help to reduce the incidence and severity of concussions by diminishing the force transference

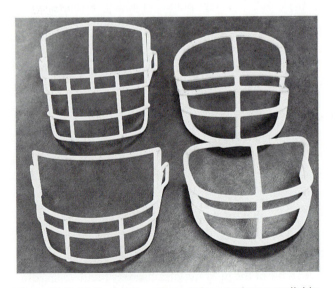

Figure 17-6. Various styles of helmet facemasks are available.

through the temporomandibular joint (TMJ) and into the cranium. Prior to face guards and mouth guards being used, 50% of injuries in high school football were to the mouth.[17] With mandatory use in the 1980s, the occurrence dropped to between 0.35% and 0.45%,[18] a dramatic decrease. In a 1984–1985 study of 626 Texas high schools, Duda reported that other sports are now the principal culprits.[19] Mouth injuries were twice as frequent in basketball as in football, and in soccer were three times higher.[20]

Baseball has the highest incidence of head and facial injuries in athletes under the age of 14 years.[21] If a tooth avulsion should occur, it should be replanted and splinted within 1 hour to potentially save the tooth.[22] One should *not* wash off the tooth, but clean off foreign debris, and place it back into the socket immediately. This is better than transporting it in milk,[23] as is commonly done.

THREE MAIN TYPES OF MOUTH GUARDS

TYPE	COST	COMMENT
Stock	$1	Readily available, potential poor fit
Mouth formed (boil and bite)	$3–$4	Often too small; need strap to hold in, better fit
Custom	$30–$40	Better retention, fit, speech, breathing ability

The mold should cover to the back teeth; and, of course, the most comfortable mouth guard is made of a resilient, flexible material.[23a]

Only amateur football, ice hockey, and boxing require mouthpieces. They seem very necessary in lacross, baseball, basketball, soccer, and even volleyball, however. A national report by the US Department of Health and Human Service Public Health Services listed as one of its objectives the use of a mouth guard in all secondary contact sports by 1990.[24]

Again, be aware of the potential liability if a performer is *not* wearing a mouthpiece. A $3000 dental bill versus $3 to $30 seems reasonable (Fig. 17-7).

Controversy surrounds the area of repositioning the TMJ and strength variations. An entire chapter could be written on this fascinating topic. This area needs more subjects and scientific trials. Moore et al compare numerous studies showing varied, and sometimes opposing, results in comparing strength with mandibular repositioning.[25]

A poorly fitting mouth protector can cause an inflammatory fibroma of the gingiva.[26] This, plus poor breathing ability and the overall feeling that they are not needed, are the complaints given by the 34% of professional football players who do not use them.[27]

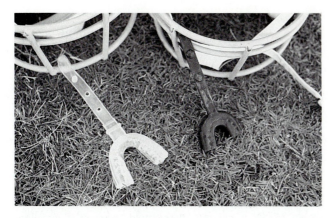

Figure 17-7. Heat-form mouthpieces should not be cut too short to allow for back teeth protection.

Smith and Sutton encircled a football helmet with straps running over the cranium anterior-posterior to the ear to stabilize a helmet for a player with a mandibular fracture.[28] They also used a large "cage" face mask and double collars to minimize penetration of forces. The player was able to finish the last half of the season without problems. It is important to note, however, that one must always be cautious of any alteration of equipment and the implications of such.

Ear Protection

Damage to the ear is most common in sports such as wrestling or boxing. Water polo, sharpshooting, and trap-skeet shooting can also be hazardous.

Although headgear is mandatory for competition, many athletes think it is not important for practice,

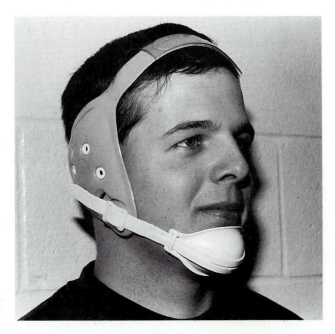

Figure 17-8. Wrestling headgear protects the ear from trauma and "cauliflower" appearance from scarring.

which of course involves the bulk of time devoted to the sport. "Cauliflower ear" is extremely common, and very preventable with headgear in wrestling. The outer superior rim of the ear is traumatized from shearing forces on the mat and the resulting edema and scar tissue changes its appearance. Other sections of this text address trauma and protection of the two other areas of the ear—middle and inner ear (Fig 17–8).

Eye Protection

The International Federation of Sports Medicine's position statement on eye injuries brings out an important point: an athlete with poor vision in one eye is at more risk, and needs the protection to minimize the loss of the "good" eye.[29] Addresses of organizations (listed by specification number) who have standards for protection devices are also provided.[30]

To compare how eye injuries can vary, contrast an 11-year study of Michigan State University[31] and a 5-year study in Quebec[32] showing some interesting results of eye injury percentages in various sports.

MSU 1975–1985	Quebec 1982–1986
Wrestling	Ice hockey
(18.4% of all wrestlers)	(32% of all injuries)
Basketball	Baseball
(10.7% of all players)	(10% of all injuries)
Ice hockey	Badminton
(8.3% of players pre–1980)	(9.5% of all injuries)
Football	Tennis
(4.1% of players)	(9% of all injuries)
	Racquetball
	(7% of all injuries)
	(Fig 17–9)
	Note: Racquet sports = 28% of all injuries collectively in Quebec study of racquet sports

Quite simply, the popularity of a sport and the type of equipment used will undoubtedly vary in incidence regionally.

Without question the eye is one of the most important and easily protected areas of the body. Racket sport eye protectors that have openings frequently do *not* protect the eye. These "lensless" guards failed tests and allowed balls to get through or shatter the protector upon impact.[29]

Two studies showed that most of the 13 open eye guards evaluated were not effective in protection.[33,34] A squash ball often travels 140 mph, and the racquets used in this type of sport travel at 85 to 110 mph themselves. Canada and the United States now have standards that must be met for their certification of an eye guard. Easterbrooks lists seven eye guards that have

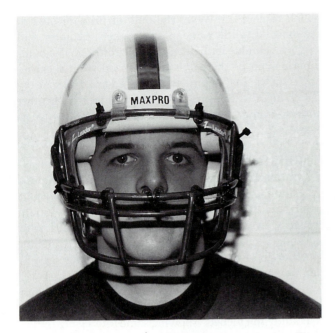

Figure 17-9. Tinted eye shield help protect ocular, maxillary, and nasal areas along with sun glare.

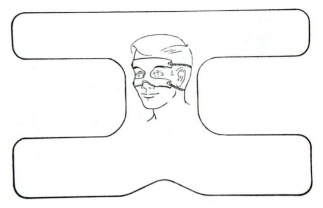

Figure 17-10. A custom thermomold nasal-orbit-maxillary guard can be padded from comfortable protection (fit with headgear).

met stringent criteria, all costing $25 or less.[35] Most YMCAs, the military, universities, clubs, and the US Squash–Racquet Association (USSRA) now have mandatory rules for eye guards. Experience, prescription lenses, contacts, or open eye guards do not prevent injuries; the data prove it.

The annual estimate of 35,000 sports/recreational eye injuries is significant; at least 25% of all injuries result in serious complications or even loss of vision.[36] Even more sad is the fact that probably 90% of all eye trauma could be avoided by use of protective eyewear and adherence to simple safety rules.[37]

Of the hockey players injured in the Quebec study, 89% did not have any face protection at all, and the other 11% were not wearing an adequate protector (full face/certified). It is projected that the National Hockey League (NHL) will make face protectors mandatory in the near future.[38]

Soccer and volleyball, which are growing in popularity, are considered "high-risk" sports for eye injuries because of the high-speed ball and the potential of collisions.[39,40]

Controlling sunlight exposure is extremely important in swimming, snow-related sports, and biking.[41,42] Intraocular cancer was found in three long-distance swimmers. Athletes with fair skin and blue eyes need ultraviolet screening glasses/goggles. Blue tint supposedly reduces snow glare; yellow, ice glare.

Maxillary Nasal Protection

Secondary to commercially available nasal–facial protection, custom guards can be molded quickly and inex-

pensively (Fig 17–10). Tracing the pattern onto an old x-ray film uses material with character that will mold easily to the curve of the face but stand out from the nasal area easily. Keep in mind that the forehead/cheek bone surfaces are the padded areas which will raise the contact area off the nose.

The stages of preparation are as follows:

1. Trace or draw pattern.
2. Check the fit on the athlete.
3. Trace onto molding material and cut.
4. Heat to material specifics (usually 160 degrees; using a hydroculator is easiest).
5. Mold to face of athlete; allow to cool and harden.
6. Pad with high-density ½-in adhesive foam or suitable padding.

Have the athletes bring their headgear (helmet, wrestling headgear, etc) and confirm the clearance on all sides prior to step 7.

7. Attach elastic straps to both side panels above and below the ear—an extra strap over the superior aspect helps tremendously with slippage. (Fig 17–11).

Aside from almost every full face mask, custom protection can be hand-made, padded with orthoplast[43] or similar heat-mold materials. Full face guards can be purchased for wrestlers if a fracture occurs in the face.[44]

Throat Protection

Wisely, baseball/softball catchers' masks have Velcro-attachable anterior throat shields (Fig 17–12). Hockey goalies' face masks often extend inferiorly to overlap the shoulder pad area; however, almost no other hockey player or athlete uses such protection. This appears to be another area where utilization is ex post facto.

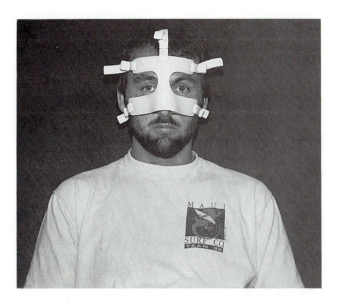

Figure 17–11. The superior strap helps stabilize shifting.

SHOULDER PROTECTION

Shoulder pads are used for a variety of sports, including football, hockey, lacrosse, and so forth. Understanding their function is the key to safe utilization. The arch is one of the strongest weight-supporting architectural

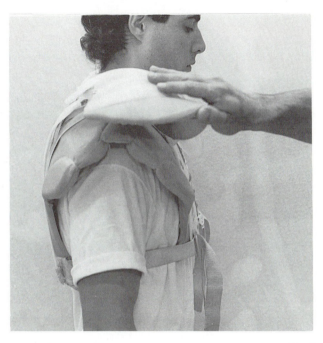

Figure 17–13. If the side straps are not kept tight, the arch of the shoulder pad can be lost.

designs known. The straps that come under the axilla hold the height of the arch at its peak. If these straps break, stretch, or become too loose, force can easily be transmitted to the underlying structure, namely the bony acromioclavicular (AC) joint (Fig 17–13).

Injury to the AC prominence is common and may require a custom shell fabrication (see custom orthosis).[45] Underliner pads are often used for increased shock absorption (Fig 17–14).

Another potential problem is when the underneath seam of the jersey sleeve has been cut (often for ventilation or movement), allowing the pad covering the deltoid to flip up freely. Direct forces from a fellow

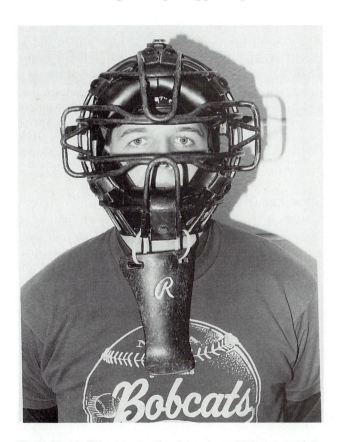

Figure 17–12. Throat protection is a wise addition, especially for foul tips.

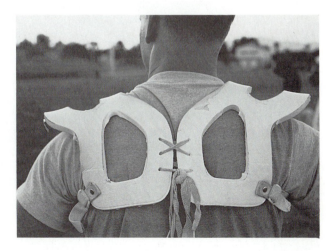

Figure 17–14. Padding under shoulder pads can be effective for extra shock absorption, especially for the AC joint.

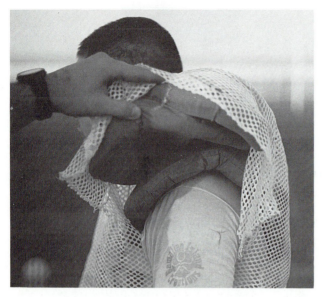

Figure 17-15. Jerseys with the sleeves slit may allow the deltoid flap to flip up.

athlete's equipment, or the ground, can cause an axillary nerve contusion. Loss of the deltoid naturally prohibits further participation (Fig 17–15).

Short-tie string jerseys, or outercoatings, that do not tuck in the pants allow for excessive shifting of shoulder pads occasionally. Players do not realize that the reason their neck liner irritates the scalene area is because the axilla strap is not being stabilized below or possibly because of poor initial fit.

No specific list of fitting instructions can cover all types of pads. Certain elements are universal, however (Fig 17–16):

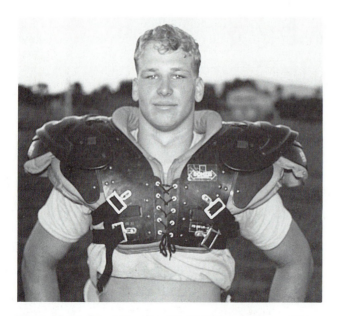

Figure 17-16. Shoulder pads with dual lateral straps and long descending anterior padding offer increased protection.

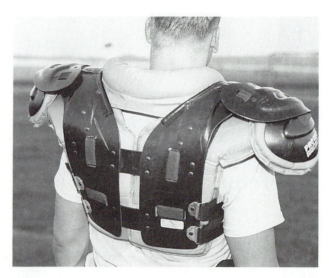

Figure 17-17. Pads that descend posteriorly offer improved spinal–rib protection.

1. The tip of inside pad covers the lateral shoulder.
2. The flap covers deltoid.
3. The neck opening allows full shoulder flexion/ abduction.
4. The axillary strap maintains a dome and controls anterior-posterior shift.
5. The scapula is covered (Fig 17–17).

The fitting instructions of the manufacturer should be carefully followed to avoid possible liability. Chest circumference at the nipple line or shoulder width are the two most common baseline measurements used.

Special pads for receivers and quarterbacks have a rotational axis approximately at the zyphoid to allow better overhead arm motion. Often they are more flat than the cantilevered blocking/tackling types.

Shoulder Dislocation Devices

Caution is the first step necessary when attempting to control motion at any joint, especially the most mobile, least stable joint in the body. Altering a shoulder pad with drill holes and attaching a check-strap to limit abduction again raises issues of legality and liability. Manufacturers now have vests,[46,47] which perhaps are a better investment because stability of the shoulder, once dislocated, is extremely compromised, even after long healing times (Fig 17–18).

NECK PROTECTION

In the discussion of helmets, legal areas were involved because a strap had been attached from the face mask to the shoulder pads to limit extension of the neck. Fur-

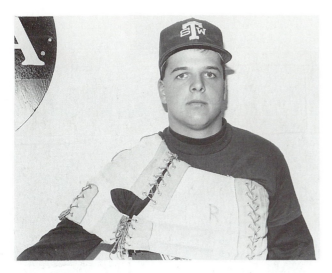

Figure 17-18. Shoulder abduction/external rotation control can be helpful for anterior dislocation problems.

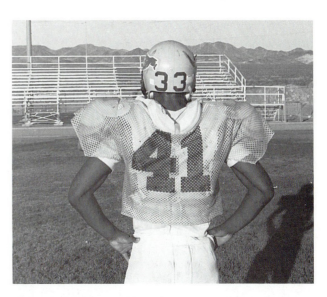

Figure 17-20. A protective collar that is too low for flexion protection.

ther understanding of how a neck roll/bag is to function should lead to proper fit and safety. The brachial plexus (C5–T1) is often stretched when the head is forced into lateral flexion away from an upper extremity that is being posteriorly abducted simultaneously. This "lightning bolt" or "stinger" sensation is intense and causes severe loss of upper extremity function, although it is usually short lived (minutes). A myotomal and cervical strength-motion examination is essential prior to further participation and a neck-roll may be desired.

Horseshoe-shaped rolls, with lace attachments anterioposteriorly, are used to check hyperextension and undesired forced lateral flexion. If properly secured to the shoulder pads (checking lateral flexion of helmet to neck roll while securing), they work very well (Fig 17–19).

Nevertheless, coaches, players, and medical per-

sonnel must not understand their function, or these rolls would not be draped down the back and applied like a shawl on an evening dress! (Figs 17–20, 17–21). Rolls that are too tight can limit rotation because the face mask will hit it, and they may function as a dangerous fulcrum rather than a limitation when forced lateral flexion occurs. The air bags often seen posterior to the helmet only limit hyperextension; recall also that the chin strap mentioned earlier may help to limit cervical hyperflexion.

If a player needs protection prior to an injury, the sports physical therapist must thoroughly understand the function of the preventative equipment. If a player is already injured, the injury should be analyzed:

Is it

1. a brachial plexus injury?
2. a muscular strain?

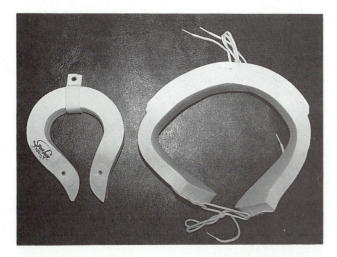

Figure 17-19. Neck rolls come in various sizes and should be fitted with shoulder gear and headgear.

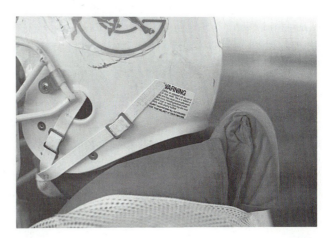

Figure 17-21. Neck rolls must fit properly to function well.

3. a ligamentous/capsular sprain?
4. facet pathomechanics?

Can the athlete safely return to practice/full participation, and what type of neck protection is needed? Recall, no amount of muscular strength or neck protection can transfer forces applied directly onto the spine from above (or if ramming into something). Thus, there is the necessity for intelligent tackling rules. It is essential to constantly remind players and coaches of these. Documentation of a preseason demonstration of undesired and dangerous techniques could be extremely helpful to the athlete as well as protective of the coaches and schools with regards to potential litigation.

BREAST PROTECTION

Recent court cases have allowed young women to participate in contact sports such as hockey and football. Basketball, racquet sports, and other contact sports can also cause trauma to the breast secondary to the expected repetitive trauma of running and jumping.

Authors of articles in this area agree that specifically designed "sports bras" should be worn.[48] Even though definitions/standards are being established by the American Society for Testing and Materials (ASTM), testing methods and standard specifications are still being formulated. Categories that were mentioned by Haycock divide sports bras into (1) supportive, (2) binding, and (3) simple modification of standard styles (not truly a sports bra).[49] Recommendations or designs to look for include padded seams (or no seams) over the nipple, covered hooks, material of at least 50% cotton, and nonelastic shoulder straps. Women larger than size C cup should be advised to wear a supportive bra designed to especially limit vertical motion. A pad that can fit into the cup of the bra should be worn for all contact sports as well.

Lorentzen and Lawson directly compare eight manufacturer's models or the basis of price, fabric, features, and their ability to control motion.[48] Baeyens[50] and Haycock[49] discuss management of specific breast problems.

ABDOMINAL/RIB PROTECTION

Rib shields should be customary and mandatory equipment for all contact sports. Donzi has rib protectors that are advertised by hitting them with a baseball bat.[51] BIKE has Rib Lite, all-sports models, as do many other manufacturers.[52] Running backs, quarterbacks, receivers, and any player who is aggressive or is predisposed to rib trauma should use this protection (Fig 17-22). Anyone who has suffered a severe rib injury

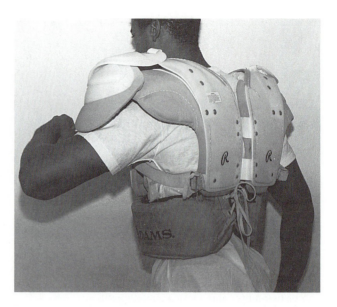

Figure 17-22. Rib-abdominal pads suspended below shoulder pads.

and awakened every day for 6 months with pain will have no difficulty understanding the need for this protection. Rib belts do assist with intercostal support, and are basically an elastic wrap, an example being the PROCARE rib belt.[53]

ABDOMINAL INJURIES

Haycock reminds us that although abdominal injuries are only 10% of sports trauma, they are potentially life threatening.[54] Cycling, horseback events, and skiing are examples where children, more often than adults, compromise the spleen, kidneys, liver, and related organs. Falling on a football, colliding in soccer, and competing on the uneven parallel bars are also common micro-macro trauma events. Pain persisting longer than 5 to 6 minutes, signs of shock, severe pain with palpation, or hematuria are indicators that immediate further testing and examination are necessary. A player must not eat or drink before a definitive diagnosis. Thus, firm, force-dispersing abdominal protectors are equipment that should be used more frequently, and definitely after any initial trauma.

ELBOW PROTECTION

Today's protective foam pads for elbows have excellent contoured designs and comfortable superior–inferior straps. The ulnar nerve is extremely exposed to hard surfaces and requires protection, as may be painfully evident to diving volleyball players and falling skateboarders.

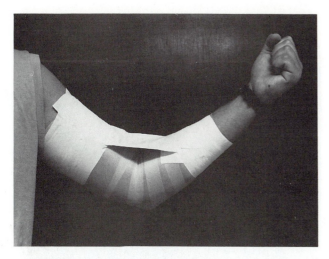

Figure 17-23. Elbow hyperextension wraps can be covered wtih an elastic wrap for competition.

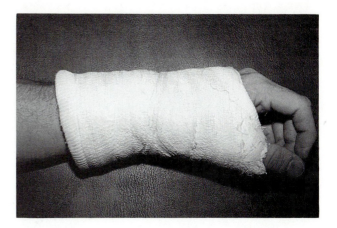

Figure 17-24. A soft, semirigid splint can be effective in wrist, metacarpal (navicular) stabilization.

Hyperextension injuries, common to wrestlers, can be supported with commercial braces[55] or tape (Fig 17–23). Circulation concerns should be constantly monitored, and never compromised.

Tennis elbow, compression, and extension check straps are used widely. Rarely are they done so preventively, and there are no data to show that they would perform as such. Lateral epicondylitis is frequently an overuse injury and requires changes in technique, treatment, and rest, as well as supports. Hinged, cast brace-type devices may be used if varus/valgus instabilities are present.[56] The specific tissue one is trying to protect needs to be stressed while the brace is worn in order to verify its integrity. Again, slippage, loosening, and monitoring alteration needs are important in both practice and competition.

FOREARM/WRIST/HAND

Various combinations of elbow/forearm/wrist/hand pads are available to dissipate compression type forces. In high school athletics, at present, no hard shell pads are allowed on the upper extremity, whether custom or commercial. Some soft-shelled splints may be allowed. Collegiate NCAA rules are different and allow certain splints (Fig 17–24).[57,58] The sports physical therapist should be aware of the rules in his or her state or setting.

Friction-dispersing shields are common to archery and gymnastics. Thumb and wrist stabilizers are also seen in bowling. High-impact materials are needed for protection in hockey, lacrosse, and football, and an elastic polymer, Sorbothane, has been used in baseball gloves with reported success.[59]

Medial thumb collateral ligament sprain is common in skiers, and is often called "gamekeeper's" thumb because of the trauma to the metacarpal phalangeal joint suffered when Old World gamekeepers would snap rabbits' necks. Splints, or customized orthoses, can help this problem, regardless of one's occupation/activity (Fig 17–25 through 17–26).[60]

Buddy-taping for the fingers is a commonly used method of support. In stabilizing the thumb/wrist, follow three basic rules of controlling the undesired motion:

1. Place joint in painfree functional position.
2. Apply anchor strips proximally–distally to the joint.
3. Apply tape to diminish painful motion.

For the six most common fractures of the metacarpals and their splinting possibilities for competition, refer to the article by McCue, which also demonstrates a silicone cast.[58] Recall, the navicular (snuff-box) frac-

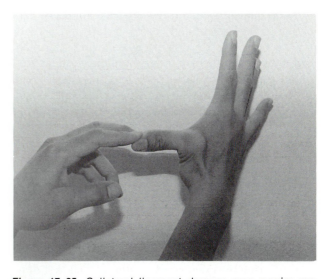

Figure 17-25. Collateral ligament damage may require surgical repair, but can be splinted.

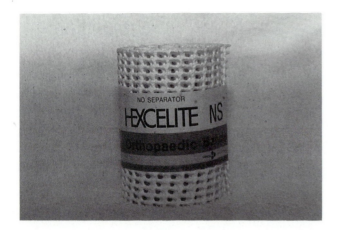

Figure 17-26. Thermomold webbing can be used for a custom splint by cutting the required amount, heating, and applying to the patient.

ture is very difficult to heal, and prone to necrosis; therefore, many therapists are hopeful that high schools will allow soft casts to be used in participation in the near future.

BACK-HIP PROTECTION

"Girdle pads" help to cover the lumbosacral area and iliac crests. "Hip pointers" are extremely painful and are due to muscular detachments of the insertions off the lateral iliac crests or anterior superior iliac spines. Frequently, belts at the waist stabilize the pads, but the pads do not ascend sufficiently high or remain in place once forces are applied. Hip pads with loops that interlock with the belt, or a new "body jacket," are recent designs that address the problems of pad shifting.

Players who do not wear hip–sacral padding because it "slows them down" emit an air of invulnerability that is dangerous to impressionable team peers. Education of the athlete and coaching staff and parents may be necessary to alter such behavior. Warm-N-Form type moldable firm inserts, and the elastic wraparound support into which they slip, have been used successfully to pad over the low back, iliac crests, and abdominal areas that need protection.[61] One's customizing imagination and secondary padding is all that is required (Fig 17–27).

The capability of lateral flexion, rotation, and especially flexion/extension should be verified. Rounding the superior and inferior edge away from the body can help to minimize skin irritation if simultaneous hip and back extension occur (Fig 17–28) or if trunk flexion is used anteriorly.

Soccer shorts now have padding built into the material covering the greater trochanter, as well as sliding pads that belt onto the waist. These are excellent shear

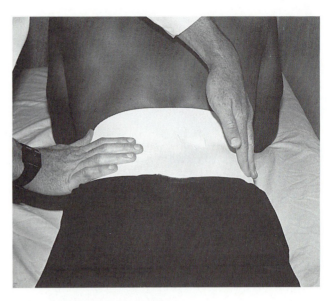

Figure 17-27. A thermomold lumbar support can be padded for lumbar, rib, or abdominal protection.

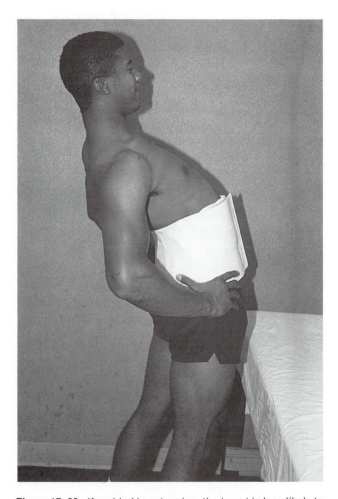

Figure 17-28. If molded in extension, the insert is less likely to irritate soft tissue.

force dissipators for baseball, softball, lacrosse, and soccer.[52]

QUADRICEPS/HAMSTRINGS PROTECTION

Repeated trauma to the quadriceps can lead to myositis ossificans. Any measurable hematoma must be guarded with protective pads, and possibly treated with full rest. Many players will tape their quadriceps and patellar pads in place if their jersey pants are too big; this allows the pads to rotate out of position.

Custom turtle shell–shaped pads[62] can help to dissipate forces to the outlying areas; however, this can also potentially enlarge the area of bleeding. Thus, monitoring the player is essential. Range of motion, circumference, and radiological consultations, are all important.

Basketball and soccer are both common sports in which a player will get "kneed in the thigh"; therefore, objective documentation of strength and functional skills should accompany all protective padding efforts.

Ironically, the hamstrings are rarely affected by hematoma/osteoblast activity. A product that shows interesting possibilities is a resilient assist for hamstring strains, and can be used for a hip flexor aid also.[63] The waist strap has rubber straps that attach proximal or distal to the knee relative to upper–lower hamstring needs. It can reportedly be used for adduction and external rotation problems.

KNEE PROTECTION

The capability of a knee brace to prevent injuries is under investigation. The following are the principal types of braces: (1) prophylactic/protective knee brace; (2) rehabilitative knee brace; and (3) functional knee brace.

Prophylactic/Protective Knee Brace

Studies being conducted on prophylactic knee braces are usually of three types[64]:

1. Epidemiologic, braced versus unbraced, same team several seasons, or many teams, one or more seasons
2. Cadaver, braced with forces applied
3. Surrogate; artificial knee model, braced lateral forces applied (allows force absorption information)

McCarthy's recent article brings out some other important facts about the last 5 to 10 years of research.[64] The braces have changed almost yearly, and there are now more than 30 types on the market. Comparing apples to apples becomes even more challenging in the face of such variables as (1) daily wear of the brace, (2) previous injuries, (3) shoe type, (4) turf/grass, (5) in a game/or at practice, (6) position played, (7) rule changes, (8) coaching style, (9) formations used most, (10) changes in surgical procedures, (11) speed, strength, size of athlete today (versus 5 to 10 years ago), (12) changes in rehabilitation procedures, (13) new stability testing equipment, (14) players' personal feelings about a particular brand of brace, (15) financial incentives, and (16) grading severity of injury.

One major study, being orchestrated by Dr. Kenneth Albright, of the University of Iowa, involves the medical personnel of the Big Ten Teams, and multiple areas of analysis using as many as 14 brands of braces.[56] Preliminary information of 3 years looking at 110 players showed conflicting data. More braced versus unbraced players were injured, but the players' and the teams' medical personnel all think the braces were and are effective. When they analyzed "survival" (how many games or practices it took for the average player to be injured), braced players took 3 times as many exposures before medical collateral ligament (MCL) injury occurred (i.e., 51 exposures versus 16 for unbraced).

Other large scale studies by Teitz et al[65] of more than 6300 players at 71 NCAA Colleges, and Grace et al,[66] in Albuquerque high schools, both found the braces to be "ineffective," or that there was a higher incidence of injury in the braced players. Studies by Rovere et al,[67] Baker et al,[68] and Paulos et al[69] all bring out questions of "true protection" against an MCL, anterior cruciate ligament (ACL) sprain. Concerns that braces may have led to preloading, and thus actually increased the potential of an injury, are still being examined. Nevertheless, reported initial concerns are not as strong as in the past years.

The American Orthopaedic Society for Sports Medicine (AAOSM) is expected to publish a position postfinal tabulation of the Big Ten Study, and a West Point Military Academy study. At this time, however, the American Academy of Orthopaedic Surgeons (AAOS) has a position statement that warns:

> "Routine use of prophylactic knee braces currently available has not been proven effective in reducing the number and severity of knee injuries; . . . in some circumstances, those braces may even contribute to an injury. There is no credible, long term, scientifically conducted study that supports using knee braces on otherwise healthy players."[64]

Estimates show that if 1 million high school players alone used two braces, the cost would be over $69,000,000.[70] Some feel that this is money better spent on strength machines, padded equipment, shoes, and

field maintenance,[71] all of which may lead to potential injuries if not done properly as well.

Assessment/Summary. No conclusive evidence exists to completely prove or disprove the efficiency of prophylactic braces at this time.

Rehabilitative Knee Braces

There continues to be questions whether rehabilitative braces (which now largely replace casts during ligamentous protection phases), truly control medial, lateral, anterior, posterior, or rotational forces. The 1985 AAOS Sports Committee looked at six braces on the market, and found little background data. The study by Hoffmann et al showed cadaver work that indicated that medial–lateral support gave more stability versus other braces without it.[72]

Functional Knee Braces

Ironically, the term "functional" is used to describe braces that are often used to help support joint stability usually due to a ligament loss, most commonly ACL deficiency. Electrogoniometers with six degrees of freedom and analysis machines that can accurately describe millimeters of laxity are the big steps forward in both design and "function." Recall that someone can have a partial tear, and yet be "functionally unstable" due to a pivot shift or giving away of the knee. Refer to chapter 22 to further understand the complexities of this area.

SHIN (TIBIOFIBULAR) PROTECTION

Neurovascular protection, especially of the anterior compartment, is directly approached by the National Federation of State High Schools and Soccer Rules Committee, who have stated that by the fall of 1990, all soccer players must wear shin guards.[73] Sensory–motor nerve loss to the foot should be prevented in other contact sports, as well. Baseball and softball players may also need commercial or custom guards if an injury occurs (Fig 17–29).

Analysis, classification, and treatment of the "shin splints" syndrome are covered by Wallensten and Erikson[74] and Detmer.[75] Complete understanding of the biomechanics of the forefoot, rearfoot, and tibiofibular joints and musculature are vital to understanding symptomatology in this area, and thus, proper protective equipment. An example of additional protective equipment for the shins is orthotics.

Stress fractures of the tibia and fibula in women were treated successfully with pneumatic leg braces (Fig 17–30).[76] This 2-year study on 13 women, some with bilateral symptoms and stress fracture diagnoses, were all able to return to competition asymptomati-

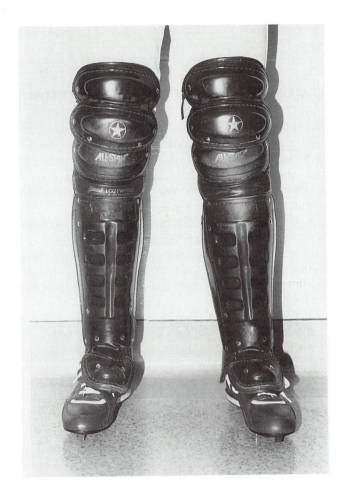

Figure 17-29. Catcher's leg protection has wisely been extended to the quadriceps and talus.

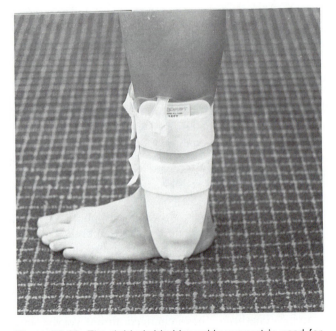

Figure 17-30. The rigid air bladder ankle support is used for sprains and has been shown effective for stress fractures.

cally in 1 month. The Air-Stirrup Leg Brace (Aircast Inc., Summit NJ) was used, and can be used in conjunction with orthotics. One is immediately reminded of Sarmiento,[77] and the numerous articles on fracture bracing that elaborate on the theories of soft tissue support around the bones through specific compression.

ANKLE PROTECTION

Ankle sprains can be extremely painful and alter performance capabilities tremendously. Often our athletes are told, "Because ankle sprains are so common, they are looked upon lightly relative to other injuries." Recent reports are showing interesting comparisons between taping and orthoses for support and injury prevention. Gross suggested that a semirigid orthosis may be more effective than taping for ankle sprains (Figs 17–31 through 17–33).[78] Rovere et al[79] showed that low-topped shoes and lace-up stabilizers were more effective in preventing ankle sprains than taped stabilizers with high-top shoes (perhaps because the low-tops allowed for periodic tightening). Refer to chapter 23 on the ankle for further information.

HEEL (CALCANEAL) PROTECTION

As stated earlier, heel spur pain (medial–anterior–inferior) can be caused by excessive stress to the corresponding support tissues from pronation phase abnormalities. Thus orthotics, stretching, or training terrain and distance should be analyzed. Doxey reviews some causes of calcaneal pain.[80]

Stress fractures should not be forgotten in the evaluation. Organic polymer shock absorbency materials (i.e., Sorbothane) have shown excellent results in sending forces laterally versus vertically. Heel cups (which come in various forms) keep the natural fat pad under the calcaneus versi allowing it to splay laterally.[81]

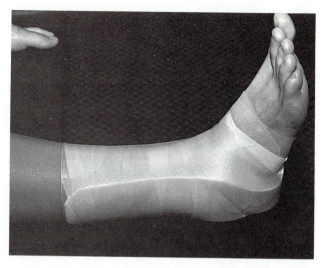

Figure 17–32. Mold the heated thermomold custom orthosis, wrap to cool, and apply to patient over protective tape.

FOOT PROTECTION

Beyond the common sense necessities of steel toes for baseball catchers' and pitchers' push-off toe, specialization seems to be the name of the game. *Runner's World* does an annual evaluation of running shoes. Control of the rear foot is of major interest to biomechanists like Barry Bates, of the University of Oregon. He co-authored an article that showed that a certain amount of cushion loss will improve foot control; thus the feel of a shoe at first may be misleading.[82]

Caution should be exercised when applying a material to the worn sole of a running shoe. If the exterior is worn, the internal shock attenuation is probably also

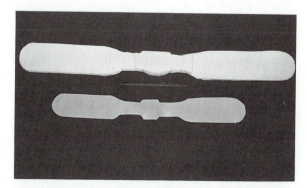

Figure 17–31. A padded template for thermomold ankle support can be made for various sizes.

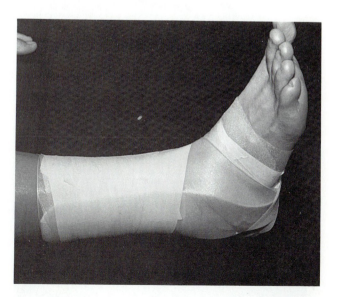

Figure 17–33. The thermomold is then taped in place (1/2 stabilized is shown).

gone. Therefore, it is probably time for a new pair of shoes.

Athletes should take the following recommendations into account when purchasing shoes:

1. The court surface and sole should be compatible (rough terrain nobby–bottom shoes offer minimal control on a smooth floor).
2. Rear foot stability counteracts excessive calcaneal motion.
3. Arch support can minimize multiple problem areas.
4. Malaligned "seconds" (which are less expensive blemished shoes) can cause undesired force vectors if the base and shell of shoe are not perpendicular when manufactured. This can be a major concern in the rear foot.

Abnormal wear patterns may indicate biomechanical shear forces versus congruency (lateral heel and medial toe are desired wear patterns).

CUSTOM PAD

Fabrication of a force-dispersing pad, or support orthosis, follows the basic principles of all medicine: (1) do

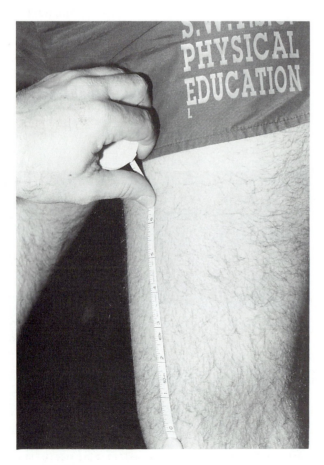

Figure 17–34. Through palpation and circumference measurements, plot the size of the area to be protected.

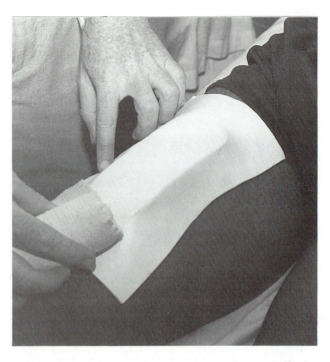

Figure 17-35. To form a dome, cut a size/shape of the "dome" according to the size/shape of area to be protected. Cut a larger size piece of thermomold to fit the area and use the "dome" to create the "relief dome." Remove dome and pad the outer edges.

no harm, (2) consider anatomic factors, and (3) consider biomechanical factors. Whenever on limits a joint's normal range of motion, be aware of possible undesired effects. Common support orthoses can be molded for the thumb, wrist,[82] Jones's fracture,[83] or even turf toe.[84]

If one is designing an extra pad to disperse force away from an injured area, the two simple facts to remember are (1) build a dome (turtle shell) over the area, and (2) transfer the force to the surrounding tissue. A removable felt pad, for example, should be used

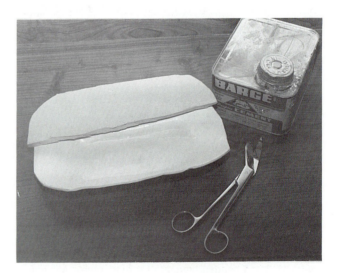

Figure 17-36. Remove the central pad, creating a "relief dome," and pad the outer trimmed edges.

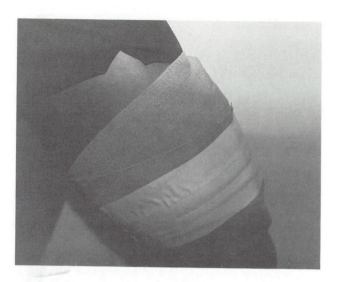

Figure 17–37. Secure the pad over the area to be protected, which can be worn under other commercial padding.

to form the dome. The surface area of dispersion should be as large as comfortably possible and well padded with layers of foam (Figs 17–34 through 17–37).

Many materials are on the market that can be thermomolded to retain a new shape and have excellent strength–density when firm again. As stated earlier, Multifoam,[85] Orthoplast, and Hexalite (perforated webbing) are excellent starters. Two other materials that are extremely inexpensive and have multiple uses are packing bubbles, and heel-lace pads. Packing bubbles are light, easily cut, folded, and taped into a pad, and can actually be jumped on without popping if folded three to four times and secured. Heel-lace pads[86] are adhesive 2×4 in foam designed for under support tape jobs, but can be layered for fast-effective pressure requirements (Fig 17–38).

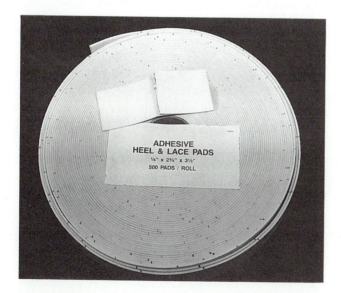

Figure 17–38. These pads can be used on thermomold custom pads, or for taping.

SUMMARY: SPECIFIC SPORT INJURY PROTECTION

Throughout this chapter, there has been a continual theme of three main points:

1. *Do no harm.*
2. Understand the intent of the equipment and its biomechanical advantages versus dangers.
3. Be aware of legal liability issues and use as a positive influence over decisions.

One's professional judgment should always be based on good intent and sound knowledge. Many judges and attorneys agree that law suits may be damaging to the "public good." A recent article states that 80 % of surveyed judges favored changes in the tort system that would reduce costs and increase the fairness of trials.[87] The article gives multiple examples of manufacturers who are deciding against new product lines and discontinuing product research based on liability concerns.

As we look at our role in the athletic environment, as clinicians, we must be acutely aware of the need for proper research methods in planning, calculating, and publishing data on injury incidence. These data are the foundation for change, whether they are in the form of altering rules, techniques, or protective equipment.

Noyes and Albright served as editors for a 220-page supplement to the *American Journal of Sports Medicine* that goes through grants, designs, populations, and statistical anlayses.[88] With numerous examples, this publication is an extremely valuable reference for anyone planning this type of research.

At the end of this chapter, after the references, is a list of associations involved in collecting data on injury prevention and protective equipment. As mentioned earlier in the chapter, injury rates can be reflective of both the protective equipment and the amount the sport is played in that geographical location. In conclusion, the following is a short synopsis of specific sports and protective equipment.

Aerobics. The flooring,[89] shoes, orthotics, and possible knee/hip padding are important aspects to look at in this ever-increasing activity.

Baseball/softball. Aside from the helmets, face protection, catchers' equipment, and gloves, breakaway bases showed positive findings in research.[90]

Boxing.[91] Facial lacerations followed by hand and eye injuries suggest the need for more enclosure-type of head gear, perhaps using high-shock absorbency materials.

Equestrian Riding. New headgear able to withstand 300g without transmitting forces will be the new standard. This is three times the former requirement.[92]

Gymnastics. According to NCAA statistics, women's gymnastics has an extremely high injury rate. Men's gymnastics is roughly equal to that of men's wrestling and higher than football.[93] Neck, wrist, palm, knee, and ankle protection are all areas of concern. Of course, suspension outriggers and padding are a high priority.

Golf. Wrist, back, and elbow injuries[94] are cited as common areas of injury and overuse syndromes.

Stretching programs, strengthening, and stabilization wraps, as well as club grip shock absorbency materials, are all protective potentials.

Rodeo.[95] A 4-year study showed the need for elbow protection specifically, and padding for contusions.

Rugby.[96] With the minimal amount of protective equipment used in this sport, head, neck, face, and lower extremity injuries are common. A change in philosophy will be necessary before equipment can be utilized. Ankle supports, mouthpieces, and proper cleats are perhaps a beginning.

Skiing. Tibial fractures and ankle sprains appear to be declining with equipment advances; however, the medically significant knee injuries have increased.[97] Bindings, boots, and ski brakes have all led to changes. The type of pole grip that is best for prevention of skier's thumb is still being analyzed. Cross-country skiers may wish to add masks to their equipment to prevent upper respiratory infections possibly caused by the cold lowering salivary antibody levels.[97]

Skating. Elite figure skaters often plagued by overuse injuries might benefit from simple stretching programs,[98] whereas outdoor skaters need elbow, knee, and wrist protection from falls.

Swimming. Shallow-water diving continues to be the number one cause of spinal injuries.[99] Protective equipment needed here is educational signs and enforcement.

Snowmobiling. Racing and recreational usage both predispose one to injury. A 10-year study shows that improved headgear and machine design, along with potential legislatively backed safety programs, are preventive potentials.[100]

Surfing.[101] Protective eye wear, sunscreen, ear plugs, and wet suit hoods could prevent the type of common injuries seen in surfers. A new soft helmet is also available.

Volleyball. Almost 90% of volleyball injuries seen at an outpatient metropolitan clinic were to the lower ex-

tremities, about 60% to the knee and 25% to the ankles. This suggests the need for support to the ankle and a review of the efficacy of knee braces for ligament sprain prevention.

REFERENCES

1. NATA, Inc. The injury factor. Dallas, Tex: National Athletic Trainers Association. 1988.
2. Powell J. 636,000 injuries annually in high school football. *J NATA.* Spring 1987; 22(1):19–22.
3. Duda M. Sports medicine education at San Diego State University. *Physician Sports med.* 1988; 16(4).
4. McMahon Publishing. NCAA statistics. *Sports Medicine News.*
5. Gerberich SG. Child's nervous system. Minnesota School of Public Health, University of Minnesota. 1987; 3:59–64.
6. Sports injury equality, athletic business. *Spectrum Sports Medicine.* Aug 1988.
7. Sports care and fitness. *Sports Fitness News.* Sept/Oct. 1988: 8.
8. Mueller F, Schindler D. Annual survey: High School Football Death Rate Declines 1987. University of North Carolina, Chapel Hill, NC. *Sports Care and Fitness.* Sept/Oct 4:9. 1988.
9. Thomas Jefferson University. SCI causes. *Sports Care and Fitness* Philadelphia, Pa; Sept/Oct; 4:10 1988.
10. Arnheim D. *Modern Principles of Athletic Training.* 6th ed. St Louis, MO: Merior/Mosby College Publishing. 1985; 180–182.
11. Houston J.T.: Helmet makers seek better product tests. *Phys Sportsmed.* issue 3 1982; 10: 197.
12. Hodgson VR Director, Gurdjian-Lissner Biomechanics Laboratory, Department of Neurosurgery, Wayne State University, Mich.
13. Available through Cassemco Inc, PO Box 354, 728 East 15th Street, Cookesville, Tenn 38501 615–328–6588.
14. BSN Sports PO Box 7726, Dallas, TX 75209.
15. Burke ER. Safety standards for bicycle helmets. *Phys Sportsmed.* 1988; 16(1):151.
16. Mintom J. Ahead of the game. *Bicycle Rider.* Spring 1985:110–117.
17. American Association for Health, Physical Education, and Recreation and American Dental Association. *Report, Joint Committee on Mouth Protectors.* Chicago; 1960.
18. Heintz MD. Update in mouth protection for athletics. *NATA.* 1987; 16:111–112.
19. Duda M. Which athletes should wear mouth guards? *Physician Sports med.* 1987; 15(9):179–183.
20. Morrow RM, Kuebkes WA Sports dentistry, a new role. *San Antonio Dent School Qu.* 1986; 2(2):10–13.
21. Castaldi CR. First aid for sports related dental injuries. *Physician Sports med.* 1987;15, (9):81–89.
22. Spangberg LS. Endodontics. In: Castaldi CR, Bran GA, eds. *Dentistry for the Adolescent.* Philadelphia, Pa: W B Saunders Co: 1980:433–486.
23. Smith L. *Pedodontics:* personal information interview. San Luis Obispo, Calif. 1989.
23a. Smith S. Sports dentistry protection and performance

from mouth guards and bite splints. *Athlet Training.* 1981; 16:100–106.

24. US Department of Health and Human Services. *Promoting Health/Preventing Disease: Objectives for the Nation.* Washington, DC: US Government Printing Office; 1980.

25. Moore TJ, et al. The mandibular orthopaedic repositioning appliance and its affect on power production in conditioned athletes. *Phys Sportsmed.* 1986; 14(12): 137–145.

26. Schmidt MA, and Medford HM. An inflammatory fibroma of the gingiva secondary to a poorly fitting athletic mouth protector. *Phys Sportsmed.* 1986; 14(2):85–88.

27. Macik J. NFL players survey. *Physician Sportsmed.* 1986; 14(12):34–35.

28. Smith CC, Sutton GS. Stop taking it on the chin: A mandibular fracture and one method of protection. *Athlet Training.* 1981; 16:2 113–116.

29. Wertenbaker L. *The Eye: Window to the World.* US News Books: 149–168.

30. International Federation of Sports Medicine Position Statement. Eye injuries and eye protection in sports. *Phys Sportsmed.* 1988; 16(11):49–57.

31. Marton K. Presentation, American College of Sports Medicine, Las Vegas, May 1987. *Physician Sportsmed.* 1987; 15(10):64.

32. Labelle P., Mercier M, Podtetener N, Trudeau F. Eye injuries in sports: Results of a five year study. *Physician Sportsmed.* 1988; 16(5):126–138.

33. Easterbrook M. Eye injuries in squash, racquetball players: An update. *Phys Sportsmed.* 1982; 10(3):47–50, 53, 56.

34. Bishop P. Performance of eye protectors for squash, racquetball. *Phys Sportsmed.* 1982; 10(3):63–64, 67–69.

35. Easterbrook M. Eye protection in racket sports: An update. *Phys Sportsmed.* 1987; 15(6):180–192.

36. National Society to Prevent Blindness and Sandusky JC. Field evaluation of eye injuries. *Athlet Training.* 1981; 16:254–258.

37. American Academy of Opthalmology. The athletic eye. In: *Opthalmology and Sports.* 1982:7, 20–30, 33–37, 39–43, 55–56.

38. Duda M. Mandatory face shields in the NHL? *Phys Sportsmed.* 1986; 14(4):33.

39. Orlando RG. Soccer related eye injuries in children and adolescents. *Phys Sportsmed.* 1988; 16(11):103–106.

40. Burke MJ. Sanitato JJ, Vinger PF, et al. Soccerball-induced injuries. *JAMA.* 1983; 249:2682–2685.

41. Green JJ. Intraocular cancer in swimmers. *Phys Sportsmed.* 1988; 16(10):15.

42. Weinstock FJ. Preventing eye injury with protective eyewear. *Sportscare Fitness.* May/June 1988:12–13.

43. J.J. Products, Inc. Orthoplast splint patterns.

44. Cliff Keen Athletic: Faceguard. Ann Arbor, Mich 48106.

45. Steele BE. Protective pads for athletes. *Phys Sportsmed.* 1985; 13(3):179.

46. Denison CD: Duke Wyre shoulder vest. Denison Orthopaedic Appliance Corporation, 220 West 28th Street, Baltimore, MD 21211; (301) 235-9645.

47. SSI (Shoulder Subluxation Inhibitor) Physical Support Systems Inc, 6 Ledge Road, Windham, NH 03087; (800) 222–5009.

48. Lorentzen D, Lawson LJ. Selected sports bras: A biomechanical analysis of breast motion while jogging. *Phys Sportsmed.* 1987; 15(5):129.

49. Haycock C. How I manage breast problems in athletes. *Phys Sportsmed.* 1987; 15(3):89.

50. Baeyens L. Breast problems in athletes. Sports Medicine Forum, *Phys Sportsmed.* 1987. 15(8):25–26.

51. Donzi's Protective Equipment, 4600 Post Oak Place Suite 315, Houston, TX 77027; (800) 231-7273.

52. BIKE Athletic Company, PO Box 666, Knoxville, TN 37901; (615) 546–4703.

53. Procare Professional Care Products, San Marcos, CA 92069.

54. Haycock C. How I manage abdominal injuries. *Physician Sportsmed.* 1986; 14(6):86.

55. Physical Support Systems, 6 Ledge Road, Windham, NH 03087; (800) 222–5009.

56. Albright J. Big Ten injury surveillance. University of Iowa, Iowa City, Iowa 52242; and Rudner M. Football players who wear knee braces show fewer incidents of serious injury. *Big Ten Conf News Serv Bur.* 1988: 2(6).

57. Bassett FH III. A protective splint of silicone rubber. *Am J Sports Med.* 1979; 7:358–360.

58. McCue F. How I manage fractured metacarpals in athletes. *Physician Sportsmed.* 1985; 13(9):83.

59. Sorbothane, Sorboturf Enterprises, 13963 Boquita Drive, Delmar, CA 92014.

60. Gamekeeper's Thumbsplint, Alimed Inc, 297 High Street, Dedham, MA 02026.

61. Warm-N-Form Back Brace, Jerome Medical, 309 Fellowship Road, Mt. Laurel, NJ 08054; (800) 257-8440.

62. Steele BE. Protective pads for athletes. *Phys Sportsmed.* 1985; 13(3):179.

63. The New Functional Brace Company Inc, 113 East 4th, Box 305, Imperial, NE 69033.

64. McCarthy P. Prophylactic knee braces: Where do they stand? *Phys Sportsmed.* 1988; 16(12):102, 115.

65. Teitz CC, Hermanson B, Kronmal R, et al. Evaluation of the use of braces to prevent injury to the knee in collegiate football players. *J Bone Joint Surg.* 1987; 69:2–9.

66. Grace TG, Skipper B, Newberry J, et al. Prophylactic knee braces and injury to the lower extremity. *J Bone Joint Surg.* 1988; 70:422–427.

67. Rovere GD, Hughson C, Mendini R, Wang J. Prophylactic knee bracing in college football. *Am J Sports Med.* 1986; 14:262–266.

68. Baker BE, Van Hanswyk E, Bogosian S, et al. A biomechanical study of the static stabilizing effect of knee braces on medial stability. *Am J Sports Med.* 1987; 15:566–570.

69. Paulos LE, Franz E, Rosenberg T, Jayarman C, et al. The biomechanics of the lateral knee bracing. Part I: Response of the valgus restraints to loading. *Am J Sports Med.* 1987; 15:419–429.

70. Garrick JG, Regua RK. Prophylactic knee bracing. *Am J Sports Med.* 1987; 15:471–476.

71. Drez D Jr. AAOS-Statement braces may not prevent knee injuries. *Phys Sports Med.* 1988; 16(1):57.

72. Hofmann A, Wytte D, Bourne M, et al. Kenne stability in orthotic knee braces. *Am J Sports Med.* 1984; 12:371–374.

73. Duda M. Knee brace, kids, placebos and water. *Phys Sportsmed.* 1988; 16(9):3.

74. Wallensten R, Erikson E. Is medial lower leg pain (shin splints) a compartment syndrome? In: Mack RR, ed. Symposium on Foot–Leg in Running Sports. St. Louis, Mo: American Academy of Orthopaedic Surgeons; 1987.

75. Detmer DE: Chronic shin splints: Classification and management of medial-tibial stress syndrome. *Sports Med.* Nov/Dec 1986; 3:436–446.

76. Dickson TB, Kichline PD. Functional management of stress fractures in female athletes using a pneumatic leg brace. *Am J Sports Med.* 1987; 15:86–89.

77. Sarmiento A. Functional bracing of tibial fractures. *Clin Orthop.* 1974; 105:202.

78. Gross MT. Comparison of support provided by ankle taping and semirigid orthoses. *J Orthop Sports Phys Ther.* 1987; 9(1):33–39.

79. Rovere GD, Giel D, Ankle stabilizers more effective than taping. *Physician Sports Med.* 1988; 16(1):59–60.

80. Doxey GE. Calcaneal pain: A review of various disorders. *J Orthop Sports Phys Ther.* 1987; 9(1):25–32.

81. Heel cup, M-F Athletic Company, PO Box 8188, Cranston, RI 02920-0188; (800) 556-7464.

82. Hamill J, Bates B. A kinetic evaluation of the effects of in-vivo loading on running shoes. *J Orthop Sports Phys Ther.* 1988; 10(2):47–53.

83. Lowry R. Functional splint for Jones fracture. *Athlet Training* 1988; 23(3):247.

84. Visnick AL. A playing orthosis for "Turf toe." *Athlet Training.* 1987; 22(3):215.

85. Multiform Splinting Materials, Ali Med Inc., 297 High Street Dedham MA 02026-9990 (hand splint text available; Hand Atlas).

86. APT. Heel-lace pads. Arlon Division of Keene, 2811 South Harbor Boulevard, Santa Ana, CA 92704.

87. Athletic Business. Liability/Sports: Judges concerned that lawsuits damage "public good." *Athlet Bus.* Oct 1988:18.

88. Noyes FR, Albright JP. Sports injury research. *Am J Sports Med.* 1988; 16(1):1–228.

89. Fitness Centers, getting floored. *Athletic Bus.* Apr 1988: 48–53.

90. Breakaway bases proposed to avoid softball injuries. *PT Bull.* 1988; 5:3.

91. Jordan BD, Cambell EA. Acute injuries among professional boxers in NY state: A two year study. *Phys Sportsmed.* 1988; 16(1):87–91.

92. Scanning sports: A new standard for headgear. *Phys Sportsmed.* 1989; 17(6): 28.

93. Testing the olympic spirit. *Sports Med News.* 1988: 17.

94. Duda M. Golf injuries. They really do happen. *Phys Sportsmed.* 1987; 15(7):191–196.

95. Griffin R, Peterson K, Halseth J, et al. Injuries in professional rodeo: An update. *Phys Sportsmed.* 1987; 15(2):105–115.

96. Tomasin JD, Martin M, Curl W, et al. Recognition and prevention of rugby injuries. *Phys Sportsmed.* 1989; 17(6):114–126.

97. Legwold G. Cross country skiers may be susceptible to U.R.I.'s. *Phys Sportsmed.* 1982; 10(4):42.

98. Brock MB, Striowski CS. Injuries in elite figure skaters. *Phys Sportsmed.* 1986; 14(1):111–115.

99. Tator CA, Edmonds VE. Sports and recreation are a rising cause of spinal cord injury. *Phys Sportsmed.* 1986; 14(5):157–167.

100. Wenzel FJ, Peters RA. A ten year survey of snowmobile accidents, injuries. *Phys Sportsmed.* 1986; 14(1):140–149.

101. Renneker M. Medical aspects of surfing. *Phys Sportsmed.* 1987; 15(12):97–105.

Appendix

Associations to Contact for More Information

NATIONAL ATHLETIC TRAINERS ASSOCIATION

2952 Stemmens, Suite 200
Dallas, TX 75247

NATIONAL ASSOCIATION TO PREVENT BLINDNESS

500 E. Remington Road
Schaumberg, IL 60173

NIKE SPORT RESEARCH REVIEW

The Editor/NIKE, Inc.
9000 S.W. Nimbus Drive
Beaverton, OR 98005

BIKE ATHLETIC COMPANY

PO Box 666
Knoxville, TN 37901–0666
Attn: Patti Broyles

AEROBICS AND FITNESS ASSOCIATION

15250 Ventura Boulevard
Suite 310
Sherman Oaks, CA 91403

AMERICAN AEROBICS ASSOCIATION

Box 401
Durange, CO 81301

AMERICAN ALLIANCE FOR HEALTH, PHYSICAL EDUCATION, RECREATION, AND DANCE

1900 Association Drive
Reston, VA 22091

CANADIAN AEROBICS AND FITNESS

692 Mount Pleasant Road
Suite 202
Toronto, ON M4S 2N3

RECREATION SAFETY INSTITUTE

Box 392
Ronkonkoma, NY 11779

US AEROBIC ASSOCIATION

Box 414
Baraboo, WI 53913

AMERICAN SOCIETY FOR TESTING AND MATERIALS

1916 Race Street
Phildelphia, PA 19103

INSTITUTE FOR AEROBICS RESEARCH

12330 Preston Road
Dallas, TX 75230

INTERSCHOLASTIC ATHLETIC INJURY

Surveillance System
1199 Hadley Road
Morresville, IN 46158

NATIONAL HEAD & NECK INJURY

Weightman Hall E–7
235 South 33rd Street
Philadelphia, PA 19104

NATIONAL HIGH SCHOOL ATHLETIC INJURY REGISTRY

Box 3548
Oak Park, IL 60303

NATIONAL INJURY INFORMATION CLEARINGHOUSE

5401 Westbard Avenue, Room 625
Washington, DC 20207

NATIONAL SAFETY COUNCIL

444 North Michigan Avenue
Chicago, IL 60611

INTERNATIONAL DANCE EXERCISE ASSOCIATION

2437 Morena Boulevard
Second Floor
San Diego, CA 92110

NATIONAL ACADEMY OF SPORTS VISION

200 South Progress Avenue
Harrisburg, PA 17109

REGIONAL SPINAL CORD INJURY

University of Alabama, Birmingham
University Station
Birmingham, AL 35294

WATER SAFETY SERVICES

1882 Tachny Road
Northbrook, IL 60062

18

Head, Neck, and Spine Injuries

Kenneth Rusche and Peter Zulia

INTRODUCTION

Head, neck, and spine injuries in sports by athletes can range from mild sprains or strains to catastrophic or disabling injuries. This chapter discusses these injuries, important signs for which the sports medicine team must be alert, and proper treatment techniques. Of all injuries sustained by athletes, these have to be looked at most carefully to prevent further injury.

HEAD INJURIES

An athlete who sustains an impact blow to the head is susceptible to a wide variety of intracranial injuries. These may vary from a mild headache to a life-threatening epidural hematoma. The necessity to administer prompt and appropriate care is a must. Bruno et al[1] point out that the initial examination of an athlete who has sustained an injury to the head must include the evaluation of facial expression, orientation to time and place, amnesia (posttrauma or retrograde), and gait pattern. Vegso and Lehman[2] have stated that this initial examination, due to the high risk nature with regard to the nervous system, demands a proper diagnosis.

In a study done by Zariczny et al[3] head-related injury had the highest incidence of any injury to school-aged children, with approximately 20% of all these injuries being head related. In another study, 39% of the soccer deaths involved traumatic injuries to the head.[4] Injuries in this study included skull fractures, subdural and epidural hematomas, and cerebral hemorrhages. Kruse and McBeath[5] reported that 18% of all bicycle injuries were to the head. Guichon and Myles[6] reported that 67% of all bicycle-related injuries were head trauma, of which four resulted in death, due to trauma to the intracranial contents.

ANATOMY

The brain and nervous system are extremely complex systems. This must be understood when we examine head injuries.

The cranium receives its static support from the bones that form the skull. There are also inner cranial supports that work in unison with the skull to protect the brain. These structures include the dura mater, the arachnoid, and the pia mater (Fig 18–1).

The outermost membrane, the dura mater, is two-layered. The outer layer, the endosteal, attaches to the inside surface of the cranium. The inner layer, the meningeal, covers the brain itself and protects the fissures of the brain. The dura mater projections also form the venous sinuses and sheaths that house the nerves that continue downward out of the skull. The dura, which continues around the spinal cord, is a single meningeal layer. The meninges extend past the spinal cord (L2–L3) and attach at the second or third sacral vertebra. There is a potential cavity between the dura mater and the next layer, the arachnoid, that is called the subdural space.

The arachnoid lies below the dura mater. This is a very delicate membrane that loosely covers the brain and the spinal cord. The arachnoid follows the general outline of the brain except for the longitudinal fissure. There is a delicate connective tissue that extends through the subarachnoid space and attaches to the pia mater. The subarachnoid space, which is between the pia mater and the arachnoid, contains spinal fluid that functions against mechanical insult or injury.

The pia mater is the innermost covering of the brain. This layer is extremely vascular and attaches close to the brain. The brain has a vast blood supply. It receives approximately 17% of the cardiac output, even though it is only 2% of the total body weight. The extensive network comes from two main pairs of

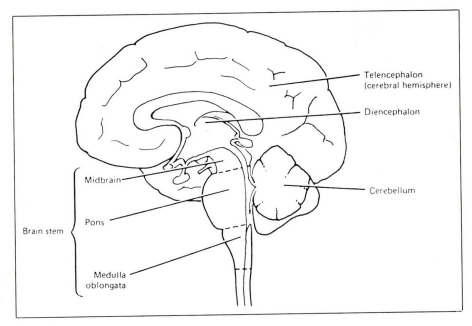

Figure 18-1. Anatomy of the brain. *(Modified from Lindner HH.* Clinical Anatomy. *East Norwalk, Ct: Appleton & Lange. 1989; 108.)*

arteries. The vertebral and the internal carotid arteries originate from the aorta. These will form the circle of Willis, which will lead into the smaller branches and enter the brain.

INJURIES TO THE HEAD AND NECK

Head Injuries

A common injury mechanism with a head injury is a direct blow to the head. Newton's third law of motion states that for every action, there is an equal and opposite reaction.[7] When the head receives a blow, the intracranial material will absorb the shock by shaking within the confines of the cranium. This is how the brain reacts with the initial blow.

Whenever there is significant trauma to the head, a skull fracture must be ruled out. When evaluating a skull fracture, palpate over the skull for any type of deformity. Other symptoms to look for with a skull fracture are soft tissue discoloration under the eyes, clear fluid exiting the ears or nose, Battle's sign (which is discoloration over the mastoid process), loose or missing teeth, or increased swelling about the cheek or jaw. A great deal of force is needed to fracture the skull, so intracranial pathology needs to be ruled out in these types of injuries.

Intracranial injury can occur with or without a skull fracture. With a blow to the head, the intercranial contents can be injured. A hematoma will increase the pressure on the brain and the brainstem, which can become a medical emergency due to its progressive nature.

Mueller and Blyth[8] state that 433 of the 643 (67.3%) fatalities in football between 1945 and 1984 resulted from head injuries. The majority of these (337)

involved subdural hematomas, although 18 suffered fatal skull fractures. The majority of the fatal head blows occurred when the athlete was in the process of tackling or being tackled.

Hematomas. An epidural hematoma is a pooling of blood between the skull and the dura mater. This occurs when there is a tearing of the arteries of the dural membrane. The middle meningeal artery is the most commonly involved artery. This injury will usually cause a temporary loss of consciousness. The athlete will regain consciousness and appear normal, with this lucid period lasting a few minutes or even hours. The athlete will then lapse into lethargy or unconsciousness. This relapse is due to the growing intracranial pressure on the brain. Brain function will be distorted, and a common sign of this injury is pupil dilation homolaterally. This occurs as the increased pressure compresses the third cranial nerve causing the dilation.[9]

Rimel et al[10] noted that a lacrosse player was found unresponsive several hours after being hit with a lacrosse stick. When the injury occurred, the player sat out for approximately 5 minutes, then returned to play until the conclusion of the match. When found in his dorm room several hours later, he had a reading of 12 out of 15 on the Glasgow Coma Scale.[11] This scale measures motor, verbal and eye response to certain commands. With the help of computed tomography (CT) an epidural hematoma and skull fracture were diagnosed at the left temporoparietal region. Surgical evaluation of the epidural hematoma was done and followup treatment, for 6 months, cleared the athlete to compete again.

An epidural hematoma is a true medical emergency that warrants fast medical treatment. The general rule is the longer the lucid period, the greater the

chance to recover because blood accumulation is slower. This gives the medical specialist the time to recognize and treat the injury. The on-the-field medical team must refer the injury to the emergency room so that the injury can be properly monitored.

A subdural hematoma occurs between the dura mater and the arachnoid in the subdural space. This injury is due to a tearing of cerebral veins running from the cortex to the dural sinuses. Acute subdural hematomas can follow a relatively minor head injury or can occur in a state of unconsciousness. Mortalities have reached 70%.[9] As a result the epidural and the acute subdural hematomas are medical emergencies.

Subacute and chronic subdural hematomas will not bleed profusely. Intercranial pressure will build over time in these injuries and the brain will try to adjust and adapt to the changes. With this type of injury a headache may be severe one day and nonexistent the next. Due to the frequent fluctuation in symptoms, the diagnosis may be missed. Medical attention to this injury is important and reevaluation of this head injury is vital due to the fluctuating patterns or continual decrease in cerebral function. If symptoms do not improve, definitive diagnostic steps, such as CT, may be deemed necessary.

Intercerebral hematoma occurs within the brain itself. There may be a rapid decrease in neurological function, and increase in pressure to this area will show signs of disorientation and consciousness. Intercranial pressure can cause numerous signs and symptoms. Pupil irregularity and amnesia can appear. Persistent and increasing headache, nausea, vomiting, increased systolic blood pressure, with a decreased dyastolic pressure, nystagmus, leakage of cerebrospinal fluid (CSF) from nose or the ears, respiratory difficulty, and papilledema are other signs and symptoms that can be a result of this injury.

If an athlete is suspected of a hematoma, he or she must be transported to the emergency room. An injury to the neck must be ruled out and the athlete should be treated for shock. Under no circumstances should an athlete return to play following this injury.

Concussions. Many athletes suffer head injuries that are not as severe as a hematoma. Concussions are common in contact sports. Rimel et al[10] define a cerebral concussion as a clinical syndrome characterized by immediate and transient posttraumatic impairment of neurological function. This involves alterations of consciousness and vision and equilibrium disturbances due primarily to brainstem involvement. A suspected concussion may be one of the following:

1. The athlete has been "dinged."
2. More severe injury has occurred, with headache, inability to concentrate, or irritability.
3. The injury is life threatening.[11]

According to Vegso and Lehman there are six grades of cerebral concussion, discussed in the following paragraphs.[2]

A grade I concussion will cause signs of confusion, vertigo (mild), headache, and disorientation. The athlete will describe the injury as "My head is ringing" or "I had my bell rung." The symptoms are reversible with no sequelae. Return to play is determined by continual monitoring of symptoms. Vegso and Lehman state that the confusion suffered in a grade I concussion is "short lived."[2] After a period of 5 to 15 minutes, the athlete will be lucid. Once the athlete is clear-headed with the absence of vertigo, confusion, headache, photophobia, and labile emotions, he or she can return to play.

Functional progression tests should also be performed before returning the athlete to competition. The athlete should go through a walk, jog, run, cut, and change of direction test. This test is a necessity because of the importance of the sports simulation to the athlete. His or her reaction time and orientation to time and place as well as activity is essential. Tasks that are asked of the athlete will help the doctor, physical therapist, or athletic trainer decide whether to allow him or her to return to play.

A grade II concussion is described as the confusion of a grade I concussion with the addition of posttrauma amnesia. The athlete will be unable to recall events from the moment of the injury. There is no loss of consciousness. The athlete should not be permitted to continue participation for that day. Follow-up evaluation is required before return to play. These athletes will possibly develop "postconcussion syndrome." This is described as inability to concentrate, irritability, and a "throbbing" headache. Postconcussion syndrome can be present for several weeks after injury.

A grade III concussion is characterized by grades I and II with accompanied retrograde amnesia. Retrograde amnesia is described as the inability to recall events prior to the injury. These athletes will not be permitted to return to play until observation and follow-up treatment is rendered. The athlete may be disoriented and suffering from vertigo. It is felt that the athlete should be transported by stretcher for precautionary reasons of cervical spine or intercranial trauma.

A grade IV concussion is characterized by a period of unconsciousness of no more than a few minutes. Following this paralytic coma, the athlete will suffer from the symptoms of grades I through III concussion. It is recommended that this patient be hospitalized if signs of prolonged unconsciousness or other signs persist.

A grade V concussion is associated with paralytic coma with secondary symptoms of loss of cardiopulmonary function. If cardiopulmonary resuscitation (CPR) fails, grade VI concussion will occur. This grade of concussion is when the athlete expires.

A concussion is an injury that needs immediate at-

tention due to the possible neural involvement. Proper assessment of the injury is needed before returning to play. Evaluation of the injury, grading the injury, followed by observation and reevaluation is imperative. Upper quarter screens, direct and consensual pupillary constriction to light, questions on short- and long-term memory, balance activity, and full orientation and emotional stability should be tested before the athlete is permitted to return to competition. With any suspected head injury evaluation of possible cervical spine injury is essential. All unconscious athletes should be treated as having a cervical injury.

Protective Equipment. Prevention of head injuries is important when considering the safety of the sport and its participants. The number of fatalities have sharply decreased during the past 10 years due to the rule changes for the player's protection. Proper techniques also need to be taught. The athlete must possess the necessary strength and proprioception and use the proper equipment. Equipment is defined as both what is worn by the athlete and the protective barriers on the field of play (padding around the goalpost or at end of gym).

In football, the advances in headgear since the turn of the century are revolutionary. From the non-padded helmet to the technologically advanced padding and shell, helmets have been proven to be better energy absorbers. The face mask of today also has absorbing capabilities. The National Operating Committee on Standards for Athletic Equipment (NOCSAE) was founded in 1969. Since then, NOCSAE has set standards for headgear in sports that have played a major role in making sports safe. The National Collegiate Athletic Association (NCAA) and the National Federation of State High School Associations make it mandatory that all participants in sports that require helmets wear NOCSAE approved equipment. At the same time, coaches are spending more time on skills for the sport they coach and medical care has improved for the athlete. The helmet has specific fitting rules which are to be strictly enforced for a proper fit. For more information, see Chapter 17.

The design of the helmet has advanced in other sports. Feriencik[12] reported a case study of a hockey player who received a depression fracture to the skull. This was due in part to a helmet that was lacking in padding and shell design. Bishop et al[13] studied the safety of hockey helmets and recommended that helmets be effectively padded, have fewer openings, and increased protection to the temporal region. These suggestions were made to increase the surface area of the helmet for better energy absorption to a blow.

Face Injuries

In addition to the head, the face is susceptible to a variety of injuries.[14] Use of mouth guards and face masks

has reduced greatly the number of injuries seen by the medical specialist.

Mouth Injuries. For safety of the mouth, mouth guards and face masks are essential. Heintz[15] believes that the use of a mouth guard can prevent facial, mouth, and teeth injury. Mouth guards were recommended in the 1950s and mandatory in high schools by 1962 and by the NCAA in 1973 for football.[16] The feeling has been that in addition to protecting the mouth, the mouth guard helps to absorb shock from a head blow.

Eye Injuries. Eye injuries are common in all kinds of sports whether contact or noncontact. When there is a foreign object in the eye, precaution should be taken in removing the object from the eye. When an object is embedded in the lower lid, first ask the athlete to remain calm due to the gentle nature of the procedure. Gently pull the lower lid out of the way and use a sterile gauze pad to excise the object. If there is an object under the upper lid, have the athlete first look downward, then pull the upper lid down. This will produce a "tear wash" and this may expose the object. When the object still remains under the upper lid, pull the lid back using a cotton swab and use sterile gauze to locate and remove the foreign object from the eye. (Figs 18–2, 18–3, 18–4).

The retina is the light-sensitive inner layer of the eye that translates light waves into an image. A detached retina occurs when the retina is peeled off the choroid, which is responsible for vascular supply of the eyeball.[17] The mechanism of injury is a blow to the eye that produces "curtain dropping" or "light flashes" followed by darkness in the affected eye. This can occur acutely or manifest over a period of time. Symptoms

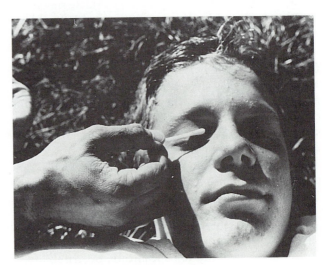

Figure 18–2. Removal of object from eye.

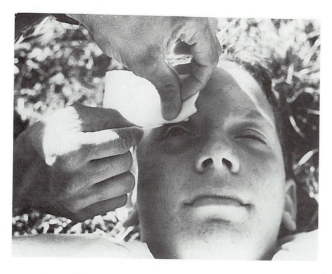

Figure 18-3. Removal of object from eye.

include blurred vision, flashes of light, or "dots" flashing before the eye. The athlete should be referred to an ophthalmologist for further evaluation when one or all of these symptoms occur.

Corneal abrasions can occur in numerous sports. An object can be lodged or scratch the cornea and have an abrasive type of action to the eye. Treatment consists of antibiotic drops and an eye patch over both eyes to prevent excessive eye motion. This athlete should be referred to an ophthalmologist for further evaluation.

A "blowout" fracture occurs when an object strikes the eye or orbit of the eye. Due to the increase in the internal pressure of the eye, the thin bone inferior region of the orbit can fracture. Symptoms of an increase in eye pressure, pain with the eye movements, or an abnormality along the orbital rim on palpation

can indicate a blowout fracture. Application of an eye patch on both eyes to prevent movement and transporting the athlete to an ophthalmologist is indicated when such symptoms are present. If there is a fracture, surgery is indicated to correct the injury within 7 to 14 days.

Hyphena shows hemorrhage to the anterior chamber of the eye due to a contusion or blow to the eye or face. Vision may be blocked or impaired. Due to the potential serious nature to other structures of the eye, an ophthalmologist's intervention in care is required.

With certain eye injuries, it is important that they be dressed carefully. At times, when stabilization and rest is required for the eye, due to injury, an eye patch pressure dressing can be placed on the athlete. It is important that the lid is not allowed to move. This is to help rest the eye. Both eyes should be covered, as movement of the uninjured eye will cause movement of the injured eye. When there are objects embedded in the eye such as splinters, a loose dressing is indicated. This is done by the use of a paper cup and a stockinette doughnut as its base. Then wrap a dressing of roll gauze or elastic wrap so the dressing is secure and then transport the person to a hospital[18] (Figs 18-5, 18-6, 18-7, 18-8).

Protective Equipment. The eye is a vulnerable organ. In sports, eye protection is a definite concern. From football players who wear a glass shield to basketball players with goggles, eye protection with minimal restriction of sight is essential. Easterbrook[19] noted that open eye protectors were not satisfactory for protection. There was no protection between rims and these could cause serious eye injury. In another study, Easterbrook[20] rated eye guards. It was felt the glasses with a thickened plastic construction were very good

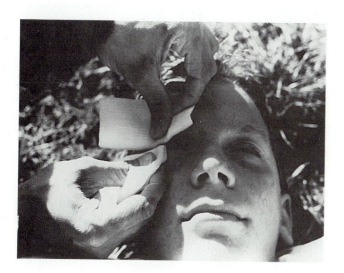

Figure 18-4. Removal of object from eye.

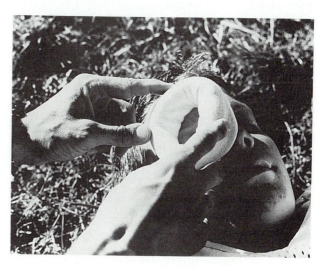

Figure 18-5. Eye protection.

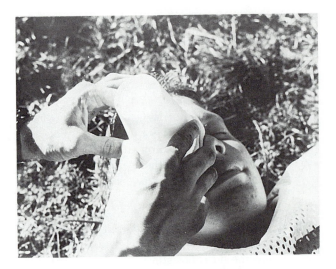

Figure 18-6. Eye protection.

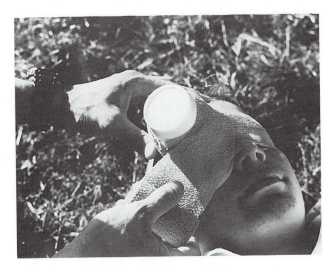

Figure 18-8. Eye protection.

in protecting the eye. Vinger[21] took the eye protection one step further when he stated that eye considerations must be taken into account in the designing of a helmet for high-collision sports. He noted the energy that is absorbed must be transmitted through the face mask as well as the helmet. This will in turn dissipate energy that can ultimately prevent head injuries.

Scalp hematomas occur when an athlete is cut on the head. In the head and face, lacerations bleed profusely even though a major vessel has not been lacerated.[22] The most effective and safest way to treat a wound is to *not* clean the wound. Clean debris from the wound but do not wipe away due to potential contamination of the brain. Control the bleeding with a sterile dressing and *gentle* pressure, not forceful compression and ice over the area. Increased pressure is contraindicated due to potential of fractures.

Nose and Jaw Injuries. When there is a blow to the jaw or temporal mandibular joint complex, there is concern for a fracture. Check for deformity throughout the region and note any painful areas. Check for the opening and closing of the mouth. Evaluate bite down and overbite. With a fracture to the jaw, the athlete's ability to communicate will be impaired.

A nasal fracture is the separation of the nasal cartilage from the bone. Immediate swelling and deformity along with profuse bleeding will be the common sign. A blow laterally will show more deformity than a blow straight on the nose. Control of the bleeding by gentle compression is needed first, followed by splinting of the nose. Arnheim[23] demonstrates that splinting the nose on either side of the nose and using adhesive tape will protect the nose until the athlete is transported to the team physician (Figs 18-9, 18-10, 18-11).

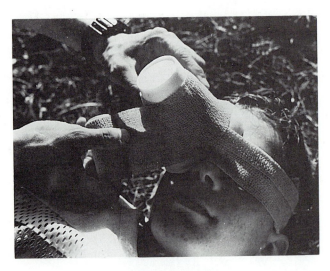

Figure 18-7. Eye protection.

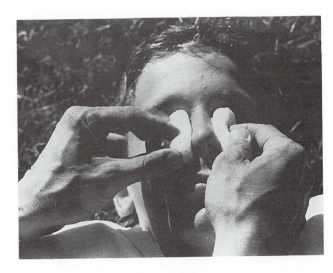

Figure 18-9. Splinting nose.

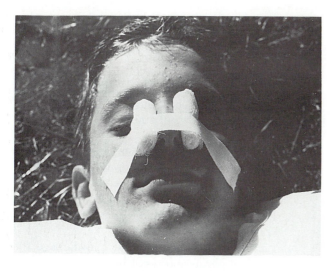

Figure 18-10. Splinting nose.

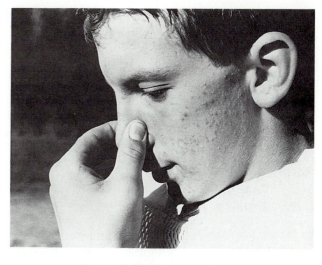

Figure 18-12. Stop nose bleed.

To stop a nosebleed, place the head forward so the athlete will not swallow blood (Fig 18–12). Put your thumb on the outside portion of the nostril that is bleeding and the index finger on the opposite nostril. Increase the pressure to decrease the bleeding. A clot will form and bleeding will cease. Use ice to pack the nose and decrease the metabolic rate to the tissues.

During competition, when time is of the utmost importance, packing the nose with a rolled up sterile gauze pad or a tampon will stop the bleeding temporarily and the athlete can continue to participate.

Ear Injuries. The ear is a delicate organ with injuries brought on by some form of pressure changes. Due to the importance of the ear in balance and proprioception, vertigo is the main symptom of ear pathology.

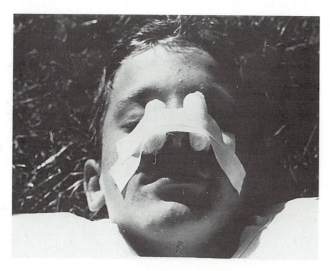

Figure 18-11. Splinting nose.

Other symptoms such as pain or hearing deficits may be present.

A ruptured eardrum is caused by a direct blow to the ear. An increase in pressure will cause a rupture of the ear's tympanic membrane. Swimmer's ear is an infection of the external auditory canal, caused by water in the canal. Burnois solution with antibiotic drops is used to treat this problem. It is important to keep the ear dry and clear after exiting the pool. Barotrauma is a condition where there is an increased pressure in the eustachian tube. This occurs in diving situations due to disorientation while the athlete is diving and can be life threatening. Caloric labrynthitis is a condition of cold water filling the external auditory canal. Drowning can occur due to disorientation and lack of eye control. Friction can cause cauliflower ear, a condition where the pinna will hemorrhage and swell the subperichondral area. Treatment of aspiration and collodian casting is indicated acutely.

CERVICAL SPINE INJURIES

Acute injuries of the cervical spine are among the most common causes of severe disability and death following trauma, and yet the diagnosis of these injuries is often delayed and the treatment inadequate.[24] The cervical spine is vulnerable to injury in all contact sports, especially football, diving, wrestling, ice hockey, and gymnastics. Spinal injuries comprise some of the most serious sports injuries but in total number they constitute only a small percentage.

Cervical spine injuries can be very misleading. Risks are high because the nervous system is so complex and the margin of error low. A brachial plexus injury

(nerve stretch syndrome) may present with paresthesia or paralysis, which would lead medical personnel or coaches to suspect spinal injury, but in minutes the injury can completely resolve itself. Severe spine injuries in sports are not common, but unfortunately trainers and team physicians have little experience in dealing with them.

In the sport of football as well as others, cervical spine injuries have been yearly problems. In 1904 President Roosevelt ordered that football be made safer or else banned as a college sport. This led to the formation of the NCAA, which today remains the governing body of collegiate sports. With development of the football helmet over the years and the protection it provided the head, players began using the head as a weapon. This technique places the cervical spine under a tremendous load.

There has been much documentation on spine injuries in sports. During 1959 to 1963 there were 78 cervical spine injuries in tackle football.[25] Thirty resulted in permanent quadriplegia and 16 in deaths. One of the few long term studies was done by Blyth and Arnold during the period of 1931 to 1976.[26] There were an average of 18.6 direct fatalities per year, which is less than 2 of 100,000 participants per season. Of the direct fatalities, 19% involved spine-related injuries. In a study by Torg et al[27] of 12 severe neck injuries that occurred in Pennsylvania and New Jersey during the 1975 football season, 8 of the injuries resulted in quadriplegia, 3 in cervical spine fracture, and 1 in death.

Good statistics were kept on spine injuries during the early 1970s. Of those cervical spine injuries resulting in quadriplegia between 1971 and 1975, at the high school level, 72% were a result of tackling. This corresponds to 78% at the college level. With regard to position played, at the high school level, 52% were defensive backs, 13% special teams, and 10% were linebackers, and at the college level, 73% were defensive backs. Fifty-two of all cervical spine quadriplegia from 1971 to 1975 were the result of spearing or direct compression, where initial contact is made with the top or crown of the helmet.[27]

In 1974, Albright et al[28] described roentgenographic changes in the cervical spine of 75 college freshman who were playing football at the University of Iowa. In one third of the freshman they observed vertebral compression fracture, abnormal range of motion, narrowing of the disc space, and fracture of the neural arch in those who participated in high school football.

Due to the incidence of quadriplegia and fatal head and neck injuries alone, the National Football Head and Neck Injury Registry was established in conjunction with the Sports Medicine Center at Temple University. Data have been collected there since 1971 in regards to head and neck injuries in sports in order to better monitor sports safety.

According to Funk and Wells there are five mechanisms of injury that can result in cervical spine injuries in athletes[29]:

1. Extension. Funk and Wells feel this is an uncommon mechanism, as they have never seen death, serious cord damage, dislocation, or fracture directly attributable to hyperextension.
2. Violent flexion is the most dangerous mechanism, and can result in flexion dislocation with or without a fracture. The area most commonly involved is C4–C5 or C5–C6.
3. Impaction where the head is driven downward.
4. Lateral stretch injuries that can damage the brachial plexus and result in nerve stretch syndrome.
5. Congenital instability.

In looking at the majority of injuries to the cervical spine the classic mechanism of injury resulting in fracture dislocation is that of accidental forced hyperflexion. Within the registry there have been two factors found in variance from the normal mechanism, the first being that it was not accidental and the second that it was not cervical spine hyperflexion.[27] In the majority of the injuries documented the athlete was using his head as a weapon and the initial contact point was the top of the helmet or crown.

During the course of a football game the cervical spine is exposed to many forces that could cause injury. Due to the anatomic composition of the spine (elasticity of the disc, mobility of the spine, and impact-absorbing capabilities of the muscle), these forces are dissipated. Injury can occur when force occurs to the top of the helmet while being transmitted along the axial alignment.

With the normal amount of cervical lordosis, the spine is in extension when the neck is in a resting position. If the neck is in forward flexion, the cervical spine is extended, and if the force is great along the axial aligned cervical spine there is no protection. This can result in disc injury or fracture. Torg et al postulate that this is a commonly unrecognized mechanism of injury.[27]

There are many types of athletic injuries that can occur to the cervical spine[2]:

- Nerve root–brachial plexus neuropraxia
- Stable cervical sprain
- Muscular strain
- Brachial plexus axonotmesis
- Intervertebral disc injury (narrowing–herniation) without neurological deficit
- Stable cervical fracture without neurological deficit
- Subluxation without neurological deficit

- Unstable fractures with or without neurological deficit
- Dislocation with or without neurological deficit
- Intervertebral disc herniation with neurological deficit
- Quadriplegia
- Death

Severe neck injuries consist of direct fatalities, cervical spine fracture dislocation, and cervical spine fracture–dislocation with permanent quadriplegia.

A more common nonsevere injury to the neck is a cervical sprain/strain. There will be a loss of range of motion but there is no paresthesia. Athletes will say that they "jammed" their neck and pain will center in the cervical area. It may be hard to identify the exact nature of the injury. Neurological examination and x-rays are negative and it is assumed that the injury occurs to the disc, ligament, muscle, or joints. Treatment of sprain/strains depends on their severity. A collar may initially be worn for comfort and anti-inflammatory medication prescribed. Physical therapy is started and the athlete can return to play when strength and motion are normal.

Nerve stretch syndrome, or as more commonly referred to as stingers/burners, are common in sports such as football and wrestling. This syndrome represents a neuropraxia of the brachial plexus.[30]

The symptoms of a nerve stretch are burning and numbness either in the shoulder or extending down the limb. There is a sensation of deadness or radiating shock like pain with an inability to lift the arm, forearm or hand. The temporary paralysis of the arm can last several hours to 10 to 15 minutes. A residual neurological deficit may persist for days or months. Most of the time these are peripheral injuries so involvement is in branches of the brachial plexus and individual nerves. Root injuries are rare in athletes and peripheral lesions common.[31] Motor power has to be assessed to rule out damage. Sensory changes take longer to develop, and in the early postinjury period are not as good of a guide as motor assessment.[31] Muscles that need to be checked are the deltoid, tricep, bicep, wrist extensors and flexors, and intrinsics of the hand as well as the trapezius and serratus anterior. Sensory function should not be overlooked.

The athlete who experiences repeated episodes of burners should have cervical spine x-rays and EMG studies performed.[32] If the studies are negative the athlete should be put on a year-round conditioning program for the neck and shoulders and even wear a neck collar to play.

Brachial plexus injuries may be divided into three categories[33]:

- *Category 1.* This is the typical, most common burner. There is a transient loss of motor power

and transient pain that resolves within minutes without actual injury or anatomic damage to the nerves. Complete resolution extends beyond 5 to 8 minutes in a moderate category 1. In a severe category 1, there is no anatomic damage, but weakness and paresthesias continues for 24 hours.

- *Category 2.* This is less common than category 1. There is some axonotmesis and injury to the nerve. Muscle weakness and manifestations of the nerve injury persist for 10 days to 2 weeks with a mild category 2.
- *Category 3.* There is neurotmesis and the weakness and evidence of nerve injury may persist for as long as 1 year. This is very uncommon.

Nerve lesions about the shoulder/neck can occur as a result of different mechanisms of injury. Bateman classifies them as follows[31]:

- *Projectile falls.* Headlong falls in which an outstretched arm provides protection. Contact is made on the point of the shoulder with the head and neck tilted in the opposite direction. These can be seen in riding, polo, diving, skiing, and football.
- *Shoulder–angle blows.* There is a force, usually to the top of the shoulder or across the supraclavicular area, but to a considerable degree the force is applied to the posterior aspect of the neck. These can be seen in hockey, lacrosse, riding, and rowing.
- *Frontal force.* Injury to the anterior aspect of the shoulder and upper part of the arm. Nerve problems can arise from forces in these areas in football, wrestling, gymnastics, and trampoline.
- *Axillar injuries.* Forces that drive into the armpit.
- *Twisting trauma.* The shoulder is exposed to extreme rotatory or twisting forces.

Chrisman et al studied 22 cases of lateral flexion neck injuries resulting in nerve stretch syndrome.[34] After the initial injury they found that neck and shoulder ache was usual and neurological changes in the arms was common. In some of the cases numbness and decreased reflex activity lasted several months. Some muscle weakness in the extensor–supinator or flexor pronator group lasted more than 1 year. There was also limitation of lateral flexion of the neck toward the affected side.

Chrisman et al[34] feel this injury is a sprain of the cervical spine with a mild stretch of the nerve root. The mechanism of injury in the majority of cases was neck lateral flexion and weakness persisted in some for more than 1 year. Several other authors have mentioned weakness lasting from weeks to months.[31,35,36]

Poindexter and Johnson studied 20 nerve stretch syndrome patients and found that the mechanism of injury was hyperextension in 4 cases, hyperflexion in 3, and lateral flexion in 3, with the remaining patients unable to recall.[37] Electromyographical findings in this study suggested a C6 radiculopathy rather than a brachial plexus stretch. Differential diagnosis with nerve stretch syndrome consists of spinal cord contusion, brachial plexus injury, radiculopathy, or a combination of the above.

Watkins did a detailed review of 12 players sustaining burners in football.[38] In each case he found the mechanism of injury to be head compression, extension, and rotation toward the involved arm. Numerous reports site the mechanism of injury to be lateral flexion of the neck and a blow to the top of the ipsilateral shoulder. He was able to reproduce the pain in compression, extension and rotation to the involved arm (Spurling's maneuver).

If the EMG studies show involvement of the deltoid, infraspinatus, supraspinatus, and bicep, then the nerve stretch would be an axonotmesis. These athletes must be kept from contact sports until they achieve full motion and strength and EMG shows axon regeneration. This can take a minimum of 4 to 6 weeks.

Axial compression–flexion injuries can occur to the cervical spine. These are incurred by striking an object with the top of the head, which can result in disruption of the posterior soft-tissue supporting elements with angulation and anterior translation of the superior cervical vertebrae.[32] The patient will have no neurological deficit.[32] Instability will usually develop, and if there is more than a 20% subluxation of the vertebral body, fusion is recommended.

Fractures/Dislocations

Fractures or dislocations of the cervical spine may be stable or unstable and may or may not be associated with neurological deficit. These injuries need medical attention as soon as possible because certain management and treatment principles are imperative. Vertebral body compression fractures can happen as a result of axial loading. These can be classified into types 1 through 5 and can be treated conservatively or surgically depending on the type.[39]

Peripheral Nerve Injuries

Peripheral nerve injuries can occur in athletes usually as a result of a blow. Injury can occur to

1. Spinal accessory nerve (trapezius)
2. Suprascapular nerve (supraspinatus, infraspinatus, and teres major)
3. Axillary nerve (deltoid, teres minor)
4. Long thoracic nerve (serratus anterior)

The spinal accessory nerve can be injured anteriorly just proximal to its entrance into the trapezius about 1 in above the clavicle. Force from a punch, hockey or lacrosse stick, or elbow can injure this area. There will be weakness lifting the arm, shrugging the shoulder or there may be a winging of the scapula.

The suprascapular nerve is purely motor and an injury may result in weakness to the supraspinatus and infraspinatus. A blow to the base of the neck may cause weakness in abduction and rotation.

A direct blow to the axillary area or an anterior shoulder dislocation will involve the axillary nerve. There is a loss of sensation in a small area of the lateral aspect of the shoulder.

On the Field Management of Spine Injuries

Rarely does the team physician, sports physical therapist, or athletic trainer have to provide care for an emergency spine injury. The successful management of this problem is of utmost importance so as not to endanger the athlete's life. When attending to an athlete who is suspect of a spine injury, remember not to act too quickly. Torg feels the most important point is to prevent further injury.[32] Adequate preparation will help prevent second guessing. An athlete may walk off the field and have a significant neck injury.

Any unconscious athlete must be assumed to have a spinal injury. Spinal injuries can be hard to detect. Grant et al suggest the following in determining spinal injury[22]:

1. What was the mechanism of injury? Could it have produced spinal injury?
2. Observe the position of the athlete.
3. Question the patient, players, and officials about the injury.
4. Do a head-to-toe examination. Are there any injuries that can be associated with a spine injury (facial, head or neck wounds)? Are there signs or symptoms of a possible spinal injury? Does a neurological survey indicate any nerve function problem.
5. Monitor the athlete to note any changes associated with spinal injury (numbness, tingling or paralysis).

Symptoms and signs of spinal injury are as follows[22]:

1. Pain without movement. Pain is not always constant and can occur anywhere from the top of the head to the buttocks. Pain in the leg is common for certain types of injury to the lower spinal cord.
2. Pain with movement. The athlete normally will lie still to prevent pain on movement. Do

not encourage him or her to move to determine if there is pain. If the athlete complains of pain in the neck or back with movement then this should be treated as a spinal injury.

3. Tenderness. Gentle palpation along the injury may reveal tenderness.
4. Deformity. Obvious spinal deformities are rare so it is not necessary to remove equipment to check.
5. Impaired breathing. A cervical spine injury can impair nerve function to the chest muscles. Panting due to respiratory insufficiency may develop.
6. Characteristic positioning of the arms. In some cases of spinal injury, motor pathways that extend the arms can be interrupted. The athlete on his or her back may have two arms extended above the head.
7. Involuntary loss of bowel and bladder control.
8. Nerve impairment to the extremities. The athlete may have loss of use, weakness, numbness, tingling, or loss of feeling in the upper or lower extremities. Paralysis of the extremities is probably the most reliable sign of spinal injury in a conscious athlete.
9. Severe shock may occur.

There are assessment procedures that need to be performed by the person who is rendering care. Once the symptoms and signs are looked at in a conscious athlete, the lower and upper extremities need to be assessed. In assessing the lower extremity in conscious athletes, the provider of care needs to see if they can respond to sensation by touching the toes. Range of motion can be checked to see if the athlete can plantar and dorsiflex the foot. Muscle function can be tested by resisting plantar and dorsiflexion.

The same sequence of tests can be performed in the conscious athlete to the upper extremity using the fingers, wrist and hand. If the athlete is able to do the upper and lower extremity tests without difficulty, then there is little chance of damage to the spinal cord. Remember, however, that these tests do not rule out all injuries such as a fracture to the spine.

In unconscious athletes make sure they are breathing, remove the mouthpiece if they have one, and maintain the airway. Keep the helmet on and if they have a pulse, maintain them until they regain consciousness or the life squad has arrived.

An unconscious athlete who is breathing and has a pulse, should be tested for spinal injury by pinching the hand and toes or ankles and noting the response. If there is a reaction to painful stimuli, then the cord is usually intact. If there is no reaction, then there is possible spinal cord damage. It can be difficult to survey the unconscious athlete as, at times, he or she will not respond to painful stimulus. These athletes need to be treated for spinal injury. It is not important on the field to know exactly what level is involved but to be able to know whether there is neurological involvement and the proper treatment.

Remember that paralysis, pain, pain on movement, and tenderness anywhere along the spine are reliable indicators of possible spinal injury in the conscious patient. If any of these are found then immobilize the patient before finishing the examination. For any athlete that is suspect for a spinal injury the following steps should be carried out by trained personnel[22]:

1. Provide manual traction for the head and neck.
2. Apply a rigid collar and continue to maintain traction.
3. Secure the patient to a long spine board.
4. Administer oxygen in high concentration. Edema to the cord may impair oxygen delivery to the cord.

In a football game, the only time the helmet should be removed from an injured athlete is if the face mask interferes with restoring an airway or if the helmet is so loose it is unable to go on a spine board correctly. The majority of the time, the helmet should not be removed.

If the face mask of a football helmet is interfering with ventilation then the face mask can be removed. Most football face masks are attached by four rubber clips. These can be cut by a sharp knife or scissors. The chin strap can also be loosened to help with the chin-lift or jaw-thrust part of CPR. If these steps do not allow proper ventilation then the helmet should be removed. Two people are required to remove a helmet. According to the AAOS, the proper procedure for removing the helmet is[40]:

1. Person 1 should kneel above the patient's head and support the head by placing a hand on each side of the helmet with the fingers on the mandible.
2. Person 2 cuts the chin strap while person one maintains head support.
3. Person 2 places one hand on the athlete's mandible with a thumb on one side and third and second finger on the opposite side. The other hand is placed behind the athlete's neck with firm pressure to the occipital region. This transfers head support from person 1 to person 2.
4. Person 1 removes the helmet remembering to expand it laterally to clear the ears. The jaw pads need to be removed.

5. Person 2 continues in-line support from below, not tilting the head.
6. Person 1, after removing the helmet, places hands on both sides of the head firmly grasping the mandible and base of the skull to provide support until the athlete is splinted.

An athlete who suffers a minor neck injury during a game may walk to the sideline and seek help from the trainer or team physician. In this case a sideline evaluation should be carried out progressing as follows:

1. Ask the athlete if there is any weakness, numbness, burning, or tingling.
2. Localize the painful area.
3. Check sensation and reflexes.
4. Check grip and leg strength.
5. The helmet can be removed if the above examination is normal. With the helmet off, check for tenderness in the neck. Check active neck range of motion. If there is full range of motion with little pain, then check neck strength and shoulder strength.
6. Perform the compression test.[41] With the chin directed toward the supraclavicular fossa, apply a compressive force downwards on the head; any pain in the neck or any radiation of pain down the arm produces a positive test, suggesting a cervical disc protrusion or rupture.

An athlete can return to play if neck muscle strength is normal, there is full range of motion, there is no pain with any test, and no tingling, burning, numbness, or weakness of any limb.[41]

Prevention of Cervical Injuries

There are a certain number of serious injuries that cannot be avoided in contact sports. Coaches, players, equipment makers, and parents can do several things to make sports as safe as possible.

Preparticipation physicals are very important to pick up any problems that an athlete may have. An athlete who complains of tingling, numbness, weakness, or sore neck should be evaluated by a physician. Athletes with prior neck injuries should also be evaluated prior to the start of sports.

In football, coaches need to be sure to teach proper technique in blocking and tackling. Skilled professionals do not rely on their helmets to block. Reaching with the neck to make a tackle needs to be discouraged. The neck muscles need to be kept on guard at all times, anticipating a blow.

Proper falling techniques need to be taught in all sports so they are routine. Gymnastic apparatus and mats need to be placed strategically to prevent the chance of serious injury.

Conditioning exercises for the neck and spine needs to be done by all athletes participating in contact sports. This is necessary both in the preseason and during the season and is discussed later in the chapter.

Well-trained officials are needed, whether the sport be football, basketball, hockey, or wrestling. They need to know the rules and enforce them to prevent spinal injuries.

Good equipment that fits properly is a must. Table 18–1 describes the correct way to fit a football helmet.

Watkins feels the primary rule for preventing burners is wearing properly fitted shoulder pads.[38] Shoulder pads have four basic functions:

1. Absorb shock.
2. Protect the shoulders.
3. Fit the chest.
4. Fix the mid-cervical spine to the trunk.

In order to fit, the chest pads need to be more of an A-frame type with rigid, long anterior and posterior panels. They should fit snugly around the chest.

Educational programs for the coaches are an important area to help prevent injuries. As coaches learn more about injuries, they are better able to communicate this knowledge to their athletes. Moreover, the best medical care needs to be available to sports programs.

Rehabilitation of Neck Injuries

Rehabilitation of neck injuries is crucial to athletes. Several injuries that can benefit from exercise to the cervical spine are strains, sprains, nerve stretches, stable fractures and peripheral nerve injuries. The goals of the program are to increase range of motion and to strengthen the neck and surrounding musculature. If the diagnosis is one of nerve stretch, or peripheral nerve injury, then the entire upper extremity may be exer-

---

TABLE 18–1. PROPER FITTING OF A FOOTBALL HELMET

1. The hair should be cut and wet to mimic playing conditions as much as possible.
2. The crown of the helmet should be one to two fingerbreadths above the eyebrows.
3. There should be at least ¾ to 1½ in of space between the athlete's head and the outer shell.
4. The helmet should turn only a little (side to side).
5. Put pressure on the top of the helmet and pressure should be felt on the top of the head.
6. Make sure the helmet does not rotate up and down so the shell does not hit the bridge of the nose.
7. Jaw pads are used to prevent side-to-side movement and should make slight contact with the cheeks.
8. Chin straps should be four point to prevent further movement of the helmet.
9. Athletes should check their helmets periodically for cracks and loose screws.

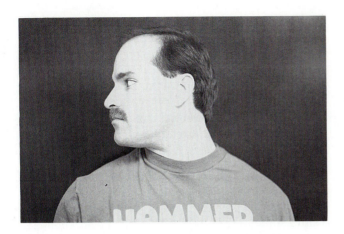

Figure 18–13. Right rotation.

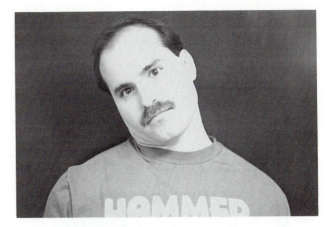

Figure 18–15. Side bend right.

cised. For an acute injury, physical therapy is used in conjunction with anti-inflammatory medications, which decrease pain and spasm. Once the athlete starts feeling better, range of motion exercises can be started, followed by isometrics. This is in turn followed by manual resistance exercise, through a full-range or pain-free range of motion. This will lead up to isotonic exercises. The entire rehabilitation program needs to be followed and under the care of a physician, therapist, or trainer.

Range of motion exercises are started once the physician permits. Each position is to be held 5 seconds and each one repeated ten times. They should be done in a pain free mode:

- *Right rotation.* In a sitting position take your chin and turn it to the right (Fig 18–13).
- *Left rotation.* In a sitting position take your chin and turn it to the left (Fig 18–14).
- *Side bend right.* In a sitting position take your right ear and try to touch your right shoulder (Fig 18–15).
- *Side bend left.* In a sitting position take your left

ear and try to touch your left shoulder (Fig 18–16).
- *Flexion.* Try to touch your chin on your chest (Fig 18–17).
- *Extension.* Extend your head back so your nose goes towards the ceiling (Fig 18–18).

Isometric strengthening exercises can be started once range of motion returns and the neck is pain free. Hold each exercise for 10 seconds and repeat ten times. The head should be held in a neutral position for all these exercises[23]:

- *Right rotation.* Place your right hand on the right side of your head and resist right rotation (Fig 18–19).
- *Left rotation.* Place your left hand on the left side of your head and resist left rotation (Fig 18–20).
- *Side bend right.* Place your right hand on the right side of your head and resist side bend right (Fig 18–21).

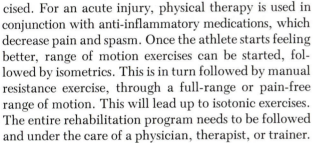

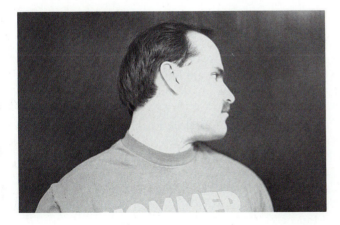

Figure 18–14. Left rotation.

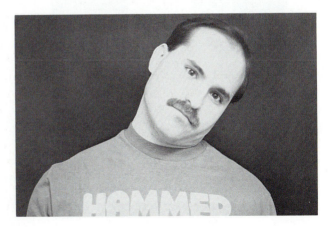

Figure 18–16. Side bend left.

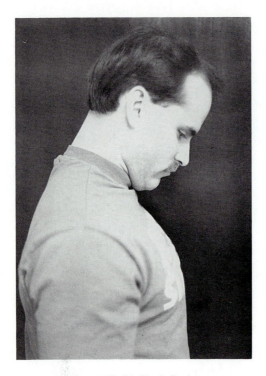

Figure 18-17. Neck flexion.

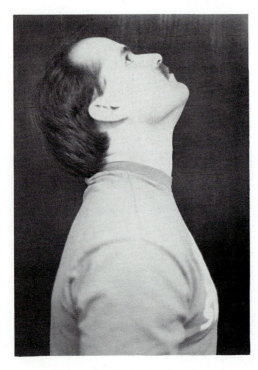

Figure 18-18. Neck extension.

- *Side bend left.* Place your left hand on the left side of your head and resist side bend left (Fig 18–22).
- *Flexion.* Place both hands on your forehead and resist putting your chin on your chest (Fig 18–23).
- *Extension.* Place both hands on the back of your head and resist extending your head back (Fig 18–24).

Manual resistance exercises can be started next as you can vary the amount of resistance to the neck. This should be done pain free and repeated ten times. This is also a superior form of conditioning the neck muscles for the noninjured athlete. This is far superior to isometrics and can be done without the expense of machines. The neck should never be exercised before practice or a game. It should be stretched before and exercised after. With manual resistive exercises, the helper must learn to vary the resistance. In the case of rehabilitation the helper should be a trainer or physical therapist.

Neck Flexion. The performer sits with the back and arms resting against the spotter's legs (Fig 18–25). He or she totally relaxes the neck and looks skyward at the beginning of each repetition. He or she then brings the chin to the chest (taking 5-7 seconds from start to finish) and pauses momentarily in that position (Fig 18–26).

The spotter then removes his or her hands so that the lifter can recover to the starting position immediately. The spotter does not apply any resistance while the lifter is recovering to the starting position.

The lifter must then relax the neck so that the spotter can gently apply some resistance to stretch the muscles at the beginning of each rep.

From this position, the lifter begins to bring the head forward, completing the entire exercise in 5 seconds and to totally relax all of his muscles (including his face) while performing the exercise!

Spotting. The spotter interlocks his or her fingers and places his or her hands around the lifter's forehead (Fig 18–25, Fig 18–26). As the lifter slowly brings the head forward, the spotter applies as much resistance as is needed to stimulate an all-out effort.

Neck Extension. The athlete assumes an all-fours position with the chin on the chest (Fig 18–27). He or she then extends the head upwards and backward until the neck muscles are fully extended with the head looking skyward (Fig 18–28). He or she must hold this extended position momentarily before the spotter releases the resistance.

The removal of the spotter's hands will enable the

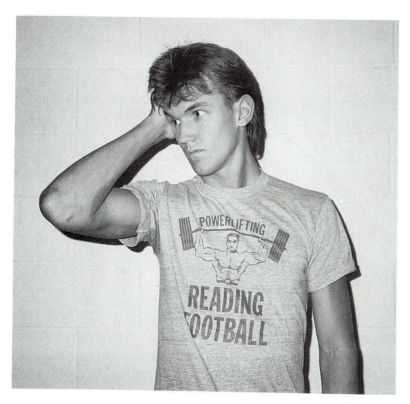

Figure 18-19. Right rotation–Isometric.

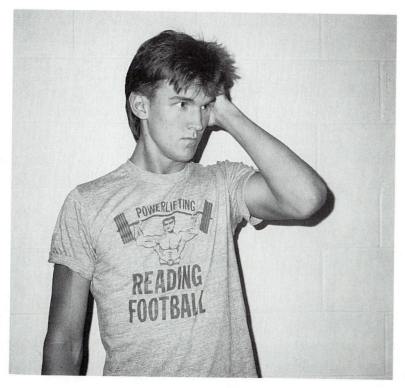

Figure 18-20. Left rotation–Isometric.

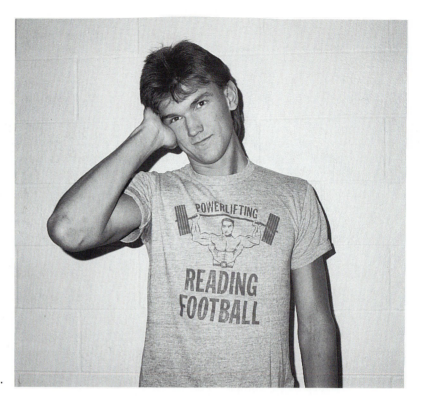

Figure 18-21. Side bend right–Isometric.

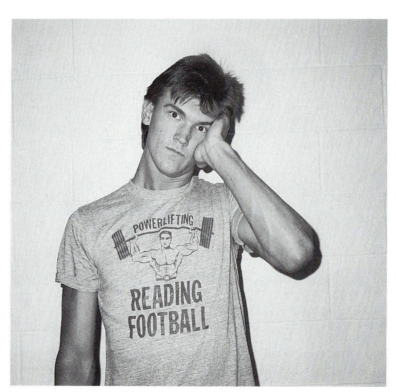

Figure 18-22. Side bend left–Isometric.

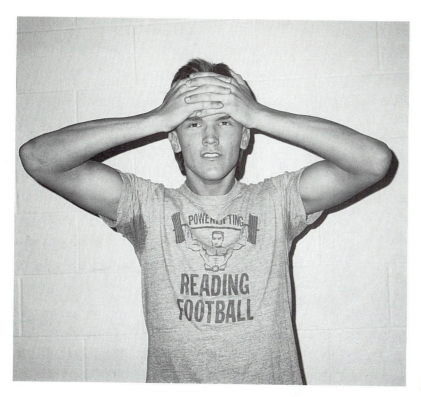

Figure 18-23. Flexion–Isometric.

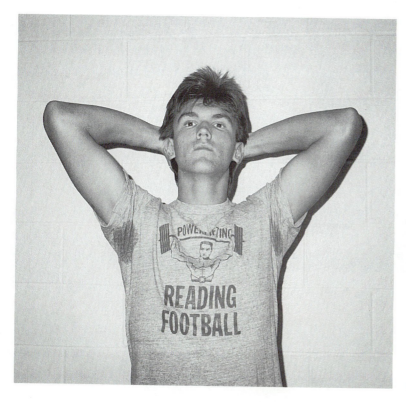

Figure 18-24. Extension–Isometric.

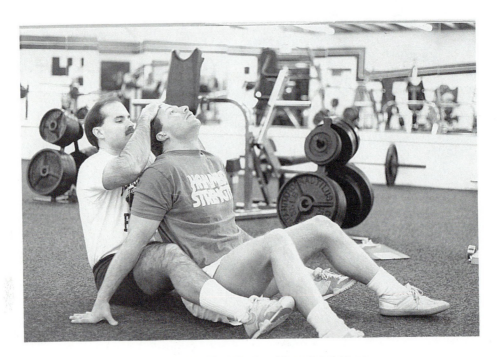

Figure 18–25. Neck flexion–Manual resistance.

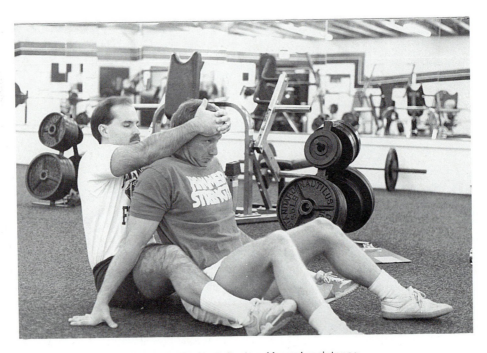

Figure 18–26. Neck flexion–Manual resistance.

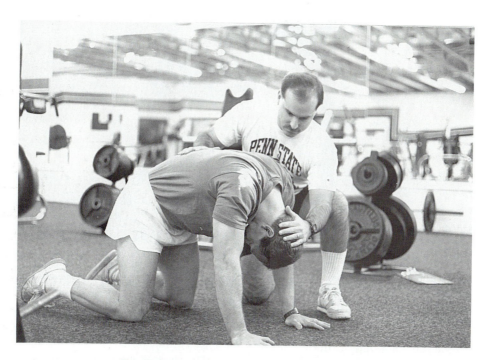

Figure 18–27. Neck extension—Manual resistance.

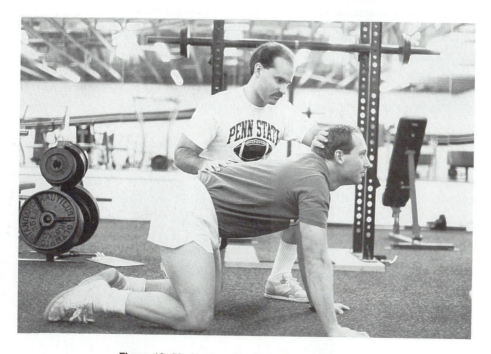

Figure 18–28. Neck extension—Manual resistance.

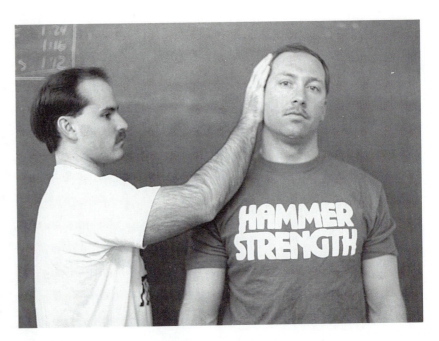

Figure 18–29. Side bend right–Manual resistance.

lifter to immediately recover to the starting position. As before, the exercise must be performed in 5 seconds from start to finish.

The spotter must not apply any resistance while the lifter recovers to the starting position. In the starting position, the lifter must relax completely so that the spotter can gently apply some resistance to provide a prestretch at the beginning of each repetition.

Spotting. The spotter kneels beside the lifter and places one hand near the top of the lifter's head. As the lifter slowly extends the neck, the spotter applies only as much resistance as is needed to stimulate an all-out effort. The amount of resistance and the angle at which the resistance is applied will vary with the range of movement.

The spotter continues to apply resistance in the extended position before removing the hand from the lifter's head.

The spotter does not apply resistance during the recovery. He or she just makes sure that the lifter extends only the neck and does not allow the lifter to lean back with the torso.[42]

Side Bending Right. In a standing position, a spotter stands behind the person's head. The spotter's hand is placed on the right side of the head (Figs 18–29, 18–30) and applies resistance as the right ear tries to touch the

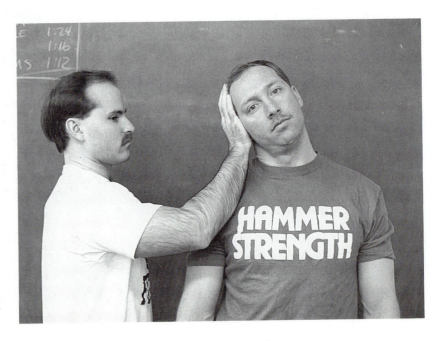

Figure 18–30. Side bend right–Manual resistance.

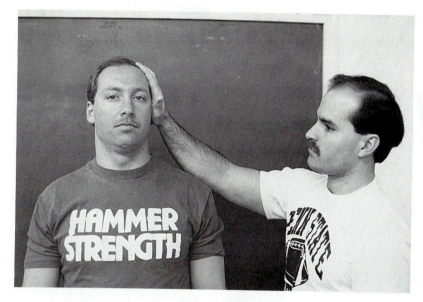

Figure 18-31. Side bend left–Manual resistance.

right shoulder. The rules as above apply to the spotter and athlete.

Side Bending Left. In a standing position, a spotter stands behind the person's head. The spotter's hand is placed on the left side of the head (Fig 18–31, 18–32) and applies resistance as the left ear tries to touch the left shoulder. The rules as above apply to the spotter and athlete.

Special Equipment. If Nautilus machines are available, these can be used to strengthen the neck musculature. The manual resistance exercises can be augmented with a piece of Nautilus equipment or if all three neck machines are available, manual resistance

can be omitted. Three machines will be discussed that will strengthen the neck muscles.

Nautilus Four Way Neck

  Anterior Flexion (Fig 18–33)

  1. Face machine.
  2. Adjust seat so nose is in center of pads.
  3. Stabilize torso by lightly grasping handles.
  4. Move head smoothly toward chest.
  5. Pause.
  6. Return slowly to stretched position and repeat.

Posterior extension (Fig 18–34)

  1. Turn body in machine until back of head contacts center of pads.

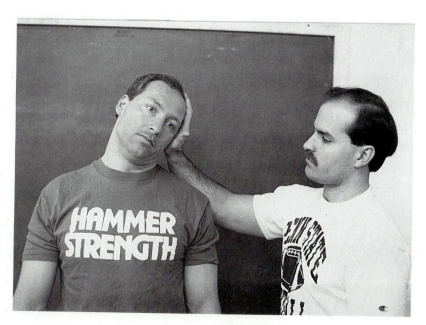

Figure 18-32. Side bend left–Manual resistance.

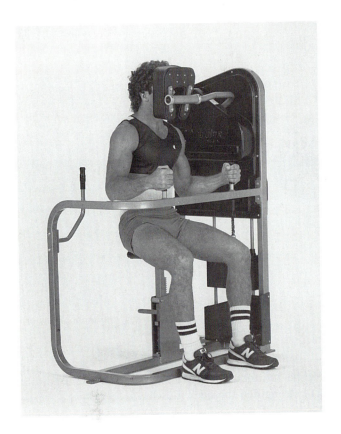

Figure 18-33. Flexion Nautilus.

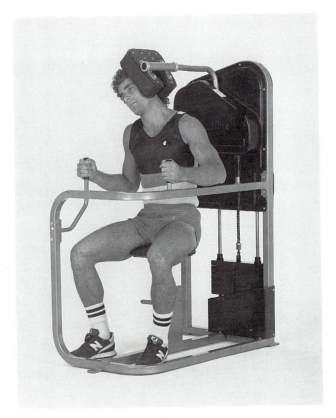

Figure 18-35. Side bend right Nautilus.

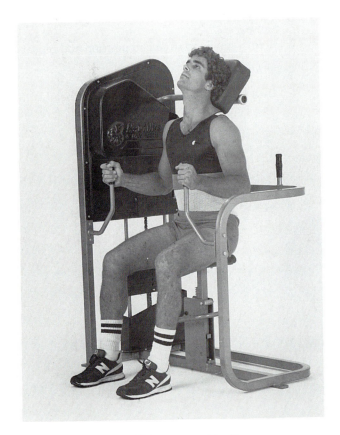

Figure 18-34. Extension Nautilus.

2. Stabilize torso by lightly grasping handles.
3. Extend head as far back as possible.
4. Pause.
5. Return slowly to stretched position and repeat.

Side bend right and left (Fig 18–35)

1. Turn body in machine until left ear is in center of pads.
2. Stabilize torso by lightly grasping handles.
3. Move head toward left shoulder.
4. Pause.
5. Keep shoulders square.
6. Return slowly to stretched position and repeat.
7. Reverse procedure for right side.

Shoulder shrug (Figs 18–36, 18–37) This can also be done with a barbell.

1. Place forearms between pads while seated.
2. Keep palms open and back of hands pressed against bottom pads.
3. Straighten torso until weight stack is lifted. The seat may be raised with elevation pads.
4. Shrug shoulder smoothly as high as possible. Keep elbows by sides. Do not lean back.

In a nerve stretch or if an athlete receives a peripheral nerve injury then an exercise program is needed to strengthen the upper extremity. The following exercises

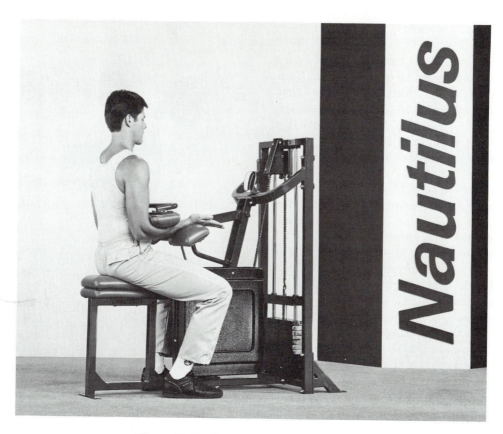

Figure 18-36. Shoulder shrug Nautilus.

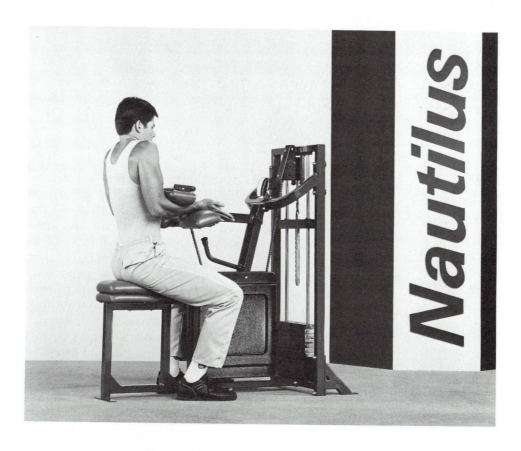

Figure 18-37. Shoulder shrug Nautilus.

can be done with barbells to rehabilitate this injury. Other weight equipment can be used (Universal Gym, Nautilus, Isokinetic) if the athlete has access to them.

Shoulder flexion (Fig 18–38, Fig 18–39). Standing or sitting: Keep elbow straight, palm turned down then lift the arm straight out in front and up by ear. Lower back down. Do not hike the shoulder or throw the arm up.

Shoulder abduction (Figs 18–40, 18–41). Standing or sitting; bring the arm straight out to the side and up by ear, leading with your thumb so that the arm rotates somewhat as you raise and lower the arm.

Shoulder extension (Figs 18–42, 18–43). Lying on your stomach, arm straight at your side with the palm turned down, lift the arm straight up.

Shoulder horizontal abduction (Figs 18–44, 18–45). Lying on your stomach, arm straight out to the side and hand turned so that thumb points upward, lift the arm straight up without allowing the body to turn up too.

Shoulder external rotation (Figs 18–46, 18–47). Lying on your stomach, arm 90 degrees away from your

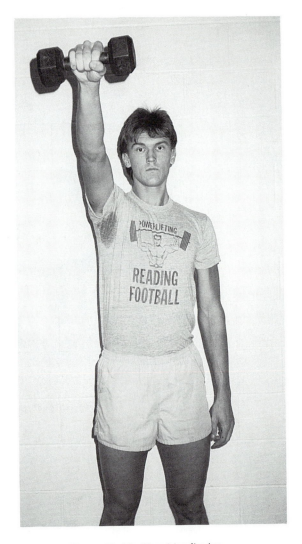

Figure 18-39. Shoulder flexion.

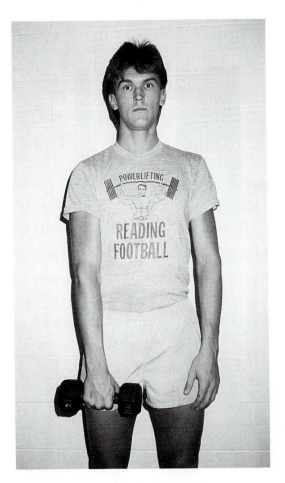

Figure 18-38. Shoulder flexion.

side and lower part of arm hanging over the edge of the table, then rotate hand up and return back down.

Bicep curl. (Fig 18–48, 18–49) Standing or sitting, work on bending the elbow up, bringing the hand towards the shoulder then lower back down.

Tricep curl. (Fig 18–50, 18–51) Standing with the arm bent so that the elbow points up towards the ceiling (can support the arm with your other hand), then straighten the hand towards the ceiling and lower back down.

Sitting dip. (Fig 18–52, 18–53) Sit on edge of chair with hands by your side and lift buttocks off surface.

Pushup. (Fig 18–54, 18–55, 18–56) Start with pushup into wall. Gradually progress to table top and eventually to floor. Do as tolerated.

Wrist flexion. With the arm on a flat surface with your palm up, bend the elbow to 90 degrees. With a dumbbell in your hand, slowly flex the wrist up.

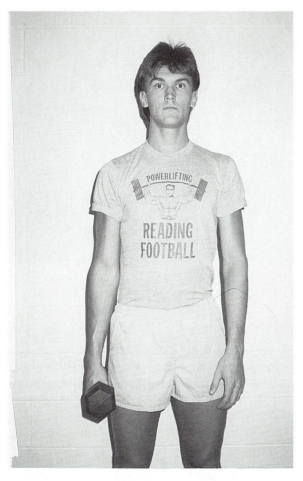

Figure 18-40. Abduction.

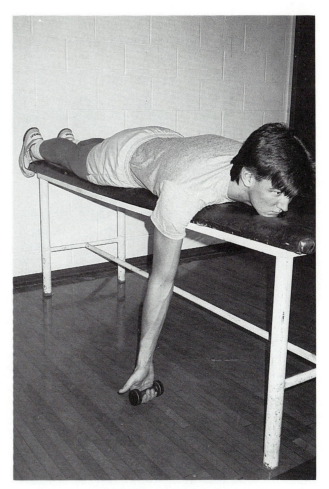

Figure 18-42. Extension.

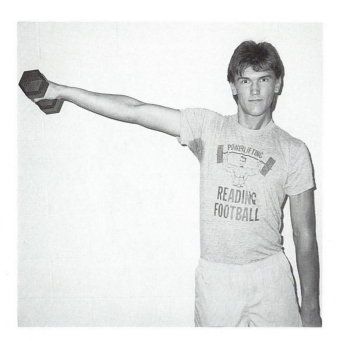

Figure 18-41. Abduction.

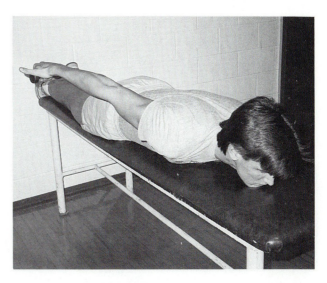

Figure 18-43. Extension.

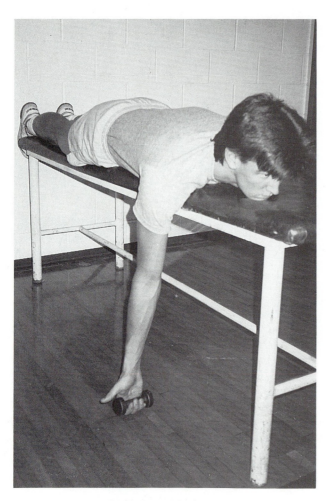

Figure 18-44. Abduction.

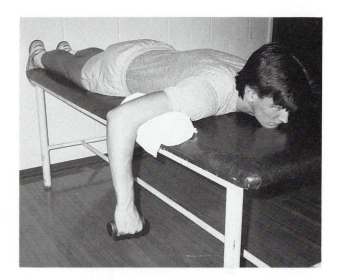

Figure 18-46. External rotation.

Wrist extension. With the arm on a flat surface with your palm down, bend the elbow to 90°. With a dumbbell in your hand, slowly extend the wrist up.

Thoracic Spine

Athletic injuries can occur to the thoracic spine. The most common injuries are sprains, strains, and contusions. Thoracic spine and dorsolumbar fractures occur infrequently in sports. If a fracture happens from T1 to T10 it is usually stable and no surgery is needed.

The most common serious injury is a compression fracture to the body of one of the thoracic vertebrae.[43] Forward flexion is usually the mechanism that com-

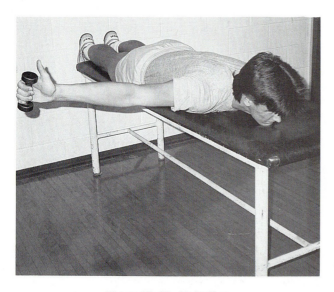

Figure 18-45. Abduction.

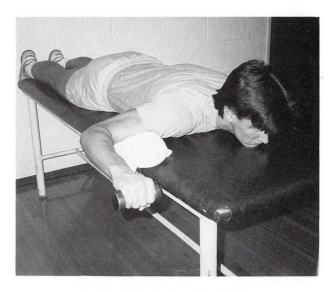

Figure 18-47. External rotation.

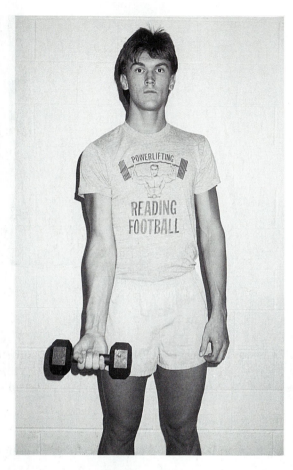

Figure 18-48. Bicep curl.

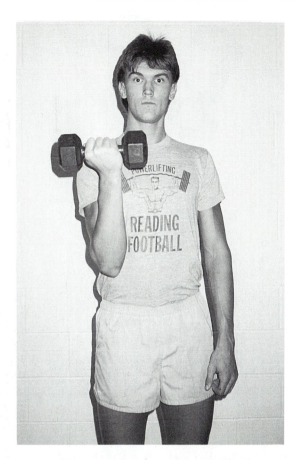

Figure 18-49. Bicep curl.

presses the anterior portion of the adjacent vertebral bodies with this injury. There are usually no neurological problems and at times the athlete will walk without any difficulty. There will be constant localized pain, which may increase with movement. Bracing may be required with these injuries.

The numerous thoracic facet and costovertebral articulations are subject to frequent trauma.[41] The chest can be compressed when athletes fall on a ball or an opponent falls on them. There will be localized tenderness and this injury can be very sore for quite some time.

Juvenile epiphysitis (spinal osteochondrosis or Scheuermann's disease) is a condition that can affect teenagers.[41] The etiology of this condition is unknown, and where the growth plate becomes unequal as a result of juvenile epiphysitis, wedging occurs in a number of the dorsal vertebrae. If left untreated, this may lead to kyphosis.

Back contusions rank second to strains and sprains in incidence.[44] The large surface area of the back makes it vulnerable to trauma in contact sports, especially football. The history will be simple as the athlete will describe being hit. Vertebral fracture must be ruled out and then the injury can be treated with physical therapy modalities.

The spine is particularly susceptible to muscular strain because of the multiplicity of muscles involved in holding the body erect.[45] It may be hard to distinguish a strain from a contusion at first. The mechanism of injury will help as it is usually caused by a violent contraction beyond the strength of the muscle.

Lumbar Spine

Due to the increased number of athletes 18 and younger participating in year-round sports and conditioning programs, the number of complaints of low back pain has increased. The majority of these cases resolve in 2 to 3 weeks.

The differential diagnosis of back pain in the athletically active child or adolescent can be complex.[46] In addition to the mechanical, metabolic, neoplastic, and infectious etiologies to be entertained in any adolescent, the potential for overuse injuries from repetitive microtrauma, including tendinitis, fasciitis, and stress fracture, must also be considered.

In a study of young athletes who had low back

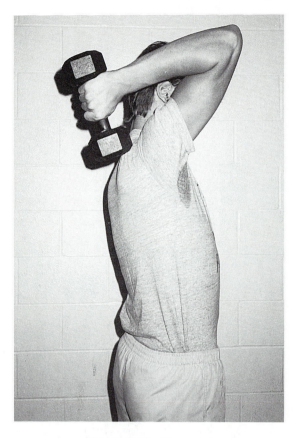

Figure 18-50. Tricep curl.

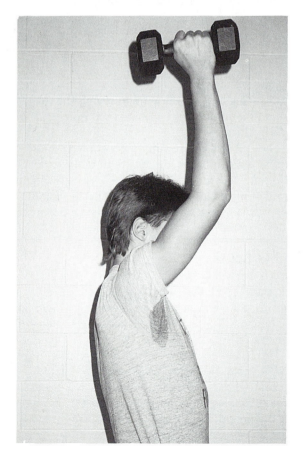

Figure 18-51. Tricep curl.

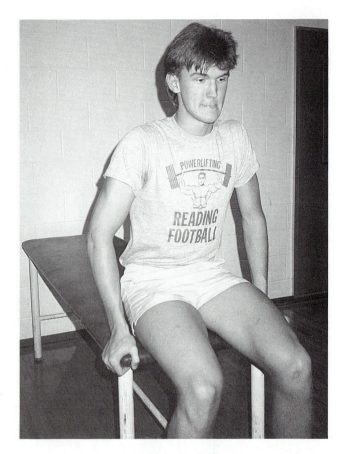

Figure 18-52. Sitting dip.

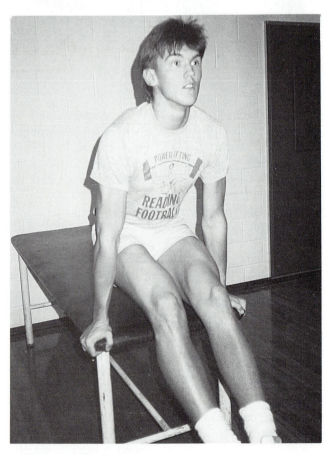

Figure 18-53. Sitting dip.

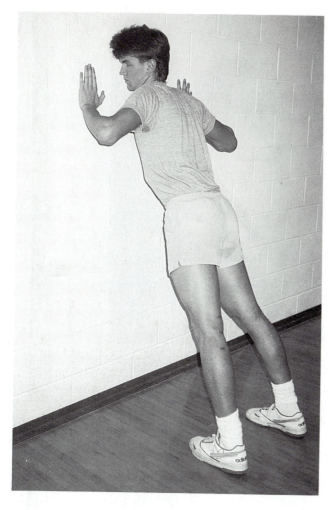

Figure 18-54. Push up.

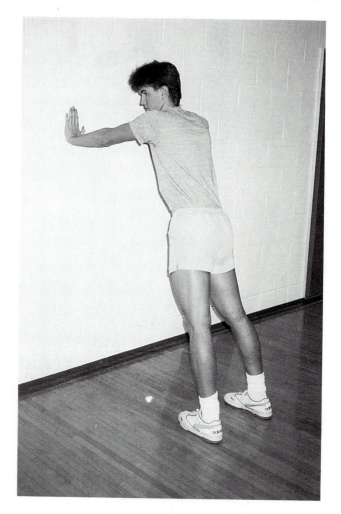

Figure 18-55. Push up.

pain for longer than 3 months, 40% had a symptomatic process related to their pars interarticularis in the lumbar spine, 10% had spondylolisthesis and segmental instability, and 10% had a symptomatic disc, with the remaining 40% having end plate fractures, growth plate injuries, altered disc spaces, and neoplasms.[46]

Low back pain is common in both athletes and nonathletes. There are a variety of opinions as far as causes of low back pain, but there is no general agreement. One theory is that the pain is due to disc degeneration involving the hyaline cartilage and annulus fibrosus.[47] Another theory is joint dysfunction of the facet and sacroiliac joints.[48] If normal motion of these joints do not take place, then there will be pain.

A frequent etiology of back pain in athletes is mechanical, resulting from acute or chronic musculotendinous or ligamentous injury.[46] This is usually associated with a functional hyperlordosis of the lumbar spine.

Young athletes can damage the vertebral growth plate in the spine. This injury can occur from the midthoracic to midlumbar region but most frequently is seen at the thoracic–lumbar junction. This can be easily confused with Scheuermann's disease. Athletes who are involved in repetitive flexion and extension activities, as in gymnastics, rowing, and diving, and who have tight lumbar lordosis can receive multiple growth plate fractures.

Spondylolysis is a stress fracture through the pars interarticularis of a lumbar vertebrae. This structure can be injured due to trauma or minor repeated trauma. The athlete will complain of back pain and tenderness for weeks. This can be seen in gymnasts and high divers. In spondylolisthesis there is actually a forward slippage of the vertebrae. Younger athletes with a slip of grade II or more should not participate in contact sports.

Many of the athletes with low back pain have tight musculotendinous and ligamentous structures about the low back, hips, and knees.[46] They also have weak abdominals and tight hip flexors. A number of steps may be taken to prevent back pain:

1. Appropriate training techniques with slow progression of technique

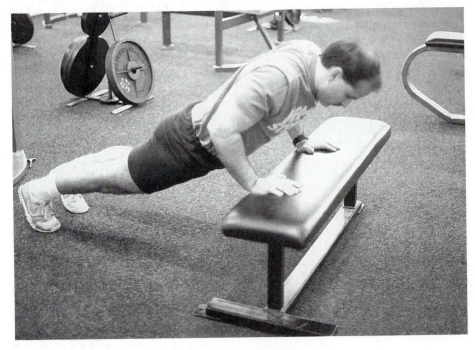

Figure 18-56. Push up.

2. Use of proper equipment as in gymnastics, with proper thickness and placement of mats and proper training techniques
3. Emphasis on stretching of the hamstrings and lumbodorsal fascia
4. Strengthening of the abdominal and pelvic muscles
5. Proper sitting, standing, and lifting posture

Spine injuries can be prevented with the use of well-fitted, safe equipment; good conditioned athletes; coaches with awareness of correct playing techniques and rules of competition; and good medical care. The sports physical therapist, as an integral part of the medical care team, can help return the injured athlete to top performance levels.

REFERENCES

1. Bruno LA, Gernarelli TA, Torg JS. Management guidelines for head injuries in athletics. *Clin Sports Med.* 1987; 1:17–30.
2. Vegso JJ, Lehman RC. Evaluation and management of head and neck injuries. *Clin Sports Med.* 1987; 1–16.
3. Zariczny B, Shattuck CJ, Mast BA, et al. Sports related injuries in school-aged children. *Am J Sports Med.* 1980; 18:318–324.
4. Smodlaka VN. Death on the soccer field and its prevention. *Physician Sports med.* 1981; 19(8):101–107.
5. Kruse DL, McBeath AA. Bicycle accidents and injuries. *Am J Sports Med.* 1980; 18:342–344.
6. Guichon D, Myles ST. Bicycle injuries: One year sample in Calgary. *J Trauma* 1975; 15:504–506.
7. Arya A. *Introductory College Physics.* New York, NY: Macmillan Co; 1979.
8. Mueller FO, Blyth CS. Fatalities from head and cervical spine injuries occurring in tackle football: 40 years experience. *Clin Sports Med.* 1987; 6:185–196.
9. Jackson FF. *Ciba Symposia, The Pathophysiology of Head Injuries.* Summit, NJ: Ciba-Geigy; 1966:196.
10. Rimel RW, Nelson WE, Persing JA, June JA. Epidural hematoma in lacrosse. *Phys Sportsmed.* 1983; 11(3): 140–144.
11. Teadsale G, Jennett B. Assessment of coma and impaired consciousness: A practical scale. *Lancet* 1974; 2:81–84.
12. Feriencik K. Depressed skull fracture in an ice hockey player wearing a helmet. *Physician Sportsmed.* 1979; 7:107.
13. Bishop PJ, Norman RW, Pierrynowski M, Kozey J. The ice hockey helmet: How effective is it? *Physician Sportsmed.* 1979; 7:96–106.
14. Frackelton WH. Facial injuries in sports. *Am J Surg.* 1959; 98:390–393.
15. Heintz WD. Mouth protection in sports. *Phys Am Sports Med.* 1979; 7:45–47.
16. Heintz WD. Mouth protectors: A progress report. *JAMA* 1968; 77:632–636.
17. Seelenfreund MH, Freilich DB. Rushing the net and retinal detachment. *JAMA.* 1976; 235:2723–2726.
18. DeVoe AG. Injuries to the eye. *Am J Surg.* 1959; 98:384–389.
19. Easterbook M. Eye injuries in racquet sports: A continuing problem. *Physician Sportsmed.* 1981; 9:91–101.

20. Easterbrook M. Eye protection for squash and racquet-ball players. *Physician Sportsmed*. 1981; 9:79–82.

21. Vinger PF. Sports related eye injury. A preventative problem. *J Ophthalmol*. 1982; 25:47–51.

22. Grant HD, Nurry RH, Bergeron JD. *Emergency Care*. 4th ed. Englewood Cliffs, NJ: Prentice Hall; 1986.

23. Arnheim D. *Modern Principles of Athletic Training*. St. Louis, Mo: Times Mirror/Mosby College Publishing; 1985.

24. Bohlman HH. Acute fractures and dislocations of the cervical spine. *J Bone Joint Surg*. 1979; 61A:1119–1142.

25. Schneider RC. Serious and fatal neurosurgical football injuries. *Clin Neurosurg*. 1966; 12:226–236.

26. Blyth CS, Arnold BC. Forty-fifth annual survey of football fatalities, 1973–1976. Proceedings of the American Football Coaches Association; 1977.

27. Torg JS, Quedenfeld TC, Burstein A, et al. National football head and neck injury registry: Report on cervical quadriplegia, 1971 to 1975. *Am J Sports Med*. 1979; 7:127–132.

28. Albright JP, Moses JM, Feldick HG, et al: Nonfatal cervical spine injuries in interscholastic football. *JAMA* 1976; 236:1243–1245.

29. Funk FJ, Wells RE. Injuries of the cervical spine in football. *Clin Orthop Relat Res*. 1975; 109:50–58.

30. Clancy WG, Brand RL, Bergfield JA. Upper trunk brachial plexus injuries in contact sports. *Am J Sports Med*. 1977; 5:209–216.

31. Bateman SE. Nerve injuries about the shoulder in sports. *J Bone Joint Surg*. 1967; 49A:785–792.

32. Torg JS. Management guidelines for athletic injuries of the cervical spine. *Clin Sports Med*. 1987; 1:53–61.

33. Torg JS. Symposium: Athletic injuries to the cervical spine and brachial plexus. *Contemp Orthop*. 1984; 9:65–94.

34. Chrisman OD, Snook GA, Stanitis JS, et al. Lateral flexion neck injuries in athletic competition. *JAMA* 1965; 192: 117–119.

35. Hoyt WA Jr. Etiology of shoulder injuries in athletics. *J Bone Joint Surg*. 1967; 49A:755.

36. O'Donoghue DH. *Treatment of Injuries to Athletes*. Philadelphia, Pa: W B Saunders; 1970.

37. Poindexter DP, Johnson EW. Football shoulder and neck injury: A study of the stinger. *Arch Phys Med Rehabil*. 1984; 65:601–602.

38. Watkins RG. Injuries to the spine. *Clin Sports Med*. 1986; 5:215–246.

39. Vegso JJ. Head and neck injuries. *Clin Sports Med*. 1987; 6:135–158.

40. American Academy of Orthopaedic Surgeons. *Emergency Care and Transportation of the Sick and Injured*. Park Ridge, Ill: AAOS; 1987.

41. Roy S, Irvin R. *Sports Medicine Prevention, Evaluation, Management and Rehabilitation*. Englewood Cliffs, NJ: Prentice Hall; 1983.

42. Riley DP. *Strength Training for Football: The Penn State Way*. West Point, NY: Leisure Press; 1978.

43. Booker JM, Thibodeau GA. Athletic Injury Assessment. St. Louis, Mo: Times Mirror/Mosby College Publishing; 1985.

44. Clafs CE, Arnheim DD. *Modern Principles of Athletic Training*. St. Louis, Mo: C V Mosby; 1981.

45. O'Donoghue DH. Treatment of Injuries to Athletes. Philadelphia, Pa: W B Saunders; 1984.

46. Clancy WG. Low back pain in athletes. *Am J Sports Med*. 1979; 7:361–366.

47. Levine D. *The Painful Low Back*. Philadelphia, Pa: Lea & Febiger; 1979.

48. Cyriax Jr. *Textbook of Orthopaedic Medicine: Diagnosis of Soft Tissue Lesions*. New York, NY: Macmillan; 1978.

19

Shoulder Injuries

Diane Slaughter

INTRODUCTION

The shoulder is the site of many painful conditions. The sports physical therapist plays a unique role in the delivery of health care to athletes. The therapist is specifically responsible for rehabilitation of the shoulder after injury or surgery and for the design of a program to return the athlete to his or her chosen sport. This chapter discusses rehabilitation of specific nonsurgical injuries, with an overview of rehabilitation protocols and regimens used clinically as well as those presented in the scientific literature. For each injury, the common problems related to that injury, the goals of rehabilitation, and the measure for accomplishing those goals are discussed.

It is apparent that successful rehabilitation requires an individualized approach. Although the problems for each injury may be fairly common, a rehabilitation program will not be successful without accounting for differences among individuals. Certain factors such as age, musculoskeletal design, prior level of function, prior injury status, and constitutional predisposition of the individual to injury are fixed, cannot be controlled, and must be taken into consideration.

Variable factors that assist in designing a rehabilitation program include the athlete's level of conditioning, the intensity of the activity, and the frequency and duration of the activity. The technique and equipment used are also important variables to evaluate and may require modification.

EVALUATION

Rehabilitation cannot begin without a complete evaluation. A number of texts provide a comprehensive review of the evaluation and special tests used in the shoulder for differential diagnosis.[1-4]

A rehabilitation program cannot be implemented until the pathology is identified. It is important to look at the magnitude of the pathology and the nature of the pain. Whether the pain is constant or intermittent in nature and how it changes throughout the course of a day are extremely helpful in assessing how aggressive rehabilitation may begin in the early stages. If there is some soreness after activity, strengthening exercises and sport-specific training may be instituted, but on the other end of the spectrum, rehabilitation will have to be tailored to the individual (Table 19-1).

The acute or chronic nature of the pathology is also considered when planning a rehabilitation program. The terms acute and chronic refer to the nature of the inflammatory condition, rather than to the length of time the condition has existed.[5]

Only after a complete evaluation of both the subjective and objective findings can problems related to physical therapy be identified. Once problems are identified, priorities should be established. This enables the therapist to concentrate on key areas with progression to long-term goals. For example, an athlete with acute rotator cuff tendinitis will have pain and loss of strength. The initial priority may be to decrease pain, with the secondary goal of strengthening the shoulder within the range as pain decreases.

Many of the conditions that are discussed have common problems. The next section discusses these general problems and some of the treatment protocols used clinically for each.

PHASES OF REHABILITATION

For the purpose of simplification and to prevent duplication, rehabilitation is divided into four phases. Phase I involves the modalities and techniques used to reduce pain and inflammation. The focus in phase II is on techniques used to improve range of motion and flexibility. Phase III presents strengthening exercises in a protected sequence, and phase IV focuses on functional activities.

TABLE 19-1. PAIN PROFILE[a]

Temporary soreness after activity
Soreness resolved with activity
Pain during activity unchanged
Activity pain which changes activity
Pain at rest
Pain disrupts sleep

[a]Identifying and analyzing pain patterns can be an important step in determining how aggressive a rehabilitation program may begin.

Phase I: Pain

Pain is a characteristic problem of many shoulder conditions. Common modalities to alleviate pain include ice, heat, diathermy, ultrasound, transcutaneous electrical nerve stimulation (TENS), and electrical stimulation (Figs 19–1, 19–2). Early range of motion is also encouraged in the reduction of pain.

Inflammation. The acronym PRICE is often used to delineate the treatment to reduce inflammation. *P*rotection from further injury, *r*est, *i*ce, *c*ompression, and *e*levation are the components of this treatment. It should be noted that rest for the majority of nonsurgical shoulder injuries is meant to be relative and not absolute. Rest taken to the extreme is often harmful to the healing process by decreasing collateral circulation and promoting atrophy. Rest can have an important role but at the same time must be integrated into the rehabilitative process. Phonophoresis may be a useful treatment for athletes with inflammatory conditions about the shoulder.[6] The most common medication used is a 10% hydrocortisone solution.[7]

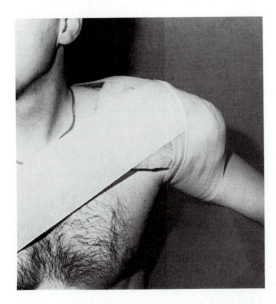

Figure 19-1. The application of ice to shoulder is used to alleviate pain.

Phase II: Range of Motion/Flexibility

Techniques about the shoulder include the use of deep heat in the form of ultrasound to increase connective tissue extensibility followed by passive stretching. Passive, active assistive, and active range of motion programs are used to regain motion throughout different phases of the rehabilitation. A technique the author has found to be particularly useful is low-intensity stretching at elevated tissue temperatures and cooling the tissue before releasing the tension. This technique makes use of the viscous or plastic properties of connective tissue.[8] Joint mobilization is also commonly used to regain both physiologic and accessory joint movements (Fig 19–3).

Phase III: Strengthening

Muscle weakness is a common problem in many of the shoulder conditions to be discussed. Therapists prescribing exercise should keep in mind the many different modes of strengthening. Isometric exercise is useful in the early phases of strengthening when joint motion is not desired. Isometric exercise can be performed at a variety of angles to begin strengthening in the nonpainful ranges. Isotonic exercise can be performed with free weight or with variable resistance machines like Nautilus and Universal. Isokinetic exercise allows accommodating resistance through the ROM against a fixed speed (e.g., Biodex, Biodex Corp, Shirley, NY 11967; and Cybex, Cybex, Division of Lumex Inc, Ronkonkoma, NY 11779). Isokinetic devices allow the practitioner the flexibility of training specific motions at specific speeds that may be tailored to the individual's sport.

Eccentric exercise or lengthening contractions are important to total shoulder rehabilitation. It is not uncommon to find weakness in the muscles responsible for eccentric deceleration of the shoulder. The deceleration forces imposed by many sports activities may put the musculotendinous unit under duress, which can lead to overuse and tendinitis.

The concept of stabilization in order to have mobility is particularly important with regard to the shoulder, where the majority of the stabilization is supplied by the shoulder musculature. The shoulder functions in an open kinetic chain and the trunk, scapulothoracic, scapulohumeral, and distal arm musculature should be addressed in the rehabilitation. Proximal stabilization exercises may be performed in the initial stages of strengthening when pain may be a factor. Manual resistance provided by Proprioceptive Neuromuscular Facilitation (PNF) is an invaluable technique for developing timing and coordination of muscular activity.

A comprehensive strengthening protocol using all modes of exercise will enable the therapist to tailor

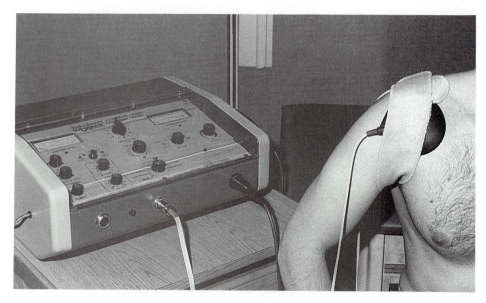

Figure 19-2. Electrical stimulation applied in the treatment of rotator cuff tendinitis.

strengthening and rehabilitation activities to the athlete's individual needs.

Phase IV: Functional Activities

Rehabilitation programs should be designed to be as relevant as possible to the nature of the athlete's chosen

sport. An exercise prescription must be based on a thorough understanding of the mechanics of the activity and the injury status of the athlete.[9] A needs analysis evaluating the athlete and the sport should be incorporated in the design of a rehabilitation program. As described by Falkel and Murphy, the needs analysis ad-

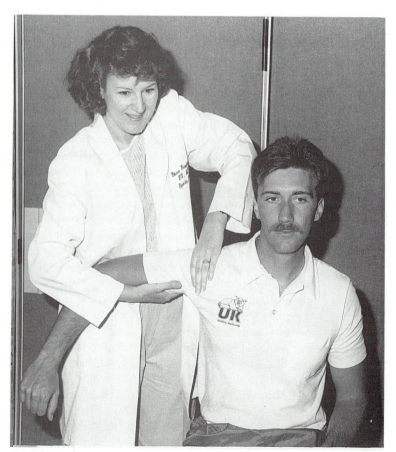

Figure 19-3. Joint mobilization is recommended for increasing range of motion. The caudal glide of the humerus is essential before progressing to overhead activities.

dresses the muscles and movements involved in the sport, the basic energy systems used in the sport, the training required in the sport, and the activities that can be performed to prevent injury. A biomechanical evaluation of the athlete's performance of a specific sport skill may illuminate problems with technique that can be addressed in the rehabilitation program.

ESTABLISHING GOALS

Following identification of the problems related to physical therapy, goals are established. Goals need to be identified that are both behavioral and measurable. A behavioral goal is based on observed performance and completion of tasks. For example, when the athlete demonstrates the ability to achieve full external rotation, he or she may begin throwing from short distances. Establishing goals based on performance aids in the progression of the rehabilitation and diminishes the need for timetables, which are often unrealistic and do not take individual differences into account. Assuring that a goal is measurable provides the therapist with objective data that can be documented, and aids in the modification of treatment protocols (Table 19–2).

COMMON INJURIES

Rotator Cuff Impingement/Tendinitis

Impingement syndrome results from painful impingement of the rotator cuff and adjacent biceps tendon against the fibrous structures that form the roof of the suprahumeral space. Jobe and Jobe describe shoulder impingement syndrome as being the most common shoulder problem in sports medicine.[10] Athletes most frequently affected are those who are engaged in repetitive throwing activities such as baseball, football, or other activities such as swimming and tennis where repetitive overhead reaching is performed.

The function of the rotator cuff is to stabilize the glenohumeral joint and at the same time to aid in the

TABLE 19-2. GOALS FOR THE REHABILITATION OF COMMON SHOULDER INJURIES

The athlete will:
- State that he or she is free of pain
- Have an absence of swelling
- Demonstrate a full range of motion actively and passively
- Demonstrate strength through a full range of motion
- Demonstrate coordination of neuromuscular timing by completing specific agility drills
- Demonstrate correct technique for his sport
- Wear and/or use properly fitted equipment
- Be instructed in the protection/prevention of reinjury

abduction and rotation of the joint.[11] The shoulder impingement syndrome manifests itself in the joint of the suprahumeral space. This space is located between the head of the humerus and an arch formed by the coracoacromial ligament. Impingement syndrome usually involves the supraspinatus tendon of the rotator cuff, but the adjacent biceps tendon may also become impinged in forward flexion because of its close proximity to the coracoacromial ligament.[12,13] Impingement may occur against the anterior edge and undersurface of the anterior third of the acromion, the coracoacromial ligament and at times the acromioclavicular joint.[14]

With overuse as the etiologic factor, it is recognized that impingement is a progressive process. Neer[14] classifies impingement syndrome into three stages. With the help of the examination procedures the diagnosis of injuries and their magnitude has become more accurate. This better understanding of the pathology of the injury gives us improved rehabilitation programs that incorporate individualized exercise protocols. Stage I involves a simple tendinitis of acute onset characterized by edema and hemorrhage. This stage is generally observed in the athletic patient of 25 years or younger, although it is not limited to this group. Stage II is characterized by fibrosis and tendinitis. Its onset is usually in athletes between 25 and 40 years old but may occur at any age. Stage III lesions may present with bone spurs and tendon rupture. The patient often has had a prolonged history of shoulder problems, with involvement progressing to the adjacent tissues of the biceps and other cuff muscles. A fourth stage has also been described that demonstrates the progressive nature of the syndrome that is characterized by a complete thickness rotator cuff tear.[10,15]

In order to differentiate between stages it is necessary to perform a complete evaluation of the shoulder, correlating both subjective and objective data.[4] As mentioned previously the supraspinatus is primarily involved in the impingement syndrome. The function of the supraspinatus is to resist upward humeral migration, to counteract and counterbalance the deltoid, to assist abduction, to act as an external rotator, and to function as an eccentric decelerator. This can be a big task for a relatively small muscle. In addition, the supraspinatus becomes impinged at a site where it is especially vulnerable. The blood supply to the rotator cuff is primarily supplied by the suprascapular artery, anterior circumflex, humeral artery, and posterior circumflex humeral artery. To a lesser degree there are also contributions from the thoracoacromial artery, suprahumeral artery, and subscapular artery.[16] Rothman and Marvel demonstrated an area of hypovascularity in the supraspinatus tendon in 63% of their subjects.[17] Involvement also included the infraspinatus with the supraspinatus in 37% of subjects, with 7% showing hypovascularity in the subscapularis.[17] McNab and Rath-

bun postulated that the angulation of the cuff tendons over the head of the humerus may increase ischemia.[18] With contraction of the cuff the humeral head acts as a compressive force against the vessels coursing longitudinally through the tendon.[18] This "wringing out" phenomenon occurs as the arm is brought down and inward. The "critical zone" of vascularity is a frequent location of calcification, tears, and tendonitis involving the rotator cuff.

The Problems. The problem list for patients with rotator cuff impingement varies according to the stage of the disease. Patients presenting with stage I disease usually complain of a toothache like discomfort that occurs after an athletic endeavor. This discomfort may progress to cause pain during the activity and may affect performance. Objectively, patients with stage I impingement syndrome are characterized by point tenderness over the greater tuberosity, tenderness over the anterior acromion, presentation of a classical painful arc between 60 and 120 degrees and the presence of a positive impingement sign.[18] The impingement sign described by Neer and Welsh[12] consists of forcibly flexing the involved extremity forward thus abutting the greater tuberosity against the anteroinferior surface of the acromion.

Involvement of the biceps tendon may occur in stage I disease but it is more commonly associated with stage II impingement. Patients presenting with stage II pathology will have similar subjective complaints as patients in stage I with a few exceptions. Patients with stage II impingement syndrome may have symptoms that progress to cause them to restrict movement and to refrain from the particular maneuver that causes the impingement. The hallmark of stage I, relief of symptoms with activity avoidance, is no longer a feature. The objective signs from Stage I will remain positive. There may now be increased tenderness over the acromioclavicular joint. The patient may complain of a painful catching sensation as well. Manual muscle testing will produce pain and sometimes weakness, especially when isolating the supraspinatus in the "empty can" position.[19] During this maneuver the subscapularis, infraspinatus, and teres minor are comparatively electrically silent.[10,20]

In stage III impingement, the clinical signs and symptoms are the same for the earlier stages, but they are more involved and frequently have other complications. These patients are generally prohibited from any athletic endeavor and as this stage is seen more often in patients older than 40 years many will be unable to continue with their activities, athletic or occupational. Objectively all signs of stage I and II are present, particularly the positive impingement sign.[15]

In stage IV disease patients will present with a prolonged history of shoulder problems. Objectively

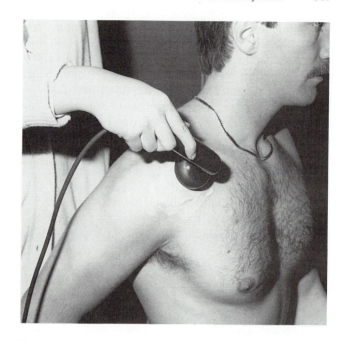

Figure 19-4. Position for phonophoresis treatment to the supraspinatus. The arm is extended and internally rotated to expose the greater tuberosity.

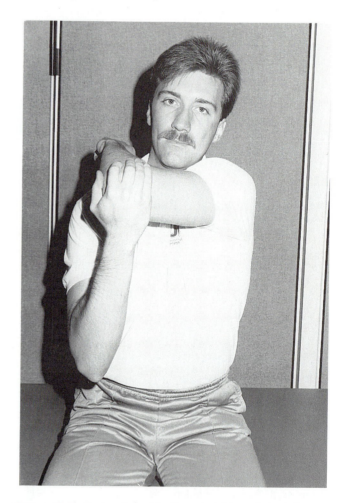

Figure 19-5. Horizontal adduction stretching of the infraspinatus, teres minor, and posterior capsule.

the examiner will see weakness and muscle atrophy. Active range will be limited particularly abduction and external rotation. The patient may have difficulty initiating abduction.[21] Frequently the biceps tendon is involved. It may have been involved at earlier stages or not at all. Tears of the supraspinatus occur before biceps ruptures in a 7:1 ratio.[14] Positive findings will be present on both roentograms and arthrograms.

Treatment Protocols. Treatment of impingement syndromes can be discussed in terms of stages of impingement. Conservative management is stressed for those patients in stage I and II. Taking a problem-oriented approach to rehabilitation the goals of the treatment are to (1) diminish the inflammatory response, (2) maximize shoulder function, or (3) correct or modify abuse.[19]

Phase I Treatment. As discussed earlier, phase I treatment focuses on the reduction of pain and inflamma-

tion. With impingement syndrome this generally consists of modalities and anti-inflammatory medication. A variety of physical agents are commonly used with impingement including electrical stimulation, cryotherapy, and TENS. Ultrasound or phonophoresis with 10% hydrocortisone is commonly used. A clinical suggestion is to position the arm slightly extended and internally rotated behind the back to better reach the supraspinatus as the greater tuberosity is brought out from under the acromion (Fig 19–4). To reach the infraspinatus and teres minor the arm may be externally rotated and horizontally abducted.

Steroid injections may be used in the early stages but should be used with caution. Kennedy and Willis[22] found that injection into a normal tendon can weaken it significantly for up to 14 days and may lead to collagen necrosis. It is prudent for patients who have received injections to be limited to light work activities for at least 2 weeks. Repetitive injections should be avoided. Relative rest is imperative to diminish the in-

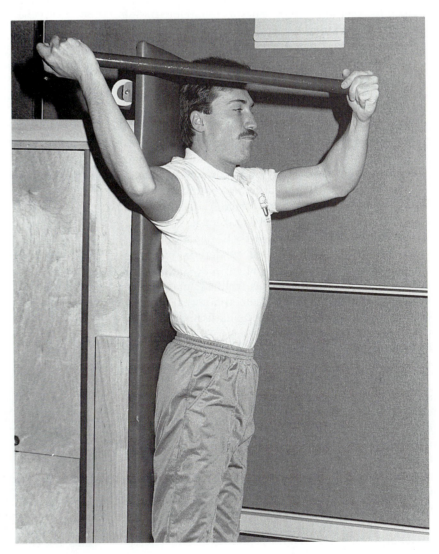

Figure 19-6. External rotation stretching supine with 90 degrees abduction, 90 degrees elbow flexion using a stick.

flammatory response. The athlete must stop the overhead activity that produced the symptom of impingement.

Phase II Treatment. Exercises for ROM should be performed, taking care to avoid the area of impingement. Mobilization may be necessary to allow the joint to regain its complete range in a functional mode. In the early phases of rehabilitation, grade I and II mobilizations will be most effective at decreasing pain and increasing range. Maintaining normal joint arthrokinematics is a primary goal when initiating ROM exercises. The caudal glide of the humerus is necessary to allow the humeral head to clear the acromion, and must be restored before elevation beyond 90 degrees is initiated. Stretching can be directed specifically to the rotator cuff and capsule (Figs 19–5 through 19–9).[23]

Phase III Treatment. A strengthening program for the rotator cuff should be implemented following a protected sequence of activities to restore function. Ini-

tially the strengthening program should be geared to the proximal musculature including the trunk. Specific strengthening of the cuff is performed, avoiding any positions of impingement. Initially, activities such as military press, lat pull downs, and full range bench pressing should be avoided. Dumbbell exercises and light resistance theraband exercise are recommended using a program of high repetitions. Exercises to the rotator cuff as a whole can be instituted early in the strengthening program. Allman[24] describes several exercises that may be used when the rotator cuff is subacute or postsurgical: (1) A gripping exercise performed at multiple angles in a PNF pattern brings the rotator cuff into synergistic contraction. (2) A modified bench press may be initiated to work stabilization and synergistic motion of the cuff. The athlete holds a barbell in a "locked out" position beginning with a narrow grip. The exercise is progressed by widening the grip from about 20 to 30 in to pain tolerance. (3) Deadlift supports where the athlete performs a 10-second shrug with the barbell held with an overhand grip at the

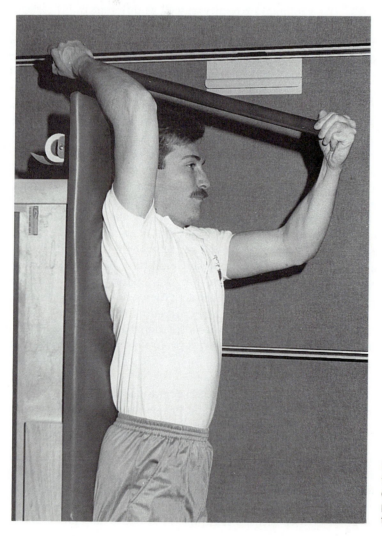

Figure 19–7. External rotation stretching may be performed at multiple angles of elevation, specific to the demands of the sport. Generally stretching is repeated at 90, 135, and 180 degrees of forward elevation.

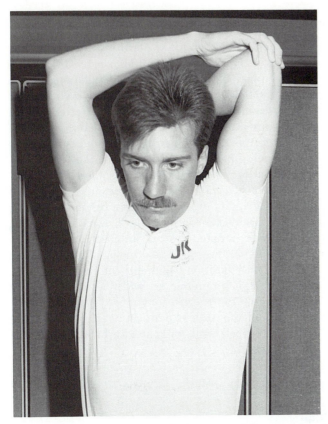

Figure 19-8. The inferior capsule is stretched by positioning the arm overhead and applying pressure posteriorly.

front of the thighs. Progression is accomplished by widening the grip and increasing the resistance (Fig 19–10).

Strengthening is advanced by gradually increasing resistance and by increasing ROM in the early exercises performed. The bench press is progressed by allowing the athlete to bend the elbows until a full-range bench press is possible. The deadlift supports progress to upright rowing. These exercises must be closely monitored to ensure that the athlete is avoiding any painful arcs.

Separate exercises for each of the cuff muscles must be included in the strengthening program.[23-25] The supraspinatus may be isolated in the empty can position (Fig 19–11). The infraspinatus and teres minor can be exercised with the athlete on his or her side, taking care to slightly abduct the arm from the side to avoid the wringing-out phenomenon discussed earlier (Fig 19–12). The subscapularis, which is responsible for internal rotation, can be strengthened in sidelying or standing (Figs 19–13, 19–14).

The rotator cuff must be able to perform its functions of stabilization before further exercise to the shoulder musculature is initiated in order to allow the shoulder to move without abnormal mechanics.[26] The serratus anterior, latissimus dorsi rhomboids, trapezius, and levator scapulae should all be included in the strengthening program. These muscles formulate the basis for the force couples that occur with scapular and glenohumeral motions. Specific sequencing of exercise to the shoulder is recommended by Davies when rehabilitating rotator cuff tendinitis and impingement.[27] It is recommended that exercise begin with internal and external rotation to promote the dynamic function of the rotator cuff to depress the humerus. The sequence continues with flexion and extension and concludes with abduction and adduction, as these motions are directly in the plane of injury.

Isokinetic strengthening of the external rotators and scapular musculature especially below the level of impingement is indicated (Fig 19–15). Ivey et al reported strength ratios when testing normal subjects on the Cybex II.[28] They demonstrated internal rotation strength greater than external rotation by a ratio of 3:2, extension strength greater than flexion by a ratio of 5:4, and adduction strength greater than abduction by a ratio of 2:1. Therapists are advised to use care when applying normative data to their patients. Unlike symmetrical comparisons of torque in the knee, studies have demonstrated statistically greater strength in the dominant extremity as well as different ratios for specific sports.[29] Ellenbecker and Derscheid[30] reported on the isokinetic testing of pitchers and elite tennis players to have ratios of internal rotation to external rotation exceeding 3:2. The increase in internal rotation strength is proposed to be the result of the specific demands of the throwing and serving motions. These individual differences should be considered in the use of isokinetics and the functional strengthening of the athlete to return to competition.

An upper body ergometer can be employed to increase the muscular endurance of the shoulder complex. In impingement the seat should be raised to keep elevation of the shoulder below the level of impingement. Retrocycling can also be added to the program to work the scapular retractors (Fig 19–16). Plyometric drills for the upper extremity are being implemented into strengthening programs when function dictates their use. Plyometric activities involve an eccentric contraction immediately preceding a concentric contraction. The eccentric contraction loads the noncontractile connective tissue with prestretch of the muscle tendon structure.

Phase IV Treatment. A gradual and functional return to activities should be stressed to prevent reoccurrence of the syndrome. In this way the rehabilitation program can proceed in a safe and logical manner. If the athlete is unable to progress to a more intense performance level, the rehabilitation program can be easily modified to conform to his or her tolerance, for example, the swimmer may progress to return to swimming with strokes least likely to aggravate the impinge-

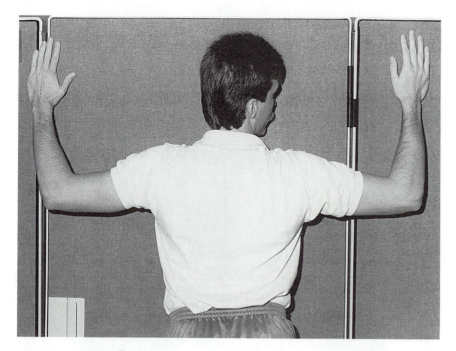

A

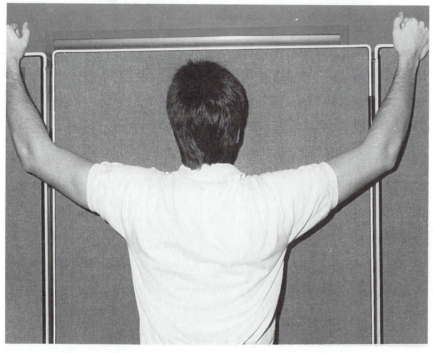

B

Figure 19-9(A,B). Pectoral stretching may be performed at different angles of shoulder elevation. To progress the stretch the athlete may stand in an open doorway and lean forward.

ment—first the breast stroke, followed by the free style, the backstroke, and the butterfly. A biomechanical evaluation of technique should also be implemented. In this type of assessment the athlete is observed while performing the sports activity. Alterations in his or her performance technique may then be made in order to lessen the risk of reoccurrence. A tennis player, for example, should be instructed to use an ele-

vated technique, with the shoulder at 135 degrees of flexion compared to 90 degrees of flexion. This elevated technique decreases the shear forces on the shoulder as well as reduces forces to the medial elbow (Fig 19–17).[31]

Improper ball toss may be another technique error. The server may toss the ball too high in the air and too far behind him or her, increasing the stress to the

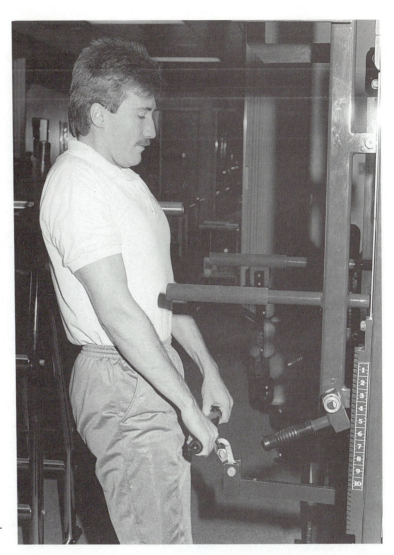

Figure 19-10. Deadlift supports for synergistic motion of the rotator cuff.

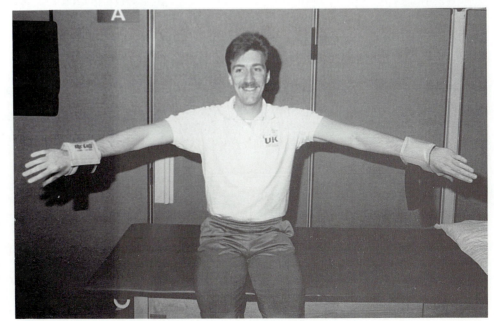

Figure 19-11. The supraspinatus can be isolated in the empty can position of 90 degrees abduction, 30 degrees horizontal flexion, and internal rotation with thumbs pointing towards the floor. Hand-held weights should be avoided to prevent deltoid contraction.

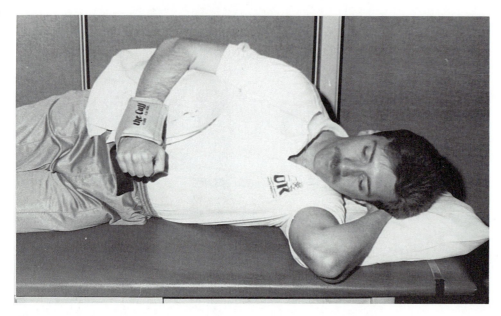

A

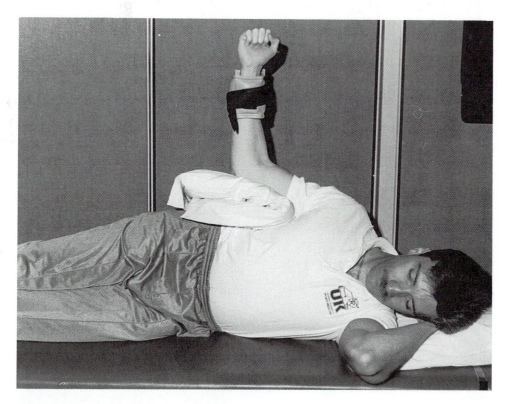

B

Figure 19-12(A,B). Sidelying infraspinatus and teres minor strengthening exercise with cuff weight. Note position of slight abduction to prevent vascular impingement.

rotator cuff. Videotape may be helpful in analyzing service technique. In the follow-through the examiner should watch that the shoulder comes across the body rather than off to the side, which requires increasing internal rotation. When returning to tennis the athlete may begin by hitting ground strokes, then hitting the ball from the baseline to the rear fence and finally into the service area. The last mentioned requires increasing stroke speed and shoulder internal rotation.

In later stages of impingement, where rotator cuff degeneration has already occurred and conservative treatment has failed, surgery is often considered. The most common surgical techniques in the athlete include anterior acromioplasty with or without repair of the

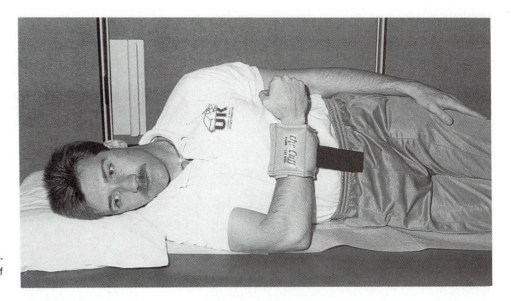

Figure 19-13. Side-lying internal rotation exercise with cuff weight.

cuff.[13] Arthroscopic debridement is also an option when conservative management is unsuccessful. In the athlete, anterior acromioplasty is reported as satisfactory for pain relief but may not allow the athlete to return to his or her former competitive status.[32]

Bicipital Tendinitis/Subluxation

Bicipital tendinitis presents as an irritation to the biceps tendon in the bicipital groove. The groove has wide variance in the angle of its walls, and anatomic variations in the prominence of the tuberosities may predis-

pose some athletes to injury. The condition is generally related to overuse. It is predominantly seen in activities that involve overhead motions and is commonly seen with the impingement syndrome described earlier. Biceps tendinitis occurs primarily as a secondary disorder.[11,33] Baseball pitchers, catchers, football quarterbacks, javelin throwers, shotputters, tennis players, and racquet ball players are most frequently affected, as throwing motions are involved in their activity.[34] Bicipital tendinitis may also be associated with a partial subluxation of the tendon or laxity of the transverse hu-

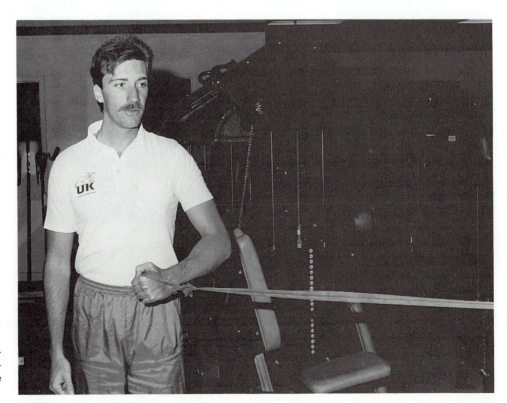

Figure 19-14. Standing internal rotation exercise with theraband using modified base position of the arm.

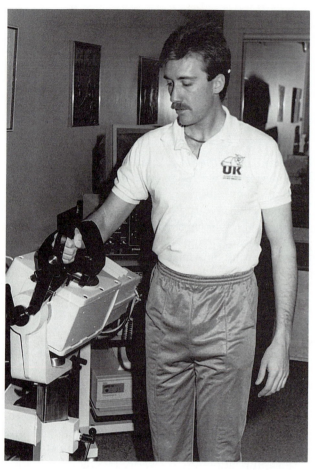

Figure 19-15. Isokinetic internal/external rotation strengthening. Note modified base position of slight abduction of the arm.

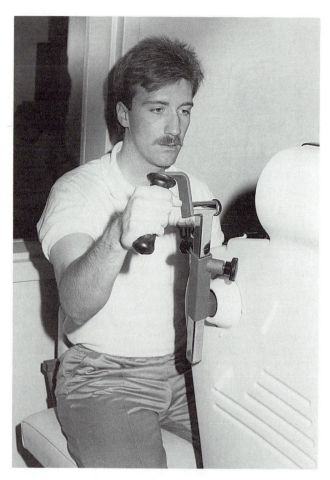

Figure 19-16. Upper body ergometer may be used for scapular protraction/retraction exercise. Arrows indicate protraction and retraction.

meral ligament, and these two conditions must be differentiated in the clinical examination. The integrity of the transverse humeral ligament is easily tested with the Yergason's test. The subluxation of the tendon can be demonstrated when the shoulder goes from internal rotation to external rotation and back again.[35] If the tendon is found to be stable in the groove, tests such as Lippmans', Ludingtons, and the straight arm raise may be performed.[3] Bicipital tendinitis can progress to a complete tear of the biceps at its musculotendinous junction, and this injury may require surgical intervention.

The Problems. The problems most frequently seen in this injury are anterior shoulder pain, pain with shoulder rotation, increased pain with resistance, and the possibility of the presence of a painful arc. The painful arc can usually be elicited with resistance of shoulder flexion with the palm facing upward at approximately 80 degrees.[15]

Pain is most pronounced when the athlete rotates the shoulder internally and externally. There may also be pain with passive stretching of the biceps in shoulder hyperextension with elbow extension and forearm pronation.[36]

Treatment Protocols.

Phase I Treatment. The initial phase treatment for bicipital tendinitis includes relative rest in the form of restriction of rotational activities that reproduce or exacerbate the symptoms. Ice, nonsteroidal anti-inflammatory medications, and TENS may be used in the acute phase to decrease pain and inflammation. Injections around the biceps tendon should be avoided. Transverse friction massage may be helpful over the bicipital groove but may exacerbate acutely or chronically inflamed tissue.[6] Transverse friction massage is performed for approximately 5 to 10 minutes in 30-second intervals.

Phase II Treatment. Loss of ROM is generally not a problem with isolated biceps injury, but stretching, as described in rotator cuff impingement, may be helpful

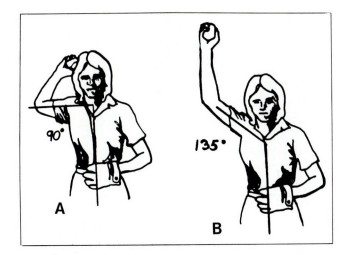

Figure 19-17. Elevated technique to protect shoulder and medial elbow. **A.** The 90-degree-angle position is most derogatory because the shoulder shear forces are greatest in this position. In addition, forces on the medial elbow are great. Therefore, this position increases the chances of injury to both the shoulder and medial elbow. **B.** High arm elevations are more protective to the shoulder tendon cuff. Higher elevations also diminish medial elbow force load. *(From Nirsch RP. Prevention and treatment of overuse injuries of the shoulder.* Clin Sports Med. *1989; 8:296, with permission.)*

because bicipital tendinitis is often secondary and associated with impingement. A long axis stretch to maintain biceps length can be a useful procedure for range and for relief of pain.[23]

Phase III Treatment. After pain and inflammation have been managed, strengthening may be initiated so that the endurance of the shoulder complex will improve and prevent future tendon irritation. Exercise may be directed to the entire shoulder complex, with emphasis on the rotator cuff, elbow flexion, and shoulder flexion. A strengthening program may begin with isometrics, and progress with isotonics, isokinetics, and eccentrics. Care should be taken to avoid any painful arcs that may be present.

Phase IV Treatment. A gradual and progressive return to sports as well as an evaluation of technique will prevent many reinjuries. For those athletes who are anatomically predisposed to bicipital irritation or subluxation a clinical suggestion postulated by Falkel and Murphy is the use of a tennis elbow strap over the upper arm just proximal to the belly of the biceps.[36] They report good clinical improvement and speculate that the strap assists in stabilizing the biceps tendon in the groove (Fig 19–18).[36]

Acromioclavicular Sprains

The acromioclavicular joint is frequently injured as the result of direct trauma. A fall on or direct blow to the top of the shoulder are the most common mechanisms of injury.[37,38] A fall on an outstretched arm may also cause injury by driving the humerus up into the acromion and tearing the capsular structures.[38] The nature of the injury to the acromioclavicular joint can be described in relationship to severity by grades. A grade I injury is characterized by a sprain of the acromioclavicular ligament, but there is no deformity. In a grade II injury the acromioclavicular ligament is torn, allowing subluxation. The coracoclavicular ligament may be

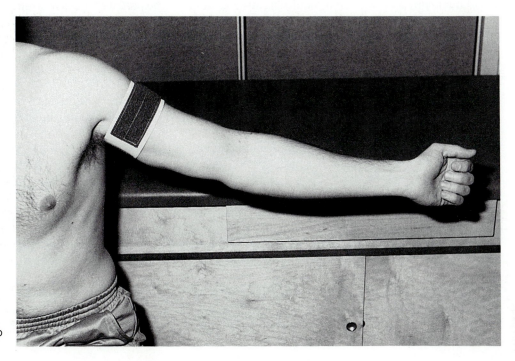

Figure 19-18. Upper arm strap for subluxing biceps tendon.

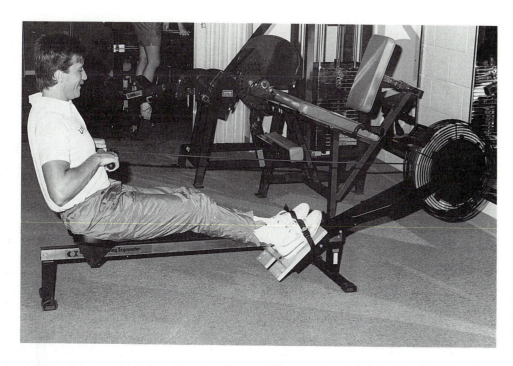

Figure 19-24. The rowing ergometer is useful for overall shoulder strengthening and cardiovascular conditioning.

3. Positive apprehension test.
4. Positive radiographic findings, often including Hill Sachs lesions.

The athlete is most commonly affected in activities such as throwing, forceful serving in tennis, and working with the arm in an overhead, strained position.

Posterior Instability. Posterior instability occurs in the athlete when motion places the humeral head against the posterior capsule and cuff tendons. Injuries associated with throwing, training, lifting, or trauma that affect the posterior shoulder (glenoid cavity, labrum, capsule, infraspinatus, teres minor, and humeral head) can lead to posterior instability and symptoms during throwing.[47] The pull-through phase of freestyle swimming and the backhand stroke in tennis may also affect the posterior shoulder.[48] The mechanism of injury is usually a posteriorly directed force on the adducted, internally rotated arm with the hand in a position below shoulder level.[41] True posterior dislocation is extremely rare, whereas subluxation is a more common condition.[49,50]

Multidirectional Instability Subluxation or dislocation may occur in more than one direction. This may be due to trauma but more commonly is atraumatic or voluntary.[41] The combination of instabilities may be anterior and inferior, or posterior or all three. The instability may be associated with an initial overuse or a predisposition to such a problem as occurs with a congenitally relaxed shoulder.

The Problems. Anterior dislocation is characterized by pain, disability, and pain with movement. The apprehension test is usually positive. The athlete with posterior instability may be unable to abduct or externally rotate the arm. The patient who has a posteriorly dislocated shoulder cannot supinate with the arm extended, as the shoulder is locked into internal rotation.[41] Posterior subluxation may or may not be associated with pain, and the athlete may not remember when the shoulder first "came out." As time progresses the athlete is usually aware of changes in the performance of the shoulder.[49] An athlete suffering from multidirectional instability may not experience pain. One third of the athletes will remember significant trauma leading to instability, such as in hyperextending and abducting the arm in a football tackle. Another third will recall only minor trauma with chronic aching and weakness, and the final third will have insidious onset of laxity.[51]

Treatment Protocols

Phase I Treatment. Treatment of a dislocated shoulder begins with reduction. Traditionally, immobilization was the basis for managing shoulder dislocations; however, studies have found the length of immobilization to have no effect on the rate of recurrence of injury.[41,43] Treatments of ice and medication may be used as symptoms dictate.

Phase II Treatment. Full range of motion is mandatory prior to return to sports activities. With a loss of

motion, abnormal stresses are generated in an attempt to compensate for the loss in power, resulting in rotator cuff inflammation.[52] Motion should be achieved by means of active exercise and progress to active/assistive motion. Gentle passive stretching exercises are added only if a serious motion inadequacy exists, and stretching is done specifically only to recover specific losses of motion. For example, an athlete who has anterior dislocation or subluxation should avoid passive stretching exercises that force the glenohumeral joint into an abducted and externally rotated position. Flexibility exercises may be contraindicated in a patient with a multidirectional instability or general joint laxity.[53] Gentle mobilization may be used after immobilization. Care should be used when mobilizing a shoulder following surgery. Depending on the surgical procedure the anterior glide should be avoided so as not to stress the surgically repaired tissue.[6]

Phase III Treatment. The shoulder girdle has very little static or ligamentous stability. Stability is primarily dynamic and requires almost perfect synergism of all of the periarticular muscles.[11] The overall goal of strengthening exercise for the unstable shoulder is the strengthening of muscles that have a role in protecting the shoulder from further episodes of instability.[53] Muscle strengthening in the midrange is preferable initially. The use of PNF for shoulder instability is invaluable. The therapist may begin working with the proximal musculature while controlling rotation and providing proprioceptive awareness.

Strengthening for anterior instability emphasizes the subscapularis, anterior deltoid, pectoralis major, coracobrachialis, and long head of the biceps. The antagonists should not be overlooked, as they play a significant role in the containment of the shoulder and may help to prevent instability. The rhomboids, latissimus dorsi, and serratus anterior should be included in the exercise regime (Fig 19–25).[52] Moynes et al[54] recommend that the shoulder position of 90 degrees abduction with external rotation be avoided. They electromyographically demonstrated the inability of the subscapularis to restrain forward motion of the humeral head in the position of 90 degrees abduction with external rotation.

The function of the rotator cuff muscles should not be overlooked in shoulder instability. The shoulder functions as a complex including the scapulothoracic, glenohumeral, acromioclavicular, and sternoclavicular joints. When the scapular rotators are functioning optimally, they are largely responsible for positioning the scapular platform accurately under the humeral head so that motions can be accomplished with maximum stability.[53] Strengthening of the rotator cuff is especially emphasized in the treatment of dead arm syndrome. The use of surgical tubing to accomplish internal and external rotation is often helpful and is easily incorporated into a home program (Figs 19–26, 19–27).

Isokinetic exercise is also valuable in the treatment of instability. In anterior laxity it is desirable to increase external rotation strength to increase the ratio of internal rotation to external rotation similar to the concept

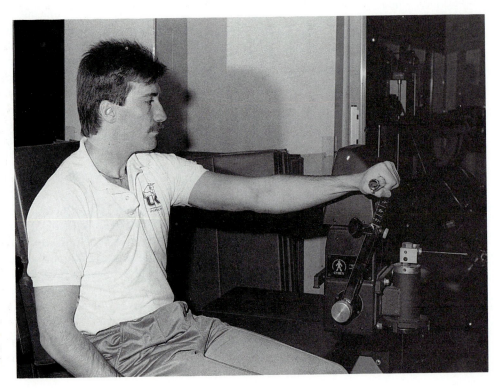

Figure 19-25. Scapular protraction/retraction exercises on the orthotron. Exercises may be performed isometrically or through a velocity spectrum.

of increasing hamstring/quad ratios for the Anterior Cruciate Ligament (ACL)-deficient knee. Isokinetics can be performed in short arc patterns and in multiple angles. Isokinetics can be used to improve the timing and neuromuscular balance needed to stabilize the shoulder. This neuromuscular balance was studied by Glousman et al,[55] who demonstrated the pectoralis major, subscapularis, latissimus dorsi, and serratus anterior to have decreased activity in a group of throwers with instability compared to a group of healthy throwers and concluded that the imbalance accentuates stresses on the anterior restraints of the shoulder in throwing and was a factor in producing or maintaining the anterior instability.

Another device that has implications in neuromuscular reeducation and timing is the Impulse Inertial Exercise System (E.M.A., Newnan, GA). It is especially valuable in the advanced stages of rehabilitation when an eccentric deceleration force is preferred and the therapist wishes to modify exercise to sport-specific positions (Fig 19–28).

Strengthening for posterior shoulder instability emphasizes the posterior rotator cuff. The posterior deltoid should also be addressed. The athlete should avoid full horizontal adduction and internal rotation.

Care should be taken to accomplish posterior rotator cuff exercises without placing the shoulder in the subluxated position. Norwood[47] recommends that exercise be performed with the elbow at the side. Rotation activities from 45 degrees of abduction to neutral should be stressed, with external rotations greater than 45 degrees avoided. The trapezius and deltoid should not be overlooked. Bench pressing is contraindicated while the arm is symptomatic, as bench pressing is the most frequent nonthrowing cause of injury. Norwood[47] also recommends restricting pushing and pulling.

With multidirectional instability the emphasis for strengthening is placed on the side of the major instability. Limiting exercise to midrange and the use of isometrics is recommended.[53] For multidirectional instability specific resistive exercise to restore muscle tone and strength of the supporting tissues is indicated and may prove more successful than surgery.[41]

Phase IV Treatment. Early return to activity generally involves a motion that is less stressful to the shoulder than the athlete's ordinary style until the muscles are sufficiently strengthened. Taping, wrapping, or a commercial checkrein device may be used to provide the athlete with feedback to help avoid end ROMs.[36]

Full return to sport requires loss of apprehension in all positions. Rigid restriction of activities until goals of rehabilitation are met and strict adherence to an aggressive strengthening program after primary anterior dislocation is reported to prevent recurrent episodes in 75% of patients.[56] Matsen and Zuckerman[42] state that, ideally, the athlete should be able to perform internal and external rotation against isotonic muscle loading equal to 20% of the body weight before returning to competition.

Athletes who fail conservative care may be treated surgically. For recurrent anterior dislocation, procedures such as the Bankart, Bristow, Putti-Platt, Eden–Hybbinette, and Magnuson–Stack may be used, depending on the specific diagnosis and pathology. Zarins and Rowe[41] feel a Bankart procedure is advisable in the

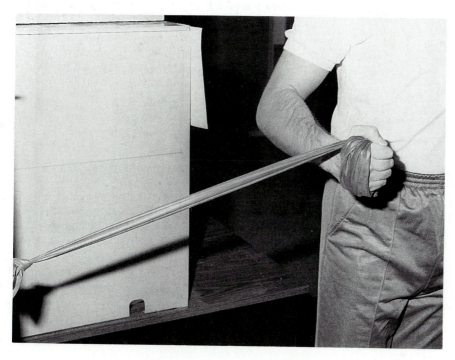

Figure 19–26. Internal rotation strengthening with rubber tubing.

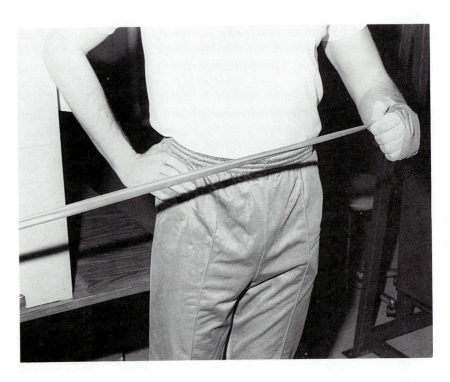

Figure 19-27. External rotation strengthening with rubber tubing.

athlete who will require a full range of motion with all muscles working in unison to perform at their optimal level. A Bankart procedure involves suturing the lateral capsule to the glenoid rim and then suturing the medial capsule to the rim so as to provide a double-breasted support along the entire glenoid rim.[46] For recurrent transient anterior subluxation, a Bankart procedure is

used when a Bankart lesion is present. In the absence of a Bankart lesion a capsulorrhaphy was preferred.[46]

Surgical repair for recurrent posterior instability is not as successful as repair of anterior instability, and athletes should be counseled that it is difficult to return to throwing at a highly competitive level following posterior reconstruction. Return to contact sport would be expected among athletes whose shoulders are neither congenitally loose nor habitually dislocated.[47] The surgical repair of instability may result in a loss of the flexibility needed for athletic participation, particularly in the thrower and the gymnast. Treatment must optimize both joint stability and joint flexibility. These considerations are particularly important for the professional athlete, whose livelihood depends on his or her ability to maintain a peak level of performance.[42]

Subacromial Bursitis

Bursitis in the athlete is rarely a primary condition. It is commonly seen in individuals with grade III impingement where the degenerative changes in the cuff progress to involve the bursa.[57] The onset of the symptoms may be gradual or sudden. Pain may begin after strenuous activity, especially with the arm in an overhead position. Prolonged immobilization, working in a slumped position, and making sudden movements in an abnormal direction or normal movements but with tension or anxiety are some of the causes of bursitis.[57]

The Problems. Pain is generally the initial symptom and is associated with limitation, if not prevention of motion. There may be difficulty initiating motion, especially abduction. The limitation of motion occurs in

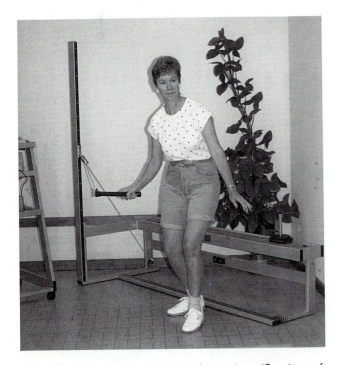

Figure 19-28. Impulse inertial exercise system. *(Courtesy of Steve Davison, E.M.A.)*

a noncapsular pattern and the end feel of passive range of motion is empty. Rotations of the shoulder in a neutral position may be relatively free. The athlete is usually unable to sleep on the affected side and may complain of popping in the shoulder. There is tenderness to palpation anteriorly and laterally and the pain is often diffuse down the lateral aspect of the arm.[58] A painful arc is often present between 70 and 120 degrees. Pain is associated with manual muscle testing especially in abduction.[36]

Treatment Protocols

Phase I Treatment. Treatment should be directed at the subacromial tissues, including the associated tendinitis. Rest for a short period of time may be helpful if pain is severe. Cryotherapy should be initiated to decrease pain and spasm. Anti-inflammatory medication and injection of corticosteroid may be used at the discretion of the physician.

Phase II Treatment. Initiating movement is paramount to preventing loss of motion. Pendulum exercises and grade I and II mobilization are useful early. As the irritation in the subacromial space decreases, range of motion exercises may be increased. The use of ultrasound has been reported in the treatment of bursitis, but a controlled double blind trial of ultrasound therapy found no significant differences in pain, range of motion or function.[59] It should be noted that the subjects treated were not athletes.

Phase III Treatment. Strengthening can be implemented as range of motion returns to normal, but the athlete should avoid movements that require abduction past 90 degrees, particularly in a position of internal rotation. The use of the upper body exercise table (UBE) with the seat raised is useful for total arm strength. Strengthening exercises for associated tendonitis should be incorporated into the rehabilitation program. Rotator cuff strengthening should be addressed to improve glenohumeral stability and to prevent the humeral head from riding up into the bursa with overhead movement.

Phase IV Treatment. Return to function is based upon symptomatic improvement and the ability to perform sport-specific drills and activities comfortably.[36] The athlete should be instructed in preventive measures that include avoidance of shoulder motions that may have led to the condition.[6]

Adhesive Capsulitis

Adhesive capsulitis, or "frozen shoulder," describes a condition affecting the shoulder capsule. It can be defined as the spontaneous onset of gradually progressive shoulder pain and limitation of movement.[60] It involves the capsule and synovium, and the inflammation leads to the formation of adhesions, specifically in the axillary fold and in the attachment of the capsule at the anatomic neck of the humerus.[61] Adhesive capsulitis is extremely rare in the athlete and is most prevalent in the age group between 40 and 60 years but may develop in the athlete as the result of trauma, prolonged immobilization, or disuse.

The Problems. Pain and stiffness are the predominant features of this disorder. The athlete has pain present during activity and rest and frequently sleep is affected. There may be diffuse soreness with tenderness over the bicipital groove. The hallmark symptom, loss of range of motion in a capsular pattern, is usually present. The capsular pattern is external rotation restricted greater than abduction, which is restricted greater than internal rotation. The end feel is capsular.[60] Subsequent loss of strength is also a feature of this condition.

Treatment Protocols. Prevention is the best treatment of adhesive capsulitis. If the condition does develop, physical therapy for the athlete is complementary to the treatment in the general orthopedic population and should be directed towards decreasing pain and improving range of motion. Gentle range of motion exercises and mobilization to regain physiological and accessory motions of the shoulder are indicated.

PREVENTION OF INJURY

Identifying and recognizing injury patterns is an important component in preventing injury. Preseason screening should be performed as recommended by the Ad Hoc committee of the Sports Physical Therapy Section of the American Physical Therapy Association (APTA) in such a way as to quantify any deficiencies that may predispose the athlete to injury during sports participation.[62] Examination about the shoulder should include an assessment of prior injuries, asymmetry, range of motion, stability, strength, and function (Chap. 3). With such a screening, potential problems may be detected and a corrective exercise program implemented prior to the start of the season. Many programs currently emphasize year-round training, which may help to prevent injury or prevent reoccurrence of preexisting problems.[63] This type of exercise is considered to be prehabilitative.

Prehabilitative exercises are defined by Falkel and Murphy as those exercises designed to strengthen and improve performance prior to the injury based on the specific demands of the sport skill.[36] The sports physical therapist is aware of the common injuries associated

with a given sport and must strive to better understand the nature of the injuries associated with particular actions or sport. As the mechanism(s) causing damage to the soft tissue structures of the shoulder are understood, we can better tailor our rehabilitative and prehabilitative exercises to address the specific forces placed upon the shoulder joint.[64]

CONCLUSION

This chapter has outlined common injuries to the shoulder, the associated problems, and the treatment protocols. Further longitudinal and prospective studies to track clinical outcomes and incidence of recurrence of injuries are needed to justify the treatment protocols commonly used in sports physical therapy.

REFERENCES

1. Falkel JE, Murphy TC. Clinical evaluation of the shoulder complex. In: Malone TR, ed. *Sports Injury Management: Shoulder Injuries*. Baltimore, Md: Williams & Wilkins; 1988; 13–35.
2. Bowling RW, Rockar PA, Erhard R. Examination of the shoulder complex. *Phys Ther*. 1986; 66:1866–1877.
3. Halbach JW, Tank RT. The shoulder. In: Gould JA, Davies GJ, eds. *Orthopaedic and Sports Physical Therapy*. St. Louis, Mo: C V Mosby; 1985; 497–517.
4. Davies GJ, Gould JA, Larsen RL. Functional examination of the shoulder girdle. *Phys Sportsmed*. 1981; 9:82–104.
5. Kessler RM, Hertling D. *Management of Common Musculoskeletal Disorders: Physical Therapy, Principles and Methods*. Philadelphia, Pa: Harper & Row Publishers Inc; 1983.
6. Nitz AJ. Physical therapy management of the shoulder. *Phys Ther*. 1986; 66:1912–1919.
7. Kleinkort JA, Wood F. Phonophoresis with 1 percent versus 10 percent hydrocortisone. *Phys Ther*. 1975; 55:1320–1324.
8. Sapega AA, Quedenfeld TC, Moyer RA, et al. Biophysical factors in range of motion exercise. *Phys Sportsmed*. 1981; 9:57–65.
9. Falkel JE, Murphy TC. Principles of rehabilitation and prehabilitation. In: Malone TR, ed. *Sports Injury Management: Shoulder Injuries*. Baltimore, Md: Williams & Wilkins; 1988:42–54.
10. Jobe FW, Jobe CM. Painful athletic injuries of the shoulder. *Clin Orthop*. 1983; 173:11–19.
11. Hughston JC. Functional anatomy of the shoulder. In: Zarins B, Andrews JR, Carson WG, eds. *Injuries to the Throwing Arm*. Philadelphia, Pa: W B Saunders; 1985: 43–50.
12. Neer CS, Welsh RP. The shoulder in sports. *Orthop Clin N Am*. 1977; 8:583–591.
13. Penny JN, Welsh MB. Shoulder impingement syndromes in athletes and their surgical management. *Am J Sports Med* 1981; 9:11–15.
14. Neer CS. Impingement lesions. *Clin Orthop*. 1983; 173: 70–77.
15. Hawkins RJ, Hobeika PE. Impingement syndrome in the athletic shoulder. *Clin Sports Med*. 1983; 2:391–405.
16. Rothman RH, Parke W. Vascular anatomy of the rotator cuff. *Clin Orthop*. 1965; 41:176–186.
17. Rothman RH, Marvel JP, Heppenstall RB. Anatomic considerations in the glenohumeral joint. *Orthop Clin Am*. 1975; 6:341–352.
18. Rathbun JB, McNab I. The microvascular pattern of the rotator cuff. *J Bone Joint Surg*. 1970; 52B:540–553.
19. Brunet ME, Hadda RJ, Porche EB. Rotator cuff impingement syndrome in sports. *Phys Sportsmed*. 1982; 10:86–94.
20. Jobe FW, Moynes DR. Delineation of diagnostic criteria and a rehab program for cuff injuries. *Am J Sports Med*. 1982; 10:336–339.
21. Bechtol CO. Biomechanics of the shoulder. *Clin Orthop*. 1980; 146:37–41.
22. Kennedy JC, Willis B. The effects of local steroid injections on tendons. *Am J Sports Med*. 1976; 4:11–21.
23. Moynes DR. Prevention of injury to the shoulder through exercise and therapy. *Clin Sports Med*. 1983; 12:413–422.
24. Allman F. Impingement, biceps, and rotator cuff lesions. In: Zarins B, Andrews JR, Carson WG, eds. *Injuries to the Throwing Arm*. USOC. Philadelphia, Pa: W B Saunders; 1985:158–172.
25. Mulligan E. Conservative management of shoulder impingement syndrome. *Athlet Training*. 1988; 23:348–353.
26. Pappas AM, Zawacki RM, McCarthy CF. Rehabilitation of the pitching shoulder. *Am J Sports Med*. 1985; 13: 223–235.
27. Davies GJ. *A Compendium of Isokinetics in Clinical Usage and Rehabilitation Techniques*. 3rd ed. LaCrosse, Wisc: S&S Publishers; 1987.
28. Ivey FM, Calhoun JH, Rusche K, Bierschenk J. Isokinetic testing of shoulder strength: Normal values. *Arch Phys Med Rehabil*. 1985; 66:384–386.
29. Perrin DH, Robertson RJ, Ray RL. Bilateral isokinetic peak torque, torque acceleration energy, power, and work relationships in athletes and nonathletes. *J Orthop Sports Phys Ther*. 1987; 9:184–189.
30. Ellenbecker TS, Derscheid GL. Rehabilitation of overuse injuries of the shoulder. *Clin Sports Med*. 1989; 8: 583–604.
31. Nirschl RP. Prevention and treatment of elbow and shoulder injuries in the tennis player. *Clin Sports Med*. 1988; 7:289–308.
32. Tibone JE, Jobe FW, Kerlan RK, et al. Shoulder impingement syndrome in athletes treated by an anterior acromioplasty. *Clin Orthop*. 1985; 198:134–140.
33. Neviaser TJ. The role of the biceps tendon in the impingement syndrome. *Orthop Clin N Am*. 1987; 18: 383–386.
34. O'Donoghue DH. Subluxing biceps tendon in the athlete. *Clin Orthop*. 1982; 164:26–29.
35. McCue FC, Gieck JH, West JO. Throwing injuries to the shoulder. In: Zarins B, Andrews JR, Carson WG, eds. *Injuries to the Throwing Arm*. Philadelphia, Pa: W B Saunders; 1985; 95–111.

36. Falkel JE, Murphy TC. Common injuries of the shoulder in athletes. In Malone TR, ed. *Sports Injury Management*: Shoulder injuries. Baltimore, Md: Williams & Wilkins; 1988; 66–108.

37. Torg JS, Vegso JJ, Torg E. *Rehabilitation of Athletic Injuries: An Atlas of Therapeutic Exercise*. Chicago, Ill: Year Book Medical Publishers Inc; 1987.

38. Wickiewicz TL. Acromioclavicular and sternoclavicular joint injuries. *Clin Sports Med*. 1983; 2:429–438.

39. Stewart MF. The acromioclavicular joint in the throwing arm. In Zarins B, Andrews JR, Carson WG, eds. *Injuries to the Throwing Arm*. Philadelphia, Pa: W B Saunders; 1985; 128–143.

40. Larsen E, Bjerg–Nielsen A, Christensen P. Conservative or surgical treatment of acromioclavicular dislocation. *J Bone Joint Surg*. 1986; 68A:552–555.

41. Zarins B, Rowe CR. Current concepts in the diagnosis and treatment of shoulder instability in athletes. *Med Sci Sports Exerc*. 1984; 16:444–448.

42. Matsen FA, Zuckerman JD. Anterior glenohumeral instability. *Clin Sports Med*. 1983; 2:319–338.

43. Henry JH, Genung JA. Natural history of glenohumeral dislocation revisited. *Am J Sports Med*. 1982; 10:135–141.

44. Fowler PJ. Shoulder injuries in the mature athlete. *Adv Sports Med Fitness*. 1988; 1:225–238.

45. Rowe CR. Anterior subluxation of the throwing shoulder. In: Zarins B, Andrews JR, Carson WG, eds. *Injuries to the Throwing Arm*. Philadelphia, Pa: W B Saunders; 1985:144–152.

46. Rowe CR. Recurrent transient anterior subluxation of the shoulder. The "dead arm" syndrome. *Clin Orthop*. 1987; 223:11–19.

47. Norwood LA. Posterior shoulder instability. In: Zarins B, Andrews JR, Carson WG, eds. *Injuries to the Throwing Arm*. Philadelphia, Pa: W B Saunders; 1985:153–157.

48. Warren RF. Subluxation of the shoulder in athletes. *Clin Sports Med*. 1983; 2:339–354.

49. Hawkins RJ, Koppert G, Johnston G. Recurrent posterior instability (subluxation) of the shoulder. *J Bone Joint Surg*. 1984; 66A:169–174.

50. Schwartz E, Warren RF, O'Brien SJ, Fronek J. Posterior shoulder instability. *Orthop Clin N Am*. 1987; 18:409–419.

51. Foster CR. Multidirectional shoulder instability. *Clin Sports Med*. 1983; 2:355–368.

52. O'Brien SJ, Warren RF, Schwartz E. Anterior shoulder instability. *Orthop Clin N Am*. 1987; 18:395–408.

53. Jobe FW, Moynes DR, Brewster CE. Rehabilitation of shoulder joint instabilities. *Orthop Clin N Am*. 1987; 18:473–482.

54. Moynes DR, Perry J, Antonelli DJ, Jobe FW. Electromyography and motion analysis of the upper extremity in sports. *Phys Ther*. 1986; 66:1905–1911.

55. Glousman R, Jobe F, Tibone J, Moynes D, et al. Dynamic electromyographic analysis of the throwing shoulder with glenohumeral instability. *J Bone Joint Surg*. 1988; 70:220–226.

56. Aronen JG, Regan K. Decreasing the incidence of recurrence of first time anterior shoulder dislocations with rehabilitation. *Am J Sports Med*. 1984; 12:283–291.

57. Calliet R. *Shoulder Pain*. Philadelphia, Pa: F A Davis Co; 1978:33–57.

58. Cogen L, Anderson LG, Phelps P. Medical management of the painful shoulder. *Bull Rheum Dis*. 1982; 32:54–58.

59. Downing ES, Weinstein A. Ultrasound therapy of subacromial bursitis, a double blind trial. *Phys Ther*. 1986; 66:194–199.

60. Wadsworth CT. Frozen shoulder. *Phys Ther*. 1986; 66:1878–1883.

61. Neviaser RJ, Neviaser TJ. The frozen shoulder diagnosis and management. *Clin Orthop*. 1987; 223:59–64.

62. Sanders BR, Eggart JS. *Guidelines for Pre-season Athletic Participation Evaluation*. 2nd ed. Sports Physical Therapy Section, American Physical Therapy Association.

63. McCue FC, Gieck JH, West JO. Throwing injuries to the shoulder. In: Zarins B, Andrews JR, Carson WG: *Injuries to the Throwing Arm*. Philadelphia, Pa: W B Saunders; 1985; 95–111.

64. McLeod WD, Andrews JR. Mechanisms of shoulder injuries. *Phys Ther*. 1986; 66:1901–1904.

20

Elbow, Wrist, and Hand Injuries

Steve Dickoff

INTRODUCTION

The elbow, hand, and wrist, as an extension of the upper extremity, are vitally important anatomic regions for the success of the athlete. Although it is a non-weight-bearing body segment (excluding some sports such as wrestling and gymnastics), the upper extremity is active in most sports, thereby leaving it quite susceptible to injury.

Without proper use of the upper extremity, an athlete cannot swing a racket or bat, throw a ball, swim, or, because of the importance of the arm to generate propulsive power, run at maximum efficiency. Statistically, the upper extremity is one of the most frequently injured anatomic regions in the athlete. In a study of 100,000 people, Zariczny et al[1] noted that 30% of the athletic injuries sustained by children were to the hand and wrist. Ho and Dellon[2] note that the hand was injured in 50% of skateboarding accidents and the thumb was the most often injured joint in the skier. The highest incidence of traumatic injury to the upper extremity was found to occur in basketball and football, and "overuse" injuries occurring most frequently in baseball and tennis.[3]

Because of the significant impact that an injury to this region can have in disabling an athlete, the sports physical therapist must have an appreciation for the types of injuries that occur to the upper extremity, their management, and, most important, the rehabilitation considerations aimed at restoring function to permit safe return to competition.

This chapter describes the most common types of injuries that occur to the elbow, wrist, and hand. As the sports physical therapist is the primary audience of this text, specific implications regarding the protection, rehabilitation, and prevention of these injuries are discussed. Although medical management such as surgery, immobilization, and pharmacology are mentioned, these skills are within the domain of the physician rather than the physical therapist.

ANATOMY AND BIOMECHANICS

To understand the types of athletic injuries that occur to the elbow, wrist, and hand, anatomic and kinesiological function must be appreciated. The following description is intended to highlight the important anatomic and biomechanical considerations as they apply to athletic injury. For a complete review of the anatomy and function of the upper extremity, the reader is urged to consult an anatomy text.[4]

Elbow Osteology

The elbow joint comprises the articulation between the distal humerus and proximal ulna. The proximal forearm is a combination of two articulations—the proximal radioulnar joint and the humeroradial joint (Fig 20–1). The radial head, because of its concavity, articulates with the convex surface of the capitellum of the distal humerus. The proximal radioulnar joint is articulated via the annular ligament. The combination of the round radial head, and its articulation with the humerus and ulna, facilitates the proximal forearm to pivot and rotate, thereby performing pronation and supination (Fig 20–2).

The humerus articulates medially and laterally with the radius and ulna, respectively, via collateral ligaments. The medial or ulnar collateral ligament comprises three bands, two of which are functional and the other which is nonfunctional. The functional bands are the anterior and posterior oblique bands. The transverse band is the nonfunctional section of the medial collateral ligament. The anterior and posterior oblique bands originate on the medial epicondyle of the humerus and both insert onto the ulna, the anterior oblique on the medial aspect and the posterior oblique on the olecranon (Fig 20–3). Jobe and Nuber have noted that the anterior oblique portion of the medial collateral ligament is the prime medial stabilizer of the elbow and is implicated in the valgus stress injuries so often seen in throwing athletes.[5]

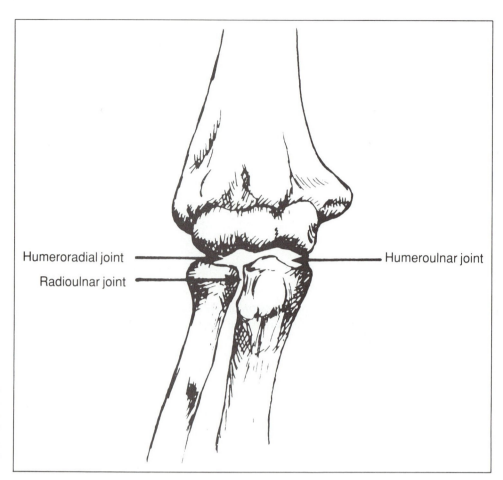

Humeroradial joint

Radioulnar joint

Humeroulnar joint

Figure 20-1. Anatomy of the elbow joint and its articulations. *(From Micheli LJ.* Pediatric and Adolescent Sports Medicine. *Boston, Mass: Little, Brown, and Co; 1984:64, with permission.)*

The lateral collateral ligament is infrequently involved in athletic injuries. It is composed of a thick collagenous band of connective tissue originating on the lateral humeral epicondyle extending across the lateral joint space and inserting onto the proximal head of the radius and the annular ligament.

Wrist and Hand Osteology

Because of their intimate relationship, the wrist and hand are considered as if they were a single functional unit. The distal radioulnar joint forms the beginning of the wrist complex. For simplicity in description, the radius is wider at its distal end than the ulna. The base, or proximal row of carpal bones, articulates with the radius and ulna via ligamentous connections and not bony contact. The important implication here is that if any ligamentous support is lost, the wrist can become unstable. There are two rows of carpal bones—proximal and distal. In the proximal row, moving medial to lateral, are the pisiform, triquetrum, lunate, and scaphoid, sometimes referred to as the navicular. The distal row consists of the hamate, capitate, trapezoid, and trapezium. The proximal and distal rows of carpal

bones articulate via interosseous ligaments and also direct bony contact (Fig 20-4). Culver describes support of the wrist dependent upon two main groups of ligaments: (1) the intracapsular ligaments and (2) the interosseous ligaments.[6] He states that the strongest stabilizer of the wrist is offered by palmar intracapsular ligaments, which are most often injured in "hyperextension" movements.

The carpometacarpal joints form the proximal ends of the fingers and beginning of the hand. The metacarpals attach to the carpal bones by small ligamentous articulations (Fig 20-5). The lumbrical tendons and collateral ligament support give these joints extreme stability; therefore dislocation is relatively uncommon. The metacarpalphalangeal joint of the thumb is the one joint quite commonly injured, particularly the ulnar collateral ligament. It attaches to the base of the proximal phalanx and distal portion of the scaphoid (Fig 20-6). Because of the lack of radial stability, this joint can easily dislocate and rupture the ulnar collateral ligament.

The phalanges articulate by collateral ligament support, medially and laterally. Proximal and distal

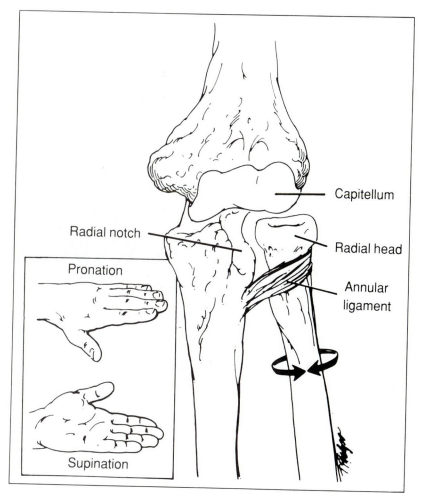

Figure 20-2. The proximal radioulnar joint.

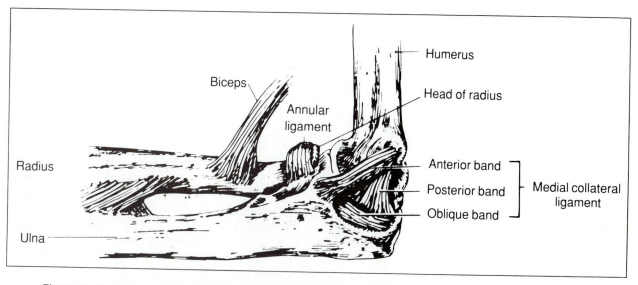

Figure 20-3. Anatomy of the medial collateral ligament of the elbow. *(From Roy S, Irvin R.* Sports Medicine Prevention, Evaluation, Management, and Rehabilitation. *Englewood, NJ: Prentice-Hall Inc; 1983:201, with permission.)*

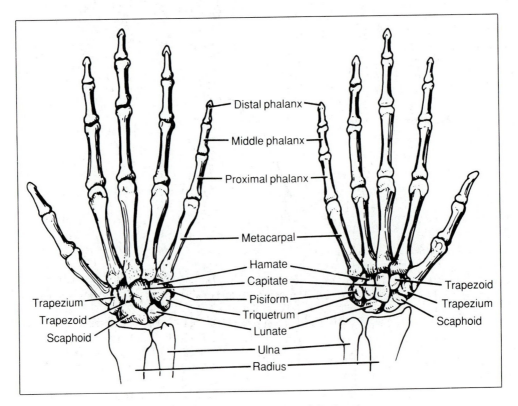

Figure 20-4. Bony anatomy of the hand.

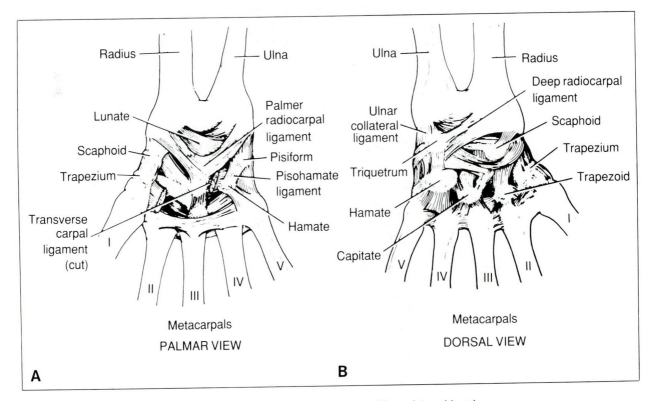

Figure 20-5. Ligamentous anatomy of the wrist and hand.

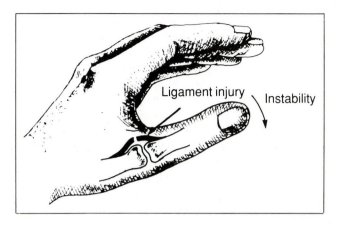

Figure 20-6. Metacarpalphalangeal joint injury of the thumb with rupture of the ulnar collateral ligament. (From Micheli L. Pediatric and Adolescent Sports Medicine. *Little, Brown, and Co; 1984:57, with permission.*)

support is offered via collateral ligaments, extensor tendon expansion, and flexor tendon articulation.

Soft Tissue Anatomy

Although a complete anatomic review of the elbow, wrist, and hand is beyond the scope of this chapter, there are certain anatomic structures that need to be mentioned to better appreciate the biomechanics of athletic activity and implication to injury.

The elbow joint is surrounded by a capsule in which the collateral ligaments blend. It offers stability to the humeroulnar and proximal radioulnar articulations. The biceps muscle attaches to the radial head, the triceps to the olecranon process, and the brachialis to the coronoid process of the ulna. Posteriorly, the olecranon bursa acts to reduce friction between the olecranon process and the skin. This structure is frequently injured in contusions of the posterior elbow. Coursing through the ulnar groove of the humerus just lateral to the medial humeral epicondyle is the ulnar nerve. Anteriorly, the important soft tissue structures lying in the antecubital space are the brachial artery, median nerve, and proximal forearm musculature. Deep to the forearm muscles are the radial nerve, pronator teres muscle, and posterior interosseous nerve. These structures are important because many nerve entrapment syndromes can occur in this region (Fig 20–7).

The wrist extensor common origin on the lateral humeral epicondyle lies in close proximity to the extensor carpi radialis longus and brevis origins. These structures are commonly involved with "tennis elbow syndrome." On the medial side, the pronator teres and wrist flexors are frequently injured during such activities as tennis, golf, and racketball.

Moving down the forearm into the hand, the flexors and extensors lead into their tendinous attachments to the distal radius, distal ulna, carpals, and phalanges.

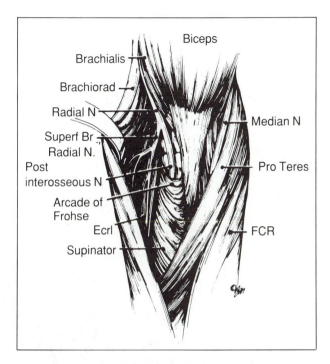

Figure 20-7. Anatomy of deep forearm structures. (*From Everson WW Jr. Entrapment and compression neuropathies. In: Green DP, ed.* Operative Hand Surgery. *Edinburgh: Churchill Livingstone, 1982:2, with permission.*)

On the volar surface of the wrist, the carpal tunnel is formed, in which the medial nerve, flexor tendons, radial artery, and ulnar artery lie directly under the volar carpal ligament. Thickening of the ligament, or injury to the flexor tendons can result in compression of the median nerve, referred to as carpal tunnel syndrome. This is a relatively uncommon entity in sports.

As previously mentioned, the hand consists of the carpal and metacarpal articulations. The most frequently injured bones of the hand are the scaphoid (or navicular) and the hamate, most often by a direct fall on an outstreched hand. An important anatomic arrangement is the position of the distal branches of the ulnar artery and nerve as they enter the hand and run around the hook of the hamate (Fig 20–8). These structures are frequently injured in cyclists who place pressure on their wrists when holding onto their handlebars. Conn et al called the frequent injury susceptibility to the ulnar artery and nerve in the hand the "hypothenar hammer syndrome," and they noted that baseball catchers and handball players are also vulnerable to this injury.[7]

The volar surface of the hand has a significant amount of anatomy that is frequently injured in sports. Superficially, the soft tissue is vulnerable to contusion, abrasion, and laceration. The thenar eminences can be injured in a fall, via direct contact, or by muscle overuse. These muscles perform a vital role in grasping objects (e.g., holding a bat or racket), and controlling fine

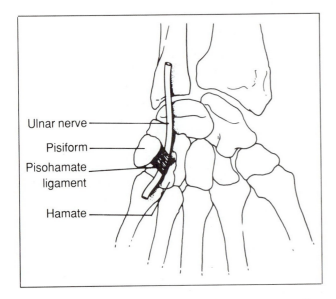

Figure 20–8. Anatomic arrangement of the ulnar nerve and artery in the wrist. *(From MaGee DJ.* Orthopedic Physical Assessment. *Philadelphia, Pa: W B Saunders Co; 1987:130, with permission.)*

coordinated hand function (e.g., throwing a baseball). Injury to these structures can render an athlete ineffective.

The fingers, particularly the proximal interphalangeal and distal interphalangeal joints, articulate via strong collateral ligaments and a synovial capsule. They are frequently sprained due to hyperextension forces that result in ligament tears, capsulitis, and restricted mobility. If not for the ligamentous support of these joints, they would be extremely unstable. Therefore, the fingers are susceptible to dislocation, fracture, and intraarticular damage.

TRAUMATIC INJURIES TO THE ELBOW

In sports requiring upper extremity function, the elbow must be able to move freely with little restriction. The speed at which the arm moves and its relative distance from the body leaves it "open" to trauma.

The most common injury to the elbow occurring from direct trauma is a contusion. These injuries occur most often in contact sports such as football and basketball and can range in severity from relatively minor to disabling. The olecranon process is susceptible to bruising because it is not protected by much soft tissue. The skin and the bursa are the only structures protecting the olecranon, therefore direct trauma to this region results in bursitis and concomitant periostitis (Fig 20–9). If the trauma is severe enough, fracture of the olecrannon can occur.

Other areas vulnerable to direct blunt trauma are the forearm, both the extensor and flexor masses. Direct contusion to muscle results in bleeding and disruption of capillary, venous, and arterial flow. When these regions are bruised, blood accumulates in these enclosed compartments. Abnormally high pressures with-

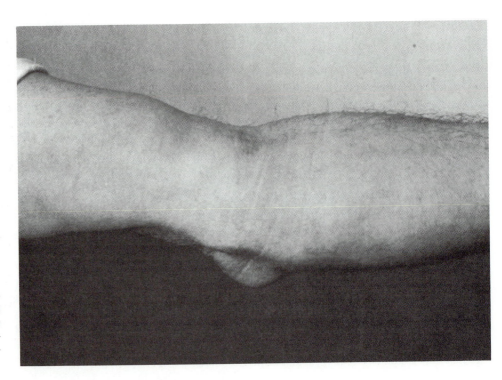

Figure 20–9. Olecranon bursitis. *(From* Athletic Training and Sports Medicine. *American Academy of Orthopedic Surgeons; 1984:214, with permission.)*

out reabsorption could result in a compartment syndrome that may be potentially limb threatening. In addition, if after the hematoma has formed, it has not been reabsorbed and dissolved, calcium deposition can occur in soft tissue, and a myositis ossificans ensues. Fortunately, the problems of a compartment syndrome and myositis ossificans in the forearm is relatively uncommon.

If managed correctly from the acute through the recovery phases, contusions result in little disability and full return to athletic function. Appropriate management of a contusion includes immediate application of ice and compression to control bleeding and initiate pain reduction. Intermittent ice application should be used for at least 24 to 36 hours, or as long as necessary to be sure that bleeding and cellular exudate is no longer accumulating in soft tissue. Other forms of ice and compression such as intermittent compression units and elastic bandages are also useful in the acute stage of a contusion.

Subacutely (36 to 48 hours after injury), gentle active motion and submaximal isometric exercise is instituted to facilitate dissemination of edema and to restore range of motion. These activities are performed through the athlete's painfree motion.

Once the bleeding has begun to reabsorb, contrast bath therapy (intermittent hot and cold soaks) is helpful to promote restoration of normal blood supply and removal of interstitial fluid accumulation. As the athlete's contusion is healing, other heat modalities can replace contrast bath therapy only if there is no evidence of an active inflammatory process. Throughout this time, submaximal range-limited isometrics can be replaced with isotonic and progressive isokinetic work. Once the range of motion is full and painfree, the athlete can be discontinued from modality treatment and concentrate on aggressive free weight and velocity spectrum strengthening. A protective pad should be constructed to protect the bruised region and dissipate force around the contusion. The athlete must wear the pad for all practice sessions and competition and should not remove the protective device unless authorized to do so by the physician, trainer, or sports physical therapist.

Humeroulnar Dislocation

The most common type of elbow dislocation occurs posteriorly, most often from a violent hyperextension force (Fig 20–10). These are relatively common in contact sports such as football and basketball, however, gymnasts are also susceptible because of the tremendous weight-bearing stresses placed on the elbow during floor events and vaulting. All elbow dislocations should be reduced by a physician. They can result in severe injury to the structures in the antecubital fossa, namely the median nerve and brachial artery. Frequently, fractures of the medial humeral epicondyle accompany posterior dislocation of the elbow.

Following reduction and immobilization, rehabilitation focuses on biceps strength, specifically the eccentric component to create a neuromuscular dynamic control to prevent excessive hyperextension stress. Once

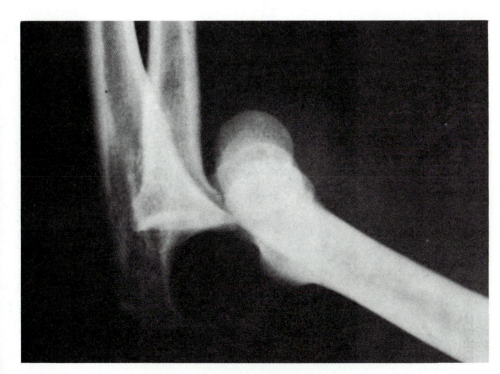

Figure 20–10. Posterior humeroulnar dislocation.

the athlete returns to competition, he or she is taped or wears a pad applied anteriorly on the forearm to prevent hyperextension.

Fractures

Fractures of the elbow are traumatic in origin and occur frequently in collision and contact sports. There are a multitude of combinations of elbow fractures, and all are amenable to physician intervention. Acute on-the-field management of a fracture or suspected fracture includes immediate application of ice, immobilization via splinting, and referral to an orthopedic surgeon. Following radiographic and other diagnostic studies, the physician may decide on immobilizing the fracture if it is stable, closed reduction, or surgical open reduction and internal fixation.

The most common regions of the elbow complex that are susceptible to fracture in the athlete are: olecranon process, humeral epicondyle, suprahumeral condyle, and radial head.

Fracture of the Olecranon Process.
The olecranon process is most often fractured by direct contact, either imparted to the elbow by another opponent (e.g., football helmet), or by hitting the elbow on a nonyielding surface such as the ground or a wall. The olecranon is

susceptible to external trauma because it is relatively unprotected and is not shielded by much soft tissue.

Avulsion fractures of the olecranon can occur from a violent contraction of the triceps muscle that can tear directly off of its attachment.[8] Fortunately, these types of fractures are not common because they are significantly more serious and require surgical restoration with prolonged rehabilitation.

Humeral Epicondylar Fracture.
The most common epicondylar fracture occurring as a result of athletic activity is associated with adolescent throwing athletes who develop an avulsion of the medial flexor muscle mass off of the medial epicondylar epiphysis (Fig 20–11). The mechanism of this injury is one of valgus stress overload, which is described in more detail later in this chapter. The point to keep in mind for the sports physical therapist is that medial elbow pain in the adolescent must be recognized early because the long-term implications of untreated epiphyseal lesions are potentially debilitating.

Supracondylar Fracture.
Another fracture common to the distal humerus and elbow joint is the supracondylar fracture. This injury occurs frequently in young adolescent athletes and is always a result of trauma. The significance of this injury is that a very complex

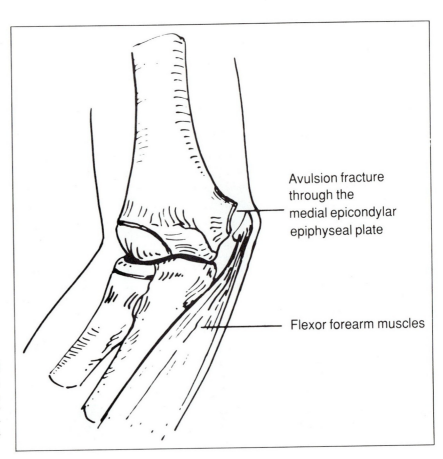

Avulsion fracture through the medial epicondylar epiphyseal plate

Flexor forearm muscles

Figure 20–11. Avulsion of the medial epicondylar epiphysis. *(From Roy S, Irvin R.* Sports Medicine Prevention, Evaluation, Management, and Rehabilitation. *Englewood Cliffs, NJ: Prentice Hall Inc; 1983:218, with permission.)*

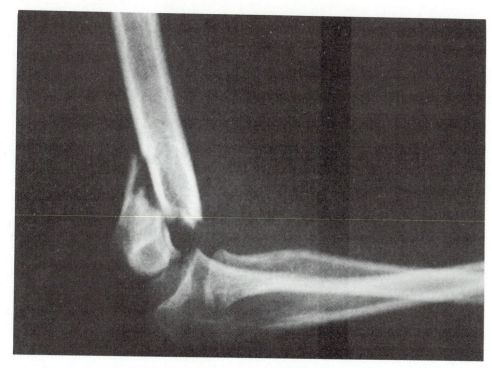

Figure 20-12. Supracondylar fracture.

anatomical network of nerves and blood vessels lie in the area of the suprahumeral condyles (Fig 20–12). These include the median and ulnar nerves and the brachial artery. Supracondylar fractures are potentially limb threatening if they result in vascular compromise of the upper extremity. It is therefore essential that these fractures be treated as absolute medical emergencies. Immediate splinting for protection and examination by a physician is the appropriate treatment for fractures of this type.

Radial Head Fracture. Fractures of the radial head and proximal radius occur quite frequently in sports. The mechanism of injury is one of indirect trauma where the athlete falls on an outstretched hand, force is transmitted up the arm, and the radial head is butted into the capitellum. Fractures can range in severity from nondisplaced, requiring immobilization for healing, to severely comminuted, which would require internal fixation or radial head arthroplasty. Clinical diagnosis of a radial head fracture includes direct pain to palpation and crepitus with forearm pronation and supination.

MICROTRAUMATIC SOFT TISSUE INJURIES TO THE ELBOW

By far the most common type of elbow injuries that will respond to the intervention of a sports physical therapist are microtraumatic. Athletic activities requiring repetitive muscular effort can result in overload, the so-called overuse syndromes. Overuse inflammatory injuries can be quite debilitating, and therefore accurate diagnosis of the nature of the problem, its biomechanical causes, and the appropriate mode of treatment is tantamount to successful restoration of function and return to painfree activity.

Throwing Injuries

Jobe and Nuber describe overuse as "when the body's physiologic ability to heal itself lags behind the microtrauma occurring with repetitive action."[5] Because the repetitive nature of throwing places tremendous soft tissue stresses on the elbow, overuse injuries are common. The adolescent and adult athlete are susceptible to elbow injury as a result of throwing, however, they are usually manifested as different clinical entities.

The act of throwing can be broken down into five phases: (1) windup, (2) cocking, (3) acceleration, (4) ball release, and (5) follow through. The acceleration phase of throwing is implicated as being the most stressful to the elbow joint. Jobe and Nuber describe the beginning of the acceleration phase as the time when the shoulder is in maximum external rotation, the trunk and shoulder are brought forward, and the forearm and hand lag behind.[5] The position of the elbow during this phase creates a valgus stress to the medial joint components (Fig 20–13). Repetitive valgus extension overload in the throwing athlete can result in a number of microtraumatic injuries. In the adolescent athlete, ulnar collateral ligament stress is the most common

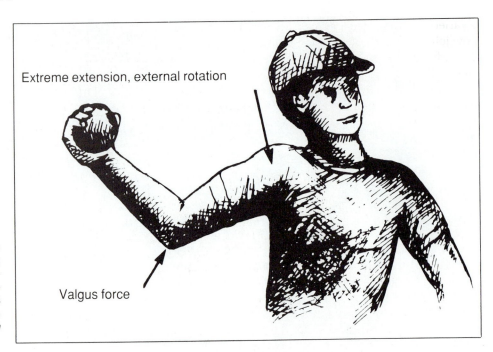

Extreme extension, external rotation

Valgus force

Figure 20-13. Beginning of the acceleration phase of throwing with valgus stress to the elbow. *(From Micheli L ed. Pediatric and Adolescent Sports Medicine. Boston, Mass: Little, Brown, and Co; 1984:71, with permission.)*

manifestation of overuse. Typically, these athletes complain of pain with throwing, ultimately progressing to the point where their elbow symptoms persist before, during, and after activity. Because of the attachment of the ulnar collateral ligament to the epiphysis of the medial humeral epicondyle, growth plate injuries are a most common finding. They need to be treated with rest, anti-inflammatory medications, and a progressively cautious return to throwing following complete remission of symptoms. Once the adolescent athlete has been medically cleared to return to throwing activity, he or she must be careful to avoid excessive stress to the elbow. Proper coaching must be implemented to ensure that correct throwing technique is employed. Common faults such as "opening up to early" where the arms lags behind the body during acceleration, and throwing curve balls with excessive forearm rotation must be addressed and corrected to avoid overuse stress. Of primary importance in the prevention of throwing injuries in the adolescent athlete is the number of pitches thrown per inning and during the span of a complete game. Repetitive pitching activity requires a synchronous firing of muscles in the lower extremities, trunk, and arm. For the distribution of muscular forces to be equal, form must be maintained through proper muscle strength, endurance, and flexibility. During the span of a baseball game, a pitcher will become fatigued, and ultimately, lose throwing control. This point of fatigue varies from individual to individual, in the young athlete, however, it is at this time that the arm, particularly the elbow, is quite vulnerable. It is therefore the coach's responsibility to watch the pitcher to detect signs of decreased performance and weakness. The athlete who is no longer throwing effectively should be re-

moved from the game, and adequate time (at least 2 days) allowed for recovery.

The adult elbow is susceptible to overuse injury, and this can be a result of valgus stress overload during the acceleration phase, or impact hyperextension stress during the follow-through phase after the ball has been released. In the younger adult, osteochondritis dissecans of the capitellum has been described by Brown et al, who felt that this injury was due to the valgus stress imparted to the elbow, leading to impingement between the radial head and capitellum.[9] Ulnar collateral ligament strain is the most common valgus stress injury in the adult pitcher. Jobe and Nuber describe four stages of ulnar collateral ligament injury: (1) edema; (2) scarring and disassociation of fibers; (3) calcification; and (4) ossification.[5] In the disassociation through ossificiation stages, ligament rupture may occur. Chronic valgus stress of the ulnar collateral ligament, hyperextension forces at the humeroulnar joint, and repetitive stress at the radioulnar articulation can also result in ossific bodies and reactive bone spur formation. When these changes take place as a result of chronic overuse, throwing a baseball is usually not possible without joint pain and swelling. Surgical removal of the spurs and ossicles is necessary for complete and painfree functional use of the elbow to be restored.

OTHER SOFT TISSUE INJURIES TO THE ELBOW

Racket sports, throwing, and other activities involving repetitive muscular effort and joint stress can result in

a variety of overuse phenomenon in and around the elbow joint. In tennis players, the most common malady of the forearm is lateral epicondylitis, or lateral tennis elbow. Gruchow and Pelltier[10] reported a 39.7% incidence of lateral tennis elbow in a study of recreational players. In a random sample of 200 players, Nirschl described a 50% ratio of players over the age of 30 who complained of lateral tennis elbow sometime during their career.[11]

Lateral Epicondylitis

Lateral epicondylitis has been described as an inflammation and local tearing of the common wrist extensor origin at the lateral humeral epicondyle.[12] Pain is usually isolated over the extensor carpi radialis brevis tendon, slightly distal to the lateral humeral epicondyle. Clinical symptoms are typically reproduced by resisted wrist extension, passive wrist flexion, and extreme passive forearm pronation. Treatment includes local application of ice, phonophoresis, passive stretching of the wrist extensors and pronators, and active strengthening of the wrist extensors (Figs 20–14 through 20–18). Other measures of treatment and prevention include the use of a counterforce brace (Fig 20–19), which has been advocated by Nirschl to alter the biomechanical stress of the extensor muscle origin, thereby minimizing frictional force between the extensor tendon origin and the lateral humeral epicondyle.[13] The tennis racket must be of proper grip width, and string tension should not exceed 50 lb for the reactional player. Measurement of grip width is determined by taking the length of the second palmar crease to the distal tip of the ring finger along the radial side (Fig 20–20). Maintenance of string tension and grip size prevent excessive impact stresses from being absorbed by the arm, and allow adequate

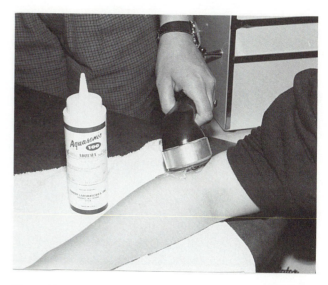

Figure 20-15. Treatment of tennis elbow with phonophoresis.

shock dissipation through the racket head. Finally, the tennis player must exhibit proper stroking form in their forehand and backhand. These techniques can be taught by an experienced coach, and should be encouraged so that each swing of the racket involves a smooth, rhythmic approach, minimizing the potential for overuse injury to occur.

Medial Epicondylitis

Medial epicondylitis occurs less frequently than lateral epicondylitis, presenting in athletes involved in racket sports and golf. Pain and inflammation are located on the tip of the medial humeral epicondyle at the origin

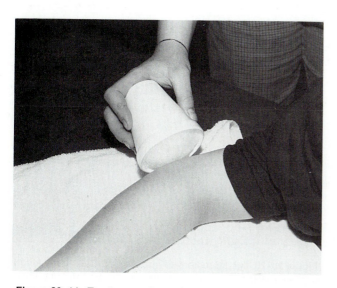

Figure 20-14. Treatment of tennis elbow with ice massage.

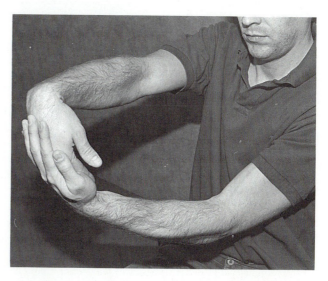

Figure 20-16. Passive stretching of the wrist extensors.

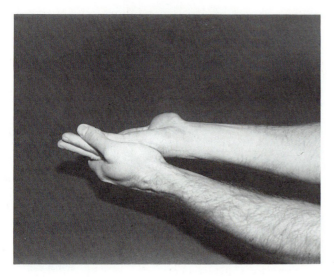

Figure 20–17. Passive stretching of the forearm pronators.

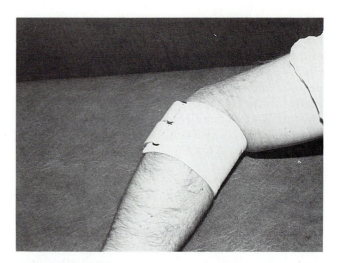

Figure 20–19. Counterforce brace for lateral epicondylitis.

of the flexor muscle mass, and also slightly distal to this region along the pronator teres muscle.[13] Treatment of this problem is the same for lateral tennis elbow, with emphasis on proper stroke technique, stetching of the forearm supinators and wrist flexors, and strengthening of the wrist flexor/pronator musculature.

Olecranon Bursitis

Olecranon bursitis frequently occurs as a result of direct trauma to the olecranon process. The "typical" golf ball appearance of the inflamed olecranon bursa makes the diagnosis relatively easy. These injuries usually respond favorably to ice, antiinflammatory medication, and

protective padding. Sometimes needle aspiration is necessary to remove synovial fluid that is not reabsorbing through the body's natural healing processess.

Biceps Tendon Strain

Biceps strain and rupture is associated with an extremely strong elbow flexion force, or, more commonly, a hyperextension force causing the biceps tendon to elongate and stretch. Injuries to the anterior joint capsule and posterior joint impingement can also occur with elbow joint hyperextension injuries.

Management of biceps tendon strain and hyperextension injuries involve immediate application of ice and compression. Protective mechanisms include compression sleeves and taping to limit elbow extension and permit soft tissue healing in a shortened position (Fig 20–21). Once adequate healing has taken place, the el-

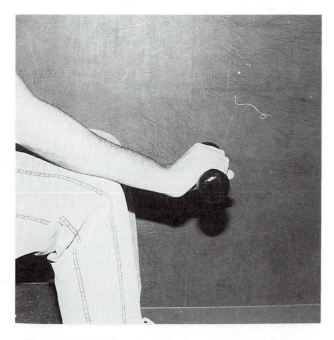

Figure 20–18. Active strengthening of the wrist extensors.

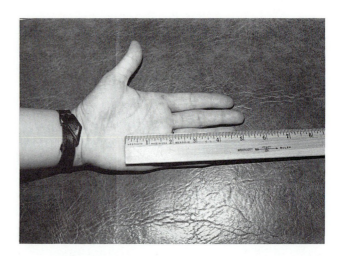

Figure 20–20. Measurement of grip width by taking the length of the second palmar crease to the distal tip of the ring finger along the radial side.

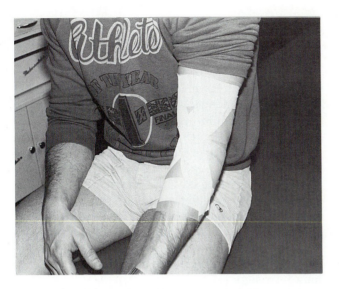

Figure 20-21. Taping the anterior elbow to limit hyperextension.

bow may be passively stretched to approach full extension, and protective splinting may be removed as long as symptoms do not persist. Strengthening emphasis is placed on early multiple angle isometric work of the biceps and supinators, progressing to isotonic and isokinetic muscular stress. Eccentric biceps strengthening is employed in an isotonic and isokinetic mode to create a neuromuscular barrier to hyperextension.

Ulnar Nerve Subluxation

The ulnar nerve lying posterior to the medial humeral epicondyle is quite superficial, and is susceptible to contusion in contact sports. In the throwing athlete, valgus stress overload can cause the ulnar nerve to stretch, and sometimes intermittently sublux. When the nerve subluxes, the athlete experiences posteromedial elbow pain, periodic sensations of tingling, burning, or even numbness into the medial half of the ring finger and entire little finger. Long-term ramifications of repetitive ulnar nerve trauma include atrophy of the hypothenar eminence with motor and sensory disturbance of all regions supplied by the ulnar nerve.

Treatment of ulnar nerve injury involves early recognition and avoidance of continued trauma. Anti-inflammatory medication, rest, and alteration of throwing technique are necessary to allow the nerve to heal and prevent further damage. In chronic cases, ulnar nerve transposition or cubital tunnel decompression have been advocated as surgical alternatives for long-term relief.[14]

Median Nerve Entrapment

Median nerve entrapment occurs most frequently in throwing athletes. The nerve is compressed at the proximal forearm and is referred to as the "pronator teres syndrome." Compression of the median nerve at the midforearm has been called the anterior interosseous syndrome, although this is a relatively uncommon phenomenon.

Typically, muscle hypertrophy from activities involving forceful gripping, repetitive forearm pronation, or direct trauma is what precipitates median nerve compression. Conservative treatment is recommended, including rest, anti-inflammatory medications, ultrasound, electric stimulation, and modification of athletic technique that may be causing symptoms. If conservative measures fail, surgical decompression of the median nerve has been advocated as an alternative.[14]

SPORTS PHYSICAL THERAPY MANAGEMENT OF ELBOW INJURIES

The sports physical therapist will be involved in the treatment and rehabilitation of injuries to the upper extremity from the point of immediate onset, through the recovery process until the athlete is ready to return to competition. It is therefore necessary that the therapist be adept at instituting on-the-field management and, once the injury has been appropriately diagnosed, be able to apply rehabilitative skills to facilitate strength, range of motion, and functional use of the injured extremity.

Soft Tissue Trauma

Initial management of all soft tissue injuries involves the immediate application of ice and compression. Once the injury has been diagnosed and the injured structures isolated, a protective pad, prophylactic taping, or some other form of restricted motion device must be applied to limit stress of the healing structure but allow painfree functional movement.

Protective Pads

Protective pads for soft tissue trauma should be designed to protect the injured area, and allow full function of noninjured structures. Materials can vary and should be light, compressible, and strong enough to dissipate impact stress. An example of a pad to protect against a forearm contusion is shown in Figure 20-22. This pad is made of foam that can cushion a blow to the extensor or flexor muscle mass. Other pads can be constructed out of more rigid material such as Orthoplast, which incorporates a "doughnut" surrounding the traumatized region and dissipates stress to the uninjured tissues.

An example of flexible casting whereby an injured structure is protected is a hyperextension taping technique shown in Fig 20-20. This type of strapping is designed to allow full flexion of the elbow and resist

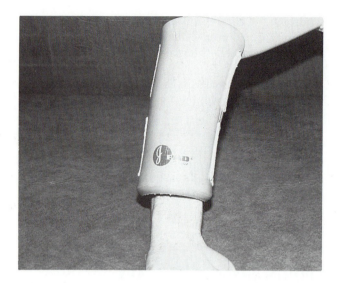

Figure 20–22. Forearm pad to protect against a contusion.

extension at approximately 20 degrees. With extension resisted, strain on the healing soft tissue is avoided and functional use of the elbow is ensured.

Protective counterforce bracing has been advocated by Nirschl and others as a means to reduce muscular forces when swinging a tennis racket (Fig 20–19).[11] Muscular support and biomechanical reduction in angular acceleration are two other advantages of using counterforce bracing in the symptomatic medial or lateral epicondylitis.

Other Rehabilitation Modalities

Traditional rehabilitation modalities assume an important role in the treatment of athletic elbow injuries. Ice

is an important anti-inflammatory and anesthetic modality that should be used whenever an inflammatory problem is present. Application of ice for 15 to 30 minutes has been shown to decrease the metabolic activity of an inflamed region, assist in removal of injurious metabolic by-products, and to decrease local pain.[15]

Other modalities such as ultrasound are useful in facilitating blood supply and nutrients, reducing local inflammation, breaking down scar tissue, and driving a medication to the injured site via phonophoresis to restore healing (Fig 20–15). Transcutaneous nerve stimulation is helpful to desensitize a region of pain via its endorphin-enhancing effects (Fig 20–23A). Electrical stimulation is another form of treatment that helps to decrease inflammation by increasing cellular permeability and also to facilitate an increase in isometric muscle strength (Fig 20–23B).

Exercise

The use of exercise in the rehabilitation of elbow injuries must be carefully implemented, judiciously prescribed, and correspond to the appropriate phase of the healing process. Exercise can take place in many forms, including passive stretching, isometric, isotonic, and isokinetic work. Each type has its merits and should be used in accordance with the type of injury, mode of treatment (surgical or nonsurgical) and ultimate goal of recovery.

Passive exercise can be of two types: (1) joint mobilization implemented by the therapist to restore physiological component mobility; and (2) passive stretching, which can be performed by the athletic patient as a means of increasing contractile and noncontractile tissue extensibility.

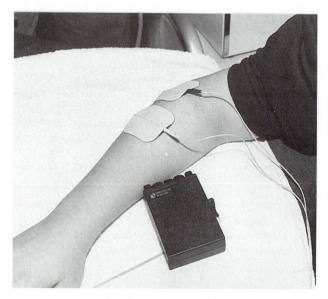

A

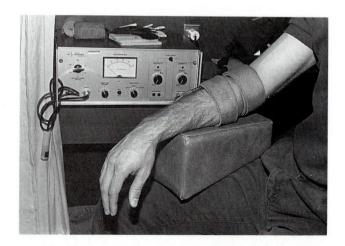

B

Figure 20–23. A. Application of transcutaneous electrical nerve stimulation to the elbow. **B.** Application of galvanic stimulation to the forearm.

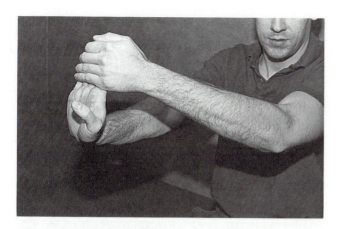

Figure 20-24. Stretching the wrist flexors.

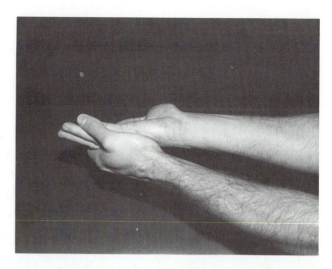

Figure 20-26. Stretching the forearm pronators.

Joint Mobilization

Joint mobilization techniques involve the passive restoration of physiological joint movement unable to be obtained by the patient. They are most frequently used after a joint has been immobilized following surgery or a traumatic injury. The reader is urged to consult other references for a complete and detailed description of mobilization principles and techniques.[16,17]

Passive Stretching

Passive stretching is advocated in the treatment and also prevention of soft tissue injuries (Figs 20-24 through 20-28). It is recommended that the following techniques be performed before, and after activity, and in the appropriate circumstance where a particular muscle group may be tight.

1. Avoid ballistic movements and hold each stretch for 10 to 15 seconds.
2. Each stretch should be performed before and after activity.
3. Each muscle group should be isolated.

4. Each stretch should be performed three to four times per session.

Strengthening Exercises

Once the ROM of the elbow has been restored, strengthening exercises can begin. Initially, isometric exercise is used through the painfree range of motion. The athlete can control the intensity of these exercises, thereby avoiding pain, and they can be performed at multiple angles through the available range of motion, providing a training effect at 5- to 10-degree intervals throughout the full range of motion. Each isometric contraction should be held for 4 to 8 seconds, relaxed slowly, and repeated six to eight times or until the athlete is fatigued (Figs 20-29 to 20-32A).

Isotonic Strength

Isotonic strengthening of the elbow is the next phase of active muscle conditioning (Figs 20-32B-E). Many

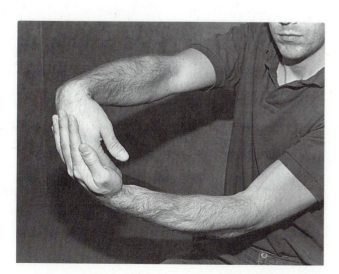

Figure 20-25. Stretching the wrist extensors.

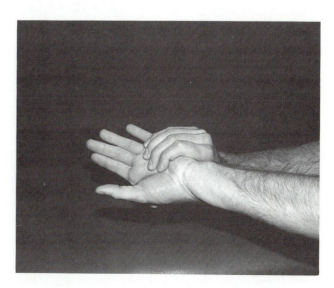

Figure 20-27. Stretching the forearm supinators.

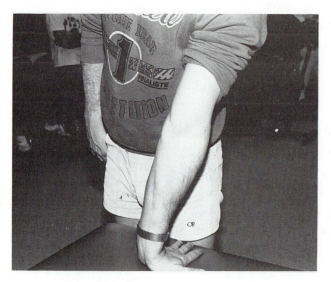

Figure 20–28. Stretching the elbow flexors.

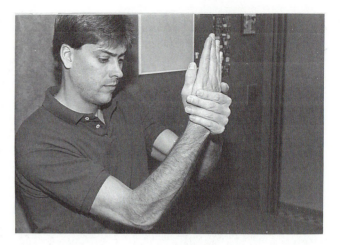

Figure 20–30. Manually resisted isometric strengthening of the elbow extensors.

variations of isotonic strength attainment have been described via the use of elastic tubing, free weights, Nautilus or Universal equipment, and a host of other resistance modalities. The goal behind isotonic strengthening is to provide muscular resistance throughout an available range of motion. Resistance should be adequate to provide muscular fatigue in a prescribed set of repetitions, depending on which training protocol is used. Muscle endurance can be trained isotonically by using resistance that is stressful enough to permit high repetition with low weight at a controlled speed.

Isokinetic Strength

Various forms of isokinetic equipment are currently available in the rehabilitation clinic. Controlled speed resistance is a valuable form of conditioning in that muscle can be strengthened at varying contractile velocities, thereby enhancing strength, power, and endurance. It has also been demonstrated that isokinetic

training is least stressful to joints and connective tissue because it is accommodating, and therefore the patient's effort, perception of pain, and weakness at certain points in their motion can result in an alteration of resistance, minimizing the chance of injury.

Recommendations regarding the method of isokinetic strengthening have been made by Davies.[18] For maximum benefit, the athlete should exercise isokinetically following this sequence (Fig 20–33):

Frequency	3 times per week
Velocity spectrum	30 degrees/sec increments
Time between reps	10–30 seconds
Number of reps	10–12 repetitions

RETURN TO COMPETITION

For virtually all sports medicine practitioners, the decision as to when it is safe to permit an athlete to resume

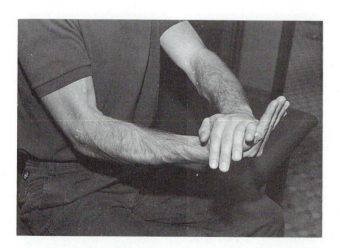

Figure 20–29. Manually resisted isometric strengthening of the elbow flexors.

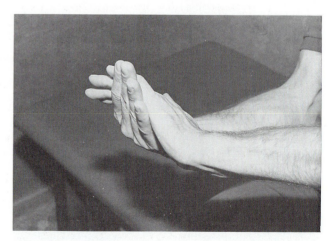

Figure 20–31. Manually resisted isometric strengthening of the wrist flexors.

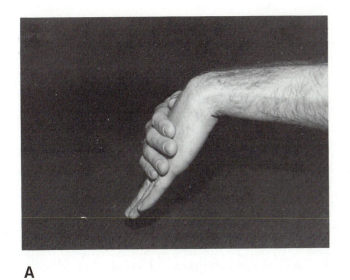

A

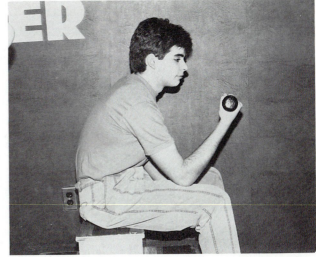

B

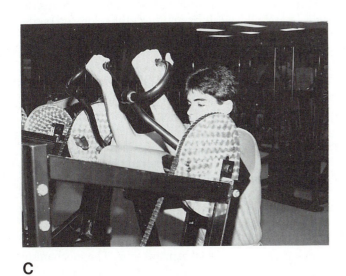

C

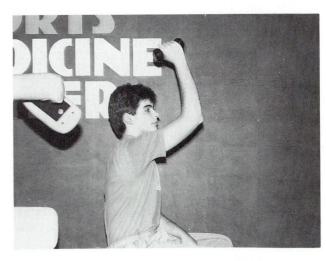

D

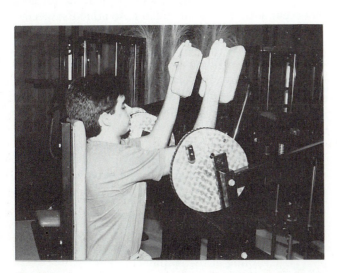

E

Figure 20-32. A. Manually resisted isometric strengthening of the wrist extensors. **B, C.** Isotonic strengthening of the elbow flexors—free weight and Nautilus. **D, E.** Isotonic strengthening of the elbow extensors—free weight and Nautilus.

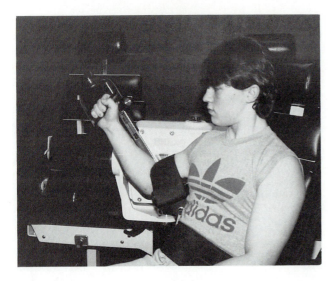

Figure 20-33. Isokinetic strengthening on the Biodex for elbow flexion and extension.

activity is a difficult one. The aforementioned treatment modalities are the prelude for restoration of normal joint function. The following is a list of "guidelines" that can serve as a protocol to determine whether it is safe to allow the athlete to begin sports competition:

1. Adequate demonstration with physician consultation that all structures have totally healed. This includes documentation by radiographs, magnetic imaging, or other studies necessary to confirm normal anatomic continuity and total healing
2. No visual evidence of soft tissue inflammation, swelling, or ecchymosis
3. Restoration of painfree normal passive joint mobility, including noncontractile and contractile elements
4. Full strength as tested manually, isokinetically, and functionally

Once the athlete has satisfied the above criteria, he or she should be permitted to gradually resume athletic activity. It is important, however, to remind patients that they must first work on functionally progressive skills to retrain the elbow neuromuscularly prior to attempting competition. For example, a tennis player must first relearn proper forehand technique and perform ground strokes for no more than 5 or 10 minutes at a time. If this activity is painless, he or she can then be coached into working on the backhand, and finally, serving technique. Usually these functionally progressive activities create a "time lag" of 7 to 10 days after discontinuance from physical therapy to a competitive event. Communication among the sports physical therapist, athlete, and coach is necessary to ensure that a

smooth transition takes place from the rehabilitation clinic to the athletic arena. Athletes who resume competition too early without adequate functional progression can suffer a recurrence of their problem, returning them to the rehabilitation stage and delaying their return to athletic activity.

INJURIES TO THE WRIST AND HAND

Because the hand is held out in front of most athletes during sports activity, it is quite susceptible to injury. According to Dobyns, 90% or more of hand and wrist injuries occur with the wrist in an extended position as it attempts to break the body's momentum during a fall.[19] A result of this mechanism is increased dorsal compression and shear forces, with concomitant tensile stress at the volar surface. Hand and wrist injuries can also occur from other mechanisms, including direct trauma. Examples include being struck by a projectile (e.g., baseball), a fall by another athlete or step on the hand, or hyperextension during an attempt at catching a ball, such as in basketball.

The wrist and hand complex is a relatively small anatomic region and has a tendency to be minimized regarding the severity of injury potential. The intricacy of its function, and importance of its use, however, have resulted in a very specialized field of study for the physician and sports physical therapist. This section describes the most common injuries to the wrist and hand that the sports physical therapist will see on the athletic field and the rehabilitation clinic.

Colles Fracture

A colles fracture is a fracture of the distal radius in which there is posterior displacement. The mechanism of injury typically results from attempting to break a fall on an outstretched hand. This is a relatively common type of injury in the general population but does not occur as frequently in athletes. An athlete suspected of having a colles fracture would exhibit visual deformity of the wrist with extreme pain on the distal radius. Treatment of a colles fracture includes radiographic studies to confirm the diagnosis, reduction (closed or open), and cast immobilization. Injuries to the distal radius in the young adolescent athlete who falls on an outstretched hand, or whose wrist is "jammed" into forced dorsiflexion include displacement of the distal radial epiphysis. Salter and Harris have classified epiphyseal injuries according to five levels of severity:[20]

1. Separation of the epiphysis
2. Fracture separation of the epiphysis
3. Fracture of part of the epiphysis
4. Fracture of the epiphysis and metaphysis
5. Crushing of the epiphyseal plate

Any injury to the adolescent's wrist resulting in dorsal pain or visual deformity should be presumed to be an epiphyseal fracture unless ruled out by a physician. Injuries to the growth plate of the distal radius respond well to immobilization, followed by progressive ROM, stretching, and strengthening exercises.

Scaphoid Fracture

The scaphoid, or navicular, bone crosses both the proximal and distal carpal rows. Kuland[21] states that the most vulnerable portion of the scaphoid lies adjacent to the styloid tip of the radius. Because the scaphoid is most often injured during a fall on an outstretched hand, the bone is forced to butt up against the styloid process of the radius and frequently fractures. Symptoms of a scaphoid fracture include a classic history of the above-described mechanism. The athlete has pain to palpation over the anatomic snuff box, and also pain with making a fist (Fig 20–34). Radiographs are frequently negative, even in the case of a fracture, but it is recommended that all athletes with the above history and symptoms be immediately casted. X-rays should be taken approximately 2 weeks after the injury to assess the status of the fracture.

Injuries to the proximal portion of the scaphoid do not heal quickly because the blood supply to this region is poor. Improper treatment or late diagnosis of a scaphoid fracture can result in a nonunion or avascular necrosis.

Following demonstration of adequate healing, the cast is removed and a protective splint can be constructed by the sports physical therapist to permit the athlete to return to competition while being adequately protected against further injury.

Hamate Fracture

Fracture of the hook of the hamate can occur from a fall on an outstretched hand, but occurs more frequently from a violent contraction of the flexor carpi ulnaris that courses through the hook along the lateral side. Activities involving a strong grip such as holding a racket or club can also result in a fractured hamate. If the compression force between the base of the wrist and handle is significant enough, a fracture results and pain is noted directly over its anatomical site. Cast immobilization is necessary to facilitate adequate healing, and if a non-union occurs, some authors advocate surgical removal of the hook of the hamate.[14]

Fracture Dislocation of the Carpometacarpal Joint of the Thumb— Bennett's Fracture

Injuries to the carpometacarpal joint of the thumb results in a frequent occurrence of fracture dislocations, the so-called Bennett's fracture. Wagner describes the Bennett's fracture dislocation as an intra-articular fracture of the carpometacarpal joint of the thumb in which the metacarpal shaft fragment displaces radially and proximally.[22]

The mechanism of injury in a fracture dislocation of the carpometacarpal joint of the thumb is usually an axial or violent impact force to the thumb. Management includes closed reduction of the dislocation, and, if stability is not maintained, open surgical reduction is sometimes necessary.

Metacarpal Fractures

Fractures to the metacarpals of the hand are relatively frequent and most often occur to the midshaft portion

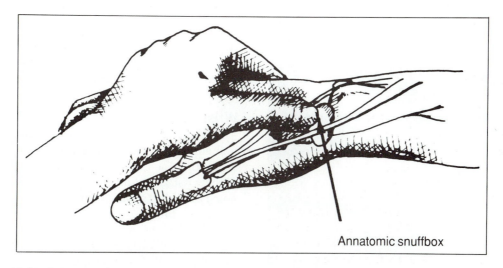

Annatomic snuffbox

Figure 20–34. Palpation of the navicular bone in the anatomical snuffbox to detect a fracture. *(From Micheli L, ed. Pediatric and Adolescent Sports Medicine. Boston, Mass: Little, Brown, and Co; 1984:64, with permission.)*

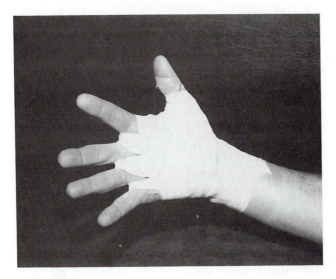

Figure 20-35. Prophylactic taping to prevent a boxer's fracture.

of the bone. A "boxer's" fracture is characterized by a break in the metacarpal neck when a closed fist displaces impact force through the metacarpophalangeal joint into the metacarpal. Boxer's fractures occur most frequently to the second and third metacarpals and respond favorably to closed reduction with the metacarpophalangeal joint in flexion. Prophylactically, taping of the hand is helpful to prevent these injuries (Fig 20–35).

Protective pads can be constructed for athletes with metacarpal fractures who are involved in contact sports, as long as the fracture is stable (Fig 20–36). These pads help to protect the healing fracture site and permit competition by dissipating impact stress and holding the fracture in a functional position.

Phalangeal Fractures

Fractures can and do occur to the proximal, middle, and distal phalanges of the fingers. Any injury to these

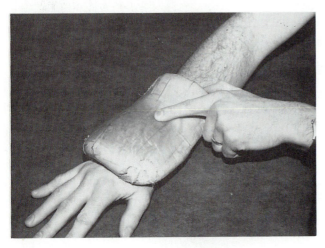

Figure 20-36. Protective pad for a metacarpal fracture.

structures should be treated as a fracture until ruled out by x-ray. Immediate treatment involves immobilization with a splint, buddy taping to the adjacent finger, and application of ice. Referral to a physician is necessary to determine the need for reduction and immobilization.

OTHER COMMON ATHLETIC WRIST AND HAND INJURIES

Avulsion of the Ulnar Collateral Ligament of the Thumb—"Gamekeeper's Thumb"

Forced abduction of the thumb results in a sprain to the ulnar collateral ligament, and the severity of this injury can range from a slight tear to an avulsion and dislocation of the metacarpophalangeal joint. Situations in which this injury has been associated include skiers who fall on their ski pole, baseball players who slide head first into a base with their arms extended outward, soccer goalies catching a ball, and hockey players involved in a fight where their thumb gets caught in an opponent's jersey (Fig 20–37).

Management of gamekeeper's thumb depends on the severity of tearing of the ulnar collateral ligament. Minor sprains without joint instability will heal if hyperabduction stress to the metacarpophalangeal joint of the thumb is avoided. Various strapping techniques including a "pancake" taping and a standard thumb spica with a strip between the thumb and index finger which helps to prevent abduction (Fig 20–38). A thumb spica splint is also useful in these injuries to shorten the ulnar collateral ligament and place it in an optimal position for healing (Fig 20–39).

Severe ulnar collateral ligament ruptures or avulsion fractures require surgical repair and subsequent immobilization to restore stability to the metacarpophalangeal joint. Following removal of the cast, the thumb is splinted with a thumb spica and the athlete is permitted to initiate strengthening of the hand and progressive athletic activity.

Wrist "Sprain"

An athlete who stretches his or her wrist beyond its normal connective tissue extensibility can tear ligaments supporting the radial, ulnar, dorsal, or volar segments of the wrist. Wrist injuries however, are often misdiagnosed as "only a sprain," when the actual severity of the problem is far worse. There are many small intercarpal ligaments in the wrist that, when torn, create pain, swelling, and variations of carpal instability that can prolong an athlete's symptoms. Healing is delayed in these types of injuries, creating a frustrating time for the athlete, sports physical therapist, and physician. Therefore, a word of caution is offered to all clinicians

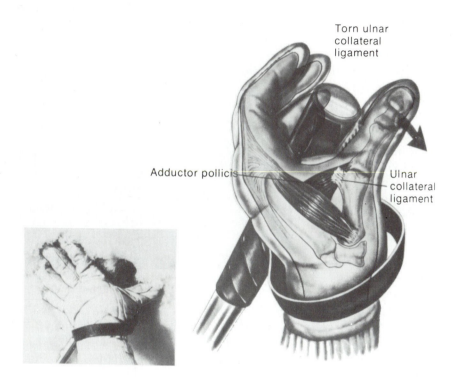

Torn ulnar
collateral
ligament

Adductor pollicis

Ulnar
collateral
ligament

Figure 20-37. Rupture of the ulnar collateral ligament of the thumb by falling on a ski pole. *(From Juland DN.* The Injured Athlete. *Philadelphia, Pa: J B Lippincott Co; 1982:312, with permission.)*

who deal with athletes susceptible to wrist injuries: "Beware of the sprain!" Wrist injuries can be quite complex, and before rehabilitation is instituted, the athlete must be examined by a hand specialist to confirm the diagnosis. It is surprising in actuality how few wrist "sprains" truly exist.

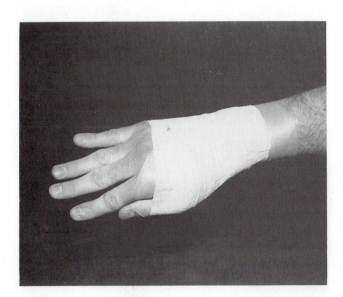

Figure 20-38. "Pancake" taping to prevent thumb abduction.

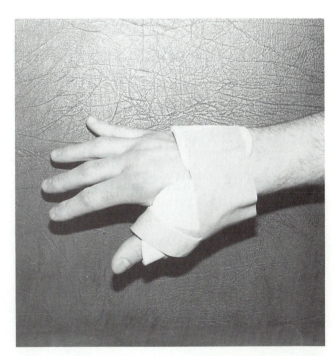

Figure 20-39. Thumb spica splint.

Dislocations and Collateral Ligament Sprains of the Proximal Interphalangeal Joint

Hyperextension forces to the fingers can result in dorsal displacement of the middle phalanx, with possible rupture of the volar plate. These injuries are quite common and must be reduced by a physician. Once reduced, the joint is immobilized in 20 to 30 degrees of flexion for 2 to 3 weeks.[22] Following removal of the splint, the injured finger is buddy taped to the adjacent finger and the athlete is permitted to return to activity (Fig 20–40). Volar plate injuries can result in flexion contractures, swan neck deformity, or boutonniere deformity if not properly treated and recognized early (Fig 20–41). Referral to a hand specialist is indicated in the event of this complication to prevent deformity.

Collateral Ligament Injuries

Injuries to the collateral ligaments of the proximal interphalangeal joint occur with a hyperextension and lateral force that usually results in rupture on the lateral side. If a partial rupture exists, there will be remaining joint stability; therefore splinting and buddy taping will be all that is necessary to facilitate healing. Complete ruptures of the collateral ligaments result in angular deformity with joint instability. In addition, volar plate rupture and avulsion fractures of the proximal and middle phalanges may occur.

Depending on the degree of rupture, immobilization for 4 to 6 weeks followed by active and passive range of motion is the treatment of choice. Complete ruptures require surgical repair, immobilization, and gradual progressive range of motion.

Mallet Finger

Mallet finger is the term used to describe a rupture of the extensor tendon attachment to the distal phalanx. Mechanically, it occurs in sports where an athlete is at-

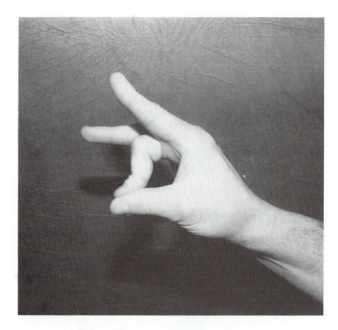

Figure 20–41. Boutonniere deformity.

tempting to catch a ball and longitudinal force is placed on the tip of the finger before it has the time to close. The extensor tendon ruptures, and the athlete loses the ability to actively extend the finger (Fig 20–42). Acute management includes a stack splint to keep the distal interphalangeal joint in full extension. This can be constructed from a tongue blade or any other material stable enough to immobilize the affected joint until it can be x-rayed (Figs 20–43 & 20–44). Sometimes, the extensor tendon may avulse a piece of

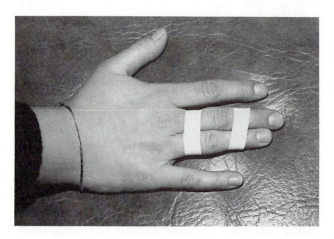

Figure 20–40. "Buddy taping" of the fingers following collateral ligament injury.

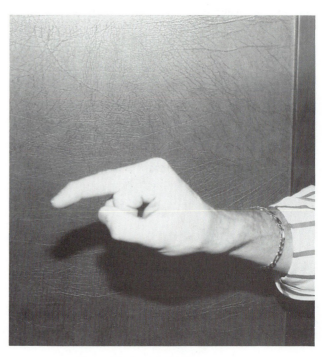

Figure 20–42. Mallet finger.

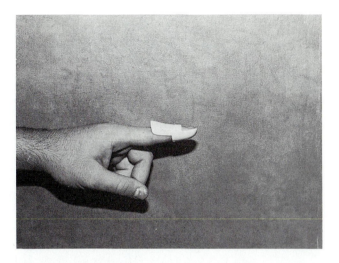

Figure 20-43. Plastic stack splint for mallet finger.

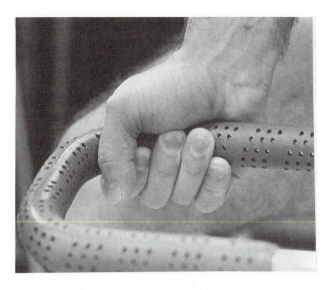

Figure 20-45. Ulnar nerve compression at the wrist from riding a bicycle. *(From Kuland DN. The Injured Athlete. Philadelphia, Pa: J B Lippincott Co; 1982:311, with permission.)*

bone off of the distal phalanx. This injury would require surgical pinning of the avulsed fragment, with splinting in full extension for 6 to 8 weeks.

Ulnar Nerve Compression

In sports such as cycling, ulnar nerve compression can occur in the hand at Guyons canal, lateral to the hook of the hamate. The hand is placed in a position where the wrist is extended and direct pressure is placed on the ulnar nerve (Fig 20–45).

Symptoms of ulnar nerve compression, or "handlebar palsy," include numbness of the ulnar half of the ring finger, little finger, and weakness of the hypothenar eminence. Treatment of this problem involves padding the handlebars on the bicycle, wearing gloves, and altering hand position when riding.

Subungual Hematoma

Trauma to the distal finger and nail can result in blood accumulation under the nail bed, which creates an ex-

treme amount of pressure and is quite painful. The hematoma must be aspirated to alleviate pressure and can be performed by rotating a sterile wide gauge needle into the nail to create a hole for the blood to escape (Fig 20–46). Following aspiration, the nail should be cleaned with betadine or hydrogen peroxide. Taping of the nail bed is helpful to prevent further subungual friction and allow the athlete to regain pain-free use of the finger.

Ganglion Cysts

Outpouching of the synovial membrane on the dorsum of the wrist can occur in the athlete who sustains direct trauma to the area or one who has a more complicated

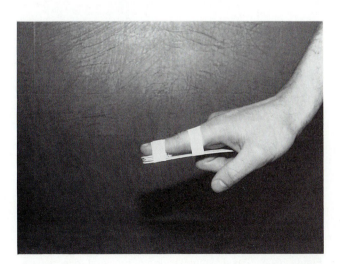

Figure 20-44. Stack splint constructed from a tongue blade.

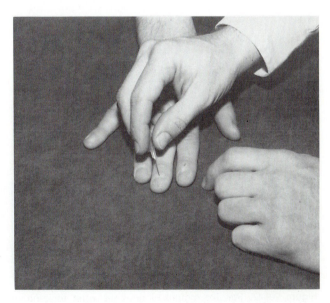

Figure 20-46. Aspiration of a subungual hematoma.

injury to the carpus. Ganglion cysts are usually benign and respond to aspiration and anti-inflammatory medication. Persistent swelling and pain may require surgical excision of the cyst and exploration of the wrist to repair soft tissue damage.

REHABILITATION OF WRIST AND HAND INJURIES

Regardless of the type of injury to the wrist or hand, rehabilitation principles remain relatively constant. Although the aforementioned injuries can be complex and may require forms of treatment ranging from nonsurgical to surgical intervention, the goals behind a rehabilitation program are as follows:

1. Restoration of normal range of motion
2. Restoration of strength
3. Return of functional use of the wrist and hand
4. Protection against further injury

Modalities for attaining the above goals vary and many combinations of stretching, strengthening, and mobilization are effective at facilitating an athlete's return to activity.

Range of Movement

After an injury has healed following immobilization, normal physiological movement of the wrist and fingers can be restored via the implementation of joint mobilization (Figs 20–47 through 20–51). These techniques are graded and progressively applied by the clinician to restore component mobility to the many joints of the wrist and hand.

Following the attainment of physiological compo-

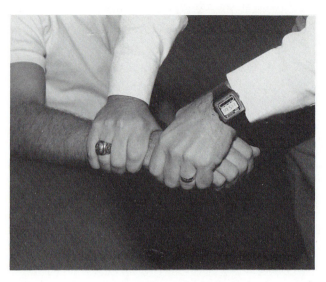

Figure 20–48. Passive mobilization of the wrist to improve extension.

nent mobility, a passive stretching program can be initiated. Each stretch should be performed before and after exercise and must be done statically. The stretch should be held for 10 seconds and repeated three to four times (Figs 20–17, 20–24, 20–25, 20–52).

Strengthening Program

A strengthening program for the wrist and hand should include wrist flexion and extension, forearm pronation and supination, finger flexion and extension, finger abduction, and coordination skills.

Rules for isotonic and isokinetic strength have been described in the previous section on the elbow. Examples of a strengthening routine for the wrist and hand are given in Figs 20–53 through 20–60.

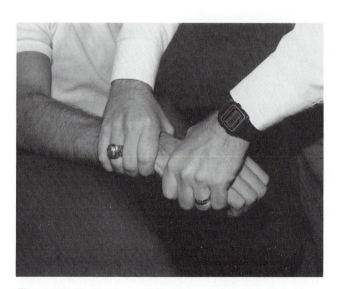

Figure 20–47. Passive mobilization of the wrist to improve flexion.

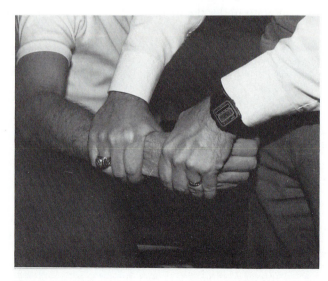

Figure 20–49. Passive mobilization of the wrist to increase radial deviation.

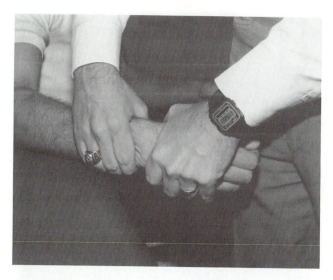

Figure 20-50. Passive mobilization of the wrist to increase radial deviation.

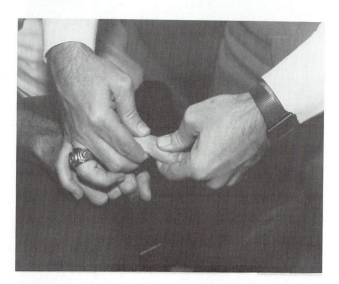

Figure 20-51. Passive mobilization of the proximal interphalangeal joint.

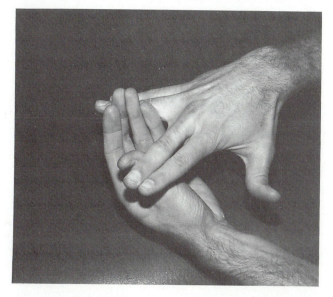

Figure 20-52. Stretching the finger adductors.

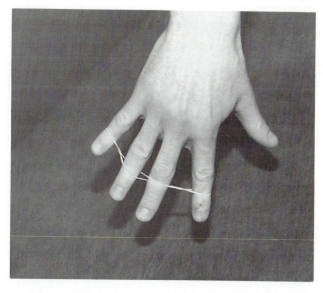

Figure 20-53. Strengthening of the finger abductors using a rubber band.

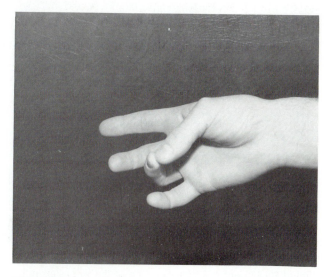

Figure 20-54. Opposition of the thumb with fingers is an excellent coordination exercise.

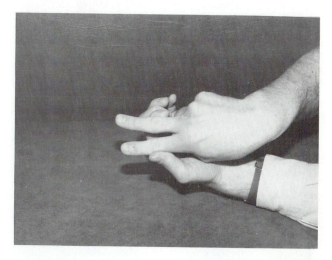

Figure 20-55. Manually resisted finger abduction strengthening.

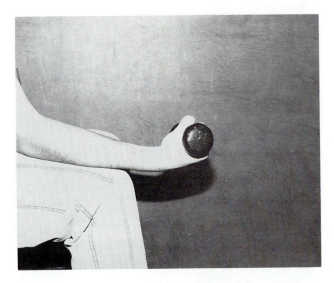

Figure 20-56. Isotonic resisted strengthening of the wrist flexors.

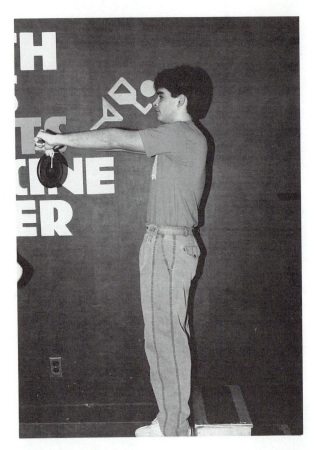

Figure 20-59. Isotonic resistance of the wrist extensors (alternative technique).

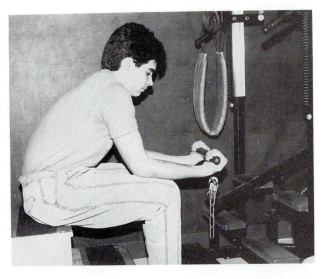

Figure 20-57. Isotonic strengthening of the wrist flexors (alternative technique).

Protection

Many techniques have been devised for taping, padding, and supporting the wrist and hand. Unfortunately, because the nature of athletic activity requires hand motion and dexterity, if the extremity is supported too rigidly, it could be nonfunctional. Care must therefore be taken to restrict the motion that has to be controlled while retaining functional mobility of non-affected segments.

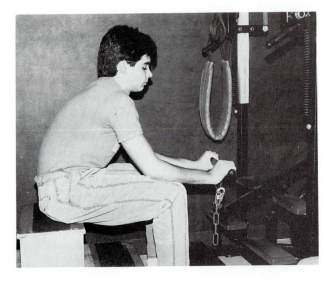

Figure 20-58. Isotonic strengthening of the wrist extensors.

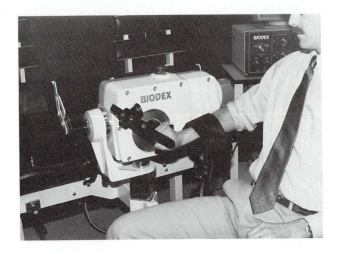

Figure 20-60. Isokinetic strengthening of the wrist flexors and extensors.

SUMMARY

The treatment of elbow, wrist, and hand injuries in the athlete runs the gamut from acute on-the-field management to functional rehabilitation. The sports physical therapist must have the knowledge of the types of injuries that athletes sustain, their biomechanical causes, and the mechanics of particular activities, so that appropriate treatment can be implemented. A close working relationship must exist between the therapist and physician so that rehabilitation of the athlete will complement medical intervention. Combining academic knowledge of functional anatomy and clinical skills will ensure that the injured athlete is not only treated appropriately but is placed on a program designed to facilitate safe and expeditious return to sports activity with a minimal risk of reinjury.

REFERENCES

1. Zaricazny B, Shattuck LJ, Mast TA. Sports related injuries in school-aged children. *Am J Sports Med.* 1980; 8:318–324.
2. Ho PK, Dellon Al, Wilgis EF. True aneurysms of the hand resulting from athletic injury. *Am J Sports Med.* 1985; 13:136–138.
3. McCue FC, Baugher WH, Juland DN, et al. Hand and wrist injuries in the athlete. *Am J Sports Med.* 1979; 7:275–286.
4. *Gray's Anatomy.*: Philadelphia, Pa: Lea & Febiger; 1975.
5. Jobe FW, Nuber G. Throwing injuries of the elbow. *Clin Sports Med.* 1986; 5:621–636.
6. Culver JE. Instabilities of the wrist. *Clin Sports Med.* 1986; 5:725–740.
7. Conn J, Bargan JJ, Bell JL, et al. Hypothenar hammer syndrome: Post-traumatic digital ischemia. *Surgery.* 1970; 68:1122–1128.
8. O'Donoghue D. *Treatment of Injuries to Athletes.* Philadelphia, Pa: W B Saunders; 1976: 269–271.
9. Brown R, Balazina ME, Kerlan RK, et al. Osteochondritis of the capitellum. *Am J Sports Med.* 1974; 2:27–46.
10. Gruchow HW, Pelltier D. An epidemiologic study of tennis elbow: Incidence, recurrence, and effectiveness of prevention strategies. *Am J Sports Med.* 1979; 7:234–238.
11. Nirschl RP. Tennis elbow. *Orthop Clin North Am.* 1973; 4:787.
12. Bernhang AM. The many causes of tennis elbow. *NY State J Med.* 1979; 79:1363–1366.
13. Nirschl RP. Soft tissue injuries about the elbow. *Clin Sports Med.* 1986; 5:637–652.
14. Cabrera JM, McCue FC. Non-osseous athletic injuries of the elbow, forearm, and hand. *Clin Sports Med.* 1986; 5:681–700.
15. Klafs CE, Arnheim DD. *Modern Principles of Athletic Training.* St. Louis, Mo: C V Mosby Co; 1977: 183–184.
16. Gould J, Davies G. *Orthopedic and Sports Physical Therapy.* St. Louis, Mo: C V Mosby Co; 1985:437–496.
17. Kaltenborn F. *Mobilization of the Extremity Joints.* Olaf Norlis Bokhandel: 1980.
18. Davies GJ. *A Compendium of Isokinetics in Clinical Usage and Rehabilitation Techniques.* 3rd ed. Onalaska, Wisc: S & S Publications; 1987.
19. Dobyns JH. Ligament injuries about the wrist. *American Academy of Orthopaedic Surgeons Symposium on Upper Extremity Injuries in Athletes.* St. Louis, Mo: C V Mosby Co; 1986; 134–141.
20. Salter RB, Harris WR. Injuries involving the epiphyseal plate. *J Bone Joint Surg.* 1963; 45:587.
21. Kuland D. *The Injured Athlete.* Philadelphia, Pa: J B Lippincott Co; 1982: 295–327.
22. Wagner CJ. Method of treatment of Bennett's fracture dislocation. *Am J Surg.* 1950; 80:230.

21 The Hip and Pelvis

John A. Romero

INTRODUCTION

The hip and pelvis play a most important role during the intricate and powerful movement patterns used in sports. Uniquely designed for the transference of shock and weight-bearing forces from the lower extremity kinetic chain to the spine, the hip and pelvis also provide the attachment of the prime movers most important for running, jumping, and cutting movements.

The Hip Joint

Each hip ball and socket joint includes a femoral head component fitting deeply into the acetabulum, deepened by a cartilaginous labrum. The hip joint's 3 degrees of freedom allow the positions necessary for activities of daily living and sports as well as the smooth translation of lower extremity movement. This mobility, however, reduces stability, which could have been provided by more restrictive bony articulation.

Muscular stability is essential for stabilization of all movements except dislocation.[1] The strong ligamentous system serves as a backup for the muscular system providing both movement restriction and stabilization.

In the kinetic chain, forces that occur upon ground contact are transferred through the foot and ankle and up the lower extremity into the pelvis through the hip socket. How the lower extremity kinetic chain reacts to these forces dictates the type and amount of force that ultimately travels to the hip. Excessive pronation, limb length differences, and abnormal lower extremity alignment all contribute to excessive force production, which the hip joint must absorb and direct through the rest of the body.

Most common injuries about the hip are sprains, strains, and contusions, followed by stress fractures, avulsion fractures, and congenital problems. Other fractures as well as hip dislocations are relatively rare. The adolescent athlete is more predisposed to hip problems involving sprains and strains due to poor muscular support, epiphyseal plate vulnerability, and Legg–Calve–Perthes disease.

This chapter reviews the anatomy, biomechanics, examination, and rehabilitation of selected hip and pelvic girdle disorders and injuries. Also addressed are the relationship of the lumbar spine, sacrum, and pelvis to the kinetic chain.

THE PELVIS AND SACRUM

The functional pelvis includes two ilia, the sacrum, and the fifth lumbar vertebrae. The bony ring of the pelvis includes the two separate ilia joined at the symphysis pubis and sacrum by strong ligamentous structures. The sacroiliac joints also have some muscular stabilization as well as a bony configuration that enhances stability and guides movement. The L5–S1 joint is the universal joint between the spine and lower body due to the attachments to the pelvis of the iliolumbar ligaments, the multifidi, and sacrospinalis musculature and its articulation to the sacrum through the facet joints and intervertebral disc. The pelvis provides the attachment of many of the powerhouse muscles which are used in locomotion and sports movements. The pelvis must also provide stability from which the prime movers can operate and distribute shock efficiently from the lower extremities to the spine. A secondary function of the pelvis is to protect the viscera, including the reproductive organs, bladder, and rectum as well as the nervous and circulatory systems.

Injuries to the pelvis and sacrum are usually sprains and strains; however, sacroiliac joint dysfunction is not uncommon, especially with female athletes and adolescents who have a much more pliable sacroiliac joint system. Sacroiliac movement is an integral part of gait and dysfunction at this joint can create significant inefficiency in gait patterns as well as shock absorption.

ANATOMY OF THE HIP JOINT

Osteology: Acetabulum

Fusion of the pubis, ischium, and ilium creates the acetabulum, with the pubis contributing 20%, the ischium 40%, and the ilium 40%.[2] The ilium is situated superiorly, with the pubis and the ischial portions more anterior and posterior. A gap in the acetabular structure inferiorly is called the acetabular notch. The transverse acetabular ligament fills this defect. The articular surface of the acetabulum, the lunate surface, is horseshoe shaped and more extensive in the superior section where there is more weight bearing.[2] Not all of the acetabulum is covered by the hyaline articular cartilage. The acetabular opening faces forward, downward, and outward to receive the femoral head and is smaller and more anterior in women. An acetabular fibrocartilaginous labrum deepens the socket and tightens about the femoral head to resist dislocation forces. This labrum blends with the transverse acetabular ligament to complete the supporting ring.

The proximal articulation of the femur is a head that has been described as spherical or ellipsoid in shape.[2-5] Moving distally there is a neck portion, a lateral greater trochanter, a more distal and medial lesser trochanter, the shaft, and the distal condyles. The trochanters provide the attachment of many hip muscles. The shaft is hollow and resists bending well. The femur is the longest and the strongest bone in the body.[2]

Articular cartilage covers the head except at the fovea centralis, a slight depression where the ligamentum teres, or "ligament of the head," attaches. The neck and shaft are angled approximately 125 degrees in the frontal plane. The frontal plane angulation is approximately 150 degrees at birth and decreases in the adult. Adult females often have a 90-degree angle due to a wider pelvis.[2,6] Deviations give rise to coxa valga, an increased angle, or coxa vara, a decreased angle. These deviations can cause dysfunction in the adolescent athlete.

Femoral anteversion in the transverse plane begins with 35 to 40 degrees at birth and decreases to 15 degrees in the adult.[2,7,8] Wolfe's law of structural remodeling and adaption is evident in the trabecular arrangement of the proximal shaft, neck, and head, which strongly resist compression, torque, and shear forces. The neck is narrower at its attachment to the head than at its attachment to the shaft.

Noncontractile Elements

Encompassing the hip joint is a thick, fibrous capsule attached to the femoral neck and the acetabular labrum including the transverse acetabular ligament. The fiber system is arranged longitudinally with some distal fiber structure circumferentially about the femoral neck. Continuous with the capsule are thickened re-

inforcing ligaments named for their attachments. The posterior aspect does not receive augmentation and is the thinnest part of the capsule. The iliofemoral ligament is shaped like an inverted Y. Its anterior placement allows it to restrict hyperextension of the hip. The pubofemoral and ischiofemoral ligaments complete the capsule and also limit extension. The pubofemoral ligament also resists abduction. The psoas muscle's tendon inserts on the lesser trochanter and complements the anterior aspect of the capsule. The ligament of the head of the femur, the ligamentum teres, does not serve to stabilize the joint, but instead carries blood supply to the femoral head in children. In the adult it serves no function and can be ruptured or absent. A well-developed intra-articular fat pad helps to maintain synovial fluid distribution, add shock absorption, and fill empty space in the acetabulum.

A number of bursa are present and act to reduce friction and shock, thus protecting other structures. Positioned over the posterolateral greater trochanter, the trochanteric bursa separates it from the gluteus maximus muscle. It is the most frequently injured bursa. The iliopsoas bursa is the largest of the hip bursa and separates the tendon from the anterior hip capsule. The ischial bursa protects the hamstring origin from the ischial tuberosity.

Angiology/Neurology

Blood supply to the hip is provided by the medial and lateral femoral circumflex arteries, the acetabular branch of the obturator artery, and the superior and inferior gluteal arteries.

Neural innervation comes from the same nerves that supply the musculature acting on the joint, namely the femoral, obturator, superior gluteal, and the sciatic nerves.

Musculature

Table 21–1 describes the action of hip prime movers and accessory muscles. Table 21–2 provides a list of average ranges of motion[9,10] Although prime movers are most important, accessory musculature is often of critical importance in long-distance running, power sports, and finesse sports. Its importance in providing proprioceptive input and stabilization cannot be underestimated. When the prime movers are exhausted, as in marathon running, muscles with minor actions in a particular direction can be asked to become prime movers, leading to injuries that can be subtle but debilitating.

The muscular system provides most of the stability for the hip joint.[1] These muscles produce all the movements of a ball and socket joint, namely flexion, extension, internal and external rotation, circumduction, adduction, and abduction. The gluteus maximus is the powerhouse for running, jumping, and lifting. The glu-

in unbalanced isokinetic scores, demonstrating a stronger long limb quadriceps and short limb hamstring.[45]

EVALUATION OF THE HIP, PELVIS, AND SACRUM

Subjective Examination

Careful examination of the patient's complaint and previous medical and exercise history can give the therapist insight to the severity, mechanism of injury, irritability, and chronicity of the problem as well as directing the objective examination and identifying the patient's attitude, goals, and personality type.

Pertinent questions should determine the

1. Chief complaint(s)
2. Behavior of the symptoms, local and referred
3. Mechanism of injury or maintenance of symptoms
4. Previous injury history
5. Previous treatment effectiveness
6. Past, present, and future activity levels
7. Realistic goals
8. Attitude toward the injury, especially responsibility and reliability
9. Total type and intensity of current activities, daily and weekly
10. Training environment: shoes, terrain, time of day, and so on
11. Medication and other medical history
12. Rating past and present pain/discomfort

During the subjective evaluation both the therapist and patient "read" each other and develop trust and confidence. The therapist should plan the type of approach that best suits the patient's personality and attitude. Most athletes prefer an examiner who conveys an understanding and concern of what they have been through without being overly critical for their obviously poor choice in training routine or poor common sense.

Objective Examination

Data collected during the objective examination helps identify the tissues at fault and the best approach for treatment. "Playing Detective" and assessing the relative contribution of each postural or alignment fault helps to put the whole picture in perspective. A small deviation that by itself would not cause dysfunction can combine with others to create a hostile environment that can produce or at least maintain the symptoms. The key questions therefore become: What is at fault? Why isn't it getting better? and How can it be rectified?

A set sequence for evaluation minimizes uncollected data and speeds the evaluation. Shortcuts in the objective evaluation process are often necessary in response to the reality of practice. Information from the subjective examination helps triage to determine which tests and areas would be most helpful to examine.

The following is a reasonably long examination sequence for the hip and pelvis:

1. Observation of gait and movement.
2. Static standing evaluation
   a. Postural deviations
   b. Symmetry of the trunk, head, extremities
   c. Pelvic alignment
   d. Limb lengths
   e. Sacroiliac joint tests (flexion, sulcus, hip drop)
   f. Lumbar spine mechanics
   g. Lower extremity alignment
   h. Weight-bearing pattern
3. Supine
   a. Posture and palpation
   b. Limb length
   c. Pelvic and femoral alignment
   d. Range of motion of the hip
   e. Sacroiliac joint clearing tests (compression, distraction)
   f. Knee clearing tests
   g. Hip clearing tests (Faber's, flex/adduction/internal rotation, scour)
   h. Muscle break tests for the hip
   i. Sacroiliac joint mechanics—long sitting iliosacral test
   j. Dural testing (neck flexion, SLR)
   k. Thomas test (hip flexion)
4. Sitting
   a. Pelvic alignment
   b. Sacroliac and lumbar mobility tests (facet tests, flexion test)
   c. Sacral mobility test
   d. Muscle break tests
5. Side Lying
   a. Pelvic mobility testing (posterior iliac rotation)
   b. Range of motion testing lumbar spine
   c. Ober's iliotibial band test
   d. Palpation of greater trochanter
6. Prone
   a. Palpation
   b. Range of motion testing hip extension, rotation
   c. Range of motion testing iliac anterior rotation
   d. Dural testing (knee flexion)
   e. Sacral and pelvic position tests (inferior lateral angles and ischial tub)
   f. L5–S1 mobility tests

Standing Evaluation

In a standing position, asymmetry and many positional faults can be determined. A schema for the observation

The therapist then moves to the side to assess weight-bearing, for example, forefoot versus heel, anterioposterior spinal curves, sacral nutation or counternutation, pelvic position, and anterioposterior head posture. Finally the posterior view provides information on calcaneal (leg–heel) alignment, pelvic position, and the spine.

Palpation in Standing. Position palpation anteriorly of the anterior superior iliac spines and pelvic crests and posteriorly of the posterior superior iliac spines should tell the therapist the difference between a true and apparent limb length posture. Limb length measurements should be qualified by testing pelvic alignment first to identify pelvic abnormalities causing apparent limb length differences. Using graduated spacers under the short foot is a reasonably accurate way to assess limb length in full weight-bearing once the pelvis is leveled. In a true limb length difference, assuming symmetrical knee extension and ankle subtalar positions, the ASIS, crest, and PSIS will all be lower on the same side. They should be level (neutral) when assessed in sitting. An

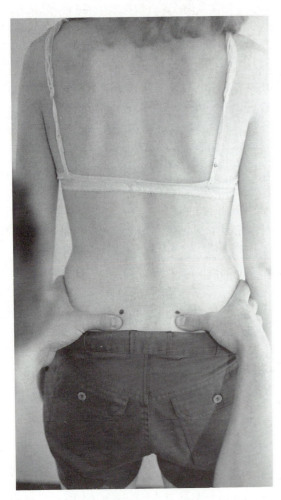

Figure 21-2. Standing flexion test. Starting position for the standing flexion test to assess iliosacral movement. The tips of the PSIS's are marked in black; palpation is along the inferior aspect.

procedure is useful. One method is to view the patient anteriorly, sideways, and posteriorly from the feet up. As viewed anteriorly, the feet should be observed for static pronation or supination. Then the patellofemoral and knee–foot alignment should be addressed. Asymmetrical weight-bearing, uneven hip heights, and deviations in the pelvis anterior to posterior can be assessed. Significant differences in shoulder and clavicle heights and signs of rotoscoliosis should be noted. Head and neck alignment should be noted.

Patients will usually assume the relaxed midtension position in the hip, while standing, that is, a balance between tensions in the internal and external rotators. Asymmetrical lower extremity rotation can identify shortened or splinted hip muscles reacting to positional faults of the pelvis and sacrum. The piriformis muscle is one of the first large muscles to react to pelvic and sacral misalignment. A patient who stands with one extremity significantly more externally rotated should receive a thorough sacro-pelvic examination.

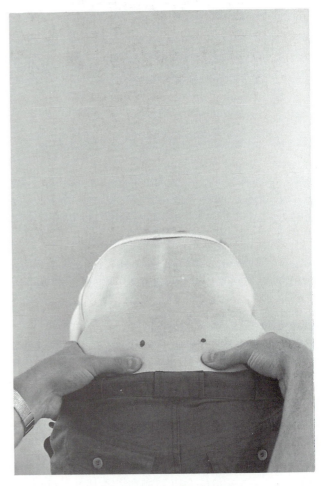

Figure 21-3. Standing flexion test. Ending position for the standing flexion test to assess iliosacral motion. Note the superior position on the right.

underdeveloped hemipelvis would be an exception but should have been noted during the observation phase. Heights of the greater trochanters can be also assessed.

Sacroiliac Joint Tests in Standing

After the pelvic position and lumbar ranges of motion have been identified, attention is drawn to the sacroiliac joints. Forward and backward bending are used to assess iliosacral movement, that is, movement of the ilia on the sacrum, and sacroiliac movement, that is, movement of the sacrum on the ilia. The feet should be acetabular distance apart and limb length should be equal.

Standing Flexion Test for Iliosacral Movement

(Figs 21–2, 21–3). With the PSISs level, using a heel lift if necessary, the patient is asked to forward bend partially (40 to 50 degrees) as the therapist palpates the bony prominences of the PSISs. Hypomobility in a sacroiliac joint will cause it to engage prematurely, caus-

ing the same-side PSIS to move sooner and often to a more superior position. Palpation contact must be maintained. Tightness of one or both hamstrings can negatively affect test results so full trunk flexion is avoided. There is flexion/extension motion of 2 to 6 degrees at the sacroiliac joints.[23] Repeating this test in sitting negates problems from tight hamstrings and limb length differences.

Sacral Sulcus Test for Sacroiliac Movement *(Fig 21–4).*

This common osteopathic test identifies the symmetry between the two sacroiliac joints as the sacrum reacts to lumbar movement. As the lumbar spine is flexed, the sacral base moves into backward bending, that is, extension or counternutation. Then the opposite movement occurs as the spine is extended.

Palpation of the sacral sulcus medial to each PSIS will demonstrate deepening with lumbar extension/sacral flexion, and it becomes shallow with lumbar flex-

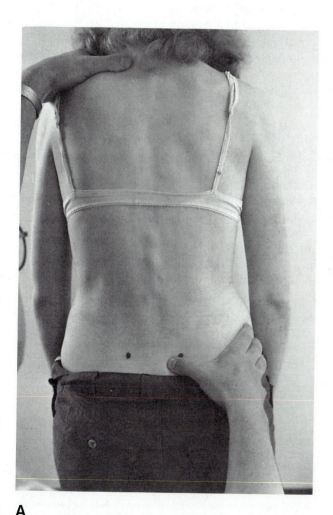

A

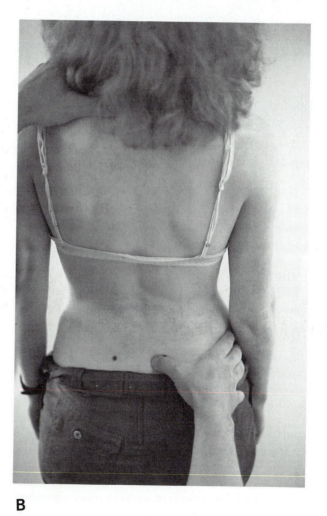

B

Figure 21-4. *A.* Testing of sacroiliac extension using the sacral sulcus test in lumbar flexion. The sulcus should become shallower. *B.* Using the sacral sulcus test to assess unilateral sacroiliac flexion with the lumbar spine in slight extension.

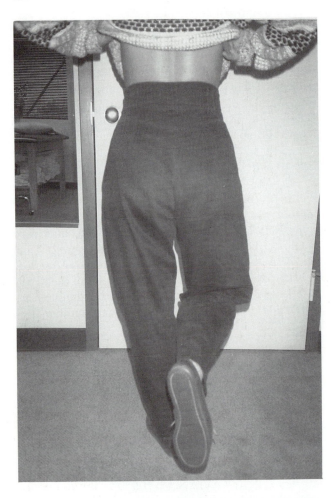

Figure 21–5. The hip drop test for lumbosacral hypomobility.

ion/sacral extension. The amount of lumbar movement required is only 20 to 30 degrees each way. A positive test identifies the hypomobile side.

Hip Drop. If the patient drops one hip while standing by bending one knee and relaxing the lower back, the unloaded PSIS should move posteriorly and inferiorly as L5–S1 side-bends away from and rotates toward the unloaded side due to the attachments of the iliolumbar ligaments (Fig 21–5). If the unloaded side does drop, hypomobility of L5–S1 would be noted. If there is a large increase in side-bending movement, backward (posterior) torsion of the unloaded innominant would be suspected. This test can also examine gluteus medius weakness if the patient is asked not to drop the hip.

The march test is a variation of the above during which the patient is asked to flex the unloaded hip to 90 degrees. Posterior rotation of the unloaded innominant is assessed for symmetry with the other side when it is tested.

Finally, gross cardinal plane movement of the lumbar spine in standing should be examined to identify problems that affect L5–S1 mobility and subse-

quently sacroiliac motion and alignment. Attention should be paid to the distribution of the movements over the segments to identify hypomobile and hypermobile joints. Identification and correction of all small spinal and lower extremity biomechanical deficiencies can help speed recovery and maintain positional corrections in the pelvis and sacrum.

Supine Examination

In the supine position, clearing tests, range of motion assessment, and limb length measurements are most commonly conducted. Observation of the rest position of the lower extremities and of the femoral condyles helps to assess muscle tightness and femoral deformities.

Pubic Symphysis Alignment Test. Palpation of pelvic landmarks including pubic symphysis alignment should be conducted carefully (Fig 21–6). A general tension balancing of the sacral base can be performed by the patient by bending the knees, bridging, and then lying down flat in a straight position. Then the examiner palpates the pubic tubercles using the thumbs to determine if they are subluxed superiorly or anteriorly. Since the pubic symphysis is the pivot area for the pelvis it should be examined and corrected first when a pelvic obliquity is suspected.

Range of Motion. Rotation range of motion testing in the supine position can be performed with the hip in neutral and also flexed. Hip rotation is often assessed with the hip and knee bent 90 degrees (Fig 21–7). To assess hip flexion range of motion, the opposite extremity must be stabilized (Figs 21–8).

The Thomas test for hip flexor tightness is important due to the iliopsoas' origin on the lumbar spine transverse processes and its effect on pelvic alignment and anterior capsule reinforcement. Iliopsoas tightness

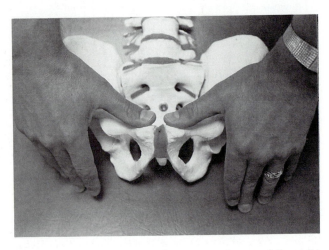

Figure 21–6. Palpation of the superior aspect of the pubic symphysis to determine alignment.

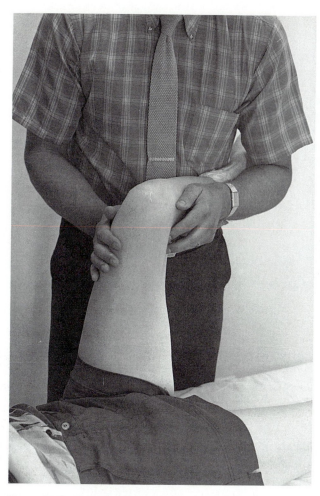

Figure 21-7. Testing range of motion and end feel for hip internal rotation. This position is best to isolate the piriformis muscle.

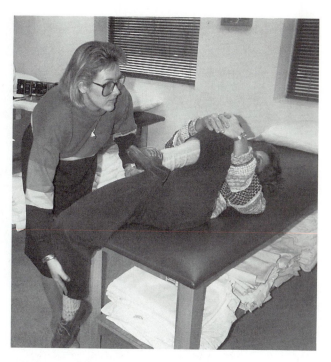

Figure 21-9. Testing rectus femoris flexibility in the Thomas hip flexor test position.

must be distinguished from rectus femoris tightness by assessing the reaction to increasing knee flexion in the Thomas test position. A positive reaction for rectus involvement will be an increase in hip flexion (Fig 21–9).

Hip joint accessory movement should also be examined. Inferior and lateral joint play can be assessed and mobilized with the hip flexed 90 degrees.

Clearing Tests. One clearing test, Fabere's test, also called Patrick's test, involves placing the hip in flexion–

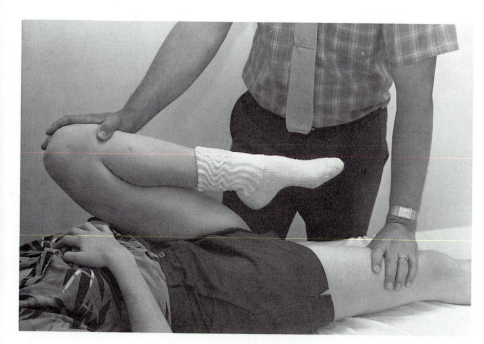

Figure 21-8. Testing hip range of motion and end feel of flexion.

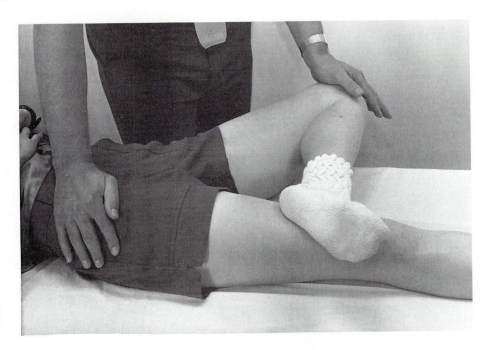

Figure 21-10. End feel testing in flexion, abduction, and external rotation (Faber's test).

abduction–external rotation and stressing the anterior and medial capsule (Fig 21–10). A positive hip joint reaction results in anterior joint pain. It also stresses the sacroiliac joint, and a positive test will elicit posterior and lateral symptoms.

Another hip and sacroiliac clearing test is the flexion–adduction–internal rotation test. Compressive pressure in the direction of the shaft of the femur stresses the inferior capsule and compresses the superior capsule (Fig 21–11).

The scour test involves flexion of the hip and compression through the femoral shaft while moving the femur in a slow circular motion. It tests the posterior and lateral capsule as well as the articular surface. A positive test will elicit pain or crepitus and named by the "clock" position of the femur.

Other sacroiliac clearing tests include compression or distraction of both ilia (Figs 12, 13). These tests are not ideally specific, and positive findings should dictate a more detailed evaluation of the sacroiliac joints and ligaments, especially sacral and lumbar mechanics.

Supine Iliosacral Long Sitting Test. Hypomobility of the sacroiliac joint can be examined by having the patient perform the tension balancing maneuver as in the pubic symphysis test. The patient's medial malleoli

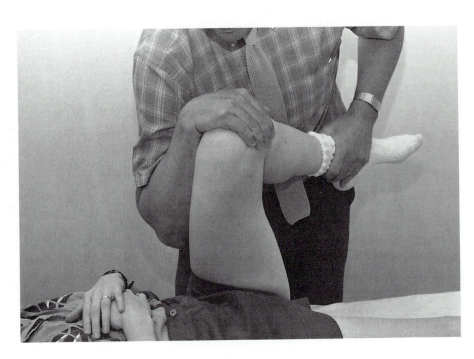

Figure 21-11. Capsular end feel testing in flexion, adduction, and internal rotation.

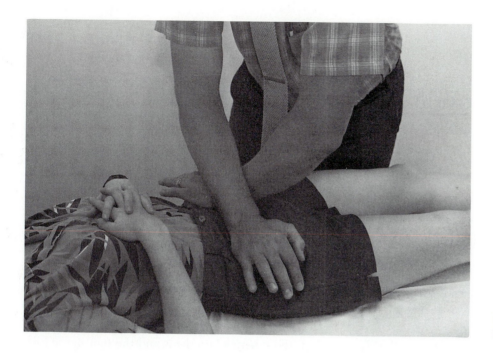

Figure 21-12. Sacroiliac compression testing.

can then be checked for position. Then the patient is instructed to sit up approximately 45 degrees with the arms propped up behind the trunk. Position of the malleoli are further examined. A lengthening of an extremity is positive for hypomobility on that side. This test should not be done to a full sitting position because acetabular mechanics will change and may affect the results, that is, the hypomobile limb will lengthen and then shorten.

Clearing tests of the knee, dural testing, and muscle strength assessment can be done easily in the supine position.

Sitting Examination

In the sitting position the hamstrings are relaxed and the pelvis is fixed on the ischial tuberosities. The seated flexion test is similar to the standing flexion test and will provide information on movement of the sacrum within the ilia. The sacrum will initially extend as the lumbar spine flexes, and then as ligamentous tension locking occurs it will flex with the ilia and spine. A positive test is indicated when a PSIS moves more superiorly and prematurely on one side, indicating reduced sacroiliac motion on that side. Palpation of the sacral inferior lateral angles as the patient extends and flexes

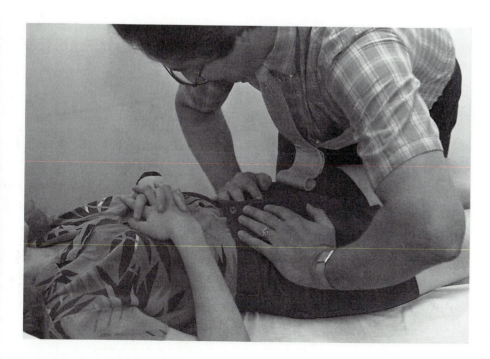

Figure 21-13. Distraction of the sacroiliac joints.

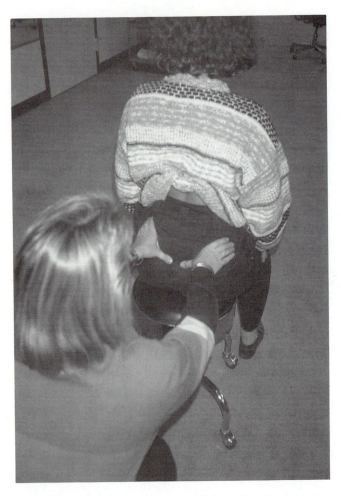

Figure 21–14. Palpation of the sacral inferior lateral angles to test sacroiliac movement during flexion and extension of the lumbar spine.

the lumbar spine up to 30 degrees helps determine sacral torsion dysfunctions (Fig 21–14). Both ILAs should move symmetrically anteriorly with lumbar flexion as the sacrum bends backward and posteriorly with lumbar extension. The ilia should be in neutral alignment because torsion of the one side will negatively affect sacroiliac movement.

L5–S1 movement should also be assessed by palpating the transverse processes and by determining vertebral rotation movement as the joint is placed in the extended, neutral, and flexed positions. A barrier to movement will cause the transverse processes to rotate. Sacral torsions will often cause counterrotation of L5–S1 to the opposite side. A posteriorly rotated ilium will create rotation of L5 to the same side through action of the iliolumbar ligaments.

Strength testing of hip musculature can also be performed in the sitting position.

Side-Lying Examination

With the superior knee bent and the foot hooked behind the inferior knee, posterior iliac motion can be assessed by grasping the ASIS and ischial tuberosity and rotating the ilia posteriorly. L5–S1 should be in ligamentous tension locking above and facet opposition below.

Iliotibial band tightness using Ober's test (Fig 21–15) can be checked by extending the superior knee, bending the inferior knee, and, while stabilizing the hip in a vertical position, dropping the upper limb to the plinth. A normal iliotibial band will allow full adduction to the plinth. A modified Ober's test can also be conducted with the upper knee slightly bent to test for flexibility of the tensor fascia lata muscle. In a nor-

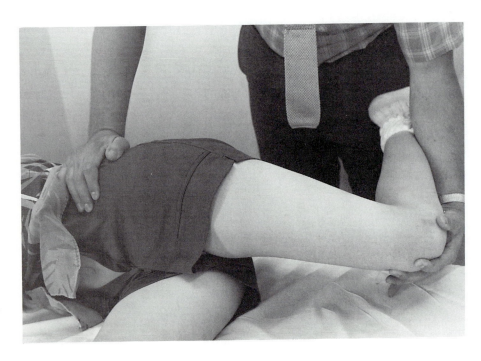

Figure 21–15. End feel testing of the hip abductors in the modified Ober's position.

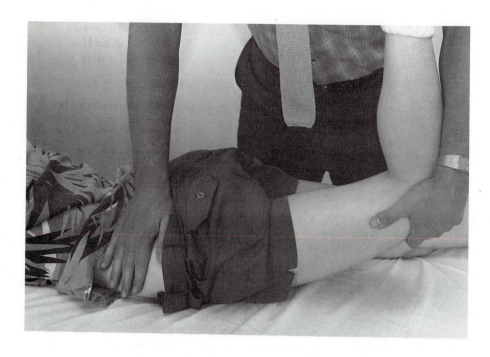

Figure 21-16. Testing unilateral iliac anterior rotation prone.

mal test the bent knee will almost touch the plinth. Lumbar spine mechanics can also be tested in a side-lying position.

Prone Examination

Range of motion testing of hip rotators is easily performed with the pelvis stabilized in the prone position. Anterior iliac movement can be examined after soft tissue slack has been taken up by stabilizing the posterior aspect of the innominant with one hand while moving the hip into extension with the knee bent 90 degrees (Fig 21–16). Other testing conducted in the prone position includes deep palpation of the iliac crests, sacroiliac ligaments, and position tests of the sacral inferior lateral angles and sacral base. L5–S1 mobility can be tested by palpating the transverse processes as the patient is positioned in neutral, extended propped-upon elbows, and flexed over a pillow. Palpation of the sacrotuberous ligaments, piriformis musculature, and sciatic notch should also be conducted. Position of the coccyx and ischial tuberosities should be noted, as should any tenderness upon palpation.

TREATMENT PRINCIPLES

Most injuries of the hip and pelvic girdle in sports are strains, sprains, and contusions. These injuries are usually the accumulation of microtrauma that exceeds the ability of the tissue to repair itself. Injuries are much less frequent to the hip joint than to the supporting musculature. Pelvic obliquities and sacral mechanical dysfunctions that can give rise to symptoms of sciatica are more common in adolescents and women and are frequently overlooked by the medical community.

Facet joint problems at L5–S1 are also common and often present with a pain–spasm–pain reaction that usually involves a myriad of primary and secondary structures in protective splinting. The lumbar spine can affect both sacral and iliac mechanics.

Hip injuries must be treated by restoring full range of motion and strength as well as lower extremity agility and proprioceptive integrity. Neurodevelopmental research has stressed the importance of proximal stability and proprioceptive reflexes. Rehabilitation must include joints above and below the area of injury because most lower-extremity injuries are just that—injuries to the entire extremity. Isokinetic research has shown the devastating effect of knee and ankle injuries on the entire limb.[46–48] As total activity level decreases, the insult involves both limbs, the cardiovascular system, and the rest of the body depending on how the training program has been modified to accommodate the injury and maintain fitness. When the injury has healed it is imperative that the rest of the system is ready to return to full activity level.

Initially reduction of pain, edema, and spasm are the focus as well as maintenance of the athlete's conditioning. Reduction of swelling through electrical stimulation, ultrasound, ice, and manual techniques is most important to minimize "down time." Even the slightest amount of edema reduces nutrient and blood flow retarding the healing process and removal of waste products and cellular debris. Pain and swelling have been shown to reflexly inhibit muscular action and baseline tone, especially when involving a joint.[49]

The exercise program must incorporate those patterns that mimic the desired activity goal when appropriate. The current trend is to use more functional positions especially using body weight and inertia and

plyometrics to train the injured areas according to the specificity of training principles. Attention should initially be paid to restoration of endurance and normal movement, and then to isotonic, isokinetic, and eccentric strength. Finally agility and coordination exercises and a graded return to the sport should be incorporated.

Treatment of pelvic and sacral disorders involves reduction of the positional fault, restoration of normal mechanics, balancing of muscular strength and length, and normalization of the kinetic chain environment. Concentrating the treatment at only one level, such as correction of the positional fault, is doomed to failure because adaptive shortening and asymmetrical weakness negatively influence maintenance of the correction.

The majority of individuals are right-handed, and some sports such as golf have been almost right-handed sports due to the equipment used. This predicts a pattern in pelvic disorders due to the repetition of one direction of pelvic torsion more than another. Throwing, serving a tennis ball, and many other activities in sports cause right posterior iliac torsion injuries among right-handed athletes. Other athletes such as hurdlers, sprinters, and soccer players will use one hip and pelvis predominantly as the power, push off, or pillar during their sport. Analysis of the mechanism of sport stress will often identify the mechanism of injury. Unfortunately, in many sports the complicated movement patterns cannot be altered so the system must be "super-tuned" to allow return to the same injury causing environment. Maintenance of conditioning, rehabilitation, and minimizing performance loss are the challenge the sports therapist faces daily.

Muscle Energy Techniques/Manipulation

Osteopathic muscle energy techniques are very useful in treating pelvic and sacral positional faults as well as spinal and extremity disorders. Direct manipulation with graded thrust techniques is also appropriate when hypomobility or positional faults are encountered. Muscle energy direct techniques, which are safer and very effective, often obviate the need for manual manipulation and can be performed by the patient athlete to maximize correction maintenance.

Muscle energy techniques can be divided into direct and indirect procedures. A direct technique involves stabilizing a muscle at one end and using its muscular action to produce movement and a positional correction at the other end. Indirect procedures such as the osteopathic strain–counterstrain and many myofascial approaches involve placing muscles on slack, which biases the Golgi tendon organs and muscle spindles allowing manual or active movement to correct a mechanical fault. Stretching using PNF type reciprocal innervation to effect relaxation and thus facilitate movement is also a muscle energy technique.

In the case of a right posterior iliac torsion with a subluxed superior right pubis, the standing evaluation would show a superior right iliac crest and ASIS and an inferior right PSIS. The supine symphysis pubis evaluation would identify a superior and slightly anterior right pubic tubercle. Hypomobility testing would also be positive on the right and side-lying and prone movement analysis would indicate a lack of posterior rotation because the available range has been taken up. Unless the innominant is locked in a posteriorly rotated position, there would be increased anterior movement available.

Treatment begins by using the adductor muscles to pull the right pubis inferiorly. The supine patient stabilizes the left innominant into posterior rotation by pulling the left knee to the axilla. Hooking the right ankle on the edge of a bed or doorway causes adduction of the right lower extremity, which in turn causes the right innominant to anteriorly rotate and the pubis to be pulled inferiorly (Fig 21–17). Contractions should be moderately strong for about 6 seconds and usually for ten repetitions. Then correction of the innominant rotation can be effected using a scissoring technique if the pubic repositioning exercise has not already reduced it. As noted previously, the rectus femoris and iliacus can anteriorly rotate an ilia and the hamstrings can produce posterior rotation torquing. Scissoring with the left hamstrings and right rectus against the therapist's body or against the ground while standing will derotate the right posteriorly rotated pelvis (Fig 21–18). Checking sacral mechanics and movement analysis of L5–S1 are followed by strength and range of motion testing. Many osteopaths suggest treatment and correction of first the pubis, then the sacral deformity, followed by the ilia, and finally L5–S1 mechanics. All of these areas must be assessed and treated to effectively correct the mechanical system.

Other manual techniques exist for moving the sacrum and pelvis and can be learned in manipulation and muscle energy courses and through muscle energy guide books.[20] Attention to posture and sitting/lying positions helps to maintain correction by enhancing motor memory.

COMMON HIP AND PELVIS INJURIES

Common Sports Injuries

Sprains and Strains. The musculotendinous unit is the most common tissue involved in overuse injuries. In the hip region strains of the supporting musculature are common and sprains of the hip ligaments are relatively rare. Due to the abundant range of motion about the hip joint, muscular stabilizers are more at risk of injury. Also predisposing the hip musculature to injury is its role as powerful prime movers and stabilizers during

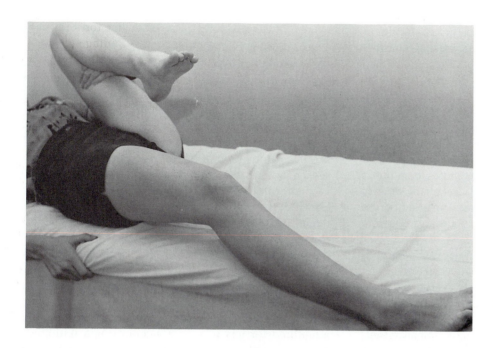

Figure 21–17. Using adductor muscle energy to reposition a superior right pubis.

the running, jumping, and cutting activities common in many sports. Mild first-degree strains of the hamstrings, rectus femoris, iliopsoas, and abductors are common. Usually the athlete does not present for treatment but instead relies on self-treatment. These injuries can become chronic and debilitating as the athlete continues training through discomfort or mismanages the self-treatment.

Second-degree strains of the hip muscles are the type most often referred for treatment. The severity of this injury precludes training and the athlete has no choice but to seek medical attention. Third-degree tears

and ruptures are not common but do occur primarily in the hamstrings, rectus femoris, and proximal abductors. Extensive hemorrhaging and contour deformity often necessitate surgical intervention.

Hamstring Strains. The four hamstring muscles originate from a common tendon at the ischial tuberosity. They are the most commonly strained muscles in sports. Any activity that requires explosive movement such as sprinting and jumping puts the athlete at risk of an injury to these muscles. Common risk factors are (1) inflexibility, (2) poor warmup, (3) neurological and

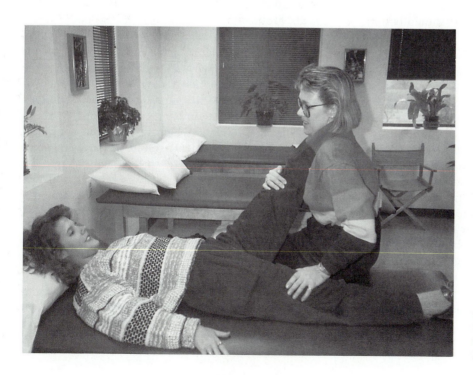

Figure 21–18. Derotation of a posteriorly rotated right ilium using rectus femoris muscle energy with counter rotation of the left side using the hamstrings.

muscular fatigue, (4) improper technique, (5) abnormal strength balance within and between extremities, and (6) poor neuromuscular control.

The short head of the biceps is the most frequently strained section.[50] It receives innervation from the tibial and peroneal divisions of the sciatic nerve, which can result in poor synchronization of contraction.

Other commonly strained areas include the proximal aspect of the popliteal fossa where the medial and lateral hamstring diverge and the musculotendinous junction at the ischial tuberosity. Like any muscle strain, hemorrhaging dissects apart the muscle fibers as a bolus of blood forms and can turn a minor tear into a major injury.

One common mechanism of injury, as the limb is accelerating forward, is inappropriately timed contractions due to protective spasm or electrolyte- or calcium-induced fatigue cramps. Sarcomere contraction requires high levels of calcium secretion, and if firing rates exceed the ability of the system to replenish itself, fatigue occurs.[51] The adjacent muscle bundles can then become overloaded as they are asked to compensate with a stronger contraction. In this state, antagonistic muscles can overpower the hamstrings. Protective reflex spasm can also be triggered by microtrauma of the lower lumbar spine and sacroiliac joints during activities such as explosive sprinting to first base or stretching out a stride running downhill.

Most athletes will report a "pop" when the muscle tears. As the severity of injury increases, intense pain and spasm increase. Often a palpable bulge is present. Ecchymosis is quite common and usually appears within a few days.

Trying to "run out" a hamstring strain increases the risk of turning a first-degree problem into a second-degree problem. Immediate treatment should be rest, ice, compression, and elevation (RICE). Prevention of a large hematoma is critical in reducing time lost from the sport activity. Active range of motion exercises can begin as soon as the area has stabilized. Collagen remodeling takes up to 3 weeks and maturation to full strength even longer. Waiting a minimum of 5 to 7 days after a mild second-degree tear before starting painfree stretching is recommended.[52] Mobilization, friction massage, and stretching after a soft tissue injury reduces edema, minimizes scar formation, prevents atrophy, and maintains range of motion. Early mobilization has been shown to reduce time lost from a sport and reduces pain, edema, and other symptoms. Often the athlete will wait many weeks before stretching, which promotes the development of a tight, weak scar that may rupture during the first vigorous activity. The healing process must be directed by judicious stretching, active range of motion and graded weight training and functional activities.

Anti-inflammatory modalities and medications can speed recovery, but second-degree tears often take 6 weeks to heal before return to full activity is allowed. In the acute period, pulsed 1 MHZ ultrasound at an intensity of 0.5 W/cm or less can help reduce edema and promote healing through molecular streaming and other effects. Most of the multitude of electrical stimulation devices are helpful in reducing pain and swelling, as is acupuncture point stimulation. The main goal is early stabilization of the injury followed by progressive (not aggressive) mobilization.

Alternative exercises must be prescribed to maintain fitness and improve nutrition and remodeling of the injury. Once the injury is stable, cross-fiber friction massage is beneficial in reducing cross-linking and random fiber alignment as collagen repairs the muscle defect.

Before a return to full activity level, the athlete should have normal flexibility, strength, endurance, agility, and power. Adjacent musculature must also be monitored for loss of function due to pain inhibition and inactivity. Graded agility and coordination exercises are a good test of the integrity of the repair. Review of the athlete's technique is always helpful in minimizing avoidable stress.

Quadriceps Strains. The rectus femoris section of the quadriceps is the most commonly strained. Due to its combined action of hip flexion and knee extension it is at risk of tearing during sprinting, jumping, and kicking. Ruptures are not uncommon at the proximal or distal ends of the muscle. As with the more common hamstring strains a "pop" or "snapping" is often reported. Treatment is the same as for hamstring tears.

Pelvic Sprains. As noted previously, the sacroiliac ligaments are possibly the strongest in the body. Acute sprains are not common, but once pelvic and sacral alignment has been altered, tearing of these ligaments due to sustained stretch will follow the pattern of the deformity. Most commonly developing a reaction to pelvic obliquities are the superior posterior sacroiliac ligaments and the iliolumbar ligaments.

Chronic overload, which fatigues the nonelastic component of the ligament, results in pain as well as cellular anoxia, as the stretched ligament collapses its capillaries. Under these circumstances, treatment will have minimal effect until the positional fault has been corrected and microcirculation restored.

O'Donoghue reports that many sacroiliac ligaments sprains in young athletes tend to be more likely sprains of the lumbosacral ligaments because the sacroiliac ligaments are so strong.[1] Referred pain from injury to these areas will project to the groin and buttocks and often laterally to the hamstrings and quadriceps. Often a diagnosis of sciatica is given, which does not identify the tissues injured or the true nature of the injury.

Many times injury to the sacroiliac joint produces paraspinal and piriformis spasm. If the hamstrings tense as a reaction to tearing of these ligaments while sprinting or kicking, the muscle may tear as it is being asked to contract to reduce iliac motion and eccentrically control motion at the same time. Many "hamstring tears" are secondary injuries caused by these inappropriate contractions, so an underlying sacroiliac or lumbar spine problem must be identified.

Acute sacroiliac and lumbosacral sprains are difficult to rest because shear or contact pressure on the pelvis is unpreventable except in a pool or outer space.

Total rest, ice, and modalities including a home transcutaneous electrical nerve stimulation (TENS) unit help get the athlete through the most painful period, often 5 to 10 days. Once calmed down, these injuries have a tendency to flare up with quick rotation movements, sprinting, jumping, kicking, and sitting crosslegged. The athlete should be instructed that the metabolism of these tissues is slow and that healing will be on the order of weeks and sometimes months rather than days.

Acute sprains are the result of violent contact with the ground or another player. An accumulation of microtears secondary to repetitive overload creates a predisposition for many of these injuries.

Pubic Symphysis/Osteitis Pubis. Since the pubic symphysis is designed to hold the anterior aspect of the pelvis together and it is the focal point of shock and weight-bearing stress on the pelvis, forceful abduction of the legs is one mechanism of injury in sports such as horseback riding, gymnastics, and water skiing. With other activities, shear forces are transmitted to the joint as it rotates and moves inferior–superior, and anterior–posterior. During single leg limb support, downward shear forces can become significant. Because of their close origin to the symphysis pubis, the adductor muscle group can both stabilize it and damage it.

Osteitis pubis, an inflammation and degeneration of the bony articulation, can be accelerated by the poor blood supply it receives.[53] It has been reported to be a more common injury in runners, karate participants, race walkers, wrestlers, and hockey and soccer players.[31,54,55] Small avulsion fractures can occur as well as inflammation of the ligaments. The pain comes on gradually with accumulation of trauma. Often the athlete ignores the symptoms as it may be confused with referred pain from the viscera or the groin and adductor muscles. X-ray changes show sclerosing of the bone and may be discernible only after a month of symptoms.[54] Koch and Jackson feel that pubic symphysitis with a positive bone scan and normal appearance on x-rays is a precursor or variant of osteitis pubis.[55]

Other evaluative findings will include point tenderness and pain with stretch or contraction of the adductors. Rest is the treatment of choice, along with anti-inflammatory medication. Modality treatment is difficult due to the proximity to the urogenital region. Swimming is the one alternative exercise using a "poor boy" float between the legs. Kicking, especially whip kicks, will aggravate the symptoms, as will cycling. Gentle stretching of the adductors may be performed to tolerance.

Piriformis Syndrome. This disorder is usually mentioned as a source of symptoms due to the infrequent perforation of the piriformis by the sciatic nerve. Some authors debate whether or not a pure piriformis injury exists.[31,54] Calliet reports that up to 15% of the population have this anomaly and that it occurs more frequently in women.[56]

Most often the piriformis muscle reacts to sacral and iliac subluxation and sprains by protective spasm. In the relaxed standing evaluation, the athlete will be positioned in more lower extremity external rotation, and internal rotation range of motion will be limited. When a sacroiliac positional fault is the underlying problem, repositioning and then PNF type stretching will restore full range of motion.

When the spasm persists or is due to local trauma, continuous 1 MHZ ultrasound is effective in relaxing the muscle. Also useful is electrical stimulation either from origin to insertion or along the sciatic nerve. Ice and heat will be superficial and cannot effectively reach this muscle but may help by relaxing the gluteus maximus. The sacrum must be examined carefully because the piriformis originates there. Often treatment directed at the insertion on the greater trochanter is effective, as inflammation from sustained tension is common there.

Contusions. Due to the nature of many sports, contact with other players, equipment, or the ground is either planned or inevitable. Direct blows to the iliac crest can result in painful soft tissue trauma called a hip pointer. This is most common in football, often resulting from contact with a helmet. Muscle fibers are crushed and separated with resultant bleeding and swelling. Usually the athlete ignores the initial symptoms and the debilitating pain occurs by the next morning.

X-rays are often taken to rule out the presence of an avulsion fracture. Trunkal movement is limited and coughing, laughing, and sneezing can be very painful. When severe, the athlete may present an antalgic gait.

Treatment of any contusion should include ice, rest, and reduction of the swelling and inflammation, followed by active range of motion and a gradual return to full function. Care must be taken to avoid aggravating the soft tissue injury by injudicious stretching. Protective doughnut padding is usually necessary.

Other common areas that become contused are the quadriceps, greater trochanter, pubis, and ischial tuberosity. Contusions of the ischial tuberosity must be differentiated from avulsion fractures.

Severe or chronic contusions can progress to myositis ossificans, a mineralization that forms in the hematoma usually within 1 to 2 weeks after a severe contusion.[57] The muscle fibers become separated by the mass and avulsion of the muscle from the bone is possible.[1] Massage and stretching are usually contraindicated, although active painfree range of motion is encouraged.[58] Isokinetic and isotonic exercise must be of low intensity and carefully graded. Ultrasound and electrical stimulation can help mobilize the mass and promote absorption.

The most common area that develops myositis ossificans is midquadriceps.[54] Surgical removal of the mass is not warranted early but may be necessary once the injury has matured, which may take up to 1 year. Excision before the mass has matured will cause reformation often larger than before.[57] Medication can be prescribed to minimize the effects of inflammation and stasis.

Fractures. Fractures of the sacrum and ilia are rare in sports. Iliac fractures are devastating because of the resultant internal soft tissue injury and damage to the attachments of trunk and hip musculature. Usually these fractures are a result of powerful forces encountered in football, skiing, ski jumping, horseback riding, and motorcycle racing. Minor injuries can be mistaken for a hip pointer. Padding used in many contact sports protects the ilia from injury. Extreme palpation tenderness and loss of function are the most important clinical signs. Treatment usually consists of rest, ice, strapping and modalities for the pain, swelling, and secondary spasm. Surgical reduction is not usually necessary.[1]

Traumatic femoral neck fractures are rare in adolescents and are often secondary to osteoporotic changes.[59] Fractures of the femoral shaft occur infrequently and are especially debilitating because the cortex of the bone is subjected to tremendous bending forces. Internal fixation and immobilization are the treatments of choice, followed by physical therapy. Exercise of the uninvolved side produces cross-training effects that help reduce atrophy of the injured area.

Avulsion Fractures. Avulsion fractures are not uncommon at the ASIS, ischial tuberosity, and symphysis pubis due to the powerful pull of the attached musculature. Usually a violent muscle contraction is the cause of this type of trauma. In the adolescent athlete open epiphyses at the ASIS contribute to the ability of the rectus femoris to cause avulsion, especially with kicking and running. Other areas that may suffer avulsion fractures are the greater and lesser trochanter.

Palpation tenderness and swelling at the avulsion site are the most significant evaluative findings and stressing the attached musculature will produce severe pain. Large fragments will need to be reduced surgically. Treatment with ice and modalities can reduce discomfort and promote healing, but rest is the most important part of treatment. Exercising around the injured area maintains conditioning; after the injury heals, in 4 to 6 weeks, a gradual return to full function should be instituted.

Stress Fractures. Brody says that the high-impact stress fracture in runners occurs when they train too fast and too long with improper shoes and over hard terrain.[31] This type of fracture is common in the young as a result of an accumulation of microtrauma. Female athletes are reported to be more prone to stress fractures.[60,61] Brody reports that these injuries can occur in the lumbar vertebrae, sacroiliac joints, and the pubic symphysis (osteitis pubis).[31] O'Donoghue describes a stress fracture across the top of the ischium.[1] McBryde's study of 1000 stress fractures in runners demonstrated a distribution of 6% at the pelvis, 7% at the femoral neck, and 5% along the proximal femoral shaft.[62] Other areas that have been mentioned are the femoral neck and pubic ramus.[63-65]

The current understanding of the etiology of these injuries is that the fracture may not be exclusively due to the accumulation of overload stress, but also due to the body's response to healing. In the past, stress fractures were described only as breakdown when the microtrauma of an activity exceeds the rate of bone repair. Recent information implicates an increase of osteoclastic activity stimulated by the microtrauma and the piezoelectric effect of the bone matrix.[66,67] Osteoclastic activity causes bone resorption, further weakening the damaged bone, and is increased when compressive forces produce the piezoelectric electrical field. In their study of basic trainees at Fort Knox, Kentucky, Scully and Besterman found that the majority of symptoms occurred between the 10th and 12th days of training.[67] They postulated that stress-damaged bone begins to be removed through osteoclastic activity by the third week in heavy training. Cycling the training by reductions in intensity and duration during the third week after beginning training facilitates remodeling of the periosteal bone. McBryde reports that 60% to 75% of clinical stress fractures are the result of training errors.[62]

Healing of stress fractures can take 4 to 15 weeks and varies widely depending on the location, body structure, and modification of training. According to Brody, healing of pelvic stress fracture can take 6 months to 1 year and running is contraindicated.[64] Any significant deviation in optimal biomechanical structure and musculoskeletal alignment must be corrected

and the training program must be evaluated and restructured.

Diagnosis by x-rays is difficult until a callous forms in approximately 2 to 3 weeks. Bone scans are most often used to provide early diagnosis when a stress fracture is suspected due to the location of symptoms and the previous exercise history.

Slipped Capital Femoral Epiphysis.

Kelsey's review of the literature on slipped capital femoral epiphysis injuries concluded that this injury occurred most frequently in males between 12 and 15 years old who were either slightly obese or lanky, with less than average skeletal maturity.[68] Lack of fusion of the epiphyseal plate at the head of the femur allows it to displace under certain conditions. Although usually unilateral, bilateral injury occurred in 15% to 20% of the cases studied by Catterall.[69] Although the exact cause of the slippage is not clearly understood, a minor injury may precipitate the actual injury.[1,54] A deficiency in calcium metabolism or dysfunction of the pituitary or thyroid may be present.[64]

The injured athlete will usually present with an externally rotated extremity and an antalgic gait. Upon evaluation, the hip will be flexed and abducted and internal rotation usually limited.

The chief complaint voiced is hip and or knee pain, so knee clearing must be conducted. X-ray diagnosis confirms the diagnosis and treatment of major slippage includes traction and internal fixation. Manipulation to reduce the deformity can damage the epiphysis and cause necrosis of the femoral head.[54]

O'Donoghue proposes bilateral pinning in the case of a unilateral problem.[1] Physical therapy should be the same as for hip fracture, with the athlete eventually progressing through appropriate proprioceptive, agility, and coordination training.

Legg-Calve-Perthes Disease.

Another cause of hip pain in the adolescent athlete can be avascular necrosis of the femoral head. It is most commonly found in children from 3 to 12 years old and occurs most often in males. Fischer reported a peak incidence at 6 years old.[70] X-ray evaluation distinguishes this disorder from simple synovitis and slipped capital femoral epiphysis. A flattening of the superior and anterolateral aspects of the head occurs as the disorder progresses.

Kuland describes a precipitating synovitis causing joint effusion pressure, which reduces blood flow.[54] This osteochondritis injury is common after hip dislocations, which are not common in sports. Clinical symptoms include muscle spasm of the ipsilateral abductors, reducing adduction range of motion and pain in the thigh, knee, or anterior hip.

Treatment involves the use of traction and rest and then immobilization in 45 degrees abduction and slight

internal rotation.[40] Treatment can last up to 2 years and surgery is often necessary. Prognosis is better for younger children who have more years of growth and thus time for remodeling.

Bursitis and Tendinitis.

Inflammation of the greater trochanter or iliopsoas bursa is common in sports and dance. The greater trochanteric bursa is positioned on the posterolateral aspect of the greater trochanter and separates it from the tendon of the gluteus maximus and iliotibial band. Anatomically the iliotibial band is a fascial extension of the connection between the tensor fascia lata and gluteus maximus. Excessive friction can be the result of limb length differences, running with the feet crossing midline, running on uneven terrain, especially banked tracks, abductor–adductor imbalance, excessive posterolateral shoe wear, and a wide pelvis with an increased Q-angle. Women are more predisposed to injury.

Chronic bursitis is often referred to as a "snapping hip" and is a common dance injury due to the factors mentioned above and increased single-limb weightbearing. The bursa thickens and the iliotibial band will snap over it as the limb is flexed and extended.

Symptoms include local pain and tenderness and an increase in symptoms with Ober's test. Pain increases with activity and continues at rest due to the inflammatory reaction. Treatment should include rest, ice, anti-inflammatory medication and modalities, and stretching of the iliotibial band and gluteus maximus when tolerated. Correction of biomechanical faults is essential to prevent reoccurrence.

The iliopsoas bursa lies beneath the pectineus muscles deep to the insertion of the iliopsoas. Since the iliopsoas muscle reinforces the anterior capsular ligaments, excessive hyperextension during activities such as sprinting and hurdling can cause pain distribution in the groin and thigh. Palpation tenderness of the lateral femoral triangle and an increase in symptoms as the hip is extended or the iliopsoas resisted reinforce the diagnosis. Hip flexor tightness can aggravate or cause this inflammation and must be reduced. Evaluation of training technique is essential.

Ischial bursitis is not common. The bursa lies between the ischial tuberosity and gluteus maximus and is occasionally inflamed when adolescent runners do too much speed work.[8] Symptoms include tenderness over the ischium and pain with sitting.

Bursitis is hard to distinguish from tendinitis, and often both are present at the same time. Tendons can become inflamed from sustained submaximal loading. Barfred found that rat tendons were more likely to be injured when a tendon underloading is subjected to rapid oblique strain.[71] Chronic microtrauma causes sustained reduction of vascularization due to swelling and edema resulting in local degeneration. The efficacy of cortico-

steroid injection should be examined considering the numerous reports of rupture following injections.[72-74]

After a tendon tear, collagen tissue forms over a 2- to 3-week period and then is remodeled.[75] Attention must therefore be given to the healing time frame before overloading the muscle tendon unit. Friction massage is useful (but painful) to reduce cross-fiber bonding.

Eccentric exercise may be useful in rehabilitating tendon injuries when significant remodeling has occurred and pain is used as a guide.[75,76]

Lateral Femoral Cutaneous Nerve Injury. Derived from the L2 and L3 nerve roots, the lateral femoral nerve courses lateral to the psoas muscle, along the iliacus, and through a tunnel under the attachment of the inguinal ligament at the ASIS. Composed of anterior and posterior branches, it supplies sensation to the lateral and posterior aspects of the thigh. Entrapment can occur just below the ASIS, affecting sensation on the lateral thigh.[77] Contusions and repetitive twisting (golf, tennis) can produce symptoms that include numbness and lateral knee pain. Treatment should include rest, ice, fascial stretching, and review and modification of training techniques. Pulsed ultrasound, electrical stimulation, and other anti-inflammatory treatments can be helpful. Pelvic obliquities can predispose this injury.

Conditioning Considerations

Since the majority of hip and pelvis injuries are sprains and strains, once biomechanical faults have been corrected, the injuries should be relatively healed in 3 to 6 weeks. More severe injuries will mean longer periods of rest and subsequent deconditioning.

Preserving strength, flexibility, and endurance in the uninjured areas is a challenge for the sports therapist. Conditioning for return to competition should begin on the first day by assessing the appropriateness of the sport for the athlete, considering age, sex, and physical and mental status. Often an athlete should not return to a particular sport and must be counseled into alternative activities that will offer the stress reduction, weight control, and the competition desired. At the same time, some athletes have such a strong desire to return to a poorly suited activity that the therapist may have to compromise. In this case, training the individual to the highest level of conditioning and allowing the opportunity to try the sport satisfies the athlete even when failure is the end result.

Discussing and setting short-term, attainable goals motivates the athlete and instills confidence. For some competitors, any injury can be devastating mentally. Weight gain is often a particular concern. The well-prepared athlete can better handle the plateaus and flare-ups that are all too common as the sports therapist pushes training to the maximum.

Normally after the acute injury has stabilized, the rehabilitation and conditioning program is designed on the basis of the sport-specific demands and the stage of healing. Holistically, the program must include maintenance or strengthening exercises for the uninvolved side for cross-training effects and adjacent muscle groups and joints to minimize delays in return to competition.

Proprioception should be fine-tuned through exercises such as weight shifting, using balance boards and agility/coordination exercises. Running or walking backwards on a treadmill can be helpful in reducing dependency on visual cues instead of proprioceptive input. Specificity of exercise and training is the key to using alternative exercises to prepare for a sport. Swimming, for instance, is a cardiovascular activity that does not "carry over" training effects to an activity such as running because it is non-weight-bearing and involves neuromuscular patterns that are not similar to running. Running in the deep end of a pool with a waterskiing belt around the waist is a better alternative for a runner with an injury such as a stress fracture.[31] Conditioning programs should include six categories of exercise:

1. Aerobic
2. Anaerobic
3. Low velocity
4. High velocity
5. Eccentric
6. Concentric

Isokinetic equipment opened the door to higher-velocity and multiple-velocity spectrum concentric and eccentric training. Normal limb velocities for sports activities are still very much greater than those provided by these devices, but the higher-velocity training is beneficial. Many isokinetic devices also provide eccentric training, which is particularly helpful in training the hamstrings, external rotators, and quadriceps muscles.

Treadmills not only allow the therapist the ability to view and videotape gait and running, but they can be used at slow speeds for agility and coordination activities such as carioca walking, sideways skipping, and backwards walking or running. Other coordination and agility exercises should be begun as soon as appropriate, such as a progression of sideways and front to back hopping, running in circles and figure eights, and zig-zag running and short sprints with fast starts and stops.

Plyometric training is an excellent way to provide

TABLE 21-4. RETURN TO RUN PROGRAM[a]

1. Warmup: 2–3 minutes and then stretch lower body muscles. Repeat five to ten times and hold 6 seconds; do not bounce.
2. Stages
   a. Slow: Run 20 steps slowly and then walk 20 steps quickly. Progress to running 3–4 minutes and walking 2 minutes for 20–40 minutes total time. Maximum three times per week.
   b. Moderate: Increase running segment to 5–10 minutes and increase the pace to a moderate pace (8–12 min/mi). Decrease the fast walking segment to 1 min. Maximum three times per week for 20–40 minutes.
   c. Fast: Phase out the walking segment and increase the pace slowly to below 8 min/mi. Maximum three times per week for 20–40 minutes.
   d. Advanced: Increase the frequency to four to six times per week and lengthen the run a desirable amount. Change pace as desired.
   e. Competition: Add hill work, fartleks, or interval training one or two times per week. Add one long run per week and mix the intensity and duration of the runs throughout the week. Try to maintain one day of rest with a maximum of under 70 mi/wk.

[a]Note: Run in new shoes on even terrain. Do not progress the program if you experience pain/swelling during the run or if any moderate discomfort is not 100% cleared in 12–24 hours.

TABLE 21-5. SPORTS PREDISPOSING HIP/PELVIS INJURIES

Collision Sports
Hockey
Football

Noncontact Sports
Running
Tennis
Gymnastics
Cross-country skiing
Swimming
Track and field
  Hurdling
  High jump
  Sprinting
  Triple jump
  Pole vault
Gymnastics

High-Velocity Sports
Skateboarding
Ice skating
Alpine skiing
Motorcycle racing
Cycling

Contact Sports
Basketball
Soccer
Volleyball
Field hockey
Baseball
Wrestling

eccentric and concentric training at higher velocities as well as training functional neuromuscular patterns. It has been used for years in Russian and European sports training institutes. Plyometric techniques provide training for jumping, running, and other explosive activities using eccentric loading and the myostatic stretch reflex to obtain optimal synchronization and intensity of muscular effort. Modifications of these techniques can be used early in the rehabilitation process. Most plyometric techniques are better suited to the athlete who is within normal levels of conditioning and is preparing for discharge. Radcliffe and Forentinos[78] and Costello[79] have described these techniques in detail.

Returning the athlete to a high-impact/stress activity such as running can be difficult. A graded return to run program is presented in Table 21–4.

To return to full competition, the athlete should be able to perform functional sport skills without pain and the injured area should be minimally tender and not swollen. Aftersoreness should not last more than 8 to 12 hours and should definitely be absent by 24 hours after the activity. Aftereffects are a much better guide to the appropriateness of an activity than symptoms during because athletes can often "block out the pain."

Sports that have a high predisposition to macrotrauma injury include collision sports such as football and hockey, and sports like skiing that involve high velocity. Other activities that involve repetitive micro-trauma such as hurdling predispose the athlete to overuse injuries. A full list of these sports is presented in Table 21–5.

REFERENCES

1. O'Donoghue H. *Treatment of Injuries to Athletes.* Philadelphia, Pa: W B Saunders Co; 1976.
2. Warwick R, Williams PL, eds. *Gray's Anatomy.* 35th British ed. Philadelphia, Pa: W B Saunders Co; 1973.
3. Steindler A. *Kinesiology of the Human Body Under Normal and Pathological Conditions.* Springfield, Ill: Charles C. Thomas: 1955.
4. Singleton MC, Le Vearn BF. The hip joint: Structure stability, and stress. *Phys Ther.* 1975; 55:957.
5. Rydell N. Biomechanics of the hip joint. *Clin Orthop.* 1973; 92:6.
6. Brunstrom MA. *Clinical Kinesiology.* Philadelphia, Pa: FA Davis Co; 1972.
7. Standish WD. Overuse injuries in athletics: A perspective. *Med Sci Sports Exerc.* 1984; 16:1–7.
8. Hoppenfeld S. *Physical Examination of the Spine and Extremities.* New York: Appleton–Century–Crofts; 1976.
9. Janda V. *Muscle Function Testing.* Boston, Mass: Butterworths; 1983.
10. Daniels L, Worthingham C. *Muscle Testing.* Philadelphia, Pa: W B Saunders; 1972.

11. Basmajian JV. *Muscles Alive.* Baltimore, Md: Williams & Wilkins Co; 1978.

12. Sashin O. A critical analysis of the anatomy and pathological changes of the SI joints. *J Bone Joint Surg.* 1930; 12:891–910.

13. Weisl H. The movements of the sacroiliac joint. *Acta Anat.* 1955; 23:80–91.

14. Walker JM. Age-related differences in the human sacroiliac joint: A histological study: Implications for therapy. *J Orthop Sports Phys Ther.* 1986; 7:325–334.

15. Bowen V, Cassidy JD. Macroscopic and microscopic anatomy of the sacroiliac joint from embryonic life until the 8th decade. *Spine.* 1981; 6:620–628.

16. Vogler JB, Brown WH, Helms CA, Genank HK. The normal sacroiliac joint: A CT study of asymptomatic patients. *Radiology.* 1984; 151:433–437.

17. Kapandji IA. *The Physiology of the Joints.* Edinburgh: Churchill Livingstone Inc; 1974; 3.

18. Don Tigny RL. Dysfunction of the sacroiliac joint and its treatment. *J Orthop Sports Phys Ther.* 1979; 1:23–35.

19. Walton WJ. *Textbook of Osteopathic Diagnosis and Technique Procedures.* Colorado Springs, Colo: The American Academy of Osteopathy; 1970.

20. Rocabado M. *Course Notes: The Pelvic Girdle.* Tacoma, Wash: Rocabado Institute; 1986.

21. Mitchell FL, Moran PS, Pruzzo NA. *Evaluation and Treatment Manual of Osteopathic Manipulative Procedures.* Valley Park, Mo: 1979.

22. Fregerio NA, et al. Movement of the sacroiliac joint. *Clin Orthop.* 1974; 100:370–377.

23. Lavignolle B, et al. An approach to the functional anatomy of the sacroiliac joints in vivo. *Anat Clin.* 1983; 5:169–176.

24. Inman VT, Ralston HJ, Todd F. *Human Walking.* Baltimore, Md: Williams & Wilkins Co; 1981.

25. Johnston RC, Smidt GL. Hip motion measurements for selected activities of daily living. *Clin Orthop.* 1970; 72:205–215.

26. Johnston R. Mechanical consideration of the hip joint. *Arch Surg.* 1973; 107:411.

27. Perry J. Kinesiology of lower extremity bracing. *Clin Orthop.* 1974; 102:18–31.

28. Slowcum DB, James SL. Biomechanics of running. *JAMA.* 1986; 205:97–104.

29. Mann RA, Baxter DE, Lutter LD. Running symposium. *Foot and Ankle.* 1981; 1:190–224.

30. Colachis JR, Warden RE, Strohm BR, Bates BT, Osternig LR, et al. Movement of the sacroiliac joint in the adult male: A preliminary report. *Arch Phys Med Rehabil.* 1963; 44:490–503.

31. Brody DM. *Clinical Symposia.* Ciba; 4, 1980; 3(4).

32. James SL, Warden RE, Strohm BR, Bates BT, Osternig LR, et al. Injuries to runners. *Am J Sports Med.* 1978; 6(2):40.

33. Clement DB. Overuse running injuries. *Phys Sportsmed.* 1981; 9(5):47–58.

34. *Course Notes. Observation Gait Analysis Workshop.* Downey, Calif: Rancho Los Amigos Hospital, Pathokinesiology Service; 1977.

35. Subotnick SI. Limb length discrepancies of the lower extremity (the short leg syndrome). *J. Orthop Sports Phys Ther.* 1981; 3:11–15.

36. Morris JM. Biomechanical aspect of the hip joint. *Orthop Clin N Am.* 1971; 2:33–54.

37. Inman VT. The functional aspects of the abductor muscles of the hip. *J Bone Joint Surg.* 1947; 29:607–619.

38. Herring SA, Nilson KL. Introduction to overuse injuries. *Clin Sports Med.* 1987; 6:225–239.

39. Woerman AL, Binder-Macleod SA. Leg length discrepancy assessment: Accuracy and precision in five clinical methods of evaluation. *J Orthop Sports Phys Ther.* 1984; 5:230–239.

40. Gould JA, Davies GJ, eds. *Orthopedic and Sports Physical Therapy.* St. Louis, Mo: C V Mosby Co; 1985.

41. Delacerda FG, Wikoff OD. Effect of lower extremity asymmetry on the kinematics of gait. *J Orthop Sports Phys Ther.* 1982; 3:105–107.

42. Cavenagh PR, Williams KR. The effect of stride length variation on oxygen uptake during distance runs. *Med Sci Sports Exerc.* 1982; 14:30–35.

43. Delacerda FG, McCrory ML. A case report: Effect of a leg length differential on oxygen consumption. *J Orthop Sports Phys Ther.* 1981; 2:17–20.

44. Brandy WD, Sinning WE. Kinematic effects of heel lift use to correct lower limb length differences. *J Orthop Sports Phys Ther.* 1986; 7:173–179.

45. Romero JA. Unpublished study of elite marathoners. Chevy Chase, Md: Sports Medicine Center Inc; 1981.

46. Gleim GW, Nicholas JA, Webb JN. Isokinetic Evaluation following leg injuries. *Phys Sportsmed.* 1978; 6:(2)74–80.

47. Nicholas JA, Strizak AM, Veras G. A study of thigh muscle weakness in different pathological states of the lower extremity. *Am J Sports Med.* 1976; 4:241–250.

48. Boltz S, Davies GJ. Leg strength differences and correlation with total leg strength. *J Orthop Sports Phys Ther.* 1984; 2:123–129.

49. Sherman WM, Plyley MJ, Pearson DR, Hablanky HA, et al. Isokinetic rehabilitation after meniscectomy: A comparison of two methods of training. *Phys Sportsmed.* 1983; 11:121–133.

50. Burkett LN. Investigation into hamstring strains: The case of the hybrid muscle. *Am J Sports Med.* 1975; 3:5–12.

51. Solomonow M, D'Ambrosia R. Biomechanics of muscle overuse injuries: Theoretical approach. *Clin Sports Med.* 1987; 2:241–257.

52. Krejci V, Koch P. *Muscle and Tendon Injuries in Athletes.* Chicago, Ill: Year Book Medical Publishers; 1979.

53. Adams RJ, Chandler FA. Osteitis pubis of traumatic etiology. *J Bone Joint Surg.* 1953; 35:685–696.

54. Kuland DN. *The Injured Athlete.* Philadelphia, Pa: J B Lippincott Co; 1988; chap 11.

55. Koch RA, Jackson DW. Pubic symphysitis in runners. *Am J Sports Med.* 1981; 9:62–63.

56. Calliet R. *Soft Tissue Pain and Disability.* Philadelphia, Pa: F A Davis Co; 1977.

57. American Academy of Orthopaedic Surgeons. *Athletic Training and Sports Medicine.* Chicago, Ill: American Academy of Orthopaedic Surgeons; 1984.

58. Hunter LY, Funk JF Jr, eds. *Rehabilitation of the Injured Knee.* St Louis, Mo: C V Mosby Co; 1984.

59. Lewinnek GE, Kelsey J, Wyte AN, et al. The significance and comparison analysis of the epidemiology of hip fractures. *Clin Orthop.* 1980; 152:35–43.

60. Micheli L. Injuries to female athletes. *Surg Rounds.* 1979; 2:44.

61. Frankel VH. Fatigue fractures: Biomechanical consideration. *J Bone Joint Surg.* 1972; 54A:1345.

62. McBryde AM. Stress fractures in runners. *Clin Sports Med.* 1985; 4:737–752.

63. *Athletic Training: Principles and Practice.* Palo Alto, Calif: Mayfield Publishing Co; 1986.

64. Brody DM. Personal communication.

65. Blatz DJ. Bilateral femoral and tibial shaft stress fractures in runners. *Am J Sports Med.* 1981; 9:322–326.

66. Markey KL. Stress fractures. *Clin Sports Med.* 1987; 6:405–425.

67. Scully TJ, Besterman G. Stress fracture—A preventable training injury. *Milit Med.* 1982; 147:285–287.

68. Kelsey JL. Epidemiology of slipped capital femoral epiphysis: A review of the literature. *Pediatrics.* 1973; 51:1042–1048.

69. Catterall A. Coxa plana. *Mod Trends Orthop.* 1972; 6:122.

70. Fisher R. An epidemiological study of Legg–Perthes disease. *J Bone Joint Surg.* 1972; 54:769–778.

71. Barfred T. Experimental rupture of the achilles tendon: Comparison of various types of experimental rupture in rats. *Acta Orthop Scand.* 1971; 42:528–543.

72. Unverth LJ, Olix ML. The effects of local steroid injections on tendon. *J Sports Med.* 1973; 1:31–37.

73. Sweetham R. Corticosteroidal arthropathy and tendon rupture. *J Bone Joint Surg.* 1969; 51B: 397–398.

74. Halpern AA, Horowitz BG, Nagel DA. Tendon ruptures associated with corticosteroid therapy. *West J Med.* 1977; 127:378–382.

75. Stanish WD, Curwin S, Rubinovich M. Tendinitis: The analysis and treatment for running. *Clin Sports Med.* 1985; 4:593–609.

76. Jensen K, DiFabio RP. Evaluation of eccentric exercise in treatment of patellar tendinitis. *Phys Ther.* 1989; 69:211–216.

77. Roy S, Irvin R. *Sports Medicine: Prevention, Evaluation, Management and Rehabilitation.* Englewood Cliffs NJ: Prentice Hall; 1983; chap 17.

78. Radcliffe JC, Farentinos RC. *Plyometrics Explosive Power Training.* Champaign, Ill: Human Kinetics Publishers Inc; 1985.

79. Costello F. *Bounding to the Top.* College Park, Md: University of Maryland.

22

The Knee

Robert Mangine and Timothy Heckman

INTRODUCTION

The knee joint is often described as the most complex joint in the body. It is one of the most frequently injured joints and one of the more difficult to evaluate. The knee is the fulcrum of the longest lever of the body and is characterized by low osseous stability and high dynamic stability provided by the ligaments and muscle groups of the leg and thigh.

Sports physical therapists must have a good working knowledge of the anatomy, biomechanics, pathologies, evaluation, treatment, and rehabilitation principles of the knee. This chapter addresses anatomy, biomechanics, pathomechanics and injuries, prevention, and rehabilitation.

ANATOMY OF THE KNEE

Femoral Component

The proximal component of the patellofemoral and tibiofemoral complex is the femur. The shaft of the femur is the longest bone in the human body and terminates as the largest articular surface to form two separate joints. Originating in the hip, it courses in an oblique, medial, and distal direction as it descends to the knee. This angle of the shaft allows for the weight-bearing condyles of the femur to align with the axis of the lower extremity, with the weight-bearing alignment falling through the tibial spine. This alignment causes a normal valgus angle between the medially oriented femur and the laterally oriented tibia (Fig 22–1). This angle is approximately 170 to 175 degrees,[1] but there is a difference, with women having a slightly increased pelvic width, allowing the angle to be less than 170 degrees. This results in a tibial valgus or knock-kneed position. An angle greater than 175 degrees is referred to as tibia varum or a bowlegged position, often associated in alignment pathologies such as in chronic anterior cruciate deficiencies.

The distal femur expands, forming a pair of large condyles that articulate with both the patella and the tibia. The articular condyles are the longest in the human, are shaped as convex in both the sagittal and frontal planes, and overhang posteriorly the shaft of the femur. Anteriorly, the condyles are divided by the trochlear groove for articulation with the patella. Inferiorly, the condyles are divided by the intercondylar notch, in which lays the cruciate ligaments. When the femur is viewed in the frontal plane and in a flexed position, the condyles form a horseshoe configuration. This configuration allows for the dual joint articulation—anteriorly with the patella and inferiorly with the tibia. The articular surfaces of the condyles are covered by smooth hyaline cartilage that ranges from 4 to 6 mm in depth to withstand compressive and shear forces placed on the surfaces during activities of daily living.

Proximal to the condyles are the femoral epicondyles that are convex in shape and easily palpable. The epicondyles serve as the site of attachment for the capsular structures, ligaments, and tendons that surround the knee and are, therefore, highly vascular. On the medial epicondyle is the adductor tubercle, which serves the dual purpose of insertion for the adductor tendon and origin of the medial collateral ligament. This tubercle is also the site of the adductor hiatus through which the saphenous nerve and vein pass. The nerve is easily involved with medial injuries. The lateral epicondyle is also easily palpable and serves as attachment for the lateral collateral ligament.

The lateral femoral condyle demonstrates several distinguishing characteristics:

1. It is more in line with the shaft of the femur due to the medial direction of the femoral shaft.
2. Its anterior-to-posterior direction is a somewhat flattened configuration.
3. In a medial-to-lateral direction, the lateral condyle is larger than the medial condyle.
4. In the trochlear groove area, the lateral con-

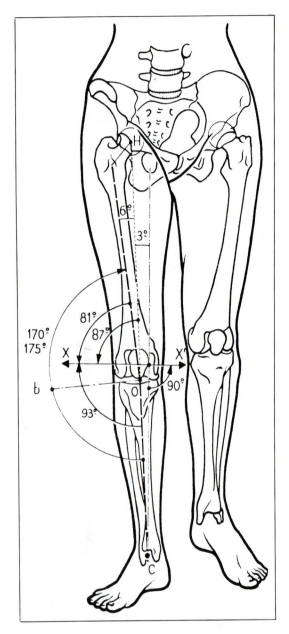

Figure 22–1. Normal alignment of the knee falls between 170 to 175 degrees. An increase in the angle above 175 degrees results in a genu varum deformity. A decrease in the angle below 170 degrees results in a genu valgum deformity. *(From Kapandji IA. The Physiology of the Joints. Baltimore, Md: Williams & Wilkins Co; 1970; II , with permission.)*

dyle increases in height to accommodate the large lateral facet of the patella and prevent subluxation or dislocation during normal patellar function.

The medial femoral condyle is distinguishable by the following:

1. It has a greater oblique angle in reference to the shaft of the femur, bringing it into line with the mechanical axis of the lower limb.

2. The anterior-to-posterior dimension is longer and is biconvexed both anterio-posteriorly and medio-laterally.
3. The longer anterior-posterior distance allows for greater rolling to occur, resulting in rotation during the terminal extension phase (Fig 22–2).

Development of the distal femur occurs from one epiphyseal growth center that is present at birth and remains active until 18 years of age. At that point, fusing occurs with the main shaft of the femur. The distal femur ossification center transects through the adductor tubercle. The distal femur has developed a trabecular system that forms a criss-crossing matrix in both the medial and lateral condyle. The design of the system changes as long stress lines run vertically up into the shaft. This system connects the articular surfaces to the cortical bone to absorb forces. A separate system of transverse trabecula interconnects the two condyles, adding to the overall strength.

Tibial Component

The distal component of the tibiofemoral joint is the proximal portion of the tibia by way of the tibial plateaus. The plateau is divided into medial and lateral compartments of two flattened shelves. Anteriorly, the plateau is even with the shaft of the tibia, but posteri-

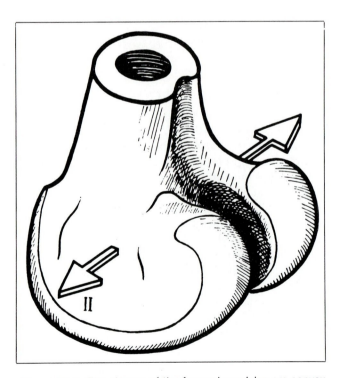

Figure 22–2. The shapes of the femoral condyles are convex, appearing as two large rocking chair rails. They overhang the shaft of the femur to accommodate the large posterior musculature and allow a large surface area for rolling. *(From Kapandji IA. The Physiology of the Joints. Baltimore, Md: Williams & Wilkins Co; 1970; II , with permission.)*

orly it overhangs the shaft. The design of the tibial plateaus at first appear as biconcaved–concaved saucers, but subtle differences are present. The articular surfaces are covered by hyaline cartilage that overhangs the plateau by 2 or 3 mm. Adjacent to the tibial plateau is the epicondylar region that is highly vascular and serves as the attachment area for the capsule and tibiomeniscal ligaments.

Differences in the medial tibial plateau include the following:

1. The medial tibial plateau is larger than the lateral in order to accommodate its counterpart on the femur.
2. It has an oval-shaped appearance that is biconcaved–concaved in both the anterior–posterior and medial–lateral planes.
3. In the lateral plane, the posterior medial plateau does not demonstrate as great a posterior overhang as the lateral.

The lateral tibial plateau differs in the following respects:

1. Its shape is circular in appearance and runs in a posterior–inferior direction to overhang the shaft.
2. The posterior lateral corner of the plateau flairs to form an articulation with the fibular head.
3. The concavity to the lateral plateau occurs in the medial–lateral plane; however, the anterior–posterior plane reveals convexity, making it a very unique structure and thereby facilitating rotation of the femur during movement (Fig 22–3).

The compartments of the tibia are divided by the intercondylar eminence. This eminence is composed of the tibial spines and several flattened regions. The tibial eminence is highly vascular and serves as a possible site of attachment of the transverse ligament and synovial tissue. The eminence is divided into medial and lateral tibial spines that can be observed as small upward projections between the plateaus. Projecting in a superior direction places the spines in the femoral intercondylar notch during flexion, making rotation easier. A second element of the inter plateau region is a flattened anterior depression that separates the medial and lateral intercondylar eminence, serving as the site of attachment for the anterior cruciate ligament (Fig 22–3).

As a continuation of the plateaus in the anterior direction there is an inferior tubercle. The tubercle serves as the insertion for the patellar ligament (quadriceps tendon) an extension of the quadriceps mechanism. Fixating the extensor mechanism on the inner margin of this triangular region is the inferiormost attachment for the capsule following the patellar tendon. Posterior to the tendon and extending from the medial and lateral border is the infrapatellar fat pad and bursa.

The ossification center of the proximal tibia remains active from birth until maturation at 16 to 18 years of age. Separate from the proximal tibia, the tibial tubercle demonstrates a separate ossification center that can be an extension of the proximal center itself or a completely separate center that initiates growth when an individual is approximately 12 years old.

The trabecular systems of the tibia resembles the pattern of the femur. The condyles have a separate system of interwoven stress lines that eventually extend to the underlying cortical bone. In addition to the segmental system is a horizontal pattern that interconnects the two plateaus, providing absorption of mechanical forces along the transverse plane.

Patella

The third compartment in the knee is composed of the patellofemoral joint. This small but complex joint is the

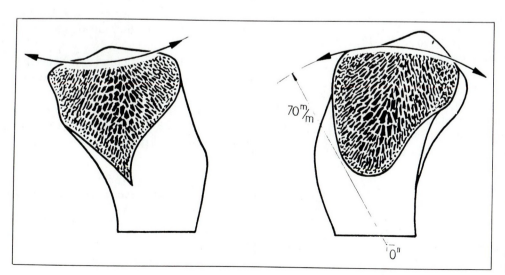

Figure 22-3. The shapes of the tibial plateaus are demonstrated. Like their femoral counterparts, the tibial compartments overhang the posterior shaft of the tibia. The medial compartment is biconcave whereas the lateral compartment is concave in the medial–lateral direction, and is convex in the anterior–posterior direction. *(From Kapandji IA. The Physiology of the Joints. Baltimore, Md: Williams & Wilkins Co; 1970; II., with permission.)*

leading cause of pain in the knee because of the unique relationship of the patella with the femur. The patella is the largest sesamoid bone in the human body and is embedded in the distal extensor mechanism. When viewed from any plane, the patella has a triangular appearance:

1. Anteriorly it demonstrates a broad superior border and a distal inferior apex.
2. Transversely, the patella reveals a broad anterior border (serving as the attachment site of the extensor mechanism) and a posterior apex, composed of the articular surfaces.
3. The lateral view reveals the same composite of the transverse view.

The anterior border of the patella is a haven of vascular foramina due to the extensive attachment of the quadriceps muscle. Initially, the tendon inserts in layers along the superior border and then continues distally along the patellar surface to eventually narrow to a 20- to 22-mm tendinous band that inserts into the tibial tubercle.

The posterior surface of the patella is divided into a medial and lateral articular facet by a central vertical ridge. These facets are further subdivided into three facets: superior, middle, and inferior, making a total of six articular regions. This division is based in contact with the femur. A seventh facet can also be identified on the far medial facet that makes contact with the femur only with the extreme range of flexion and is identified as the "odd" or flexion facet. The shapes of the articular surfaces are convexed in order to accommodate the concaved femoral trochlear groove. The articular surface of the lateral facet is wider to correspond to the femoral surface. The hyaline cartilage covering the posterior facets may be the thickest in the human body, measuring 5 mm in depth. The forces crossing this surface may exceed 12 times the body weight with daily activities.

The initial composition of the patella is cartilage cells at birth, but can be easily palpated. Ossification is generally completed by 6 years, but the posterior surface may continue to change into the second decade of life. The trabecular stress systems are quite simple, with the first system parallel and the second system perpendicular to the anterior surface. These form a criss-crossing pattern from the posterior surface to the anterior surface. The patella must resist traction forces in excess of 2000 lb that are applied through the extension mechanism.

Menisci

The next interarticular system consists of the fibrocartilage discs we term menisci. Various functions have been attributed to the menisci but perhaps its most important function is its role as a stabilizer. This is due to the poorly designed osseous system, which requires augmentation. These are two intra-articular fibrocartilage menisci that attach along the peripheral border of the tibial plateaus. The attachment of the menisci occur through the peripheral meniscotibial ligament along the epicondylar border of the plateau.

Secondary functions attributed to the menisci include

1. Increasing the integrity of the joint capsule
2. Aiding in transmission of the weight bearing forces
3. Improving lubrication
4. Aiding in the rolling of the femoral condyles during motion

The shape of the meniscus varies by compartment, but some mutual characteristics are seen. From a frontal view, they appear as wedge-shaped crescents with a rounded peripheral surface, thinning to a concave apex in the central joint. Superiorly, the sufaces are concave, matching their tibial counterparts but flattened on the inferior surface. A superior view of the menisci show that they follow the shape of the tibial plateaus on which they lie.

Medial meniscus variances include the following:

1. A semilunar shape with a wide base of attachment both anteriorly and posteriorly. The anterior and posterior segments are called the horns
2. The medial meniscus flares posteriorly and widens to a greater extent than the lateral meniscus
3. The medial meniscus has a tight connection to the medial collateral ligament by the deep layer of that ligament

Lateral meniscus differences include the following

1. It has a more circular shape.
2. Attachment of its anterior and posterior horns are closer together on the tibial eminence; the result of this is a higher degree of mobility for this meniscus than the medial during knee motion.
3. The anterior horns of the menisci are connected by a transverse ligament bridging across the depression anterior to the tibial eminence.
4. The peripheral attachment of the lateral meniscus is not as extensive and features a hiatus in the posterior lateral quadrant for passage of the popliteal tendon.

The menisci (Fig 22–4) also display dynamic features by way of attachment of tendinous expansions into the capsule alignment. Anteriorly, this occurs by the way of the extensor mechanism in the format of the meniscopatellar ligament. Posteriorly, the semimembranous inserts into the medial meniscus by attaching

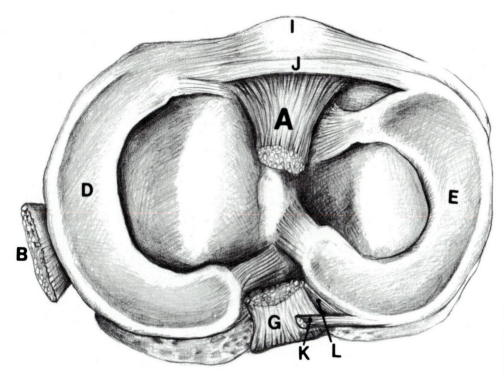

Figure 22-4. The medial (D) and lateral (E) menisci as they are connected by the transverse ligament (J) anteriorly. B represents the medial collateral ligament and its close communication to the MCL. The anterior cruciate ligament and posterior ligament are shown as A and G, respectively. The ligament of Wrisberg and Humphreys are slips of the posterior cruciate ligament shown as K and L, respectively.

to the posterior capsule. Laterally, this is accomplished by the popliteal tendon sending a slip into the lateral meniscus as it comes through the hiatus. Due to their extensive capsular attachment, the menisci receive a vascular and neural supply to the outer third termed the red zone. The inner portion is avascular and termed the white zone and is also thought to be aneural.

During flexion and extension, the dynamics of the menisci follow the path of the tibia. Therefore, extension results in anterior displacement (due to tension on the meniscopatellar ligaments) and flexion produces a posterior translation (due to the semimembranous on the medial side and popliteous muscle on the lateral side). There is a marked difference in the amount of play in the menisci, the medial meniscus having a 6-mm displacement and the lateral meniscus a 12-mm displacement. With rotation an opposite motion occurs, with the menisci following the femur as they are impinged to a particular position.

A unique feature of the lateral meniscus is that it can receive an attachment from one of three possible structures: the posterior cruciate ligament; the ligament of Wrisberg, a posterior slip off of the posterior cruciate ligament (PCL); or the ligament of Humphrey, an anterior slip off of the PCL. The ligament of Humphrey and Wrisberg is found only in 36% of the population and their function is highly questionable.

Knee Capsule

The knee joint complex is enveloped by the most extensive capsule in the human body. The function of the capsule is multifaceted and receives both static ligament support and dynamic muscular support through tendon insertion. Attachment of the capsule is along the articular borders of the patellofemoral and tibiofemoral joints and inserts peripherally to the articular margins. Due to its immense size, features of the capsule include the following:

1. A posterior recess covers both the femoral medial and lateral condyles
2. Indentation into intercondylar notch of the femur
3. Large superior patellar pouch
4. Attachment of the menisci along the peripheral border of the tibia, assisting in the stabilization of the menisci; this peripheral attachment is referred to as the coronary ligament
5. The capsule descends over the anterior crest of the tibia along the borders of the patellar tendon
6. The anterior inferior packet is filled by the inferior patellar fat pad and the infrapatellar bursa
7. The capsule is supported on the medial and lateral sides by aponeurotic expansions of the quadriceps mechanism, of which one of these expansions is termed the meniscopatellar ligament, and the second expansion is the patellofemoral ligament running from the mid-patella to the adductor or lateral femoral epicondylar respective of their name

The extensor mechanism expansions in the capsule serve vital dynamic and static functions. By attaching at the anterior third of the menisci, the meniscopatellar ligaments cause an anterior glide with extension. The second half of the expansion is the patellofemoral ligament, which serves to stabilize the patella by both static and dynamic restraint. It is unclear whether these ligaments are present at birth or develop as a result of mechanical stress associated with activities of daily living.

Medial Ligaments

The medial compartment of the knee is supported by three key structures: the collateral ligament, the posterior oblique ligament, and the capsule. The deep portion of the capsule is reinforced by the deep collateral ligament, which is divided into two segments. The superior portion originates along the peripheral border of the femoral condyles to a midpoint above the superior border of the medial meniscus. The second portion originates along the peripheral border of the tibial plateau and runs superior to the interior meniscal margin. The deep layer is reinforced by the outer superficial section of the ligament, is approximately 2.54 cm in width, and originates from a fan-shaped attachment along the lower border of the adductor tubercle, giving it a deltoid shape appearance as it descends past the joint line to a point approximately 3 or 4 cm below the tibial plateau. The insertion lies under the pes anserinus tendon and is separated from that tendon by the pes anserine bursae. From a biomechanical standpoint the significance of this shape is that tension is present in some portion of the ligament throughout the range of motion. The primary function is to stabilize the tibiofemoral joint from valgus stress; maximal tension, however, is seen in the 0–degree to hyperextension position.

Posteromedial to the medial collateral ligament is a thickness in the joint capsule inserting into the tibia along the roughened groove just inferior to the articular surface. It is supported dynamically by the tibial arm of the semimembranous tendon. The ligament formed in this corner is the posterior oblique ligament, stabilizing the knee against valgus and anteromedial rotatory instability.

Posteriorly, the capsule runs superiorly and covers the articular surfaces of the femoral condyle forming two large bags. Posteroinferiorly, it runs along the tibial plateau but descends at the central area along the inner border of the posterior cruciate ligament indenting into the intracondylar notch. Superficial to the posterior cruciate and coursing across the two femoral condyles is the oblique popliteal ligament. The ligament runs in an oblique superior direction from medial-to-lateral orientation, transversely crossing the posterior cruciate. Again, it is provided augmentation from the capsular arm of the semimembranous muscle. A point to reiterate is that, due to extensive attachment to the capsule and ligament, contraction of the semimembranous muscle will result in a posterior glide of the medial meniscus.

Posterolateral Complex

The posterior lateral region of the joint is a complex arrangement of static and dynamic support tissues. The first structure to be understood is a static reinforcement of the posterior corner that is provided by the arcuate complex. The dynamic augmentation to this area is the popliteal tendon, and the lateral head of the gastrocnemius muscle. The arcuate complex originates along the margin of the lateral femoral condyle and runs inferiorly and obliquely, converging into the fibular head by a narrow apex forming a triangular structure. As previously mentioned, dynamic support is provided by the popliteal tendons, of which fibers of the tendon blend with the aponeurosis of the posterior lateral capsule. This attachment extends into the posterior portion of the lateral meniscus. The popliteal tendon also provides reinforcement to the oblique popliteal ligament as it courses in an oblique inferior direction. The second ligamentous structure on the posterolateral corner of the knee is the fabellofibular ligament. This structure originates on the posterior aspect of the lateral condyle or the fabella, which is a sesamoid bone in the posterolateral soft tissue. It curves in an inferior oblique direction to insert into the fibula. The third structure in the lateral region that inserts into the fibular styloid process is the lateral collateral ligament. It initiates from the lateral femoral epicondyle and is a thin 12-mm structure that is easily palpable because it is the most superficial. The function of these structures is to form a posterolateral pillar that fans out, providing varus restraint and lateral tibial plateau rotation, in much the same manner as does the posterior oblique ligament.

Internal Ligamentous Structure

In the femoral notch lie two ligament structures that have received the greatest attention of all ligaments of the knee, the anterior and posterior cruciates. These structures are covered by their own synovial sheath, which separates them from the joint capsule. The name "cruciate" was derived from the fact that the ligaments form a crossing pattern that results in their rotating around each other in various ranges of motion.

The anterior cruciate ligament (Fig 22–5) originates from the depression anterior to the medial tibial eminence. It is the anteriormost structure in the femoral notch. From this position, it runs in a superior, oblique, posterior direction to insert on the medial surface of the lateral femoral condyle; the attachment orientation is a semicircular pattern at both ends and has a twisted configuration. The anteriormost fibers may

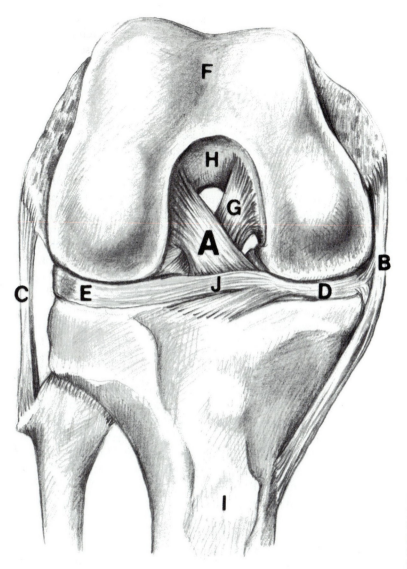

Figure 22-5. Anterior cruciate ligament (A), posterior cruciate ligament (G), lateral meniscus (E), medial meniscus (D), medial collateral ligament (B), lateral collateral ligament (C), Transverse meniscus ligament (J), intercondylar notch (H), and trochlear groove (F).

have a slip running to the anterior horn of the lateral meniscus. Girgis has not found an attachment to the medial meniscus to be common.[1] The semilunar shape of attachment to the anterior cruciate can result in it being divided into two functional portions: the anteromedial and posterior bands. The anteromedial band is described as the functional portion because there is tension in this segment in the 20- to 45-degree range of motion.

Immediately behind and in communication with the anterior cruciate ligament is the posterior cruciate ligament in the intercondylar notch. Insertion occurs on the posterolateral aspect of the medial femoral condyle, again in a semicircular pattern or pointing in the posterior direction, with the arch of the circle running adjacent to the femoral condylar articular surface. The course of the posterior cruciate is in a posterior, oblique, inferior direction to its insert site in the posterior depression between the tibial plateaus. It continues

inferiorly along the tibia approximately 1 cm, which gives it a very broad and convex configuration. Furthermore, the ligament sends a slip into the posterior horn of the lateral meniscus. The posterior cruciate is also divided into two functional units, the anterolateral and posterior functional bands. Unlike the anterior cruciate, it is the posterior portion of the ligament that becomes taut in flexion, with the bulk of the anterior portion coming under tension during extension. Both attachments in this ligament lie posterior to the mechanical axis of the knee.

The remaining two posterior ligaments are the Wrisberg and Humphry ligaments.[2] These structures are found in various combinations, most commonly attached to the posterior horn of the lateral meniscus and then running in a medial direction, inserting on the medial femoral condyle or posterior cruciate ligament. The function of these structures is to give support to the meniscus during rotational movement of the tibia.

Bursae

Surrounding the human knee is a combination of two dozen or more bursae.[3] The function of these bursae includes reducing friction, either between muscle and tendon, tendon and tendon, or tendon and bone. Four of these bursae are routinely seen to be involved in inflammatory states: the prepatellar, infrapatellar, suprapatellar, and the pes anserine bursae. The bursae surrounding the patella are generally injured as a result of direct trauma. Football, soccer, wrestling, volleyball, and baseball are sports commonly associated with injuries to these structures. The patellar bursae are located on the anterior aspect of the knee and are easily palpable. The pes anserine bursa is interposed between the medial collateral ligament and the pes anserine tendon just distal and medial to the medial joint space. This structure can become involved with overuse type of trauma such as in a longdistance runner in extremely long duration training.[1] The bursa may also become involved with injuries to the medial collateral ligament since there is close communication.

Clinically, evaluation can be quite difficult, especially in distinguishing between inflammation of a bursitis versus swelling due to joint effusion. Bursitis is localized and remains outside the knee capsule itself whereas an intraarticular swelling indicates an internal derangement.

Musculature

Muscle systems that surround the knee fill two important roles in providing normal locomotion while dynamically protecting the joint against injury.[3,4,5] The musculature support was devised as a dynamic backup to the capsular and ligamentous systems, therefore, injury reduction by muscle mechanics occurs due to its proper placement and force production. Alteration in the muscle due to congenital causes on disuse due to injury may reduce its efficiency and increase the risk of injury to the knee joint. It is now clinically acceptable to support the significance of the thigh musculature in prevention of knee injuries, masking acute symptoms and providing the ultimate function to minimize future re-injury.[4,5,6,7,8]

Anterior Musculature

The anterior thigh musculature is composed of the quadriceps extensor mechanism, sartorius, and iliopsoas muscles. The quadriceps extensor mechanism consists of the rectus femoris, vastus lateralis, vastus intermedius, and vastus medialis oblique and longus. The literature is inundated with discussion of the selective functions of the different portions of the extensor mechanism.[9] The origin of this muscle group ranges from the anterior inferior iliac spine (rectus femoris) to the anterior, medial, and lateral proximal shaft of the femur (vasti group and articularis genu). These structures are innervated by the femoral nerve and function in union upon contraction. Injury to the knee can result in palpable atrophy that affects all muscles but is first noticeable of the vastus medialis.

The vastus medialis has received a great deal of attention in the literature due to its crucial role in dynamically protecting the patella during tracking. The crucial factor of the vastus medialis is the oblique portion inserting into the patella at a 55-degree angle to support the patellofemoral ligament, thereby linking their relationship to various patellar dysfunctions. Due to this oblique orientation, there are questions pertaining to its importance in actually serving as a knee extendor at all versus purely as a dynamic patellar stabilizer. The remainder of the extensor mechanism inserts at the superior border of the patella and continues across the anterior surface to converge as the patellar tendon inferiorly. The femoral quadriceps muscles can generate and must withstand tremendous forces when involved in activities of daily living (ADLs) as well as athletic activities.

Posterior Musculature

The posterior thigh musculature is composed of the hamstrings, gastrocnemius, and popliteal muscles. All three muscle groups dynamically reinforce the posterior capsule and posterior oblique ligament. The hamstrings, however, have an additional function by an indirect effect through their biarticular attachment. The proximal attachment is the ischial tubercle in the pelvis. Weakness of the hamstring can result in an anterior pelvic rotation innominate, and tightness can result in a posterior rotational innominate. The distal insertion of the hamstring is in a "Y" pattern after the muscle divides at the midpoint. The medial attachment of the semitendinosis is by way of the pes anserine tendon and the semimembranous to the posterior medial tibial plateau capsule and sweeping across the back of the knee. The hamstrings on the lateral side insert into the fibular head by way of the biceps tendon.

The hamstrings also play a role in rotatory movement of the tibia. Through its tibial arm attachment, the semimembranous muscle can induce a medial rotation. The biceps femoris muscle provides external rotation of the tibia.

Normal function of the hamstrings does not require them to produce as much force as the quadriceps. Velocity testing studies performed by isokinetic evaluation, however, show at high speeds that torque production of the two muscle groups by the hamstrings will approach a 1:1 relationship. The importance of the hamstrings as knee stabilizers is now widely accepted, especially in the patient whose anterior cruciate ligament is deficient. Its role on stability provides the rehabilitation specialist a special challenge in knee injuries.

The gastroc muscle originates in the depression

immediately proximal to the femoral condyles. These structures can provide some stabilization to the posterior knee structures but are not well defined. After descending distally the two separate heads converge to form the Achilles' tendon. Distally, this structure easily becomes involved in pathology by developing atrophy, which may lead to an overall loss of muscular power of the lower extremity.

The final muscle on the posterior aspect is the popliteal. This originates in a small indentation superior and anterior to the lateral collateral ligament on the femoral condyle. It descends under the ligament and then moves through a hiatus in the lateral capsule, fanning out to insert on the posterior aspect of the medial tibia. When it enters the knee, it sends a slip into the posterior horn or of the lateral meniscus and capsule. The popliteus is the key that unlocks the knee during the intial phase of flexion. In the first 15 degrees of flexion, internal rotation must occur to unlock the screw bone mechanism. The popliteus is a key source of this rotation and flexion.

Medial/Lateral Musculature

The importance of medial thigh musculature to the knee joint is frequently overlooked. The medial and lateral structures may play an important role in stabilizing the knee and influencing knee function by the muscle·s influence on the pelvis. Weakness in either musculature creates dysfunction of pelvic movement, resulting in an upward movement of the innominate, affecting limb length. The medial musculature further provides stability to the femur during ADLs, preventing pelvic rotation and thereby allowing normal function. The iliotibial band on the lateral side is described as providing varus stability, patellar stability, and aiding in controlling pelvic rotation. It can easily become involved with patellar malalignment patients (excessive lateral compression syndrome) and overuse pathologies.

Biomechanics

The knee joint must be considered a tricompartmental unit composed of the patellofemoral, medial tibiofemoral, and lateral tibiofemoral joint. Movement of these three joints is coupled and influenced by the muscles, bones, ligaments, and menisci.

Adequate motion of the tibiofemoral joint requires coupling of the arthrokinematics of rolling, gliding, and rotating in an altered form of a hinge joint. Thus the tibiofemoral joint functions with six degrees of freedom. Noyes[10,11] has described a matrix of three rotations—

- Flexion/extension
- Internal/external
- Valgus/varus

and three translations—

- Anterior/posterior
- Medial/lateral
- Distraction/compression

Proper tibiofemoral function requires the freedom of motion and the control of the applied forces. During tibiofemoral motion the mechanical axis of flexion/extension falls through the femoral epicondyle and follows a constantly changing pattern described as a helicoid. A predetermined pattern results due to the shape of the femoral articular surface. Initially, with flexion from extension a rolling pattern predominates, followed by a sliding pattern at mid range and a rolling pattern again at the end range. This axis may shift slightly throughout life as the articular surfaces wear and the joint spaces narrow.

Patellofemoral Joint

The patellofemoral joint mechanical pattern is directed by the quadriceps muscle, the shape of the femoral sulcus, the patellar shape, static restraints, biomechanics at the hip and foot, and dynamic muscular restraints.[12] The patella's primary function is to increase the distance of the extensor muscle from the mechanical axis, provide a smooth articular surface, and protect the anterior knee.[13] To perform its normal function, the patella must glide in the trochlear groove, following a predetermined pattern that is influenced by the leverage force of the extensor muscles. While fulfilling its role to enhance extensor forces, however, the patella must withstand shear and compressive forces that must be absorbed by the articular surfaces.

In the extended knee, the patella lies superior to the trochlear groove, resting on the suprapatellar fat pad, capsule, bursae, and synovium. This position is slightly lateral due to the resting position of the tibial tubercle and anterior inferior iliac spine by which the rectus femoris attaches as well as the resting normal valgus position of the lower extremity. Even in the extended position, the patella will still slide superiorly approximately 1 cm with quadriceps contraction. Upon initiation of flexion, the patella is pulled into the trochlear groove.[14] By 20 to 30 degrees of flexion, the patella is now engaged in the trochlear groove and is laterally oriented. With further flexion, the patellar articular surfaces segmentally come in contact with the trochlear groove. The inferior facets of the patella first contact the superior femoral condyles, then the mid facets of the patella contact the mid femoral at the 60- to 90-degree range, and finally the superior facets of the patella contact the inferior femur at 90 to 120 degrees. The exception to this is the "odd" facet, or flexion fact, which is a smaller facet on the medial aspect of the patella.[13] With extreme flexion, the "odd" facet of the patella is contacted, with greater resultant pressure as it

contacts the inner margin of the medial femoral condyle in the region of the intercondylar groove. Lateral contact follows the same pattern and occurs in the extreme inner margin.

The primary arthrokinematic pattern the patella displays is gliding as it moves distally into femoral trochlear groove. At the end of flexion and extension, the patella also displaces a tilt that is slightly lateral. Tilts can be observed in patients performing active and resistive motions. During extension, the patella glides proximally, being pulled superiorly by the extensor mechanism. Again, at the end of extension, a lateral tilt and shift are observed.

Stabilization of the patellofemoral joint is provided by static and dynamic systems. Dynamic stability is performed by contraction of the vastus medialis oblique muscle, which was previously described. This muscle also augments the static system on the medial border of the patella and medial femoral condyle. The static stability is provided by the trochlear groove, the patellar size and shape, and the patellofemoral ligaments. Pathology to either joint can result in abnormal affects in the patellofemoral joint tracking. This is commonly seen by way of atrophy to the vastus medial oblique muscle on scarring of the lateral reticular tissues.

Lower Extremity Mechanics

Total lower extremity function requires proper mechanics of the pelvis, hip, knee, and ankle. These structures function in an open or closed kinetic chain system. The concept of open versus closed kinetic chain rehabilitation has a definite influence on knee injuries and their management. The lower extremity circles through an open kinetic chain when the foot is off the ground and a closed kinetic chain when the foot is in contact with a supporting surface. The significance in this system is the linear forces placed on closed kinetic chain, potentially prohibiting the function of the distal segment (i.e., the foot), thereby transferring forces to the remaining parts (i.e., the knee and the hip). Abnormal forces that cannot be distributed must be absorbed by all tissues in the closed kinetic chain. The inability to dispose of abnormal forces frequently leads to overuse injury to the knee, foot, pelvis, and lower limb soft tissue (Fig 22–6).

PATHOMECHANICS OF INJURY

Knee injury stems from two broad categories and results in trauma of a micro or macro effect. Generally speaking, injury is caused by an accumulation of repetitive forces (as seen in the overuse syndrome) rather than a single application of a powerful force. Forces applied to the human body must be countered internally and

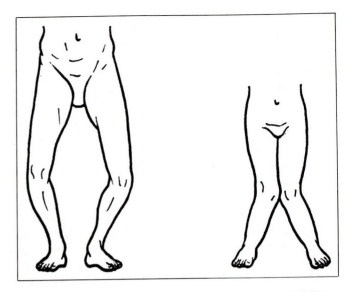

Figure 22–6. The two most common lower extremity malalignments—(4) genu varum and (5) genu valgum. (*From Kapandji IA. The Physiology of the Joints. Baltimore, Md: Williams & Wilkins Co; 1970; II., with permission.*)

any force that is not dispersed results in tissue dysfunction.

Microtrauma due to repetitive overload results in an inflammatory reaction. During growth and maturation, our bodies learn to absorb normal forces associated with ADLs. If, however, an individual increases the intensity of a force or the length of time it is applied during activity, an inflammatory process can result from this excessive normal force. Excessive normal forces include either high-repetition activities with a low load or low-repetition activities with a high load.

In microtraumatic injuries the pathology may be simple, but finding the underlying cause extremely difficult. For example, limb-length difference, pronatory problem, flexibility, strength deficit, and compensatory gait pattern all cause the lower extremity kinetic chain to lower its tolerance to absorb or disperse ADL forces, thus leading to tissue breakdown.

In some patients, however, malalignment conditions may be preexistent, for example, limb-length differences as great as three-fourths in, gross pronation, muscular tightness, muscle deficiencies, patellofemoral joint malalignment, and lower extremity malalignment. When a macrotraumatic injury occurs it may start a cycle that becomes very difficult to manage and interrupt.

Whether primary or secondary pathology occurs it can affect a multitude of tissues, including but not limited to ligament, tendon, muscle, synovium, nerve, capsule, articular cartilage, and bone. It is often a finding that several of these tissues either unilaterally or in some combination result in bizarre pain patterns. At the onset of pain, the patient usually chooses to modify

activity or attempts to compensate. Either choice often results in a more serious condition. The second most common finding by the patient is joint swelling, leading to an advancement of the condition.

The initiation of conservative management of knee pathology centers around discovery of the causal factor. If only the symptoms are treated, they frequently recur upon return to activity. The pathomechanical causes of lower extremity microtraumatic injuries were previously listed and careful assessment must be performed to determine the cause.

Macrotrauma is injury centering around a high internal or external force resulting in immediate clinical signs and symptoms. The knee joint can receive an external force by direct contact to disrupt any and all tissues. The reverse to this are individuals who can generate high internal muscular forces that cannot be absorbed or dispersed by the static system. These high-force injuries can disrupt the ligament, muscle–tendon unit, menisci, joint capsule, articular surfaces, bone, nerve, and blood vessel system. Isolated injuries are rare. Macrotraumatic injuries result from exceeding the limits of joint motion, for which there is a protective mechanism, whether by direct injury such as a valgus contact injury or an indirect mechanism such as a rotational load as in a cutting type injury.

As with microtraumatic injury, the conditon is exacerbated if predisposing factors are present. These must be identified and treated to ensure a safe return to activity.

Pathomechanics of the Patellofemoral Joint

The patellofemoral joint is probably the most common source of complaint in knee injuries. The most common patellofemoral injuries represent

1. Extensor mechanism malalignment
2. Patellofemoral chondrosis
3. Patellar contusions
4. Lateral patellar compression syndrome
5. Patella subluxation
6. Patellar dislocation

Most individuals exhibit some level of malalignment without symptoms unless the repetitive stress of activity creates an overuse situation. A moderate malalignment (e.g., increased femoral anteversion, increased genu valgum, increased tibial torsion), however, may create an environment for complaints during normal ADLs. Secondly, an abnormal patellofemoral configuration can occur. This would represent an abnormal relationship between the patella and the trochlear surface. Lastly, an imbalance can occur between the medial and lateral restraints (passive—medial and lateral retinaculum; and dynamic—vastus lateralis and vastus medialis obliques).

Patellofemoral chondrosis is usually considered a secondary diagnosis. Changes to the articular surface occur as a result of some other pathology. In the general population there is a 2:1 female-to-male ratio of patellofemoral chondrosis but among athletes the ratio approaches 1:1. Conditioning techniques such as full squats with heavy resistance, deep knee bends, and running stadium stairs increase the incidence of patellofemoral chondrosis.

The mechanism of injury for a patellar contusion is direct trauma. This will usually be the result of a fall on the anterior knee or from some direct blow to the knee. One common scenario would be a motor vehicle accident in which the knee strikes the dashboard.

Lateral patellar compression is typically the result of a patellofemoral configuration that has a lateral predominance, tight or thick lateral retinaculum, or inadequate medial restraint. Repetitive flexion–extension activities seem to increase the stress on the lateral facets, which may create a lateral pain syndrome.

Patella subluxation and dislocations have very similar mechanisms of injury. These usually result from some twisting or pivoting episode (foot planted, forcible tibial external rotation with forcible femoral internal rotation). This greatly exaggerates the lateral valgus vector forces, and the patella is forcibly shifted in a lateral direction.

Pathomechanics of the Tibiofemoral Joint

Injuries to the tibiofemoral joint are sometimes easy and occasionally difficult to assess. This is in part due to the knee joint's six degrees of freedom of motion and the fact that traumatic episodes usually do not occur in a single plane. Therefore, when taking a history from the patient, it is critical to have an understanding of how the person was injured because in many instances the diagnosis can be made by knowing the exact mechanism of injury.

Medial Collateral Ligament

Injuries to the medial knee ligament occur primarily because of a direct blow to the lateral aspect of the knee creating a valgus force. The valgus force stresses the medial collateral and capsular ligaments. This type of injury occurs frequently in a collision sport such as football.

Medial meniscus injuries can be secondarily associated with medial collateral ligament injuries due to its deep capsular attachment. These tears typically occur in the periphery.

Lateral Collateral Ligament

Injuries to the lateral collateral ligament are less common than injuries to the medial collateral ligament. The primary mechanism is a direct blow to the medial knee, creating a varus thrust to the knee. A second mechanism is a falling away situation over the fixed

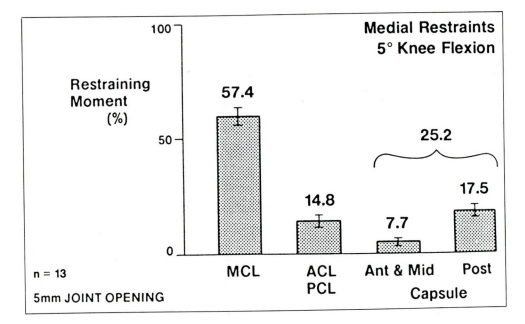

A

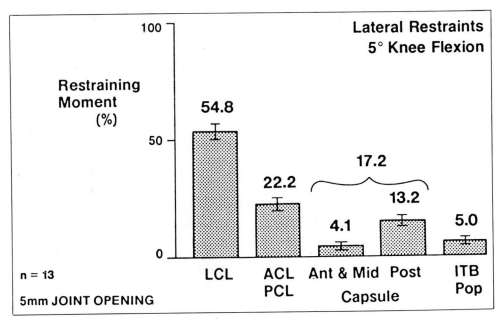

B

Figure 22–7. **A.** The primary and secondary ligament restraints from the medial compartment to resist valgus opening. **B.** The primary and secondary ligament restraints from the lateral compartment to resist varus opening. *(From Grood ES, Noyes FR, Butler DL, Suntay WJ. Ligamentous and capsular restraints preventing straight medial and lateral laxity in the intact human cadaver knee. J Bone Joint Surg. 1981; 63:1257, with permission.)*

foot that would create a varus force on the knee. In some cases, the lateral collateral ligament may tear at its origin, which would indicate an avulsion-type injury (Fig 22–7).

Anterior Cruciate Ligament

Injuries to the anterior cruciate ligament (ACL) are frequently misdiagnosed. In sports that involve pivoting, twisting, and jumping, however, the ACL is often injured. Common mechanisms include

1. Valgus—external rotation
2. Hyperextension
3. Varus—internal rotation
4. Deceleration

These injuries can occur with some direct trauma, although this is less common.

With ACL injuries that are twisting in nature, immediate swelling (acute hemarthrosis) within 12 hours, a popping or tearing sensation, immediate pain, pseudo-

locking, and an inability to continue activity are common findings.

Posterior Cruciate Ligament

The posterior cruciate ligament (PCL) is less commonly injured than the anterior cruciate ligament. The PCL is constructed to be the strongest ligament in the knee, and therefore injuries may occur as an avulsion instead of midsubstance tear. The most common mechanisms are

1. Extreme rotation associated with valgus or varus
2. Posterior displacement with a flexed knee (Fig 22–8)
3. Hyperextension

In addition to PCL injuries during athletics, it is quite common for them to occur in work-related episodes or motor vehicle accidents with direct trauma to the proximal tibia. The PCL is the primary restraint to

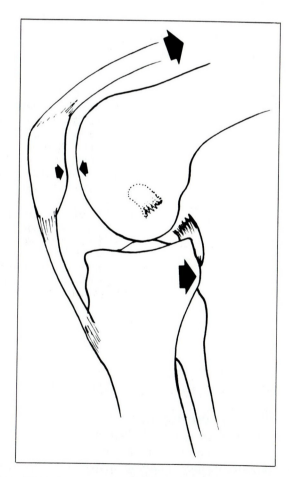

Figure 22–8. A common mechanism of posterior cruciate ligament injury. The resultant injury posteriorly displaces the tibia, increasing the forces on the patellofemoral joint. Rehabilitation often can lead to destruction of the patellofemoral articular cartilage.

tibial dropback, and therefore important from a functional standpoint (Fig 22–9).

Rotatory Instability

Because most athletic activities involve some pivoting or twisting, rotational injuries can occur. These injuries are classified by the direction of instability presented by the tibia:

1. Anteromedial rotatory instability (AMRI)
2. Anterolateral rotatory instability (ALRI)
3. Posterolateral rotatory instability (PLRI)
4. Combined rotatory instability[15]

With anteromedial rotatory instability, the injury occurs to the anterior cruciate ligament, and one third of the medial capsular ligament, at the posteromedial corner. The mechanism involves an external rotation force of the tibia superimposed over a fixed or planted foot, flexed knee, and abducted thigh.

Anterolateral rotatory instabilities are the most common and involve a twisting mechanism. The injury occurs to the ACL, lateral capsular ligament, arcuate complex, and posterolateral capsule. The mechanism of injury involves a sudden valgus force superimposed over the fixed foot, flexed knee, and internally rotating femur.

Posterolateral rotatory instability results from an injury to the PCL, the posterior third of the lateral capsule, and the arcuate complex. The mechanism for this instability involves a direct blow against the anterior tibia with the foot planted and the lower extremity in a varus and externally rotated position.

In a combined instability situation, the disability usually prevents any type of athletic activity because of the extent of the instability pattern. Careful medical supervision is warranted to ensure appropriate and timely surgical intervention.

Meniscus Injuries

Injuries occur to the meniscus primarily through either traction or compression forces associated with some degree of rotation. The most common mechanisms are a planted foot, with the knee in either flexion or extension, and rotational stress. Injury to the medial meniscus occurs primarily through an external rotation force of the tibia superimposed over a flexion to extension movement of the knee (longitudinal tear). An internal rotation stress superimposed over a flexion to extension movement of the knee would injure the lateral meniscus (transverse tear). Other mechanisms of injury to the medial meniscus include

1. Abduction force applied to the lower extremity, followed by knee extension (longitudinal tear)
2. Forced hyperflexion
3. Varus stress
4. Degenerative process

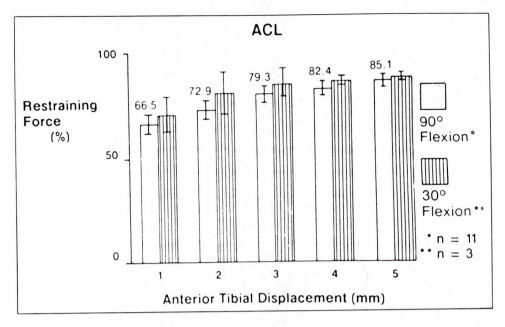

A

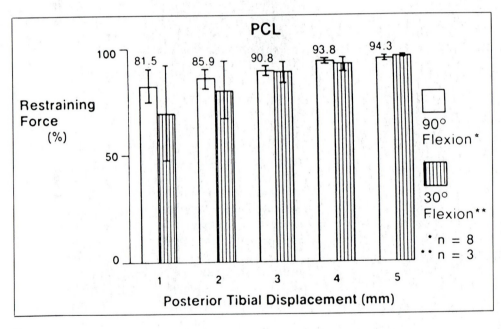

B

Figure 22-9. A. The force resistance provided by the anterior cruciate ligament (ACL) at various angles of testing, 30 degrees versus 90 degrees of flexion. B. The force resistance provided by the posterior cruciate ligament (PCL) at various angles of testing, 30 degrees versus 90 degrees of flexion. *(From Butler DL, Noyes FR, Grood ES. Ligamentous restraints to the anterior–posterior drawer in the human knee. J Bone Joint Surg. 1980; 62:259. with permission.)*

Injury mechanisms for the lateral meniscus include

1. Forced hyperflexion
2. Valgus stress to the knee
3. Degenerative process

Prepatellar Bursitis

The prepatellar bursa is a large fluid sac that is located between the skin and patella. Acute trauma or a direct blow usually creates a large effusion. A chronic prepatellar bursitis can occur after repeated direct blows or with repetitive kneeling for a prolonged period of time. The wall of the bursa will thicken over time.

Patellar Tendon Rupture

Patellar tendon ruptures result from excessive loading of the quadriceps but are rare in the normal knee. Mechanisms include jumping activities or excessive weightlifting. Rupture is usually secondary, due to weakening of the tendon as a result of chronic jumper's knee (infrapatellar tendonitis) or corticosteroidal injections into the tendon.

Osgood–Schlatter Disease

Osgood–Schlatter disease is also known as tibial tubercle apophysitis. The tibial tubercle serves as an extension of the proximal tibial apophysis and functions as the insertion of the patellar tendon. The injury appears to be growth related where an excessive traction force occurs on the tibial tubercle. Athletes involved in sports with running and jumping appear to be affected the most. The incidence of the injury is greater in men than women. A thorough differential diagnosis is needed to identify the problem.

Osteochondritis Dissecans

Osteochondritis dissecans usually involves the medial femoral condyle near the attachment of the PCL. Other locations of injury include the articular surface of the medial and lateral femoral condyles or patella. With osteochondritis dissecans, the articular cartilage separates from the subchondral bones and can do so partially or completely. If the bone separates completely, it is referred to as a loose body.

Osteochondritis dissecans appears to be age dependent. During the first decade of life, anomalies of ossification represent local areas of deficient blood supply within the epiphysis. These injuries can resolve or develop into juvenile osteochondritis dissecans. In the second decade of life, problems occur secondarily to trauma superimposed over the ischemic bone. Repeated trauma can result in a fatigue fracture, thereby creating the osteochondritis lesion. Lastly, in the adult, trauma that produces ischemia progresses to fatigue fracture and the osteochondritis lesion. Another common mechanism is a tear in the menisci, creating lesions on the articular surfaces.

Fractures

Fractures about the knee are rare but can occur in athletes. They may be a result of a direct/indirect blow, torsion, stress, compression, or leverage. Most commonly, fractures involve the distal femur, proximal tibia, or the patella. There can be other associated pathology with the fracture:

1. Ligamentous instability
2. Tears of the menisci
3. Articular cartilage damage

Fractures of the distal femur are either supracondylar, intercondylar, or condylar. A supracondylar fracture usually occurs due to either a direct linear force or torsion and creates a separation between the shaft of the femur and the femoral condyle (Fig 22–10). Intercondylar fractures are usually more severe than supracondylar fractures and are the result of a direct linear force. They typically present in a "T" or "Y" appearance (Fig 22–11). Condylar fractures usually result from a varus or valgus force. The fracture line is most

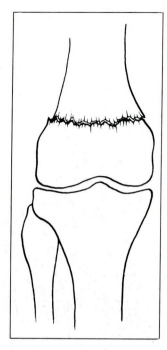

Figure 22–10. Supracondylar fracture of femur.

commonly vertical (Fig 22–12). The collateral ligaments can be injured secondarily because of the varus or valgus mechanisms.

Proximal tibial fractures are more common than the femoral fractures. These fractures usually result from a jumping sport when the knee is extended or by a varus or valgus stress placed on the knee. A vertical force can create a "Y" fracture through both the medial and lateral tibial plateaus (Fig 22–13).

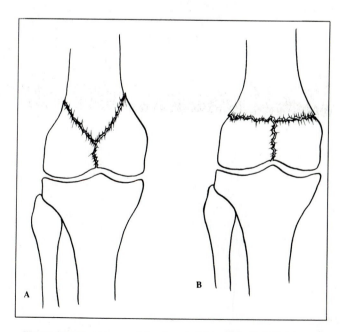

Figure 22–11. Intracondylar femoral fracture. **A.** "Y" fracture. **B.** "T" fracture.

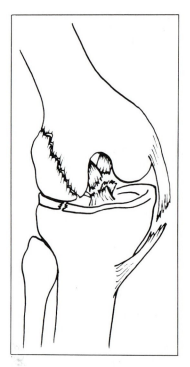

Figure 22-12. Condylar fracture of femur and associated meniscal and ligamentous damage.

Due to its anterior and unprotected position, the patella is susceptible to transverse or (comminuted) fractures due to a direct blow, such as falling onto the knee or striking the patella on the dashboard.

Avulsion fractures can occur where the bone gives way before the ligament or tendon does. Mechanisms

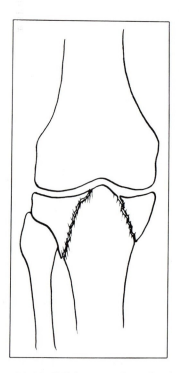

Figure 22-13. "Y" fracture of proximal tibia.

of these injuries would be similar to those of ligamentous or tendinous injuries, except that the structure has a chip of bone attached to it. Usually this is confirmed radiographically.

The last type of fracture usually associated with athletics would be an epiphyseal plate fracture. This ordinarily occurs because the epiphyseal plate is less able to dissipate the stresses imposed on it. A thorough differential diagnosis is critical to appropriate care and treatment.

Plica Syndrome
The plica represents a fold in the synovial lining that is a remnant from embryological development. The plica is present in up to 60% of the population and originates from the undersurface of the vastus lateralis, traverses to the medial femoral condyle, and continues in an oblique and transverse direction to attach along the infrapatellar fat pad. The plica is not usually pathological until directly injured.

Common mechanisms include trauma by a direct blow or by stretching or tearing due to repeated twisting or pivoting actions. This causes pain and swelling and can result in a chronic condition if not evaluated and treated in its acute stage. In chronic cases, arthroscopic evaluation and debridement are indicated.

Overuse Injuries
It is very common for injuries to the knee to occur without a traumatic incident. In prolonged, sustained activity, the repetition may create a cumulative stress situation. These types of injuries are very common in such sports as long distance running and aerobics. In many instances, mild malalignments coupled with repetitive exercise leads to a situation where the body is not able to recover and an inflammatory condition arises. This condition will, many times, progress as the warning signs of pain and swelling are ignored. This can lead to a change in the activity pattern of the athlete that will cause weakness and stiffness and help to perpetuate the injury.

Training errors are a very common source of injury with repetitive exercise. These training errors can include inadequate warm-up, sudden increases in distance, pace, or frequency, running on hills or hard surfaces or changing surfaces, inappropriate goals, and improper foot wear. Certain body characteristics may also predispose an athlete to overuse injuries, including inadequate strength, inadequate flexibility, previous orthopaedic injury, and leg length discrepancy.

Iliotibial band syndrome is a common source of knee pain in long distance runners. The iliotibial band crosses back and forth over the lateral femoral epicondyle with repetitive flexion and extension. This repetitive rubbing creates a friction syndrome and inflammatory condition. This injury can be exacerbated by a

normally tight iliotibial band, forefoot varus, tight hip adductors, leg length discrepancy, or sudden increases in the distance or mileage.

Infrapatellar tendonitis is also known as "jumper's knee." This injury is very common in basketball players due to the repetitive jumping involved in practice and games. It can also occur in weightlifters due to the continual strain placed on the patellar tendon. The pain is usually point tendon over the infrapatellar tendon or its origin at the inferior pole of the patella.

Popliteus tendonitis occurs quite frequently in runners who train on hills. The muscle arises from the posterior proximal tibia and then passes laterally and superiorly to attach on the lateral aspect of the lateral femoral condyle. Its function is to prevent excessive internal rotation of the femur. It is quite active during squatting and walking or running downhill.

The pes anserine bursa lies between the pes anserine tendons and tibia. As is true of most bursa, its function is to decrease friction between the tendons and bone. The bursa may become inflamed by repetitive forceful knee flexions. Pain is generally pinpointed over the pes anserine tendons.

Prevention of Knee Injuries

The incidence and severity of knee injuries in sports mandate that more attention be paid to prevention. Abbott[16] and Bender[4] have demonstrated that it is possible both to predict and to prevent knee injuries through appropriate intervention. Cahill and Griffin[5] have demonstrated that some types of knee injuries can be prevented at the high school level by use of appropriate exercise and preseason conditioning programs.

The knee joint is one of the most commonly injured joints of the body. It has a high incidence for temporary and permanent disability because of the number of traumatic injuries that occur during recreational and competitive athletics. The knee joint is the weak link in the lower extremity for many individuals. The knee has two separate joints which can exhibit pathology, the patellofemoral and tibiofemoral joints. There is a close relationship between these two joints, and, in many cases, an injury to one joint also causes some pathology to the other.

REHABILITATION MANAGEMENT OF SPECIFIC KNEE PROTOCOLS

The implementation of a rehabilitation protocol after injury often causes a variety of dilemmas for the rehabilitation specialist. If a scientific approach is taken, however, the protocols become less cumbersome and more customized to individual patient needs. It is crucial that the approach to the patient be holistic and not confined to a single body part. Psychological factors

must also be considered. Rehabilitation protocols are designed for the majority of patient populations, but the sports physical therapist must be cognizant of those patients who fall outside of these ranges.

The proper rehabilitation program must treat the psychological and social concerns by addressing

1. Patient motivation
2. Patient compliance
3. Verbal versus nonverbal communication
4. Patient–family interaction
5. Patient–peer interaction
6. Patient–physician interaction

These components must be carefully observed in order to identify their effects on the outcome of the rehabilitation program.

Specific protocols based on pathologies to ligamentous structures are presented in this section. It is imperative, however, that all members of the rehabilitation team discuss these protocols to guarantee their compliance. Protocols should be designed so that there is a staging of exercises based on physiological principles. The systems that must be closely monitored include

1. Muscular
   strength   length
   power   size
   endurance   dynamic capabilities
2. Soft tissues
   synovium   fat pad
   capsule   bursa
   nerve   ligament
   skin   fascia
3. Joints
   bones
   articular cartilage
   intra-articular structures

Phases to Rehabilitation

Phase I. This is the period of maximum protection where the primary emphasis is to treat pain, inflammation, and intra-articular swelling. Motion may be permitted but must be kept within a biomechanically safe range. The goal of phase I is initial healing and maintenance of structures around the joint.

Phase II. This period of moderate protection is a time to regain limited motion and initiate a re-education program to disused tissues. Pain and swelling must be controlled. Ongoing tissue modeling occurs during this period and careful assessment must assure its integrity.

Phase III. During this period of minimum protection, retraining of functional behavior occurs. Tissue realignment is still ongoing, so forces on these tissues must

be controlled. There is also an initiation of functional training to reduce risk of reinjury to tissues during ADLs.

Phase IV. This period of light activity is directed toward full functional retraining. This must account for the whole body and not just the injured segment. The evaluation must be objective so that higher levels of activity can be instituted.

Phase V. The final phase is the period of full return and maintenance. For resumption of full activity a comprehensive objective evaluation must preclude full resumption of activity. Second, a rational maintenance program needs to be outlined and implemented.

Rehabilitation protocols must be based on a sound foundation of basic science, including

- Biomechanics of joint function
- Soft tissue healing
- Physiological process of muscle
- Development of functional skills
- Objective based evaluation

A well-planned protocol will maximize the effect of the program and reduce the risk of failure.

Protocol I—Conservative Management of the ACL-Deficient Knee

An ACL tear treated nonoperatively can develop into a complicated clinical syndrome, resulting in a varied amount of functional limitations. The sequela of the syndrome includes the initial injury, repeat injuries (full giving-way episodes occurring after the initial injury), additional joint damage such as meniscal tears or chondral fractures, and articular cartilage deterioration.

Several variables affect this syndrome. The number of reinjuries statistically correlates with increased articular cartilage damage. Although some patients may experience only one to two reinjuries per year, during a 5-year period this adds up to ten additional significant reinjuries. The type of sports played and individual occupations is another important variable; activities involving twisting, cutting, or pivoting place a patient at a higher risk for reinjury than those involving single plane lower-extremity movement. Other variables include the amount of total anteroposterior translation found, secondary ligamentous damage, compliance to the rehabilitation program, and the amount of time from the original injury.

The young, highly athletic individual must be educated from the beginning that an ACL tear is a significant injury that, if not treated correctly, could result in joint arthrosis at an early age. The primary goal should be to prevent joint damage.

Our studies have shown that one third of the population compensated well for their knee condition and did not require reconstruction. Another third compensated and experienced livable but occasionally aggravating symptoms and the last third worsened over time, failed the rehabilitation and modification protocol, and required reconstructive surgery. The eight-point rehabilitation treatment program described below is still used today for patients desiring conservative treatment. Arthroscopy is used to treat meniscal problems and to appropriately advise the patient as to the correct preventative program to follow.

For an athlete considering operative treatment, the goals of surgery must be that a return to sports activities with minimal symptoms and objective stability for at least 5 to 10 years postoperative. Many athletes undergo surgery and elect, for lifestyle reasons, to diminish sports activities. Could these individuals have done just as well without surgery? For the individual who suffers symptoms with ADLs, one must ask whether reconstruction will reduce symptoms and the rate of joint arthrosis, or if the morbidity of the surgery will result in increased articular cartilage damage.

The ACL-deficient knee represents a true treatment dilemma. At present, only minimal data are available from long-term studies on both operative and nonoperative treatment. There is no unified knee rating system for assessing subjective and objective parameters for treatment outcomes between studies. Multicenter collaborative studies have not been performed to assess treatment of varied populations and varied surgical procedures.

The successful rehabilitation of the ACL-deficient knee depends on completion of the following eight-point rehabilitation protocol:

1. Correct strength/power defects.
2. Increase muscular work and endurance capabilities.
3. Implement a high-speed dynamic–functional program to control the joint.
4. Reciprocal reflex–speed is maintained.
5. A brace is used in sports activities.
6. Modify activities.
7. Weight loss or maintenance programs are instituted to minimize risk of arthritis.
8. Educate the patient regarding future damage.

The therapy program must be directed toward increasing the patient's ability to resist forces that place the joint at risk for giving way (Fig 22–14). The abnormal motion that must be restrained is anterior tibial translation. It is this abnormal motion that is coupled to an increase in anterior lateral tibial displacement, leading to rotation. Therefore, control of tibial movements by the hamstrings has become the hallmark for the chronic ACL patient. The exercise design, however, cannot be only isotonic in resistance, which is speed

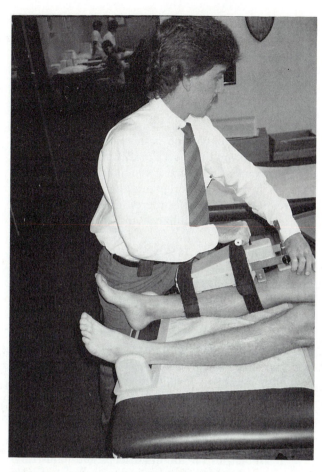

Figure 22–14. The use of the KT-1000 joint arthrometer aids in monitoring patient progress concerning increasing instability associated with anterior cruciate deficiencies.

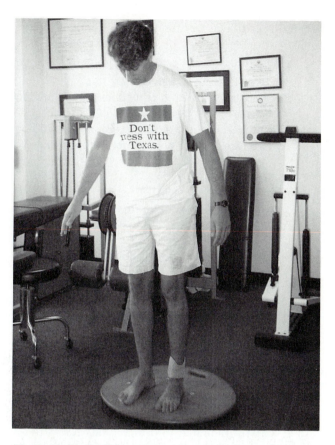

Figure 22–15. Postinjury or surgery proprioception training is crucial for activities of daily living. The use of a BAPS board can be useful in accomplishing this reeducation process.

specific at low velocity. High-speed dynamic movements in exercise may be more beneficial in muscle adaptation to respond to a protective functional mode.

The second aspect that must be considered is high-repetition duration protocols. The need for prolonged muscle action in endurance activities may decrease the risk of fatigue giving-way episodes.

The third area of rehabilitation concern is proprioception control of the joint. The neurological input from mechanoreceptors in the ligament aids in normal joint function. Injury describes this flow of information. It is crucial to reestablish this key link in protective neuromuscular protection. Much of the work done in this area is to increase work durations, coordination, speed, endurance, and strength.

An objective assessment is crucial to determine patient advancement through the program and to evaluate his or her status (Fig 22–15). Evaluation must include

1. Muscle parameters
2. Joint displacement
3. Articular cartilage status
4. Functional capability

The assessment must be performed every 3 to 6 months depending on the patient's complaints or activity level.

Protocol II—Postsurgical Management of the ACL Knee: Immediate Motion

Anterior cruciate ligament reconstructive procedures presents the physical therapist with a unique set of circumstances. The problems arise from the biomechanics of the injury, the multitude of reconstructive procedures, and the development of an early rehabilitation program that prevents ligament failure, minimizes muscle atrophy, and protects the articular surfaces.

The rehabilitation process, including progression of range of motion, weight bearing, and exercise intervention, must be gradual. Too early or too strenuous an exercise protocol can lead to forces not tolerated by the healing graft. During the rehabilitation process, the therapist must account for

1. Time frame of soft tissue healing
2. Biomechanics of joint function
3. Surgical techniques
4. Muscle forces
5. Tissue utilization in repair[17]

Days 1 to 7

1. Compression dressing
2. Continuous passive motion (CPM) 10 to 90 degrees, 12 to 14 hr/day
3. Quadriceps and hamstring isometrics following the rule of 10s. If surgical technique is mechanically weak, the quadriceps exercises should be performed at the neutral point approximately 70 degrees of flexion, or co-contractions are used
4. Straight leg raises (SLR) supine position prone are initiated when tolerated
5. Modality intervention for postoperative hemarthrosis should begin immediately until it is under control, to reduce the joints response to surgical procedure
6. Hemovac for 48 hours
7. Electrical muscle stimulation (EMS) to quadriceps to prevent shutdown
8. Patellar mobilization; aggressive superior glides are important to avoid infrapatellar contracture. This may also develop if quadricep reeducation is not completed in a specific time frame

Weeks 1 to 4

1. CPM: graduated to 0 to 110 degrees, 8 to 12 hr/day. If restricted motion problems develop, earlier increases are recommended, with the target ranges obtained by 3 weeks.
2. SLR: initiate hip adduction at week 3 unless lateral or medial repairs are performed. Weight can be added in supine and prone position at week 2.
3. Continue cryotherapy if needed based on objective evaluation (Fig 22–16).

4. Toe-touch weight-bearing is begun unless lateral or posterolateral repairs are also performed. This progresses to 25% weight bearing by 14 days and 50% weight bearing between 21 and 28 days.

Weeks 5 to 16

1. **The range of motion is increased to 125 to 135 degrees from the fourth to fifth weeks. (The therapist must realize that if a joint contracture develops, increases in motion must be accelerated. This requires monitoring progress every 3 to 4 days to assess patient compliance and scar tissue formation.)**
2. **Weight-bearing: 75% weight-bearing by week 5 initially based on a joint arthrometer measurement, showing an increase in total anteroposterior (AP) translation at 20 degrees of no more than 2 mm when compared to the opposite limb. If more than 2 mm is detected, then a careful examination of the exercise protocol and patient compliance is needed. At 6 weeks, weight-bearing is full with crutch or cane protection. This is discontinued when the patient is comfortable. In patients who demonstrate even a 1.0 to 2.0 mm increase, a functional brace is used.**
3. **Exercise program**
   a. **Isometrics for the quadriceps and hamstrings are combined with electrical stimulation in slowly developed patients.**
   b. **Cycling is initiated at 8 to 10 weeks postoperatively, with the seat in a higher than normal position to reduce anterior cruciate forces.**
   c. **Progressive resistive exercises (PREs) are initiated if certain criteria are met: the absence of**

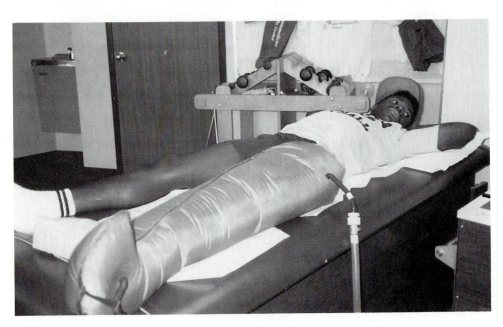

Figure 22–16. The use of a JOBST Cryotemp system can be effective in combating postsurgical swelling.

joint swelling, objective weekly measurements of AP translation, minimal patellofemoral crepitus, and a lack of pain symptoms. Progressive resistive exercises are initiated between 90 and 30 degrees and are gradually increased to full extension during a 16-week period. Flexion PREs are initiated, avoiding hyperextension to protect the reconstructed knee.

d. Swimming can be initiated at 8 weeks postoperatively. The criteria described for the PRE program are applied. The first phase consists of allowing the patient to ambulate in the water to build endurance and gradually move onto freestyle; this also aids ambulation training.

e. Toe raises are begun, progressing from flat standing to off-the-step exercises.

f. Wall sits (hold for 30 seconds), progressing by 10-second increments. These are performed at a 70 degree flexion angle to reduce ACL forces.

g. Flexibility training for the hamstrings and gastrocnemius. If range of motion is excessive after the postoperative brace is removed, training should be avoided.

h. Functional proprioception training using balance boards is implemented to aid dynamic function during the gait-weaning phase. Also PNF-type exercises should be initiated to develop patterned movement and aid functional training; surgical bands are often useful (Fig 22–17).

Weeks 17–24

1. Exercise program
   a. Continue above exercises, increasing weight and amount of time.
   b. Endurance: initiate walking and gentle hip kicking in the pool, or Nordic Track workouts. Upper extremity training can be accomplished via an air dyne or other ergometer system.

Weeks 24 to 48

1. Repeat KT-1000 at 70 and 20 degrees of flexion and measure external rotation at 70 degrees of flexion. If measurements are within normal limits, proceed as described below.
2. Function: all activities are continued in the brace if there is a suggestion of lateral or ACL dysfunction. A Cincinnati Ligament Brace is used when the ACL is reconstructed and a combined instability device by Donjoy is used if the posterolateral structures are also involved.
3. Exercises
   a. Isokinetics in the 300-to 450-degree per second

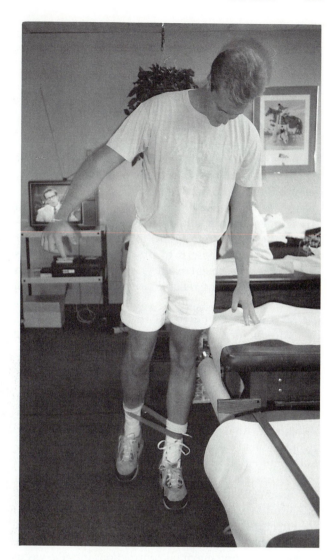

Figure 22–17. This picture demonstrates the use of an exercise band by Sports Camps International. Movement for this type of exercise is done with high speed and high repetition.

range if the patient does not have access to a pool. These exercises must be performed slowly, with constant evaluation for patellofemoral crepitus and graft healing. Lower speed submaximal training is also initiated.

b. Continue PREs, increasing weight as symptoms of pain and swelling and joint arthrometer measurements allow. Limit extension to 30 degrees; *patellofemoral crepitus must be minimal.* Flexion PREs are with light weight and limited range; the last 15 degrees of extension is avoided to protect the graft.

c. Continue all other exercises, gradually increasing the amount of difficulty.

Weeks 48 to 60

1. Gradually increase function using all previously mentioned criteria—patellofemoral crep-

itus, symptoms, and joint arthrometer measurements. Use objective functional testing as a guide for safe return to activity.

GENERAL CONCEPTS OF REHABILITATION OF THE PATELLOFEMORAL JOINT

Knee rehabilitation for the quadriceps and extensor mechanism, with reference to the patellofemoral joint, revolves around isometrics and SLR, with PRE implemented in a late phase. The process includes gains in strength, endurance, and agility; the goal of this protocol is for the athlete to return to play with no pain or swelling. Our purpose is to provide general concepts and answer treatment cliches, and not to present a "cookbook" for knee rehabilitation for patellofemoral disorders.

1. There is a time to rest and a time to rehab.

After injury or surgery, knee pain and swelling dictate the need for rest, ice, compression, and elevation, and a very light rehabilitation program. The large forces around the patellofemoral joint provide this rationale. An overly rapid rehabilitation program may result in a reflex sympathetic dystrophy syndrome development. An overly strenuous program may increase symptoms and cause a shut-down of the extensor mechanism musculature rather than increase strength.

2. Keep isometrics in their place.

Isometrics are inefficient strength builders, but they do have two important purposes: (1) they lessen the effects of disuse in the initial phase of rehabilitation after injury or surgery; and (2) they can train the quadriceps by building maximal contractions into the vastus medialis oblique (VMO). (This requires the use of an electrical muscle stimulator in the early phase.) The VMO has been found to have maximal output in the range of 60 to 70 degrees, so multiple angle isometrics are of definite value to this muscle in the early phases. The role of isometrics cannot be overemphasized.

3. Leg lifts—lift little without a shrug.

An isometric contraction in the quadriceps muscle while performing a leg lift should be done in a slightly flexed position. The patient must be instructed on proper usage of the quadriceps muscle because overuse of the rectus femorus muscle will negate the effect of the exercise on the vastus muscle group. Furthermore, SLR should be performed in multiple planes. Limited research has shown that adduction of the hip in a SLR fashion may result in a greater VMO contraction than a hip flexion with knee-flexed position.

4. Squats and patellas do not mix.

The forces on the patella can range from 1.5 times the body weight in normal walking to 3.4 times the body weight in stair climbing. In squatting activities up to 60 degrees knee flexion will result in 4 times the body weight, whereas full squatting results in 8 times the body weight. Patellofemoral forces triple with knee flexion. The body weight shifts behind the knee with flexion, and the moment arm increases from the knee to the body weight lines as further flexion occurs. The quadriceps must provide greater force to prevent the knee from collapsing, and this ultimately loads the patellofemoral joint. The increased force that is required by the quadriceps muscle, combined with its transmission into the patellar ligament, and knee flexion forces, gives a resultant compressive force on the patellofemoral joint.

The reverse is true with knee extension exercises. As the knee extends, the moment arm of the leg increases. The quadriceps force increases to balance the leg, resulting in a larger patellofemoral compressive force toward extension. The moment arm from an ankle weight or free weight is greatest with the knee extended. The increase, the length of the teeter-totter arm at 10 degrees, requires a larger quadriceps balancing force. Therefore, a greater weight or compressive force is transmitted to the patella. It is not uncommon during rehabilitation for the therapist to be faced with an extensor lag deficit. In many cases, this is the last problem that needs to be overcome. This may occur when attempting to overload the quadriceps too early, or after immobilization in a flexed position. This lag must be worked vigorously in the extended part of the range with electrical stimulation and isometrics. The lag may occur after immobilizaton which leads to patella infra. Tambrello et al[18] reported that the inferior shift of the patella results in an extensor lag situation because it does not proximally guide with muscle contraction. We cannot overemphasize the importance of immediate patellar mobilization following surgery (Fig 22–18).

5. Don't skate a patella on rough ice.

Patellofemoral contact surfaces change with knee flexion. The rehabilitation program should be oriented around the area of crepitus. This is similar to the program used for shoulder impingement in which we attempt to avoid the impinged area of the range of motion in the PRE program. Our current program for PREs for patellofemoral joints consists of a simplistic approach of preventing crepitus with the movement of weighted exercise. The patient is often comfortable in the 45- to 90-degree range, which allows for a greater area of surface contact for dispersion of the force. Furthermore, in the lower ranges we find a greater electrical output on EMG in the vastus medialis muscle group. In conclusion, we avoid exercises in the range where crepitus is prominent.

6. Fancy is not better but it is more fun.

There is a great deal of new, sophisticated machinery on the market. Many exercise programs for patellofemoral disorders are not based on a sound scien-

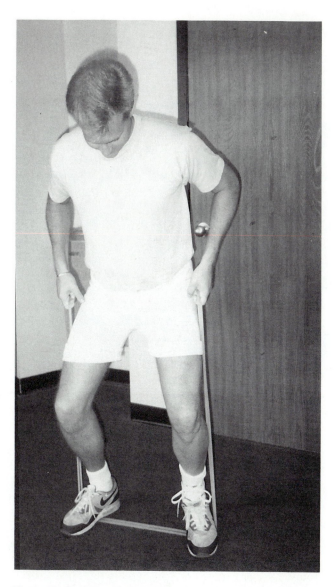

Figure 22-18. This picture demonstrates the use of surgical tubing in a squatting movement. The advantages to this exercise are that it allows reproducibility of pattern movements, can incorporate high speed, can incorporate high repetitions, and gives the clinician the ability to limit the range of motion based on patellar crepitus and pain.

tific basis. Many efforts are not being made to examine these devices as part of a patellofemoral program and implement proper changes. Many machine and brace companies are projecting the image of being able to cure patellofemoral problems without sound mechanical or physiological reasoning. Some of these devices can be used in a safe, efficient manner if the therapist and orthopaedist apply the basic principles of biomechanics, assess the pathological condition of the joint, apply the physiological basis of muscle strength programs, and use basic clinical common sense.

7. Mix, stir, and simmer all the exercises with a big stick.

This cliche refers to the time and close supervision

required by the therapist and staff to ensure patient compliance. The quadricep rehabilitation protocol is specifically designed as a patella protection program and is divided into four phases: initial, intermediate, advanced, and return to activity and maintenance. The program must be assessed according to the patellofemoral disorder in terms of flexibility, muscle strengthening, endurance exercises through biking or swimming programs, proprioceptor neuromuscular feedback, and functional training. If only one aspect of this program is missed, it could lead to failure. During the initial phase, the goals include rest, pain control, and healing of damaged soft tissue. The quadriceps are trained by VMO electrical stimulation; feedback is the key to controlling patellar dynamic stabilization.

Upon successful completion of the first three phases, the advanced program is initiated. The goals are to maximize strength, increase endurance, and obtain a normal range of motion. This phase is begun when the athlete returns to normal activity and has achieved the objective goals for isokinetic testing, flexibility testing, endurance testing, and proprioception training. It is extremely important in the return to activity phase that the process is a gradual one and that all of the objective criteria are met prior to its initiation.

MENISCUS REHABILITATION: RULES FOR POSTSURGICAL MANAGEMENT

Our protocol for rehabilitation following meniscal repair is divided into three phases—maximum protection, moderate protection, and return to activity and maintenance. These time periods are based primarily on the healing time of peripheral tissues. The rate of success in this program (> 90%) has been excellent.

The key factors in meniscal repair include:

1. Anatomic site of the tear; vascular (red) or non-vascular (white) (Fig 22–19)
2. Suture fixation—can lead to early failure if an overly vigorous program is initiated
3. Anatomic site of the tear; anterior or posterior—may affect exercise program
4. Other intra-articular pathology, for example, ACL, MCL, PCL, bilateral meniscal involvement

Maximum Protection Period: Weeks 1 to 8

Phase I: Immediate postsurgery day 1 through week 3

1. Cryotemp, or equivalent
2. EMS to quadriceps

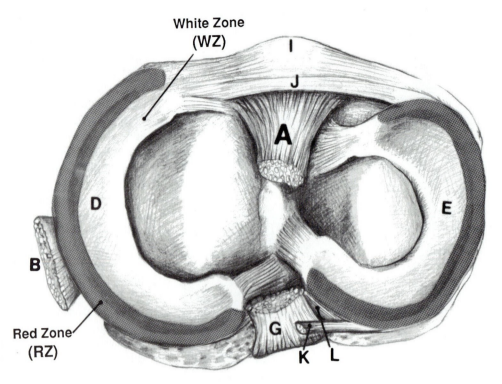

White Zone (WZ)

Red Zone (RZ)

Figure 22-19. The meniscus—(D) the medial meniscus and (E) the lateral meniscus. The outer third of the menisci are vascular and are considered the red zone. The inner two thirds of the menisci are nonvascular and are termed the white zone.

3. Brace for protected range of motion:
   a. Peripheral to midzone repairs (0 to 90 degrees)
   b. Peripheral post-zone repairs (20 to 90 degrees)
   c. Peripheral anterior zone repairs (20 to 90 degrees)
   d. White zone repairs (20 to 70 degrees)

Range of Motion. Motion is limited for the first 7 to 21 days, depending on the development of scar tissue around the repair site. Flexion is usually limited for the first 14 days and then gradually increased until full flexion is attained by four weeks postop. Patients who have extension limited to −20 degrees may increase the range to −10 degrees after 10 days and to 0 degrees after 17 to 21 days postoperatively. Careful assessment of pain in the repair area is important as range of motion is increased.

Continuous passive motion is used in the initial phase following the allotted range of motion limits. This is often only needed for 14 to 21 days.

Exercises. Quadriceps exercises are crucial to prevent shutdown. The range used is the furthest point of extension and flexion. If a total peripheral tear is repaired, the patient should perform co-contractions to prevent excessive tension on the suture line. The same concept is used for posterior horn tears, in which maximum hamstring efforts are avoided for the first 3 weeks postoperatively. Exercises include

- Quadriceps isometrics
- Hamstring isometrics

- Straight leg raises (use weights at the fifth postoperative day if tolerated)
- Passive range of motion

Patellar mobilization is initiated as soon as patient comfort allows. The key directions are superior, medial, and lateral.

Scar tissue mobilization is initiated at 7 to 10 days to avoid excessive scarring. This is used to eliminate neuroma formation in patients who underwent arthrotomy.

Weight-bearing is limited in the first 3 weeks to toe-touch to 25%.

Phase II: Weeks 4 to 8

Weight-Bearing. The factor crucial to the progression of weight-bearing is the repair site. For red-zone tears, one-fourth weight-bearing is begun at 3 weeks and total crutch time can be limited to 5 to 6 weeks. For white-zone tears, weight-bearing is limited for the first 4 weeks to toe touch and total crutch time is 8 weeks.

- *Red Zone*

Postoperative week 3	One-fourth weight-bearing
Postoperative week 4	One-half weight-bearing
Postoperative week 5	Three-fourths weight bearing
Postoperative week 6	Full (may need one crutch)

- *White Zone*

Postoperative week 4	One-fourth weight-bearing
Postoperative week 6	One-half weight-bearing
Postoperative week 7	Three-fourths weight-bearing
Postoperative week 8	Full (may need one crutch)

Exercises. At 4 weeks an aggressive program is initiated. Damage to the repair site is still possible, as maturation takes 6 months to complete.

- Straight leg raises; all planes, with gradual weight added
- Limited arc progressive resistive quads, performed in a range less likely to impinge or pull on the repair
- Proprioception training from a weight-bearing functional progression
- Flexibility to lower extremity; with avoidance of vigorous flexion
- Cycling is initiated at 3 to 4 weeks with no tension. The range will vary depending on the repair site. The initial time is 15 minutes, which is gradually increased according to pain and swelling. The main goal is to increase endurance and not to use high tension.
- Surgical tubing exercises are initiated in flexion–extension patterns and PNF patterns. Our program is oriented towards increasing endurance which does not require maximal efforts.

Goals. The goal of the first 8 weeks postoperatively is to develop endurance, rather than strength; the latter is the goal of the time period described below.

Moderate Protection Period: Weeks 8 to 20

This phase is oriented towards strength gains and functional rehabilitation. No running, jumping, or twisting activities are performed. For white-zone repairs, this period is delayed until the 12th postoperative week (and concludes at the 28th postoperative week).

Exercises

- Flexibility is now pushed in all ranges. The extreme of flexion is still avoided, as pressure on the repair site is minimized. Hamstring, gastroc, hip flexion, and abduction are pushed, however.
- Strength is developed, with PREs to the quads continued. The terminal portion of extension may be limited initially, but an increase to full extension may be permitted. Hamstring PREs can be initiated if desired.

- Toe raises are performed off of a step, progressing to one leg.
- Lateral stepups are performed in a 50- to 10-degree range, beginning with five sets for 30 seconds and working up to 5 sets for 60 seconds.
- Mini-squats with surgical tubing are performed in a 50- to 10-degree range, emphasizing speed of movement. These are performed in a three-set, 20- to 30- repetition series.
- Isokinetic exercises are begun in the 6- to 8-week time frame if desired. Our protocol includes a submaximal program, at low-velocity (120 to 180 degrees per second; 3 sets for 15 to 20 seconds) and a maximal program, at high speed (300 to 450 degrees per second; 3 sets for 20 to 30 seconds).

Endurance Program. In this phase of the rehabilitation protocol, endurance training centers around noncompressive type of activities. Excessive compression may result in tearing of the suture line:

- Swimming: freestyle, wall kicking, walking/running in the water. Begin at a 15- to 20-minute time frame and slowly increase.
- Cycling is increased in time first, with intensity increased later in the protocol. Time must reach 45 minutes before intensity is increased.
- Nordiac track is employed, working increases in time and not intensity.
- Stair machines in a short arc, for short aerobic bursts of 20 to 45 seconds at maximal efforts, can be used.

Coordination Program

- Balance training on a proprioception board is used, beginning with bilateral training and working to unilateral work.
- High-speed exercise bands in a hip flexion–extension and abduction–adduction position are used.
- Sprinting in a pool is used for both endurance and coordination training.
- Backwards walking is useful in developing awareness, especially for posterior meniscal repairs.

Polymetric Program. Towards the end of this phase, we initiate a low-level polymetric program beginning with side-to-side maneuvers and working towards forward and backwards movements. Height is also graduated, beginning with 4 in and progressing to 10 to 12 in. These exercises are performed for 20 to 30 seconds, progressing to 45 to 50 seconds.

Return to Activity and Maintenance Period: Weeks 20 and Beyond

This phase emphasizes return to skill, including both occupational and sporting activities. The program centers around increasing function and specific movement analysis. For patients with white zone repairs, this phase is not initiated until the 28th postoperative week.

Functional Protocol. Increase speed of movement in certain exercises, for example, tubing program, polymetrics, running in the water.
Running protocol:

- Jog/walk   ¼ jog/⅛ walk × 4 cycles
- Jog/walk   ½ jog/⅛ walk × 4 cycles
- Jog/straight   1½ miles
- ½ speed sprint
  20–20 yd   backward sprint 20–20 yd
  20–40 yd
  10–60 yd
- ¾ speed sprint
  20–20 yd   backward sprint 20–20 yd
  20–40 yd
  20–60 yd
  10–80 yd
- Full speed sprint
  20–20 yd   backward sprint 30–20 yd
  20–40 yd
  20–60 yd
  10–80 yd
- Circle sprint starting at 20 × 20-yd radius and closing to a 5 × 5-yd radius for ten repetitions, in both directions.
- Lateral run (cavioca). Stepover running is done in both directions for a 10- to 20-yd distance for ten repetitions.
- Figure-of-8 running. This pattern starts at a 20-yd distance and can be cut all the way to a 3-yd distance around cones.

Key Points

- Return to sports on a slow, gradual basis.
- Carefully monitor pain and swelling.
- Pain over the scar may develop if an overly aggressive program is used.
- Occasionally a brace is used to avoid swelling.

Summary

Rehabilitation of many knee pathologies can be incorporated into one of the above protocols, an example being

- Partial ligament injuries can be placed in the meniscus protocol.
- Postpatellar surgery still requires the same con-sideration as the conservative approach after the initial healing phase.
- Posterior cruciate ligament repairs are treated in a similar fashion to ACL protocol with a variation in motion.

It is important that protocol decision making is placed on a sound scientific basis when possibile. All too often, rehabilitation is based on clinical impressions without sound scientific support.

Orthopaedic care of joint injuries requires a working knowledge of anatomy, biomechanics, soft tissue healing, muscle physiology and mechanics, and neuromuscular interaction. The highest reported success rates are supportive of this approach. It is our responsibility to continually strive for advancement of basic knowledge of therapeutic intervention.

SUGGESTED READINGS

Akeson W, Woo S. The Connective Tissue Response to Immobility: Biochemical Changes in Periarticular Connective Tissue of the Immobilized Rabbit Knee. *Clin Ortho Rel Res.* 1973; 93:356–362.

Anderson A, Lipascomb AB. Analysis of Rehabilitation Techniques After Anterior Cruciate Reconstruction. *Amer J Sports Med.* 1989; 17(2):154–160.

Arms S, Pope M, Johnson R. The Biomechanics of ACL Rehabilitation and Reconstruction. *Amer J Sports Med.* 1984; 12(1):8–18.

Blackburn TA, Eiland WG, Bandy WD. An Introduction to the Plica. *J Ortho Sports Phys Ther.* 1982; 3:171.

Brewster C, Moynes D, Jobe F. *Rehabilitation for anterior cruciate reconstruction. J Ortho Sports Phys Ther.* 1983; 15(3):121–126.

Burdett R., Van Swearingen J. *Reliability of isokinetic muscle endurance tests. J Ortho Sports Ther.* 1987; 8(10):484–488.

Butler DL, Noyes FR, Grood ES. *Ligamentous restraints to anterior-posterior drawer in the human knee. J Bone Joint Surg.* 1980; 62:2.

Currier L, Mann R. *Muscular strength development by electrical stimulation in healthy individuals. Phys Ther.* 1983; 63(6):915–921.

Eriksson E, Haggmark T. *Comparison of isometric muscle training and electrical stimulation supplementing isometric muscle training in the recovery after major knee ligament surgery. Amer J Sports Med.* 1979; 7(3):169–171.

Eriksson E, Higgman. Reconstruction of the posterior cruciate ligament. *Ortho.* 1986; 9(2):217–220.

Farrell M, Richard J. *Analysis of the reliability and validity of the kinetic communicator exercise device. Med Sci Sport Exer.* 1986; 18(1):44–49.

Feiring D, Ellenbacker TS. *Test-Re-Test Reliability of the Biodex Isokinetic Dynamometer.* Lincoln Inst. for Ath Med. Unpublished. 1989.

Ficat RP, Hungerford Ds. *Disorders of the Patellofemoral Joint* Baltimore, Md: Williams & Wilkins, 1977.

Haaggmark T, Janssen E, Eriksson E. *Fiber type area and metabolic potential of the thigh muscle in man after knee surgery and immobilization. Int J Sports Med.* 1981; pp 12–17.

Hamberg P, Gillquist JA. *Comparison between arthroscopic meniscectomy and modified meniscectomy. J Bone Joint Surg.* 1984; 66 B(2):189–192.

Jenkins WL, Thackaberry M. *Speed specific isokinetic testing. J Ortho Sports Phys Ther.* 1984; 6(3):181–183.

Jurvelin J, Kiviranta I. *Partial restoration of immobilization-induced softening of canine articular cartilage after remobilization of the knee* (stifle) joint. *J Ortho Res.* 1989; 7(3):352–358.

Knapik JJ, Ramos M. *Isokinetic and isometric torque relationships in the human body. Arch Phys Med Rehabil.* 1980; 61:64–67.

Krisoff WB, Ferris WD, *Runners injuries. J Phys Sports Med.* 1979; 7:55.

Markey KL. *Rehabilitation of the anterior cruciate deficient knee. Clin Sports Med.* 1985; 4(3):513–526.

Moffroid M, Whipple R. *A Study of isokinetic measurements with test repetitions. Phys Ther.* 1969; 49:735–746.

Montgomery LC, Douglass LW. *Reliability of an isokinetic test of muscle strength and endurance. J Ortho Sports Phys Ther.* 1989; 315–322.

Rothstein J, Lamb R, Mayhew P. *Clinical uses of isokinetic measurements. Phys Ther.* 1987; 67:1840–1844.

Sisk TD, Stralka SW. *Effect of electrical stimulation on quadriceps strength after reconstructive surgery. Amer J Sports Med.* 1987; 15(3):215–220.

Thompson MC, Shingleton LG. *Comparison of values generated during testing of the knee using the Cybex II plus and the Biodex model B-2000 isokinetic dynamometers. J Ortho Sports Phys Ther.* 1989; 11(3):108–115.

Thorblad J, Ekstrand J. *Muscle rehabilitation after arthroscopic meniscectomy with or without tourniquet control. Amer J Sports Med.* 1985; 13(2):133–135.

Tibone E, Antich TJ. *Functions analysis of untreated and reconstructed posterior cruciate ligament injuries. Amer J Sports Med.* 1988; 16(3): 217–22.

Troyer H. *The effect of short term immobilization on the rabbit knee joint cartilage. Clin Ortho Rel Res.* 1975; 107:249–257.

Slocum D. *Rotary Instability of the Knee.* American Academy of Orthopedic Surgeons: Symposium on Sports Medicine. CV Mosby, St. Louis, 1969.

Smilie JS. *Injuries of the Knee Joint.* Williams & Wilkins, Baltimore, 1970.

Wilk K, Levine B. *Reliability of the Biodex B-2000 Isokinetic Dynamometer. Phys Ther.* 1988; 68(6):Abstract.

REFERENCES

1. Girgis FG, Marshall JL, Almonjem RS. The cruciate ligaments of the knee joint: anatomical, functional and experimental analysis. *Clin Orthop* 1975; 106:216–231.

2. Gray H. *Gray's Anatomy.* Philadelphia, PA: Lea & Febiger; 1974.

3. Basmajian J. *Muscles Alive: Their Functions Revised by Electromyography.* Baltimore, MD: William & Wilkins; 1962.

4. Bender JA. Factors affecting the occurrence of knee injuries, *J Am Phys Med Rehabil,*1964; 18:537.

5. Cahill BR, Griffin EH. Effect of pre-season conditioning on the incidence and severity of high school football knee injuries, *Am J Sports Med* 1978; 6:372.

6. Klein K, Allman FC. *The Knee in Sports,* Austin, TX: Jenkins Publishing; 1969.

7. Larson RL, Subluxation-dislocation of the patella. In: Kennedy J (Ed). *The Injured Adolescent Knee,* Baltimore, MD: William & Wilkins; 1962.

8. Noyes F, Torvik P. Biomechanics of ligament failure. *J Bone Joint Surg.* 1974; 56A(2):1406–1418.

9. Leib J, Perry J. Quadriceps functions, an EMG study under isometric conditions, *J Bone Joint Surg,* 1971; 53:749.

10. Noyes F, Mooar P, Matthews D, Butler B. The symptomatic anterior cruciate deficient knee. Part 1. *J Bone Joint Surg,* 1983; 65A(2).

11. Noyes F, Matthews D, Mooar P, Grood E. The symptomatic anterior cruciate deficient knee. Part 2. 1983; *J Bone Joint Surg,* 65A(2).

12. Kaufer H. Mechanical function of the patella, *J Bone Joint Surg.* 1971; 53A(1153).

13. Brattstrom H. Shape of the intercondylar groove normally and in recurrent dislocations of the patella. *Acta Orthop. Scand* 1964; 8:226.

14. Outerbridge RE. The etiology of chondromalacia patellae, *J Bone Joint Surg.* 1961; 44B:752.

15. Hughston JC. Classification of knee ligament instabilities I and II. *J Bone Joint Surg,* 1976; 58A:159.

16. Abbott HC, Kress JB. *Preconditioning in the Prevention of Knee Injuries.* Physical Medicine and Rehabilitation Association (booklet). 1969.

17. Noyes F, Mangine R. Early knee motion after open and arthroscopic ACL reconstruction. *Amer J Sports Med,* 1987; 15(2):149–160.

18. Tambrello, M. *Patella Hypomobility as a Cause of Extensor Lag* Master's thesis: Medical College of Virginia: Virginia Commonwealth University, Richmond, VA 1982.

23

Ankle Injuries

William S. Case

INTRODUCTION

The ankle is one of the most underrated joints in the human body. It is the first major joint to come into contact with the ground in any weight-bearing sport or activity. Even though the line of stability starts from the ground up, most athletes are interested in exercising from the top down to the ground. The upper extremity is considered the glamour area, from the huge shoulders to the enormous pectoralis muscles, and a small waistline and powerful quadricep muscles denote power. Injury to the ankle, however, whether fracture or ligamentous blowout, can debilitate an athlete throughout most or all of the season.

Ankle sprains are among the most frequent injury in sports, resulting in 25% of the time lost from injuries in every running and jumping sport.[1] Although head and neck injuries are more severe, ankle injuries simply occur more frequently.[1]

All health care professionals are aware of the high incidence of ankle injuries, but, other than taping, little is done in the way of prevention. The diagnosis may be differential and the treatment is usually indifferent. Therefore, for the sports physical therapist to prevent injuries he or she must be able to recognize biomechanical abnormalities and muscular and ligamentous weaknesses and understand the mechanisms of injuries to thoroughly rehabilitate the athlete to an optimum level of performance. Modalities such as heat, cold, and electricity, along with innovative exercises and external orthosis, are tools we use as practitioners to help reduce the amount of time spent in the rehabilitation process.

This chapter follows the sports physical therapist's assessment of objective findings and presents various therapeutic modalities for treating acute and chronic conditions affecting the ankle. Although the biomechanics and the anatomic structures of the ankle are important, the principal focus is on understanding the role of the sports physical therapist in returning the athlete to his or her level of competition in the shortest and safest period of time.

BIOMECHANICS

The ankle joint appears to comprise a single vertical axis, allowing up and down motions. When an athlete runs, and needs to perform twisting maneuvers, however, the motion must be from a more sophisticated joint. The joint must be capable of striking uneven surfaces, tolerating abrupt changes in direction, and withstanding impacts from all directions. Knowledge of the biomechanics and versatility in the ankle joint enables the sports physical therapist to properly assess the mechanism of injury and joint stability for an aggressive and functional recovery.

The ankle joint comprises many articulations from the tibia, fibula, and talus, forming the tibiotalar, fibulotalar, and tibiofibular joints. The joint combines many motions, one being that of dorsiflexion and plantarflexion occurring in the sagittal plane. This up and down motion occurs between the talus and the medial and lateral malleolus. In the transverse plane there is a more anterior placement of the medial than the lateral malleolus. In the frontal plane there lies a more caudal placement of the lateral than the medial malleolus. The joint axis passes from the distal end of the medial malleolus through the body of the talus, distally and posteriorly, to the distal and anterior tip of the lateral malleolus.[2] "Quantitatively the ankle joint axis measures 80 degrees on the average from a vertical reference and 84 degrees from a longitudinal axis of the foot" (Fig 23–1). Because this axis deviates from a true frontal plane orientation of the foot by 6 degrees and from a true transverse plane orientation by 10 degrees, motion around the ankle joint is triplanar rather than uniplanar.[2] The triplanar motions are those of pronation and supination. Pronation of the foot requires dorsiflexion in the sagittal plane, eversion in the frontal

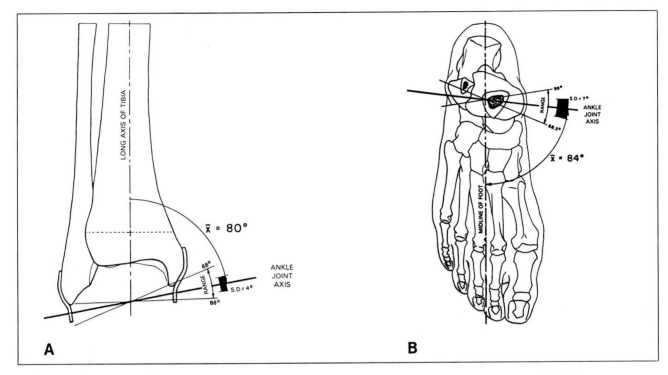

Figure 23-1. Orientation of the ankle joint axis. Mean values measure (**A**) 80 degrees from a vertical reference, and (**B**) 84 degrees from the longitudinal reference of the foot. *(From Novick A. Anatomy and biomechanics. In: Hunt GC ed.* Physical Therapy of the Foot and Ankle. *New York, NY: Churchill Livingstone; 1988; and Isman RE, Inman VT. Anthropometric Studies of the Human Foot and Ankle: Technical Report No. 58; University of California, San Francisco, 1968, with permission.)*

plane, and abduction in the transverse plane. Supination, on the other hand, includes plantarflexion in the sagittal plane, inversion in the frontal plane, and adduction in the transverse plane.[2]

THE GAIT CYCLE

The gait cycle requires specific simultaneous interactions between the joints of the lower extremity. The two phases of walking are the stand and swing phase.

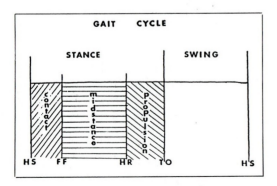

Figure 23-2. Gait cycle. Functional divisions of stance phase. HS, heel-strike; FF, foot-flat; HR, heel-rise; TO, toe-off. *(From Tiberio D. The effect of excessive subtalar joint pronation on patellofemoral mechanics: A theoretical model.* J Orthop Sports Phys Ther. *1987; 9:162, with permission.)*

The stance phase occurs when the foot is in contact with the ground and the swing phase is initiated when the foot leaves the ground to advance the body forward. The stance phase is divided into three parts—contact, midstance, and propulsion. The contact phase starts when the heel of the foot first strikes the ground and continues until the foot is flat. The midstance phase occurs while the foot is flat until the heel rises. Finally, the propulsion phase begins as the heel lifts off and continues until the push off with the toes. Then the swing phase advances the body forward before the cycle starts over (Fig 23–2).[3]

THE SUBTALAR JOINT

The subtalar joint (STJ) constitutes the articulation of the inferior aspect of the talus and the superior aspect of the calcaneus. The STJ axis is a triplanar joint revealing a mean deviation upward of 41 degrees from the transverse plane and a medial deviation of 23 degrees from the longitudinal reference (Fig 23–3)[2] There may be some differences in the longitudinal reference line measurements between researchers, but this may be due to the reference line of the toes used. Nevertheless, it is important to note that the triplanar movements of the STJ occur as a combination of motions.[2,4]

The triplanar motions of the STJ are pronation

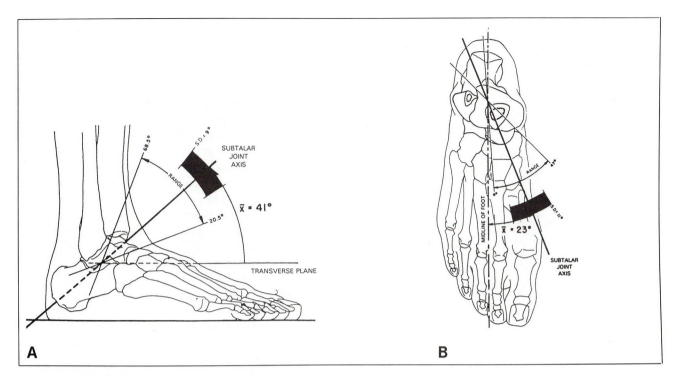

Figure 23–3. Orientation of the subtalar joint axis. Mean values measure **(A)** 41 degrees from the transverse plane and **(B)** 23 degrees medially from the longitudinal reference of the foot. *(From Novick A. Anatomy and biomechanics. In: Hunt GC ed.* Physical Therapy of the Foot and Ankle. *New York, NY: Churchill LIvingstone; 1988; and Isman RE, Inman VT.* Anthropometric Studies of the Human Foot and Ankle: Technical Report No. 58. *University of California, San Francisco, 1968, with permission.)*

and supination. The combined motions of pronation are dorsiflexion, abduction, and eversion to unlock the foot on uneven surfaces to compensate for stability.[4] Loading and compression forces are easier to accept in this position. When an athlete comes down on an extended leg, a more stable base is established when the STJ is functioning normally. When he or she is ready to push off and propel the body forward the STJ supinates combining plantarflexion, adduction, and inversion. This motion enables the foot to adjust and increase the lever for propulsion.[4]

During the gait cycle the STJ is supinated until contact is made during the heel-strike phase, after which the foot pronates. The foot pronates until full contact takes place, and then the STJ starts to supinate as continued forward movement occurs. Supination occurs through the midstance and propulsion phases until toe-off, where it peaks in motion (Fig 23–4).[3]

During the contact phase the STJ pronates, causing the calcaneus to evert and the talus to move into a plantarflexion and adduction position.[3] Because the talus has such a close approximation with the medial and lateral malleolus the lower extremity must internally rotate to achieve the full position of a closed chain pronation position. (Fig 23–5).[3] As the forward movement in the gait cycle progresses the STJ supinates, causing the lower extremity to externally rotate, while advancing the body.[3]

The normal movements of an athlete when running requires many ankle deviations. The subtalar joint is responsible for much of the compensatory action that takes place during the gait cycle.[4] The versatility of the entire lower extremity is responsible for an exceptional performance, and any alteration in the joint's structure will affect stability. The triplanar movements of pronation and supination affect the stability of the ankle on uneven surfaces and assist in the noncontrolled move-

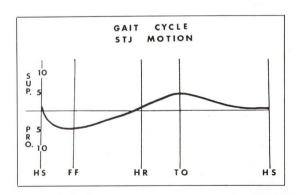

Figure 23–4. Motion of the Subtalar joint during the gait cycle. HS, heel-strike; FF, foot-flat; HR, heel-rise; TO, toe-off. *(From American Rehabilitation Network. 1984; and Tiberio D. The effect of excessive subtalar joint pronation on patellofemoral mechanics: A theoretical model.* J Orthop Sports Phys Ther. *1987; 9:162, with permission.)*

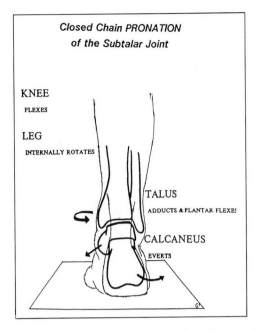

Figure 23–5. Internal rotation of the lower leg with closed chain pronation. *(From American Rehabilitation Network. 1984; and Tiberio D. The effect of excessive subtalar joint pronation on patellofemoral mechanics: A theoretical model.* J Orthop Sports Phys Ther. *1987; 9:162, with permission.)*

ments of the lower extremity when changing directions. Limited or excessive STJ motion may be a sign of instability, causing weakness in this joint and the surrounding structures.[4]

It is extremely important to be knowledgeable of the biomechanics of all the weight-bearing joints. Each joint is linked by a specific anatomic design, and the slightest deviation can create a shift, resulting in referred pain, or an instability that may go unnoticed, causing further injury.

CLOSED VERSUS OPEN CHAIN ASSESSMENT

The gait cycle consists of two weight-bearing positions: open chain (non-weight-bearing) and closed chain (weight-bearing). The anatomic structures of the lower extremity are affected differently in these positions of motion.[4] The rotational components of the ankle, knee, and hip reverse directions when changing from an open to closed chain position. Because stability starts from the ground up, the STJ joint can affect the function of each joint of the lower extremity. Weight-bearing assessment is critical when determining the level of function. The athlete may display good range of motion and strength, but when asked to perform a skilled activity may lack proprioception stability due to inactivity. This level of assessment should be an ongoing

part of the rehabilitation program to determine when practice or competition should begin.

Kantner, Gray, and Lattanza report data emphasizing the importance of an accurate assessment of eversion, as a component of pronation, measured in a functional weight-bearing or closed-chain position compared to a non-weight-bearing or open-chain position. "One of the critical motions that occur as a component of pronation is eversion."[4] Because pronation causes eversion of the STJ, the tibia will internally rotate as a compensatory reaction secondary to the eversion movement of the STJ. Therefore, the degree of tibial rotation is controlled by the movement of the STJ.[4] Excessive eversion of the STJ may be due to a forefoot varus deformity. This excessive STJ compensation may lead to medial knee pain, which may be overlooked, due to increased tibial rotation at the knee. Excessive STJ motion may go undetected when a manual passive eversion test is performed in the non-weight-bearing position, but not in the full weight-bearing position, as excessive eversion from the neutral subtalar position would be noted.[4]

Compensatory motion of the STJ when ambulating can be so nonspecific that a patient may not even be aware of the preexisting condition when complaining of chronic lower extremity or back pain. It is important to evaluate the ankle in non-weight-bearing positions, but because we are active in a weight-bearing environment, the assessment should be continued in a functional position.

Understanding the functional biomechanics of the ankle in relationship to the lower extremity chain can have profound clinical applications. Realizing the importance of open- and closed-chain STJ positions during the gait cycle offers another means by which to evaluate and formulate an exercise program. It is also important to note the triplanar motions of the ankle, which act as shock absorbers and weight distributors for the lower extremity kinetic chain, and establish a stabilizing structure at the push-off phase for efficient running. Once the biomechanics are properly assessed during the evaluation, then the specific rehabilitation can be implemented.

ANATOMY

Ligaments and Capsule

The ankle joint is encapsulated by fibrous tissue. The strong ligamentous support structures are located medially and laterally. The lateral supporting ligaments are the anterior talofibular ligament, the calcaneofibular ligament, and the posterior talofibular ligament. These ligaments provide the lateral stability required when performing an activity and are stressed individually by the position of the talus.[5] Plantarflexion is supported

by the anterior talofibular ligament and dorsiflexion is stabilized by the calcaneofibular ligament, limiting excessive inversion movements. When the leg is hit from behind the forward ankle displacement on the foot is restricted by the posterior talofibular ligament.[5] The medial aspect of the ankle is stabilized by the deltoid ligament. This ligament is very broad, having a superficial and deep component, extending down from the medial malleolus to the structures supporting the arch of the foot. Therefore, not only is the deltoid ligament important in preventing eversion movements of the ankle but it also aids in supporting the arch of the foot.[6] The lateral malleolus is anatomically situated to offer medial stability with the deltoid ligament. Impact compression forces to the medial aspect of the ankle may cause a lateral malleolar fracture along with ligament disruption. Due to the increased mobility of the ankle on the lateral aspect, however, the most common injury is the lateral sprain.

Musculature

The musculature that crosses the ankle joint into the foot provides secondary stability to the ligamentous components of the bones. The muscles for performing dorsiflexion and plantarflexion movements are found anterior and posterior to the ankle. Palpation can easily define the strong anterior tibialis (anteriorly) and gastrocnemius (posteriorly). Joint stability is also provided secondarily by the medial and lateral muscles when performing walking or running activities.

The lateral muscles offering stability are the peroneals, longus, and brevis (Fig 23–6). The muscles are found in the lateral aspect of the lower extremity passing posteriorly and inferiorly to the lateral malleolus. Palpation of the peroneal tendon can be performed by

everting the foot and noting the tendon posterior and distal to the lateral malleolus. The function of these muscles is to provide lateral stability and absorb the many stresses of inversion movements that are present in cutting and twisting movements.

The peroneals play a very important role in ankle stability and injury. A severe inversion movement of the ankle can overstretch or even tear the peroneal muscles. With time and protection the ankle injury will heal well if the ligamentous structure is not disrupted. The lateral muscles, however, will atrophy following the strain if not properly rehabilitated. Many of the chronic ankle injuries that occur on a repeated basis are not from the instability but from the weakness established after the initial injury.

Medially, the tendons of the posterior tibialis, flexor digitorum longus, and flexor hallucis longus pass posteriorly and inferiorly to the medial malleolus. These muscles are found passing posteriorly in the lower extremity and assist the deltoid ligament in medial stability. Palpation can be performed by inverting and plantarflexing the foot where the posterior tibialis is most prominent posteriorly and inferiorly to the medial malleolus.

EXAMINATION

The examination process includes many variables to consider before a plan of treatment can be formulated. The examination should include the history and subjective and objective data. A good initial assessment will enable the therapist to note changes and responses to the treatments as they occur, maintaining an ongoing performance flow sheet.

History

The history is regarded as information from the patient or athlete that leads up to the initial visit. The history should report data such as (1) trauma, (2) weight changes, (3) activities that relate to the problem, (4) occupational activities that may affect the problem, (5) mechanism of injury, (6) frequency of signs and symptoms, (7) referred or associated symptoms of pain, (8) current or past treatments, including specific procedures, and (9) present status.[2]

Subjective Assessment

The subjective data offer the sports physical therapist information described by the athlete about his or her condition. The particular pain may only be described on a scale of 1 to 10, but it is what the patient feels. If an athlete has an acute injury, the information is specific, but, if it is chronic, then asking questions pertinent to activities of daily living (ADLs) is essential. The examiner must gather as much subjective information

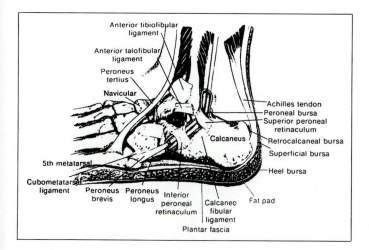

Figure 23–6. The lateral side of the ankle and foot contains many structures that may be injured during sports. *(From Kuland D: The Injured Athlete. Philadelphia, Pa: J B Lippincott Co; 1982, with permission.)*

as possible to (1) assess the problem, (2) establish criteria for an objective examination, (3) determine his or her level of disability, (4) design a treatment program, and (5) project goals for his or her rehabilitation. The subjective information provides a gauge that can be used to determine the effectiveness of the treatment and a reference to measure an ongoing assessment of his or her progress.[2]

The patient should be asked to describe specific signs/symptoms present, along with their intensity:

- Pain (specifically burning, aching, etc)
- Paresthesia
- Other associated symptoms (swelling, giving way, etc)
- Limitation of activities
- Symptoms at rest versus activity
- Onset acute or chronic

Objective Assessment

Following guidelines obtained from the history and the subjective information taken, the therapist gathers objective data on the patient. This information may be observations made by the examiner noting certain reproducible findings. Findings that can be documented due to specific characteristics are important.[2]

The objective assessment of the athlete should include the following:

- Posture
- Weight-bearing status
- Sensation and skin changes
  Areas of pain
  Areas of numbness
  Areas of hypersensitivity
  Skin color
- Measurements
  Range of motion
  Strength
  Joint play
  Stability
  Alignment
  Gait
  Balance
  Footwear

It is very important to assess the patient's posture whether weight-bearing or non-weight-bearing. Although the ankle may be the affected area, the foot, knee, hip, and trunk positions should not be overlooked, as injuries may result from compensatory actions in these areas. A gait screening examination should be performed to identify any abnormalities during the stance phase. A slow-motion video camera (if available) would enable the therapist to perform a full gait analysis.

Classification and Diagnosis

There seems to be no specific guidelines for determining the severity of ankle injuries. Some classifications are determined by the level of functional instability present and others by the mechanism of injury and the signs/symptoms present. Due to these nonspecific forms of ankle injury assessments a consensus in using x-rays is being developed for specific classifications. Stress x-rays can assist the therapist or trainer in determining exactly what ligaments were involved by the degree of instability found. The initial treatment can then be established and a functional rehabilitation program developed.

Strains and sprains are classified by the structures involved. A strain primarily involves a muscle–tendon unit and its bony attachment and a sprain suggests ligamentous involvement, usually indicating some form of instability.[2] When an athlete sustains an injury, it is considered acute from overstress. If the injury reoccurs, chronic instability from overuse is the classification. These injuries still require a structured rehabilitation program; however, the repeat injury usually involves greater instability. Preventive measures are critical once the chronic injury is present to avoid a more invasive treatment, namely surgery.

Treatment is decided by the pathology present, stress x-rays, and the objectives of the athlete or patient. A grade I sprain usually has some mild swelling without a great deal of functional loss. A grade II sprain usually notes some functional loss, but, not enough to require surgery. A grade III or IV sprain, however, results in disruption of the ligament, with complete loss of function, and surgery is usually necessary.

MECHANISMS OF INJURY

Lateral Ankle Sprain

The lateral ankle sprain (inversion injury) is one of the most common of all ankle injuries to athletes, constituting approximately 85% of all ankle injuries.[7] Usually, the position of the foot for an inversion injury is plantarflexion, where stress is placed on the anterior talofibular ligament. This constitutes a single-ligament injury. A double-ligament injury takes place when additional stress to the anterior talofibular ligament leads to a tear of the calcaneal–fibular ligament, which provides secondary stability (Fig 23–7).

In a single-ligament injury to the anterior talofibular ligament, the lateral instability present will only be when plantarflexing the foot. When a double-ligament injury occurs, however, the lateral instability of the ankle joint will usually be in all positions, except when dorsiflexing the foot, which may offer some sta-

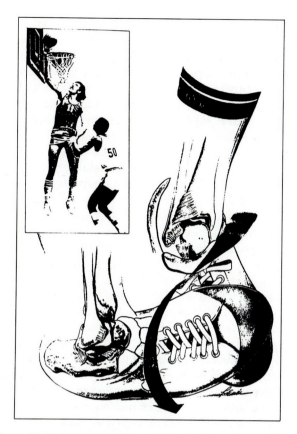

Figure 23-7. Lateral Sprains. A "single-ligament sprain" occurs when the player's plantar-flexed ankle is inverted, tearing the anterior talofibular ligament. If the inversion continues when the whole foot has reached the ground, the calcaneal-fibular ligament rips, producing a "double-ligament sprain." *(From Kuland D.* The Injured Athlete. *Philadephia, Pa: J B Lippincott; 1982. with permission.)*

bility. A third structure that reinforces the joint posteriorly, the posterior talofibular ligament, may also be affected on severe inversion twisting injuries.[5,7,8]

Anterior Capsular Sprain

An anterior capsular tear results from an athlete having an impact placed on a plantarflexed foot. The initial evaluation reveals a painful foot, at the proximal and dorsal aspect of the ankle, when passively plantarflexed. Resistance applied when the athlete dorsiflexes the foot also causes pain. The rehabilitation process usually requires a long period before full function is regained. Strengthening of the dorsiflexor muscles for stability against plantarflexion is essential and may require functional taping or strapping to prevent hypermobility into plantarflexion.[8]

Syndesmotic Disruptions

Syndesmotic disruptions occur between the distal tibia and fibula, where the bones are held together by a ligamentous attachment. An ankle injury may include

many pathologies, and, if not diagnosed properly, the athlete's recovery may be impeded. Therefore, differentiation between those ankle injuries with and without a syndesmotic disruption is important. Usually the mechanism of injury is a valgus–external rotation stress placed to the ankle when an athlete, for example, running-back, is hit from behind. The running-back is hit in the posterolateral aspect of the leg, when the ankle is in the toe-off position. With this type of injury other structures may be involved: the anterior tibiofibular ligament, interosseous membrane, posterior tibiofibular ligament, and the deltoid ligament.[9]

The initial findings are similar to those of a lateral and interosseous sprain but differ in some respects. Both injuries may reveal tenderness to the deltoid ligament; interosseous sprains, however, will be tender at the anterior tibiofibular syndesmosis and frequently up the interosseous membrane. There are two main evaluations that can be performed to determine the presence of a syndesmotic disruption. First, the examiner places the foot in a neutral position and then externally rotates it. A disruption will be present if pain is in the area of the interosseous membrane. Secondly, an athlete with a medial or lateral ankle injury will be able to toe-raise with minimal pain but the athlete with a syndesmotic disruption will have difficulty or be unable to perform a toe-raise due to pain in the syndesmosis area.[9]

Medial Ankle Sprain

Medial ankle sprains are seen less frequently, usually in contact sports. This type of sprain is an eversion injury that affects the deltoid ligament. The medial ligaments are much stronger than the lateral structures and are also supported by the length of the lateral malleolus. Stress to this bony block of eversion movement is frequently coupled with a compression fracture of the fibula. Deltoid injuries, which may also be associated with interosseous sprains, result from a valgus or valgus external rotation stress to the lower leg.[5,9]

FUNCTIONAL INSTABILITY

All of the research concerning diagnosis and treatment of lateral ankle injuries has one goal in mind, prevention of long-term functional instability. We all know there are predetermined factors that lead to instability; however, which pathological factor causes chronic instability is still unknown.[1] Secondary support structures are definitely called upon once an injury has occurred, but to what extent is hard to evaluate. Many times an athlete's symptoms have diminished and he or she has returned to activities without being able to determine his or her level of instability at that time, due to proprioception loss.

Once an injury has taken place a certain amount of instability will occur. Depending on the severity of the injury and the rehabilitation that follows, caution should be used by the therapist in returning the athlete to competition. Although the sports physical therapist has guidelines and timetables to use in rehabilitation, the only actual gauge is performance. Keeping in mind three possible causes of prolonged functional instability can help minimize further reinjury: (1) mechanical instability, (2) peroneal weakness, and (3) proprioception deficits.[1]

TREATMENT

Early diagnosis and treatment of ankle sprains is essential. If early treatment is not initiated, complications may arise due to disuse, pain and swelling. Closely monitoring the signs and symptoms during the initial evaluation can expedite the treatment process.

There are two basic forms of treatment: operative and nonoperative. The former follows the same guidelines as the latter, except that additional time is involved. I concentrate below on the nonoperative procedures for lateral ankle sprains.

Immobilization

For some physicians, immobilization is the treatment of choice for the more severe ankle sprains. The athlete is placed in either a walking cast or removable walking cast boot for 4 to 6 weeks. Weight-bearing is as tolerated using crutches. Following the immobilization period the athlete starts a program of contrast baths, electric stimulation, taping, gentle passive to active exercises, and progressive resistance exercises.

In a recent study, the effects of mobilization, cast immobilization, and surgical repair plus immobilization were compared. Surgical repair afforded the greatest amount of mechanical stability, with mobilization and cast immobilization having similar results.[1] The shortest period of disability was noted with mobilization. Approximately 55% of those treated conservatively were free of symptom after 1 year, as opposed to 25% of those who underwent surgery.[1] Therefore, regardless of the severity of the ankle injury, mobilization is the treatment of choice.[1]

Another study comparing primary repair, plaster immobilization, and strapping of ankle injuries revealed that strapping involved the shortest period of disability. The symptoms of instability were less following the surgical repair, however, than following the nonsurgical treatment (3% versus 20%). Despite the greater stability provided by surgery, it was felt that mobilization and strapping would be the treatments of choice, with surgery reserved for those young athletes with chronic ankle instabilities.[1]

Functional Method

The functional method is presently being used by sports physical therapists and is not new, but I feel that it has merit and sound guidelines to treating the acute ankle injury. Initially, there is an ice whirlpool for 15 to 20 minutes, followed by taping for compression. Several days later, after the swelling has started to subside, taping with a heel lock is applied to place the ankle in dorsiflexion and eversion. It is important to keep the ankle joint in a stable position while healing, to eliminate scarring in a stretched position. Generally, gentle passive, assisted-active, and active exercises are started as soon as possible to assist the edema in decreasing and maintaining muscle tone with joint range of motion.[7]

Partial weight-bearing with crutches is also started as soon as possible and is progressed as tolerated. Within 1 week, contrast baths are started to promote healing and decrease the swelling. Usually, this program of contrast baths plus exercise and taping is performed for 3 weeks. The athlete's weight-bearing program is progressed as tolerated and full weight-bearing is started once there is ambulation without a limp.[7]

Once the athlete's functional level of performance has been assessed by the therapist and weight-bearing is painfree with good range of motion, controlled agility activities are started. The activities may incorporate weights on a balance board or controlled running and agility drills. It is advised that protective taping be used for at least 3 to 4 months during practice and competition following an ankle injury. The athlete is usually ready to return to activity with this method of treatment in 3 to 4 weeks, depending on the severity of the injury.[7] This type of early mobilization treatment has actually shown evidence that range of joint motion assists in the healing process of torn ligaments.[7] It has also been reported that exercise stimulates and affects the strength of ligaments.[7]

Modality Application

The rehabilitative process begins the day of the injury. The initial acute goals are to immobilize the joint with compression and elevation to control the edema, by taping. The addition of cryotherapy treatment enables the athlete to perform range of motion and isometrics exercises to decrease the pain and swelling, while preventing atrophy. Limiting the weight-bearing activity, with crutches, relieves the compression forces of the ankle and prevents further ligamentous damage. Applying electric stimulation to the ankle for muscle re-education, pain management and tissue swelling also helps in the healing process.

Iontophoresis, or ion transfer, is also a new and useful modality for tissue application. It involves the "introduction of topical applied, physiologically active ions into the epidermis and mucous membranes of the body by the use of continuous direct current."[10] This

modality is becoming popular in the treatment of sports-related injuries. Iontophoresis has several advantages compared to the standard injection. It is noninvasive, painless, and sterile and avoids the tissue damage resulting from needle injection, which can often be tender for several days. It has been successfully used in the treatments of athletes and patients with a variety of conditions, including calcium deposits, softening of scar tissue and adhesions, fungus infections, musculoskeletal disorders such as arthritis, bursitis, and tendonitis, edema reduction, and slow healing wounds. It should be used in conjunction with other modalities to achieve results desired.[10]

External Supports

External support devices or taping also aid in stability as early weight-bearing increases. In the acute injury, early protected weight-bearing may assist in the stimulation of proprioceptive responses for stability. If the joint receptors for kinesthetic awareness have not been torn during injury, then their ability to return for function is favorable. Without proper rehabilitation, however, the incidence for reinjury is increased, possibly with further damage resulting from each subsequent injury. Proprioceptive deficits caused by direct trauma to articular receptors of the ankle have been proposed as a neuromuscular etiology of chronic ankle instability. Chronic ankle instability has also been postulated to result from partial deafferentation of joint receptors of the injured joint.[11] Therefore, early protected weight-bearing may assist in the continuity of proprioceptive responses.

A Four-Phase Rehabilitation Program

Every rehabilitation facility has its own protocol for returning the patient or athlete to competition. The degree of competition is not as important as the patient's level of function. Treatment and prevention can be divided into four phases: (1) acute phase; (2) protective phase; (3) functional phase; and (4) preventive phase.

Acute Phase. During competition, the athlete plants the foot to change directions or pivots sharply to retrieve a serve (while playing a racquet sport) or receives an impact playing a group sport. Then he or she hears a pop and feels a tear while falling to the ground in pain. This is the classic example of how an ankle is injured, usually the lateral aspect. Once the injury has occurred, it is the responsibility of the sports physical therapist to initiate treatment for the acute phase of rehabilitation.

Initial 24 to 48 Hours. Ice, compression, elevation, painless weight-bearing comprise the immediate treatment.

Three to Seven Days Postinjury. Contrast baths can begin 48 hours after the initial injury, depending on the degree of heat and swelling in the ankle. The ratio of heat and cold may vary, but I use a 1-minute cold and 2- to 3-minute heat for 15 minutes. The treatment always ends with cold. The temperatures for the cold and heat are 60°F and 105°F, respectively, depending on the patient's tolerance. The patient is asked to exercise the ankle in gentle range of motion movements while in the heat and cold. The contrast bath method is used for 2 to 3 weeks or until the swelling has decreased and stabilized.

Each subsequent treatment should reveal a decrease in pain, swelling, and paresthesia, and an increase in range of motion, strength, and weight-bearing. Foot and ankle exercises consist of half-circle movements, limiting the painful arc, and musculotendinous specific exercises to strengthen the muscles needed for secondary stability.

Electric stimulation may be applied to the lateral aspect of the lower extremity, along with isometric exercises, to prevent muscle atrophy. Peroneal strengthening exercises are vitally important, since many of the chronic ankle reinjuries are due to weakness and atrophy. Electric stimulation is also important for pain management where joint dysfunction is lost in response to injury.

Gentle (active–passive) range of motion exercises should begin, depending on the pain and swelling. The earlier passive exercises are implemented, the less immobility will be present. Inversion movements should be avoided entirely, with emphasis placed on dorsiflexion and eversion. Active muscular activity will assist in decreasing the edema as well as the soreness.

Seven to 14 Days Postinjury. At this stage of the rehabilitation the modality application may vary depending on desired results. Electric stimulation may be in the form of a muscle stimulator for reeducation, high-voltage galvanic stimulation for edema and tissue response, and transcutaneous electrical nerve stimulation (TENS) for pain control.

The stretching exercises should progress to standing heel cord stretches and the isometric exercises to manual resistance. With discomfort as a guide, all activities should be minimized when pain is present. The ligament injury is very susceptible to reinjury, and any increase in pain, swelling, or discoloration should be treated with caution.

Proprioceptive exercises on a tilt or balance board (sitting to standing) can be gradually initiated. Toe-raises seated to standing are also started for stability and kinesthetic purposes. When an ankle is sprained, the proprioceptive nerve endings are also disrupted. The nerves provided the necessary information for muscle and joint action. The athlete may increase ankle

joint stability by using a balance board to provide strength, balance, and coordination. The board creates a variety of passive joint angles that the athlete would find on uneven surfaces when performing a functional activity. Resistance can be applied to the board on the side of instability to increase the strength. Other activities to increase awareness of the ankle joint for motion and position would be standing or walking on a foam pad or a mini-trampoline.[11]

The exercise progression begins with passive range of motion, followed by active-assistive to active range of motion and strengthening exercises. Before any resistive work is initiated, painfree range of motion must be achieved. By following rehabilitative criteria rather than timetables the athlete will maximize his or her program to progress aggressively and safely.

Protective Phase.

Two to 4 Weeks Postinjury. After the acute phase, a more aggressive and controlled exercise regime can be started. The athletes range of motion and strength should have increased significantly, depending on the severity of the sprain. The primary muscle groups on which to concentrate are the peroneals, dorsiflexors, and plantarflexors. Any combination of these muscles or specific isolated exercises are incorporated into the rehabilitative program. Cycling, which may have already been implemented, is now stressed. Isotonic and isokinetic exercises are added for strength, power, and endurance to resist inversion (Fig 23–8). Hydraulic exercises offer the athlete an accommodating resistance to exercise in more than one plane (Fig 23–9). Eccentrically loading the foot and ankle with backwards ambulation (with increasing the stride), and up-and-down step-ups on a stool (progressing to stairs) assists the sta-

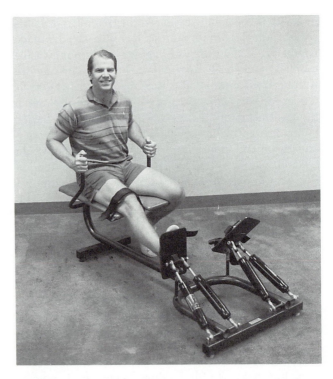

Figure 23–9. Hydraulic equipment for ankle strengthening.

bility of the ankles by incorporating a lengthening contraction. Side-to-side step-ups on a stool also aid in proprioceptive responses.

Additional proprioception exercises consist of using the BAPS (the balance board mentioned earlier), the Sand Dunes (foam pad), the mini-trampoline, and the Profitter (a functional side-to-side exerciser). These exercise apparatus offer a variable degree of difficulty, depending on use. After assessing the level of ankle dysfunction, the athlete is instructed in a progressive non-weight-bearing to full weight-bearing program.

The BAPS (circular tilt board) is a good weight-bearing device to increase range of motion, strength, and stimulate joint mechanoreceptors in a controlled fashion. The joint angle is established by the size of ball on the underside of the disc. Once the ankle motion has been increased to the desired level, weight-bearing can be increased, with standing and weights added to the periphery for resistance (Fig 23–10).

The Sand Dunes is an excellent way to start early proprioceptive responses through weight shifting on a foam pad. Activating musculotendinous structures on the lateral aspect of the ankle helps facilitate foot/ankle placement as weight-bearing increases (Fig 23–11). The mini-trampoline is more aggressive towards weight-bearing activities, enabling the athlete to perform light jogging motions (Fig 23–12). The Profitter is important in achieving lateral stresses in a structured side-to-side manner (Fig 23–13).

Protecting the ankle with external support while

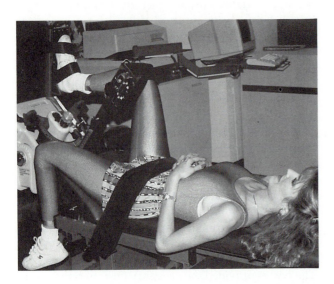

Figure 23–8. Ankle rehabilitation using isokinetic equipment.

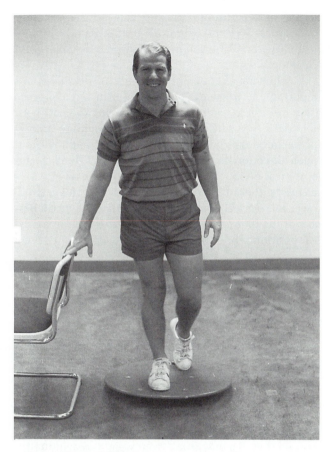

Figure 23-10. BAPS board for proprioceptive responses.

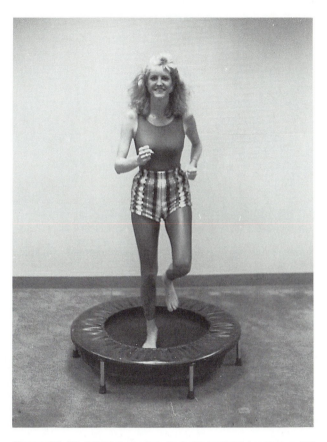

Figure 23-12. Mini-trampoline to initiate light jogging activities.

exercising may not be indicated because the athlete is strengthening the ankle in a controlled manner. The BAPS board can be modified to offer minimal to maximal joint range of motion, the mini-trampoline starts off with standing weight-shifting to easy jogging, and the isokinetic and surgical tubing exercises are limited by a manual or physical stop (Fig 23–14).

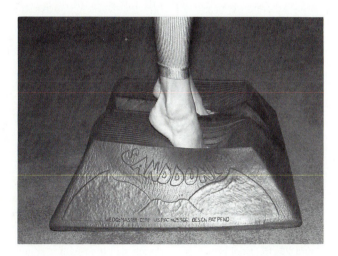

Figure 23-11. Sand Dunes enables early weight-bearing.

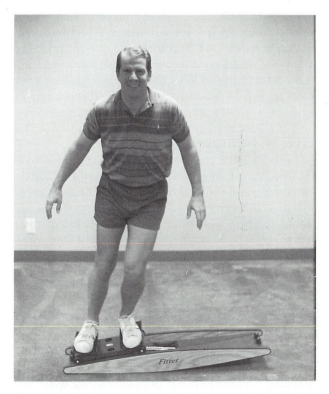

Figure 23-13. Profitter for a controlled side-to-side lateral ankle stabilizing exercise.

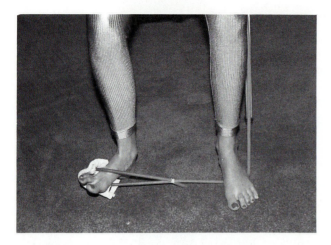

Figure 23-14. Surgical tubing for home strengthening of ankle stabilizers.

During the course of the protective phase an ongoing assessment is made to re-evaluate the areas of pain, tenderness, swelling, strength, and any loss of motion. Any combination of deficits noted must require a modification or elimination of the activity until the signs and symptoms of irritation have subsided.

Functional Phase.

Four to 6 Weeks Postinjury. This phase of the rehabilitation process can be used to prepare the athlete for functional running and agility skills. Modality application is not stressed here, but continued flexibility and joint-specific exercises are encouraged. The time when an athlete is ready to start a more aggressive running program is determined by the sports physical therapist on the basis of the athlete's progress through the previous phases. The functional phase may be delayed in some athletes, but maintaining sound principles during the early phases of rehabilitation will maximize the healing and strengthening process.

The athlete is now ready for sport-specific activities: jogging, running, figure-eights, and cutting activities. Taping and external devices should be used to restrict any unnecessary inversion movements. Once the athlete returns to practice and competition, taping with a lateral heel lock is mandatory because the collagen in the ligaments takes about 7 months to heal.

Prevention Phase.

Stretching. Calf stretching exercises have been reported to reduce ankle injuries.[2] In a recent study, athletes who exhibited less than 10 degrees of dorsiflexion were placed on a stretching program.[2] Ten degrees of dorsiflexion is necessary for normal walking when the knee is extended and the subtalar joint is in a neutral position, with running activities requiring at least 15 degrees of dorsiflexion.[2] Because calf muscles are plantarflexors as well as supinators, it appears that limited flexibility in dorsiflexion may predispose the ankle joint to a lateral sprain.[2]

Achieving the maximal amount of dorsiflexion is important in preventing ankle injuries but consideration must be given towards maximizing the best position of the foot when stretching. Most standing stretching techniques require that the knee be straight without much direction for the foot placement. The subtalar joint must be in a neutral position to offer an effective stretch to the ankle joint. To accomplish this a small towel roll or thin board is placed under the medial aspect of the foot to maintain the subtalar joint in a neutral position while stretching (Fig 23–15).[2]

Proprioceptive Training

Some athletes train with ankle weights, throwing off their coordination and agility and predisposing themselves to early fatigue and injury. Proprioceptive training on uneven surfaces allows the athlete to stimulate particular kinesthetic receptors of the ankle to discriminate joint position and motion. Joint-specific activities with specificity training far exceed weight training once the athlete has developed normal strength and range of motion. Timed agility drills and structured running programs offer the coordination, stability, and stamina that can only come from weight-bearing activities. This also enables the athlete to detect any inconsistencies in performance so that he or she can concen-

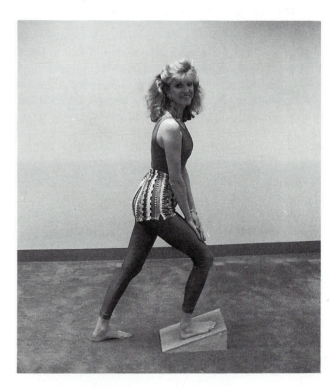

Figure 23-15. Heel cord board stretch modified with a small towel roll under the medial aspect of the foot.

trate on specific exercises already mentioned. Weight training has a place in returning normal strength, but once this has been accomplished functional activities should be emphasized.

FOOTWEAR

Chronic lateral ankle instability injuries from overuse running (on uneven or hard terrain) or from inversion instability with weekend activities can be managed with proper footwear. By looking at the heel of a worn shoe, it can be determined if abnormal pressure is being applied when running. Modifications can be made by shoe inserts or by having the shoe built up.

There are a few considerations when looking for a good athletic shoe. Running causes increased pronation.[12] Rear-foot stability is important in a shoe, reducing the amount and rate of foot pronation after heel-strike.[12] Some manufacturers have approached this by extending the shoe counter medially, reinforcing the counter, and extending the sides of the midsole to reinforce the counter.[12]

Shock attenuation is also important because athletes generate forces 2.5 to 3 times their body weight when running.[12] The midsole is the main shock-absorber of the shoe, and this must be taken into account when purchasing a shoe. The support of the shoe and the shock attenuation may vary with increased shoe wear. It is necessary to monitor the wear of the shoe and any change in lower extremity symptoms as running increases.[12]

Hard midsoles function poorly as shock absorbers but offer good mediolateral support.[13] As running increases, the shoe loses it shock-absorbing properties but increases in mediolateral support. Once the shoe loses its shock-absorbing properties, however, it fails to be an effective running shoe. The initial feel or performance of the shoe may be misleading because 300 to 400 km of wear is necessary to determine the shoe's functional changes.[13]

Following an ankle injury, the shoe of choice is a high top. This type of shoe is not designed for straight ahead running, however. Therefore, an external ankle support or taping must be administered inside the running shoes. Uniform taping of both ankles for preventive measures is discouraged due to weakening of the natural support structures of the ankle. Ligaments thicken with stress, but if the athlete remains taped for all activities the support structure weakens.

Cleats also influence the degree of stress placed on an ankle during running activities. The more narrow the cleat placement, lessening the base of support, the higher degree of ankle injury can be expected. Cleats placed towards the lateral margin of the shoe affords maximum stability.

Runners come in a wide variety of shapes and sizes, with each being anatomically and functionally different. Their needs demand that the shoe offer stability and shock attenuation for any foot or toe deformity. Even though runners may have differences in structure that cannot be changed, shoe modifications can be made to accommodate most runners' needs. Therefore, sports physical therapists should be aware of the shoe or athletic stores in their area and become familiar with their employees, who can provide assistance in finding or modifying a functional running shoe.

Due to the increasing number of running shoes available, I suggest a complete evaluation of the athlete before recommending a sports shoe. Determine the instability or lower extremity pathology present and recommend a shoe that offers the support needed. It is also necessary to consider the athlete's height, weight, and, most importantly, the frequency with which and terrain over which the athlete runs before recommending a particular shoe.

CONCLUSION

Athletes come from many walks of life—high school, collegiate, professional, and, most importantly, the weekend warrior. There are books on exercise, health clubs with qualified instructors, home videos with sound principles, and something new found in the various forms of the media nearly every day. Anyone who has participated in a sport for any length of time has twisted an ankle, perhaps not severely enough to warrant medical attention but severely enough to warrant ice and rest. That initial strain or partial tear creates a weak link for that lower extremity. Without proper function and strengthening of the ankle, then each and every joint connecting with it may be disrupted in time.

It is our responsibility as professionals in the health field to emphasize the importance of preventive medicine to our patients. Education is the key to any prevention. Once some basic principles of flexibility, strength, agility, and signs of overuse are made known, injury can be avoided or minimized.

Understanding the basic biomechanics of the ankle and the lower extremity can help you treat and prevent further injury. As a sports physical therapist it is your responsibility to stress the significance of the ankle's function to your patients because their recovery will be dependent upon your instructions.

REFERENCES

1. Balduini FC, Vegso JJ, Torg JS, et al. Management and rehabilitation of ligamentous injuries to the ankle. *Sports Med.* 1987; 4:364–380.

2. Hunt G, ed. *Physical Therapy of the Foot and Ankle.* New York, NY: Churchill Livingstone Inc; 1988; (15):4–15, 50–55, 62–70, 207–210, 227–228.

3. Tiberio D. The effect of excessive subtalar joint pronation on patellofemoral mechanics: A theoretical model. *J Orthop Sports Phys Ther.* 1987; 9:160–165.

4. Lattanza L, Gray G, Kantner RM. Closed versus open kinematic chain measurements of subtalar joint eversion: Implications for clinical practice. *J Orthop Sports Phys Ther.* 1988; 9:310–314.

5. Kaumeyer G, Malone T. Ankle injuries: Anatomical and biomechanical considerations necessary for the development of an injury prevention program. *J Orthop Sports Phys Ther.* 1980; 1:171–177.

6. O'Donoghue DH. *Treatment of Injuries to Athletes.* 4th ed. Philadelphia, Pa: W B Saunders Co; 1984: 601–609.

7. Cox JS, Brand RL. Evaluation and treatment of lateral ankle sprains. *Physician Sportsmed.* 1977; (5)b:51–55.

8. Kuland D. *The Injured Athlete.* Philadelphia, Pa: J B Lippincott Co; 1982:434–442.

9. Lindenfeld TN. The differentiation and treatment of ankle sprains. *Orthopedics.* 1988; 11:203–206.

10. Nelson RM, Currier DP, eds. *Clinical Electrotherapy.* East Norwalk, Conn: Appleton & Lange, 1987: chap 11.

11. Garn SN, Newton RA. Kinesthetic awareness in subjects with multiple ankle sprains. *Phys Ther.* 1988; 68:1667–1671.

12. McPoil TG. Footwear. *Phys Ther.* 1988; 68:1857–1964.

13. Hamil J, Bates BT. A kinetic evaluation of the effects of in vivo loading on running shoes. *J Orthop Sports Phys Ther.* 1988; 10:47–53.

24

Running Injuries

Perry S. Esterson and Dallas A. Simons

INTRODUCTION

Injuries to the runner present the sports physical therapist with a wide array of conditions, ranging from simple blisters to complex biochemical breakdowns. To assess an injury accurately, the sports physical therapist should obtain a complete history, thorough physical examination, and biomechanical analysis. This systematic approach will lead to an accurate diagnosis. Only then can appropriate and effective treatment start. Constant follow-up will provide feedback to evaluate the effectiveness of the treatment program.

Assessment of running injuries may be time consuming. Careful questioning and listening will lead to insightful analysis and proper time management with these patients.

HISTORY TAKING

Most runners will reveal the cause of the injuries if the therapist is willing to listen carefully. It is important to determine the onset of the injury. Is it acute or insidious? How long has this problem been going on? Careful review of the training schedule will often reveal the runner has broken a rule of "too fast, too soon, too often, too far":

- *Too fast:* Has the runner trained at a pace that is beyond his or her capacity? Speed workouts, namely interval training, require an adequate base before being included into the training schedule.
- *Too soon:* Has the runner increased the mileage too rapidly? A rule of thumb is no more than 10% increase mileage per week.
- *Too often:* Is the runner allowing adequate rest between runs? For some, running on alternate days will allow the body to rest. For others, daily running interchanging hard and easy workouts will suffice.

- *Too far:* Has the runner gone on a run that is significantly longer than the normal training runs?

Along with the above factors, changes in the terrain will often precipitate injuries. Running across a slope will increase the varus or valgus stress across the lower extremities. Increased hill running may exacerbate knee pain as the ground reaction forces through the legs increase on hills.

Is the athlete participating in other cross-training activities such as biking or swimming, weight training, or other sports? How do these activities affect the running program? The cumulative stress may be too great for the present level of fitness or readiness of the runner.

Evaluation of the shoe and its wear pattern often reflect the stresses present in the runner's lower extremities. Has the runner changed shoes recently? Is this pair of shoes appropriate for the runner and the foot type? Does the runner need or use orthotic devices and are they effective? Are they worn out or in need of adjustment? Running shoes are discussed later in this chapter.

Other prior injuries and their treatment, are other important considerations in the history. What effect has rest had or has other treatment been effective? The present injury may be an extension of a previous problem that was never totally resolved.

A complete and systematic history is the foundation of the treatment. This is a critical area in the treatment and management of the runner, and sufficient time must be allowed to obtain all the necessary information.

RUNNING SHOES

The running shoe is an essential piece of equipment. The day is long gone when a canvas upper and rubber-soled shoe was the standard athletic wear. Running requires that shoes provide both stability and shock

attenuation. These two characteristics may have an inverse relationship, however, producing undesirable results.[1]

To provide rear foot stability, most running shoes have a strong heel counter that is extended forward medially, and a plastic stabilizer placed between the counter and the midsole. Newer devices include the Adidas Torsion System (Adidas, Warren, NJ), which cuts a groove across the midsole of the shoe, allowing the heel and forefoot to rotate, whereas a Kevlar bar is embedded in the midsole to prevent excessive torsion. The Avia ARC (Avia Athletic Footwear, Portland OR) is a flexible platform composed of a Dupont material Hytrel that is molded into their cantilevered sole. Avia claims this combination significantly reduces impact loads as well as controls rearfoot motion. Turntec (Irvine, CA) attempts to produce stability with its Anatomical Cradle, a specially designed midsole that allows the calcaneus and midfoot to sit in rather than on it.

Several manufacturers have developed alternative methods for controlling the ground reactions forces or shock that is present in runners. Nike (Beaverton, OR) placed air chambers in the polyurethane midsole whereas Brooks (Rockford, MI) introduced the Hydro-Flow heel cushion. This two-chambered system contains silicone, which flows from the rear to the front chambers as the foot progresses from heel-stroke to toe-off.[2]

The selection of a shoe must be matched to the different requirements that runners present. A foot with excessive pronation will require more control whereas a relatively rigid or pes cavus type foot will need more shock protection. Moreover, heavier runners require materials that will not bottom or wear out prematurely.

Fitting the shoe to the foot requires more than looking at the size and width. McPoil describes three tests to determine the proper fit[3]: (1) The length of the shoe may be checked with an athlete standing and a thumb placed on the end of the vamp to determine whether $\frac{1}{2}$ to $\frac{5}{8}$ in of space is present in front of the end of the longest toe. (2) To assess the proper ball width (the widest point at the level of the metatarsal heads), the pinch test is performed. While the athlete is standing, the examiner grasps the vamp "just below the eyestay and pinch(es) the material between the index finger and the thumb. If the material cannot be pinched, it indicates improper ball width of the shoe with refitting necessary." (3) To evaluate the fit for the heel-to-ball length, the distance from the heel to the metatarsal heads is compared to the distance from the heel to the toe break in the forefoot. If these measurements are similar, then the foot is aligned with the construction of the shoe.[4]

TREATMENT APPROACHES: BIOMECHANICAL

The act of running places the body under various mechanical stresses. As the foot strikes the ground, there are reactionary forces that are transmitted through the body. Understanding these forces and their relationships in a closed kinetic chain will provide the groundwork for assessing many injuries. Newton stated that for every action, there is an equal and opposite reaction. The foot, as a mobile adapter, both absorbs and directs forces about the lower extremity. When it is functioning properly, shock is absorbed in the heel strike and midstance phase and the body is propelled forward in the toe-off phase. Malalignment of the body parts during these phases of running will create excessive forces throughout the lower extremities as well as the trunk.

The goal, therefore, of a biomechanical approach is to reduce unwanted forces on the body by maintaining the body parts in optimal functional positions while running. This is accomplished through various means, including stretching, strengthening, orthotic control of the foot, proper selection of shoes, and judicious training.

SYMPTOMATIC TREATMENT

Runners seek help when there is a problem and not when things are going well. Pain, swelling, tenderness, lethargy, and tightness are symptoms that should alert the runner to a problem.

These are the signs of potential injuries and as such should not be overlooked. The athlete should recognize the difference between the strain of training and symptoms that are not a part of normal training. Running through pain and injury is a formula for disaster. Therefore, symptoms should be treated, but their cause must be discovered. If reason for the breakdown is not found, the problem will return.

MAINTENANCE OF AEROBIC CONDITIONING

The last words a runner wants to hear is "stop running." These athletes have come to the sports physical therapist to find out how they can handle their injury while they continue to run. Rather than prescribe total rest as a treatment, the concept of "relative rest" should be applied. With this approach, the injured part may be rested while the rest of the body exercises. For example, an ankle may prevent running on land, but not in

a pool or riding a bike. Swimming may be a practical alternative to running with a stress fracture of the tibia.

Runners work hard to reach a level of fitness that allows them to compete or function in life. Therefore, alternate forms of aerobic exercise are necessary to obtain patient compliance with the treatment program.

REGIONAL AREAS

Forefoot

Blisters. Although not generally encountered in normal physical therapy practice, blisters can be a disabling injury to the runner. Blisters are caused by excessive friction about the toes and foot. Once a blister is formed, it must be treated to allow a quick return to running and prevent infection. If the blister is closed, then the surrounding area should be cleaned with an antiseptic and a "doughnut" pad placed around but not over the blister. An antibiotic or lubricant salve should be placed over the sore to prevent further rubbing and then covered with a sterile dressing. If the blister is open, the affected area should be cleaned as outlined above, loose tissue trimmed away with a sterile scissors, antibiotic ointment applied, and the sore covered with a sterile dressing. Second Skin, a sterile skinlike product made by the Spenco Medical Group (Waco, Texas), may be applied directly over the open area to serve as a cushion as well as sterile dressing. Dressing should be changed before and after each run.

Prevention is the key to blister control. Socks should be well fitting without wrinkles. New shoes should be gradually broken in rather than breaking down the feet. At the first sign of a blister, that is, a hot and sore spot on the foot, the source of friction should be removed by applying a skin lubricant or a doughnut pad to relieve pressure.

Excessive callous formation will also lead to blisters that are deep under the skin and slower to heal. This thickened skin should be kept down by filing the excessive buildup with a callous or nail file.

Ingrown Toenails. This condition is usually found on the great toe, with the nail growing into the adjacent soft tissue. Frequently, this irritation becomes infected and requires antibiotic therapy. Soaking the toe in warm water or a betadine solution may reduce the superficial infection. Trimming the nail straight across will often prevent the ingrown nail.[5]

Athlete's Foot. A fungus infection, particularly between the toes, can be quite painful. Topical treatments of fungicidal ointment readily available over the counter will generally control the infection. Adequate

drying of the toes and foot with the use of clean socks will help prevent reoccurrence.

Turf Toe. This condition usually affects soccer, football, or baseball players and is caused by the jamming or forced hyperextension of the hallux at the metatarsalphalangeal (MP) joint.[6] Acceleration off this injured toe can be disabling. Treatment consists of preventing hyperextension of the MP joint by applying a spica type wrap to the proximal first ray (Fig 24–1) and wearing a more rigid shoe. Modalities of choice can be used to control pain and swelling.

Runners Toes. Shoes with inadequate room in the toe box will cause bleeding in the nail bed, and the nails will appear black. This problem is generally more cosmetic than functional and can be alleviated by use of shoes that have sufficient space in the front. This condition is exacerbated with downhill running as the foot slides forward in the shoe. Toenails need to be trimmed short and straight across.

Sesamoiditis. Generally affecting the first ray, the sesamoids may become irritated by excessive pounding. Stress fractures may also occur at this site. Metatarsal bars or pads can be placed just posterior to the metatarsal head to relieve pressure. Orthotics with this area relieved will also protect the joint.

Midfoot

Arch Sprains. The foot has a complex of four arches that support the weight of the body and provide shock

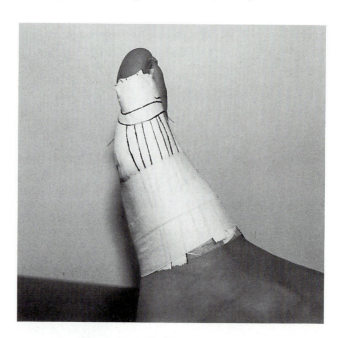

Figure 24–1. Turf Toe tape support.

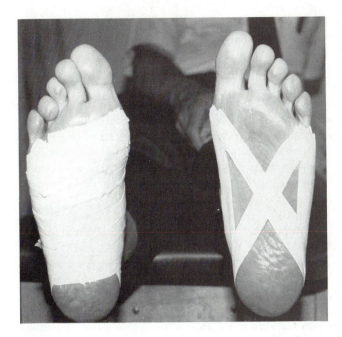

Figure 24-2. Taping for longitudinal and metatarsal arch support.

absorption. Any of these ligamentous structures—the transverse arch, metatarsal arch, or inner and outer longitudinal arch—may be weakened through overuse or overloading, which will result in pain.[7] A stretching of the transverse or metatarsal arch may lead to excessive callous buildup under the metatarsal heads, pain on the stance or push-off phase of running in this area, or compression of the interdigital nerves and pain as in Morton's neuroma. Weakening of the longitudinal

arches may place the foot at a biomechanical disadvantage to be an effective rigid lever in running. Excessive pronation will exacerbate tension on the longitudinal arch, which may lead to pain or plantar fasciitis (discussed below).

Excessive pronation can be found in several different foot structures. The overly mobile foot will excessively pronate in the stance phase due to lax ligamentous support. In the cavus or "high-arched" foot, the plantar flexors are often tight and inflexible, keeping the calcaneus elevated in the heel strike phase of gait. This in turn leads to compensatory pronation of the forefoot and additional stress placed on the longitudinal arch.

Treatment of an arch problem must be related to the cause of stress and not just focused on the painful area. Taping the arches or fabricating orthotic devices (Figs 24-2, 3) will support the foot in the neutral position[7] and reduce stress in the mobile foot. In the rigid or cavus foot, orthotic support should be more accommodative than rigid to absorb shock. Proper shoe selection will also help control the forces around the foot.

Plantar Fasciitis. Plantar fasciitis is a common overuse injury in runners. The plantar fascia at the insertion of the calcaneus becomes inflamed. In severe cases, a heel spur develops as a result of traction at this site. Treatment requires the athlete to reduce the stress in the fascia through rest, reducing speed and hill running, taping or orthotic control, and checking the running shoes for support. Stretching the gastrocnemius and soleus musculature will reduce the upward pull on the calcaneus. Physical therapy modalities and nonster-

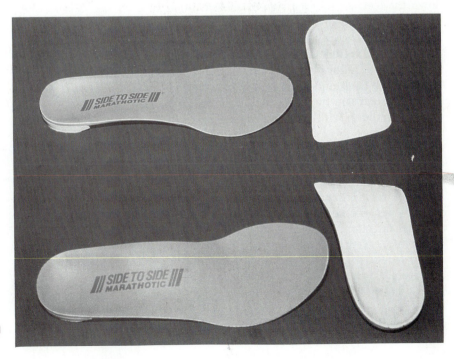

Figure 24-3. Orthotic device with full length top and two metatarsal heads.

oidal anti-inflammatory medications may be administered to reduce the initial pain and inflammation. Review of the training program is critical to find the cause of the overstress. This problem may be stubborn and in a small percent, require surgery to release the plantar fascia.

Heel Bruise. The heel is cushioned by a layer of fatty tissue. When force at the heel is too great, the protected layer is compressed and the inferior calcaneus may be bruised. Adding a heel cushion in the shoe that will not bottom out, made of either a closed cell or viscoelastic material, will prevent this type contusion. Worn-out shoes should also be replaced.

Rear Foot

Achilles Tendinitis/Tenosynovitis. Pain in the Achilles tendon affects both the untrained and the trained runner. In the former, the intensity of the running program may be at too advanced or strenuous a level. Often, a change in running surface or shoes will cause this problem in the experienced runner. Symptoms of either tendinitis or tenosynovitis will start with stiffness or pain after a workout. In acute tendonitis, there will be pain on plantar flexion, stretching of the tendon, and direct palpation. The tendon may be swollen. With tenosynovitis, the peritenon sheath will be inflamed and swollen, but stretching of the tendon does not usually cause pain. Fine crepitus or "creaking" will be palpated about the tendon. It is important to treat this condition early; otherwise a chronic problem will develop.

In acute cases, rest and stopping running until the symptoms disappear are necessary. A physician may prescribe anti-inflammatory medication. A ¼-in heel wedge will reduce tension across the tendon. At this time, stretching the Achilles tendon and soleus musculature is to be avoided, as it will increase the inflammatory process.[8] Once the symptoms are quiet, running at a less intense level than prior to the injury may be resumed. Stretching of the calf muscles as well as strengthening of the dorsi flexors with latex tubing will serve to prevent further injury. Eventually, the heel lift should be discontinued to allow for full flexibility in the Achilles tendon complex.

In chronic cases, progress to an asymptomatic state may take weeks or months. Pain and stiffness may decrease as the runner warms up, but these symptoms will return after running. Scarring in the tendon keeps the runner in the pain–inflammation–pain cycle. Cross-fiber friction massage as advocated by Cyriax[9] is often helpful at breaking down the scar tissue formed by the chronic inflammation. Orthotic control is also helpful to maintain the foot in a neutral position. Alternative forms of aerobic conditioning such as biking, swimming, or running in the pool will maintain performance while resting the injured part.

Retrocalcaneal Bursitis. Pressure over the posterior aspect of the calcaneus can lead to either inflammation of the superficial bursa between the skin and Achilles tendon (Pump bumps) or in the deep bursa between the Achilles tendon and calcaneus (Achilles bursitis). Excessive pressure from the shoe is generally the cause. In the superficial bursitis, there will be a swelling lateral to the Achilles tendon that can be quite tender. In the deep bursitis, the space between the tendon and calcaneus may feel boggy and be quite focally tender. Treatment includes padding the counter of the shoe to relieve pressure. The physician may inject the bursa with steroids in some cases. Activities that do not provide pain may be continued, but running may have to be stopped for a short period.

Calcaneal Apophysitis. In the runner whose growth areas are open, excessive traction can produce pain. Calcaneal apophysitis, like Osgood Schlatter's disease, is a self-limiting condition. Vague pain will be felt in the posterior calcaneus. X-rays will confirm the diagnosis. Inflexibility in the gastrocnemius and soleus increases the traction across the apophysis. Rest, heel lifts, ice, and gentle stretching usually resolve this problem.

Ankle Injuries

The most common injuries about the ankle include inversion sprains, syndesmosis injuries, subluxing peroneal tendons and tendinitis, and various fractures. These topics are covered in chapter 23.

Distal Leg

Shin Splints. Shin splints is an overused term to describe any pain between the knee and ankle. In the context of running, shin splints is one of a number of problems that are secondary to biomechanical imbalances or overuse conditions secondary to training errors.

Shin splints present as two different clinical pictures, either with pain along the posteromedial tibia or in the anterior compartment of the leg. The former is more frequent than the latter and is generally seen in runners that have excessive pronation. With this problem, there is increased tension at the attachment of the posterior tibialis into the tibia with the initial symptom of pain. If left untreated this often will progress to a stress fracture (discussed below). Treatment consists of two approaches—symptomatic and biomechanical. Ice and other physical therapy modalities can be used to control pain and swelling over the posteromedial tibia. Reduction of excessive pronation will eliminate the cause of the additional stress. This can be accomplished

by taping the arch as described earlier. Semirigid orthotics can be fitted to provide permanent control of excessive pronation. If there is tightness in the gastrocnemius and soleus, flexibility exercises must be initiated. Finally, the running program should be reviewed to assess whether proper progression in mileage, speed, and terrain is being maintained.

In the anterior compartment shin splint, the mechanism of injury is different. There is a relative imbalance between the plantar and dorsi flexors, with the former being much stronger. Treatment is aimed at strengthening the anterior tibialis, extensor digitorum, and extensor hallucis longus. A circumferential taping (Fig 24–4) will also support the inflamed area. Ice should be applied and hill running should be reduced temporarily.

Stress Fractures. A stress fracture can occur anywhere the bone is not sufficiently strong enough to withstand the forces around it. The most common sites are the metatarsal shafts, distal fibula, or proximal tibia.[10] Point tenderness will be present over the affected bone. Plain x-rays in the first month may not show the fracture. A bone scan can be used to make a definitive diagnosis. Healing fractures will show new periosteal bone formation.

Treatment consists of rest and a prohibition of running on land. Running in the pool is an acceptable alternative, as there is no overloading impact to the lower extremity. Running may be started when there is no pain or tenderness over the bone.

Compartment Syndromes. Caused from increased pressure within the fascial compartment, these syndromes must be differentiated from shin splints and stress fractures. Pain in any of the anterior, lateral, or posterior compartments of the leg usually starts during exercise. This discomfort may be relieved with rest, but often will be present for hours after running is finished. Weakness, tenderness, or a tight feeling of the dorsi flexors, and numbness in the anterior leg indicate involvement of the anterior compartment. The above symptoms in the peroneal musculature indicate a lateral compartment syndrome. Pain that is medial and deep to the tibia signals a problem with the posterior compartment.

The increased pressure leads to a local ischemia that produces the pain. Measuring the compartment pressures via a Wick catheter before and after exercise confirms the diagnosis.[11] Treatment to relieve excessive compartmental pressure consists of deep fascial massage, altering the running program to reduce its intensity, and ice to reduce inflammation. If conservative measures fail, then fasciotomies may be performed. After soft tissue healing, a progressive running program can be started.

Peroneal Tendonitis. Excessive pronation may cause peroneal tendonitis. Also, a chronically unstable ankle may have overly active evertors as a compensatory stabilizer. Symptoms include pain and focal tenderness about the lateral malleolus, pain with either resistance or stretching of the peroneals, and crepitus in the tendon sheaths. Treatment includes icing, anti-inflammatory medication, and a rehabilitation program to strengthen the lateral muscles. This can be accomplished with rubber tubing exercises, balance board activities (Figs 24–5 through 24–7) or moving the ankle

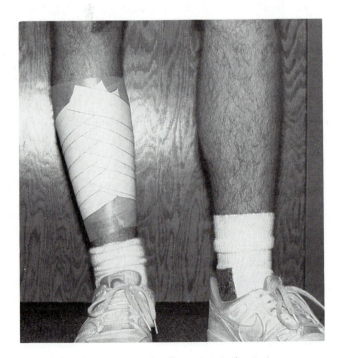

Figure 24–4. Shin splint taping for support of anterior musculature.

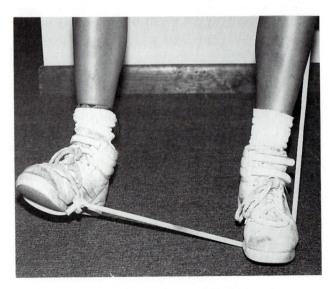

Figure 24–5. Rubber tubing exercises for eversion.

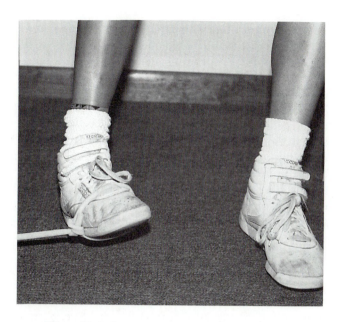

Figure 24-6. Rubber tubing exercises for inversion.

through motions in a container of rice. Orthotic control may also help reduce compensatory stresses.

Achilles Tendon Rupture. A common injury in runners over 30 years, the Achilles tendon rupture is a sig-

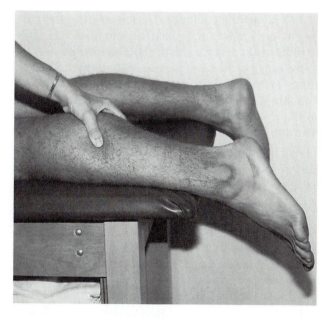

Figure 24-8. Negative Thompsen test for Achilles tendon rupture.

nificant injury. Pain in the tendon is severe, with the feeling of being struck sharply. In a complete rupture, the runner will be unable to push off on the affected foot or stand on the toes. In Thompsen's test, the examiner squeezes the calf and looks for a resultant plantar flexion of the foot (Figs 24–8, 24–9). When positive, there is no plantar flexion during the test.[12] Manual muscle testing will reveal absent or extremely weak plantar flexion. Swelling and tenderness in the area of the rupture are present.

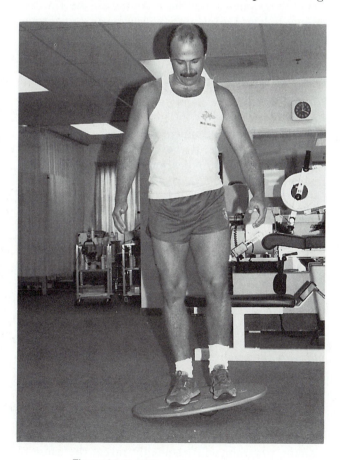

Figure 24-7. Balance board exercises.

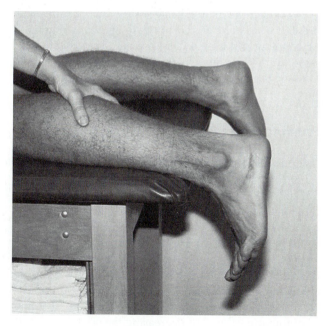

Figure 24-9. Positive Thompsen test for Achilles tendon rupture.

Orthopedic consultation is necessary, as either surgery or immobilization is the treatment of choice. After 10 to 12 weeks of casting in the equinus position, gentle active range of motion exercises may be started. Progressive return of dorsiflexion during the course of 6 to 8 months is expected. Maintaining aerobic conditioning on the stationary bike or in the pool is essential. Full return to running is not expected until 12 months.

Partial Tear of Achilles Tendon.
Less severe than a complete rupture, the recovery period for a partial tear of the Achilles tendon may be several months. Initially, the symptoms will be the same as above except that Thompsen's test will be negative. Immobilization may be used, again in the plantar flexed position to reduce the stretch on the tendon. In partial tears, there may be a residual weakness in the plantar flexors due to the lengthened tendon. Once adequate healing has taken place, vigorous strengthening of all the plantar flexors is essential to safely and effectively return to running. Heel lifts up to ⅜ in may be used to provide biomechanical support.

Partial Tear Medial Head of the Gastrocnemius/Plantaris Rupture.
Both of these injuries produce pain in the posterior calf but generally heal rapidly. The plantaris rupture will feel like the calf has been sharply hit, but active plantar flexion is present. Pain may be present anywhere along the length of the plantaris tendon. Initial treatment consists of compressive wrapping, icing, and modalities to reduce inflammation. Active range of motion and light resistive exercises may be instituted as soon as pain allows.

Tears of the medial head of the gastrocnemius will present with pain at the musculotendinous junction. Active plantar flexion will be present. Treatment is the same as for the plantaris rupture with the addition of massage over the injured site to prevent excessive scarring.

Proximal Leg

Osgood–Schlatter Disease.
This syndrome affects runners with open epiphyseal areas. Excessive hill running or sprinting may lead to inflammation in the tibial tubercle. This problem is self-limiting and will not occur after growth has stopped. Until then, however, running, sprinting, and squatting activities should be stopped until the area is painfree. Immobilization is indicated for only the most severe cases. Gentle quadriceps stretching will help reduce the traction at the tibial insertion. Compressive wraps may be of some symptomatic value, but decreasing the offending activity is most effective.

Patellar Tendinitis.
This is sometimes referred to as "Jumper's knee" and is frequently associated with downhill running, sprinting, or fartlek-type training. Tenderness is at the inferior pole of the patella or most commonly over the medial aspect of the tendon itself. Less occasionally pain is located at the distal insertion on the tibia. Generalized swelling does not exist, although there may be localized swelling. Pain in the tendon often remains after running has stopped. This condition is frequently related to microtrauma of the tendon fibers and can be resistant to treatment, especially if biomechanical abnormalties are ignored. For example, excessive pronation will increase the valgus stress on the patellar tendon and create excessive shear forces. Treatment is therefore directed to control the excessive pronation in the foot by taping the arch or using semirigid orthotics. Cortisone injections into the tendon is not indicated, as this may lead to tendon rupture.

Popliteus Tendinitis.
Popliteus tendinitis presents with vague pain in the posterolateral knee. This condition has been related to hyperpronation and downhill running because these produce traction of the popliteus tendon with the concomitant internal rotation of the tibia.[10] Careful palpation may reveal pain over the tendon of the popliteus, but this is not always present. Resistance to knee flexion with internal and external rotation may also reproduce the pain. Treatment includes changing the biomechanical problems causing excessive pronation and changing running surfaces.

Knee Pain

"Runner's Knee."
Runner's knee is a catchall phrase similar to shin splints. Rather than a specific diagnosis, it provides a general indication of the site of the pain. Knee injuries account for about 25% of injuries to runners.[13] The majority of all knee injuries from running are related to repetitive stress. They are not acute or traumatic. This section deals with the former group of problems. The reader must remember, however, to perform a complete knee evaluation if a traumatic injury has occurred. The important phase of treating runner's knee is to locate the irritated tissue and determine the cause. Usually it is biomechanical or training related.

During evaluation, the specific structure involved must be determined, that is, synovium, tendon, or bursa. A thorough biomechanical evaluation, starting with the feet and going to the hip, must be done. Relationships between pronation, tibial torsion, genu varum/valgum, and hip anteversion/retroversion must be delineated. Other important considerations include flexibility and muscle testing. Attention to the runner's training program will frequently reveal the cause of

pain. Most common is "too fast, too much, too soon." Look for any major training changes such as increase in hill running, new or old shoes, different running surface, too long a run for the established training base, or different running partner (changed pace).

Treatment of these areas is similar and based on the degree of discomfort. First, local symptoms are treated with ice, rest, and other modalities. Second, the cause, biomechanical or training, is determined. Flexibility and strengthening programs should be developed. (Quadriceps strength is very important, as running does not develop adequate strength in this muscle group.) Finally, running may begin, with a gradual increase in mileage, speed, and intensity.

Retropatellar Pain. Frequently misnamed as chondromalacia, retropatellar pain is generally diffuse around and behind the patella. It is increased on hills or stairs or with prolonged sitting with knees flexed to 90 degrees (theater sign). Symptoms are not necessarily consistent from day to day. The patellofemoral compression test can magnify these symptoms. Swelling may or may not be present.

Iliotibial Band Tendinitis. This condition presents itself with pain along the lateral side of the knee proximal to Gerdy's tubercle or over the prominence of the lateral femoral condyle. Applying compression to the iliotibial band while flexing and extending the knee will exacerbate the symptoms. Frequently there is localized effusion and occasionally crepitus over the femoral condyle. The runner with this problem will also have a positive Ober test a majority of the time. Biomechanical changes, including excessive downhill running or running on a highly canted surface, are also implicated.

Synovial Plica Syndrome. This syndrome most commonly involves the medial patellar plica, which becomes a thickened synovial fold irritating the patellar and femoral condyles. It runs along the superior and medial borders of the patella and is aggravated by repetitive extension and flexion. There is frequently tenderness on direct palpation of the plica.[14] Short of arthroscopy, however, it may be very difficult to diagnose. This condition frequently mimics a torn medial meniscus or chondromalacia in its symptoms.

Chondromalacia Patella. This is a specific condition in which the articular cartilage over the patella undergoes specific changes. Chondromalacia means "soft cartilage."[15] Its symptoms depend on how far the condition has progressed. As cartilage has no nerve supply, discomfort must come from the underlying bone.[16] This

is not a common problem in runners, but has long been misused for general knee pain.

Malalignment Syndrome. Also referred to as subluxating patellar syndrome or excessive lateral pressure syndrome, these all relate to the abnormal lateral tracking of the patella. Causes can be structural malalignment such as increased Q angle or quadriceps weakness, especially in the vastus medialis. Symptoms are similar in nature to retropatellar pain. In addition, there may be a positive apprehension test or focal tenderness on the lateral or medial facets of the patella or in the medial retinaculum. Generalized swelling is common during acute phases. Treatment programs must be specific to correct structural changes if possible through stretching, strengthening, and orthotics.[17] Patellar stabilizing braces are also useful in controlling symptoms.[18]

Pelvic and Hip Conditions

Leg Length Differences. Differences in the length of the legs can be from many causes. Correct treatment requires determining the source of the difference and taking the appropriate steps. Leg length differences can be divided into two categories: functional and anatomic. Hoppenfeld describes assessing the problem by measuring leg length from the umbilicus to medial malleolus for an apparent or functional difference and measuring from the anterior superior iliac spine (ASIS) to the malleolus for true anatomic differences.[19] Excessive pronation, which occurs with legs of equal length, will shorten the affected leg and may cause a pelvic obliquity. If this compensatory action occurs on an anatomic longer leg, however, then there will be "apparent" equal legs. It is important to assess leg length both in the standing and supine positions to include the changes that may take place in the foot and ankle.

Differences as small as $\frac{1}{4}$ in may cause problems in runners. Treatment is biomechanical, using either a heel lift or an orthotic appliance. Without correction, leg length differences can produce varied problems in various areas, ranging from the foot to the back.

Piriformis Syndrome. Spasm produced by the piriformis can cause sciatica like pain. The sciatic nerve passes through or under this muscle. Direct palpation will reveal tenderness and spasm. Treatment consists of ice, early use of ultrasound, deep massage to reduce spasm, and stretching.

Trochanteric Bursitis. Pain is directly over the greater trochanteric bursa. Tight tensor fascia lata, leg length differences, muscle weakness, or excessive running on canted roads will lead to this problem.

Treatment is aimed at isolating the cause and correcting the problem. Use modalities to reduce the local symptoms. Stretching of the ilio tibial band will reduce friction over the greater trochanter (Fig 24–10).

Ischial Bursitis. Pain is present over the ischial tuberosity and proximal hamstrings. Differential diagnosis must include avulsion fractures or traction apophysitis in the younger runner.

Symptoms are treated locally with modalities including ice and rest. A gentle stretching program for hamstrings and adductors may be started.

Pubic Symphysis Pain. This syndrome presents as lower abdominal pain or discomfort. The runner may be unable to run or walk without pain. Causes include adductor strains, stress fracture of the pubic ramus, or osteitis pubis.[10]

The treatment of choice must be rest until the symptoms subside. Attempts at vigorous stretching or strengthening only prolong the symptoms. Once the pain has subsided, a slow gradual return to activity is initiated. Gentle stretching and strengthening include the adductors, abductors, hamstrings, abdominal, and back muscles. This is typically a very frustrating problem to treat and may have lingering symptoms.

Iliac Crest Stress Fracture or Apophysitis. This problem usually develops during speed workouts, sprinting, long jumping, or high jumping. Pain is directly over the iliac crest. There is difficulty standing upright or walking. Pain is reproduced with contraction of the abdominals or hip flexors.

If a fracture is not complete, it is treated as a sprain. Modalities include icing and compression wraps to support the area. The athlete should avoid motions involving trunk extension with sprinting until asymptomatic.

Sacroiliac Joint Sprain. This injury presents as lower back pain, unilateral or bilateral. Pain may radiate into the buttocks or anteriorly into the groin. This sprain can mimic other back problems such as disc herniation. Differential diagnosis includes isolating the area of tenderness with palpation directly over the sacroiliac joint. Compression or distraction of the joint may increase the pain. Patrick's maneuver may be positive.

Treat with rest and local modalities. A compression belt may be helpful.[20] Gradual return to activities usually occurs after 5 to 6 weeks if the sprain is acute. The more typical presentation is a chronic sprain from overuse in hypermobile individuals.

Lower Back

Lower Back Pain. A condition that is present in many runners, the etiology of lower back pain is varied, ranging from muscle strains, disc or facet dysfunction, ligament sprains, to mechanical imbalances. A specific evaluation is necessary to determine the cause and is covered in chapter 18. A biomechanical approach would include the entire lower extremity, focusing on the closed kinetic links among the foot, ankle, and leg. Treatment is based on the specific findings. If the disc is suspected, further evaluation is required.

Spondylolisthesis. An anterior slippage of one vertebra on a distal vertebra, this condition most commonly occurs at the L-5 level. Clinically, the therapist will palpate a "shelf" at this L-5 spinous process. X-rays will confirm the diagnosis. Symptoms will present as persistent localized back pain and possible nerve root irritation.

Treatment is directed at reducing the shear forces across the lesion with a series of flexion exercises including hamstring stretching. The runner needs to avoid ex-

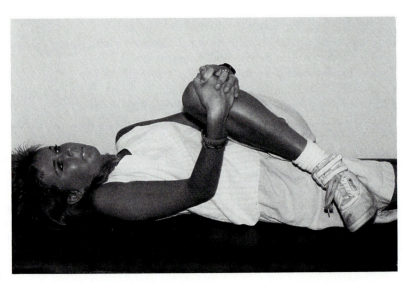

Figure 24–10. Iliotibial band stretch.

tension and hyperextension motions. Lumbar and hip flexion motions can be used for symptomatic relief.

CONCLUSION

When dealing with runners and their injuries, there is very often a fine line between overuse and abuse. Runners typically will seek help only when the pain from running becomes unbearable. Thus, even though the symptoms are acute, the problem is probably chronic. This is why two separate evaluations must take place: the physical examination to determine the structure(s) involved and an analysis of the runner's training regimen.

It is usually possible to discover when the problem started as well as why. Remember the axiom "too far, too fast, too soon, too often." Look for a major change in the surface, shoes, topography, or running partner. These clues are essential because the runner must be convinced that changes are mandatory if he or she wants to keep running. Through education and understanding the cause of the problem, the runner will be able to make his or her own modifications in the future, thereby preventing many potential problems. After all, is not "prevention" of future problems the reason most people run as part of their overall health and fitness program?

REFERENCES

1. Cook SD, Kester MA, Brunet ME. Shock absorption characteristics of running shoes. *Am J Sports Med.* 1985; 13:248–253.
2. 1989 spring shoe survey. *Runner's World.* 1989; 24(4):45–74.
3. McPoil TG. Footwear. *Phys Ther.* 1988; 68:1857–1865.
4. Rossi WA, Tennent R. *Professional Shoe Fitting.* New York, NY: National Shoe Retailers Association; 1984.
5. *Basic Athletic Training.* Garder, Kan: Cramer Products Inc; 1987.
6. Sammarco GJ. How I manage turf toe. *Physician Sportsmed.* 1988; 16:113–118.
7. Root ML, Orien WP, Weed JH. *Normal and Abnormal Function of the Foot.* Los Angeles, CA: Clinical Biomechanics Corp; 1977.
8. Curwin S, Stanish WD. *Tendinitis: Its Etiology and Treatment.* Lexington, Mass: Collamore Press; 1984.
9. Cyriax J. *Textbook of Orthopaedic Medicine: Diagnosis of Soft Tissue Lesions.* 7th ed. London, England: Bailliere Tindall; 1975.
10. Brody DM. *Running Injuries. Clinical Symposia 32, number 4.* Summitt, NJ: Ciba Pharmaceutical Co; 1980.
11. Whitesides TE, Haney TC, Morimoto K, Harada H. Tissue pressure measurements as a determinant for the need of fasciotomy. *Clin Orthop Relat Res.* 1975; 113:43–51.
12. Petertson L, Renstrom P. *Sports Injuries Their Prevention and Treatment*, Chicago, Ill: Year Book Medical Publishers; 1986.
13. Roy S, Irvin R. *Sports Medicine Prevention, Evaluation, Management and Rehabilitation.* Englewood, NJ: Prentice–Hall Inc; 1983.
14. Davies GJ, Malone T, Bassett FH. Knee examination. *Phys Ther.* 1980; 60:1565–1574.
15. Cox J. Problems in runners. *Clin Sports Med.* 1985; 4:700.
16. Pickett JC, Radin EL. *Chondromalacia of the Patella.* Baltimore, Md: Williams and Wilkins Co; 1983.
17. McConnell J. The management of chondromalacia patellae: a long term solution. *Aust J Physiother.* 1986; 32:215–223.
18. Palumbo PM. Dynamic patellar brace: A new orthosis in the management of patellofemoral disorders: A preliminary report. *J Sports Med.* 1981; 9(1):45–49.
19. Hoppenfeld S. *Physical Examination of the Spine and Extremities.* New York, NY: Appleton–Century–Crofts; 1976.
20. O'Donohue D. *Treatment of Injuries to Athletes.* Philadelphia, Pa: W. B. Saunders; 1976.

25

Swimming Injuries

Jeffrey E. Falkel

INTRODUCTION

Swimming is one of the most popular recreational and athletic activities in the world today. It is an excellent form of aerobic activity, a rehabilitative medium, an avenue for competitive endeavors, and an individual activity that can be accomplished almost anywhere there is water available. The water offers buoyancy and anti-gravity effects as well as added resistance during exercise. Due to the nature of the repetitive activities of the arms and legs while swimming, however, this activity is also prone to overuse injuries, primarily of the shoulder and knees. It was once felt that the "swimmer's shoulder" was a consequence of any prolonged swim training, and that injuries to the shoulder region were an unavoidable consequence. This is not the case, as has been documented in the recent literature. This chapter details the mechanisms of the overuse injuries to the shoulder and knee that are seen in swimmers. It also provides effective evaluation protocols to identify swimmers who are at risk for developing overuse injuries from prolonged swimming. Also presented are rehabilitative and preventative exercises that can be used in the treatment of athletes who have swimming shoulder problems and hopefully to prevent further complications associated with swimming. This chapter deals primarily with the freestyle stroke with regard to shoulder injuries and the breaststroke whip kick in reference to the overuse injuries of the knee. Although injuries do occur during the performance of the other major strokes, the vast majority of most swim training, even for the specialty swimmers, is done using the freestyle stroke.

One of the major causes for the overuse injuries seen in swimming is faulty stroke mechanics. If these stroke faults are corrected, a vast majority of the overuse injuries to the shoulder and knee could be prevented. Figures 25–1 through 25–4 show the proper stroke mechanics involved with each of the four competitive swimming strokes.[1] These figures are intended to show the proper sequence of arm and leg positions throughout each cycle of the swimming stroke. For a more detailed description of the proper stroke mechanics, Counsilman[1] and Maglischo[2] provide excellent reference material. Because the vast majority of shoulder injuries occur during the prolonged swimming of the freestyle stroke,[3–5] the shoulder mechanics of this stroke are detailed in this chapter. It is important to understand the complex biomechanical relationships involved in the movement of the shoulder, trunk position, and head position during breathing, and hand placement to enable the sports physical therapist to assist the swim coach and swimmer in correcting and preventing overuse problems in the shoulder.

DESCRIPTION OF NORMAL SWIMMING MECHANICS IN THE FREESTYLE STROKE

The propulsive power in the freestyle (and other strokes, except breaststroke) comes from the extension, adduction, and internal rotation of the shoulder during the power phase of the pull in the water[1,2,6,7] (Fig 25–5). The contributions of the hand, wrist, and elbow are all significant to the overall stroke propulsion. The greatest stresses, however, occur at the shoulder, and, thus, this is the site of most of the pathology in swimming injuries.[4]

The power of the stroke is provided by the shoulder muscles involved in adduction, external, and internal rotation. Fine-wire electromyography, however, has shown that approximately 35% of the entire stroke cycle of the freestyle is composed of recovery mechanics.[8] To date, little if any attention or specific exercise training has been directed at the recovery phase of the stroke. Research from our laboratory has shown that much shoulder pathology might be prevented when specific exercise regimes and coaching mechanics are directed at the recovery phase of the freestyle stroke.[9]

Table 25–1 provides a summary of the biomechan-

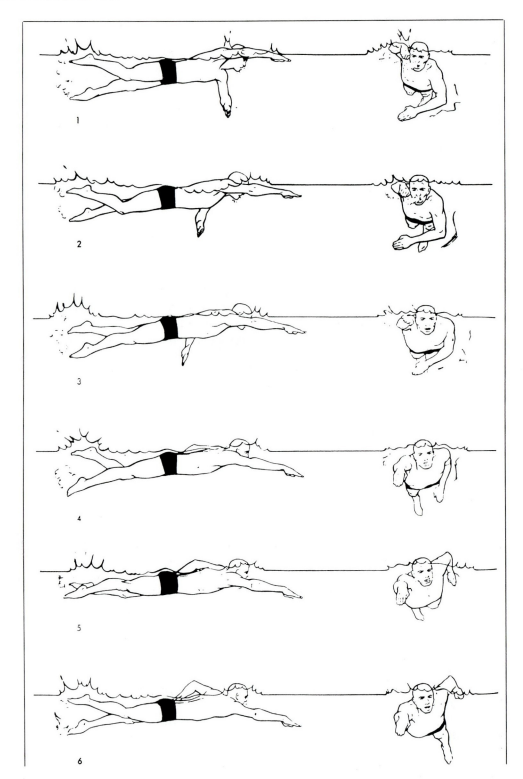

Figure 25-1. Sequencing of pull and kick during the freestyle. *(From Counsilman JE.* The Science of Swimming. *Englewood Cliffs, NJ: Prentice-Hall; 1968, with permission.)*

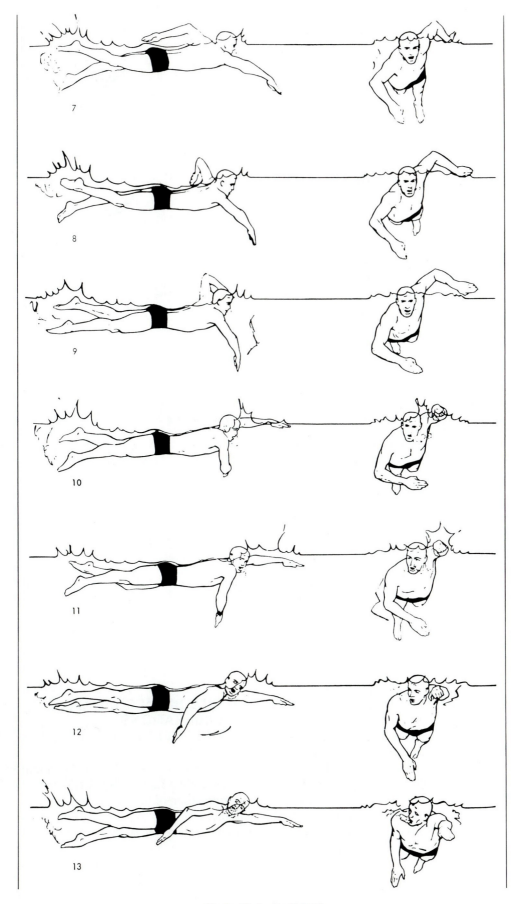

Figure 25–1. Continued

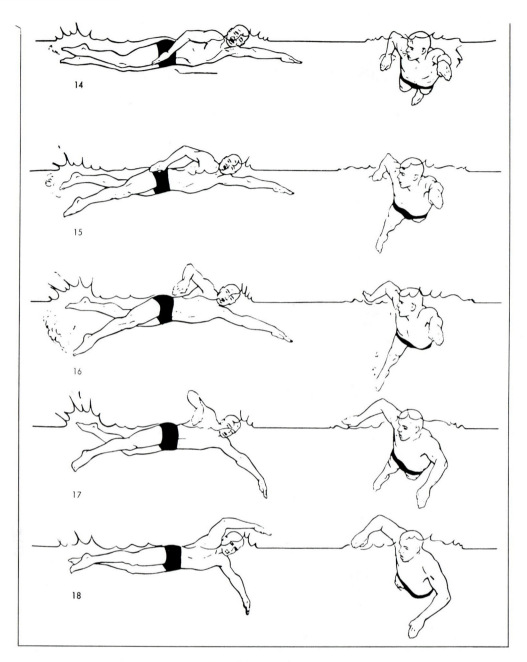

Figure 25–1. Continued

ical description of each phase of the freestyle stroke. The pull-through phase of the stroke begins with hand entry, which is also called the catch, and continues through mid pull-through. The final aspect of the pull ends with the shoulder fully internally rotated, adducted, and extended as the elbow reaches terminal extension.[1,2,6,7] The recovery phase begins with the lifting of the elbow as the hand exits the water. The shoulder begins external rotation at this point and becomes fully externally rotated just beyond the horizontal position in mid recovery. This phase is then terminated at hand entry with the shoulder in a fully externally rotated and maximally abducted position.[1,2,6,7]

SPECIAL BIOMECHANICAL CONSIDERATIONS OF THE FREESTYLE STROKE

The freestyle stroke is composed of a number of unique biomechanical movements that determine the successful completion of the swimming motion. The difficulty in observation of the entire stroke mechanics of pull-through and recovery by both the coach and the athlete, however, present a significant problem to the successful and correct completion to the stroke. The swimmer cannot truly see any component of the stroke, and must rely on his or her own proprioceptive and kin-

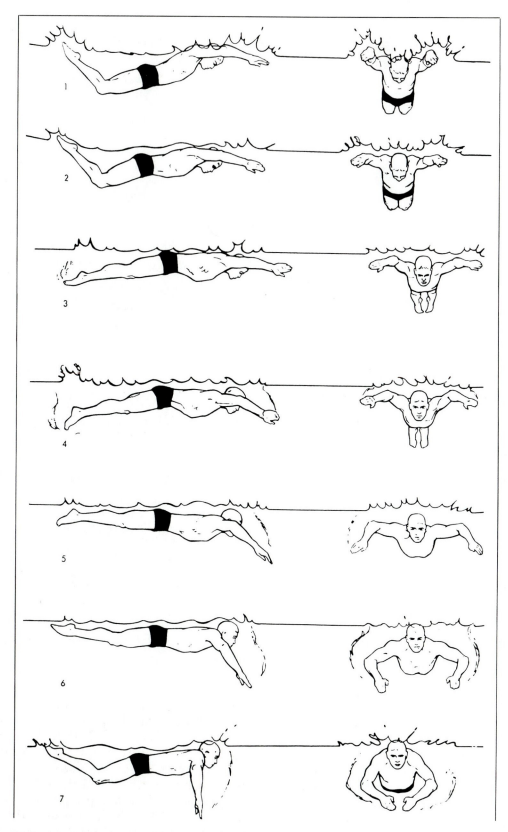

Figure 25-2. Sequencing of the pull and kick during the butterfly. *(From Counsilman JE.* The Science of Swimming. *Englewood Cliffs, NJ: Prentice-Hall; 1968, with permission.)*

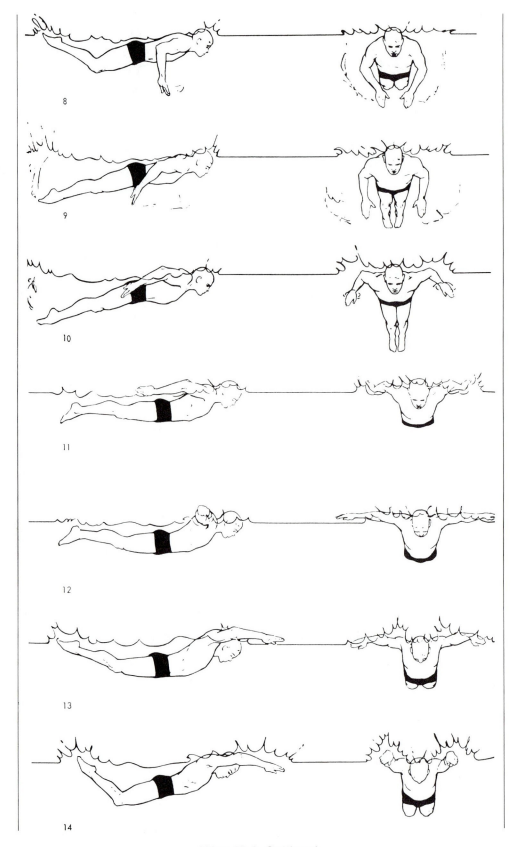

Figure 25-2. Continued

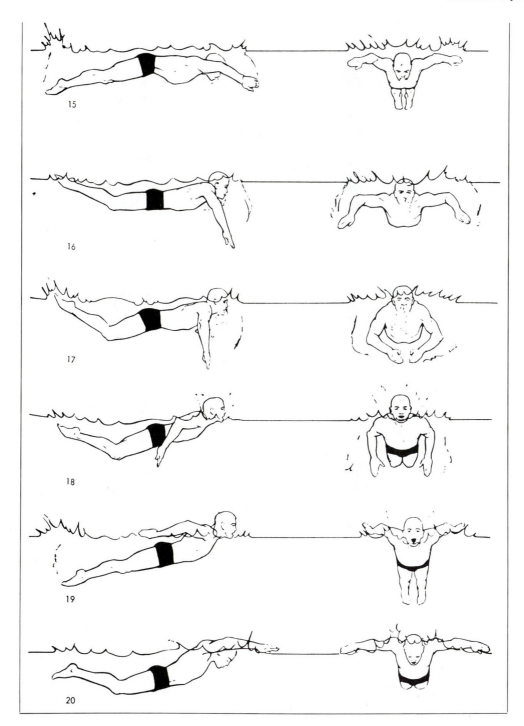

Figure 25–2. Continued

esthetic awareness to perform the stroke "correctly." The coach, on the other hand, can only view the recovery without observation from an underwater viewing area. These difficulties are coupled with the number of repetitions performed in a single practice. Therefore, the sports medicine professional who works with swimming athletes must also have a thorough understanding of the normal mechanics to assist coaches and athletes with the problems of swimmer's shoulder.

There are important rotational mechanics involved in the stroke recovery. The rotational position of the humerus with respect to the proximity of the greater tuberosity of the humerus and the coracoacromial arch is of critical importance in understanding the mechanism of impingement of the shoulder during swimming. If the glenohumeral joint is internally rotated, the greater tuberosity is in a closer approximation to the suprahumeral structures. This becomes a

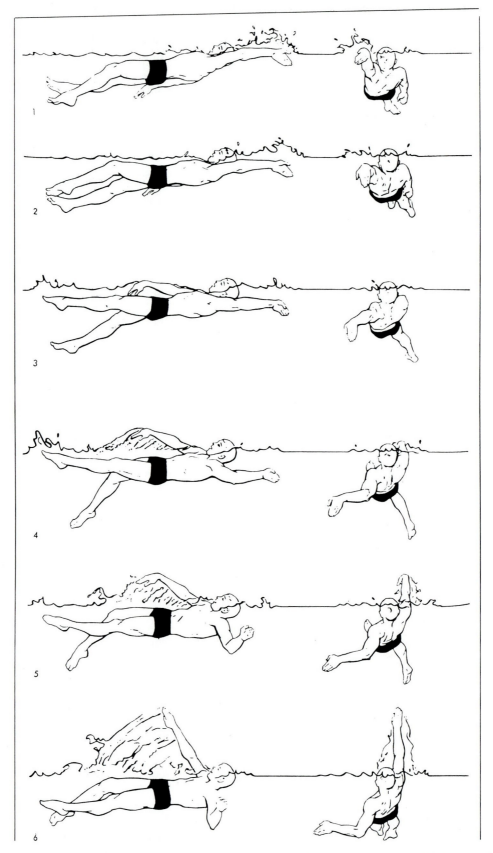

Figure 25-3. Sequencing of the pull and kick during the backstroke. *(From Counsilman JE.* The Science of Swimming. *Englewood Cliffs, NJ: Prentice-Hall; 1968, with permission.)*

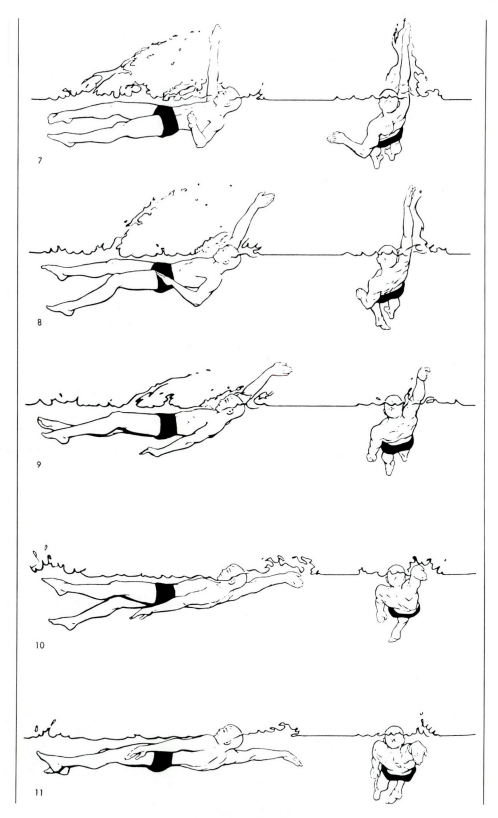

Figure 25-3. Continued

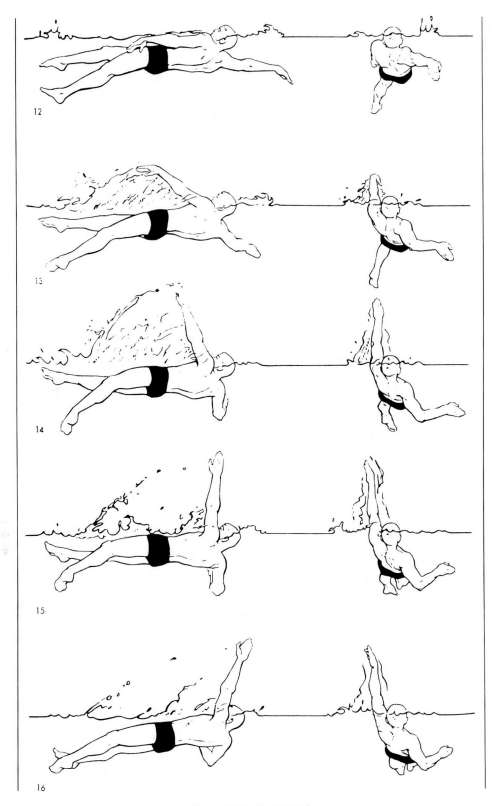

Figure 25-3. Continued

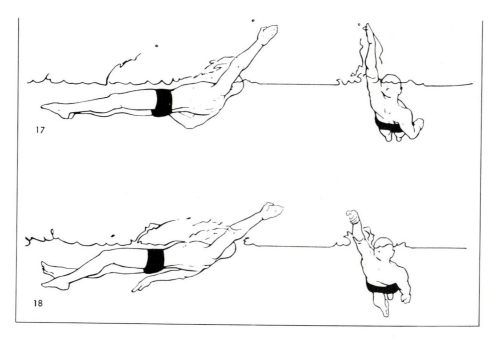

Figure 25-3. Continued

problem during abduction in the recovery phase and may lead to mechanical impingement.[10,11] Cailliet[12] has described the depression of the humeral head by the rotator cuff mechanism. This depression will act to reduce the degree of impingement by the greater tuberosity of the humerus as the overhead motion of the stroke recovery occurs. The head of the humerus may also be stabilized by a strong contraction of the biceps long head[13] The contributions of the biceps long head in this stabilization role have been alluded to with EMG studies,[8,14] although the evidence is far from conclusive at this time.

The proper placement of the hand and position of the hand allows for the correct setting of the hand at the catch. This proper catch position helps to set up the optimal elbow and shoulder position to begin the pull-through phase. If the stroke mechanics in the recovery phase are faulty, the position of the hand at the catch may be unfavorable, and will result in a reduced efficiency of the pull.[1,2,6,7] Crossover placement of the hand (moving the hand across the midline) will also place the shoulder in an improper position to begin the pull-through. Crossover results in placing the shoulder in a position of flexion, internal rotation, and horizontal adduction (Fig 25-6). This positioning of the arm in the pull-through phase creates both a mechanical impingement of the biceps long head tendon, as well as a vascular impingement of the arterial supply to the supraspinatus and biceps tendons.[15] It has been reported that the greatest discomfort in the shoulder by most swimmers occurs when the arm is in a position of midline crossing in the early pull-through phase.[5,13]

TABLE 25-1. BIOMECHANICAL DESCRIPTION OF STROKE PHASES OF FREESTYLE

Stroke Phases	Description
Pull-through	
Hand entry	Shoulder external rotation and abduction; body roll begins.
Mid pull-through	Shoulder at 90-degree abduction and neutral rotation; body roll is at maximum of 40–60 degrees horizontal
End of pull-through	Shoulder internally rotated and fully abducted; body returned to horizontal position
Recovery phase	
Elbow lift	Shoulder begins abduction and external rotation; body roll begins in opposite direction from pull through
Mid recovery	Shoulder abducted to 90 degrees and externally rotated beyond neutral; body roll reaches maximum of 40–60 degrees; breathing occurs by turning head to side
Hand entry	Shoulder externally rotated and maximally abducted; body roll has returned to neutral

Adapted from Richardson AB, Jobe JW, Collins HR. The shoulder in competitive swimming. Am J Sports Med. *1980; 8:159–163, with permission.*

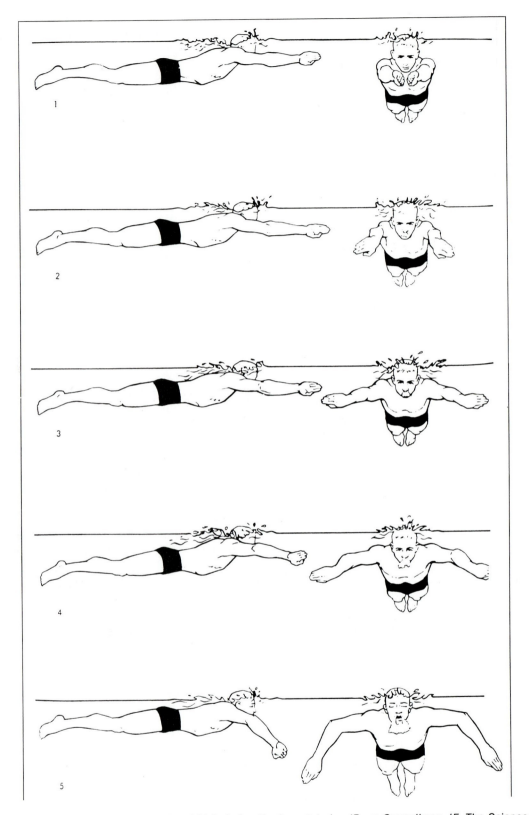

Figure 25–4. Sequencing of the pull and kick during the breaststroke. *(From Counsilman JE.* The Science of Swimming. *Englewood Cliffs, NJ: Prentice-Hall; 1968, with permission.)*

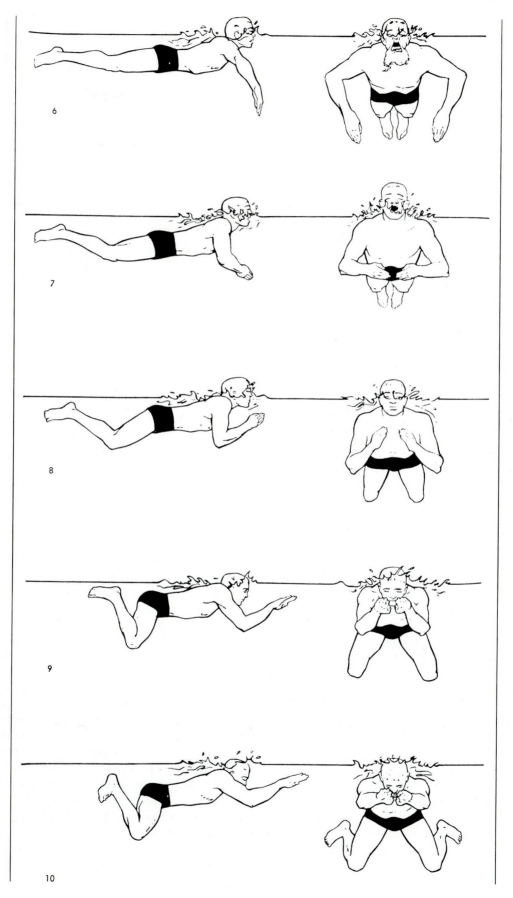

Figure 25-4. Continued

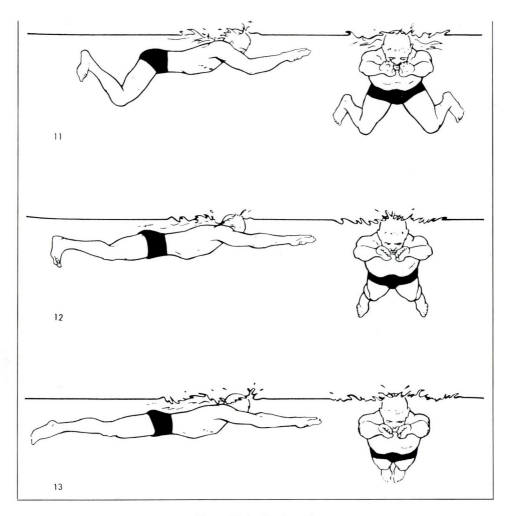

Figure 25-4. Continued

There is an extremely important consideration for body roll and rotation in the stroke mechanics of the freestyle stroke. A body roll of 40 to 60 degrees during the recovery phase will minimize the amount of horizontal abduction that is required for the initiation of the arm movement in the recovery phase.[1,2] This amount of body roll will also permit the overhead movement of the arm to occur with sufficient external rotation to avoid the potential mechanical and vascular impingement of the shoulder.[16] The degree of body roll is critical, for excessive or insufficient body roll will result in stroke deficits. An excessive body roll leads to either a crossover entry into the water at the catch, or a crossover during the propulsion phase of the pull-through. A lack of body roll during the recovery phase of the stroke will result in a restriction of full external rotation, which will not only cause an abnormal hand placement at the catch but will also increase the amount of mechanical impingement of the long head of the biceps and mechanical stresses of the shoulder joint.[16]

The final biomechanical considerations involved in the freestyle stroke mechanics are the position of the head and the breathing patterns used while swimming freestyle. If the head is in an exaggerated head-down position, the arm will have to pull deeper and the body position will be malaligned during both the pull-through and recovery phases.[1,2,6,7] An exaggerated position with the head held too high will yield a concomitant lowering of the hips and thus increase drag and water resistance.[1,2,6,7] The head should be held in a neutral position, in line with the rest of the spine, and breathing to either one side or the other should take place in a rotational plane around this neutral position of the head. There has been no consistent correlation between the side of breathing and the degree or occurrence of shoulder pain.[5,13,17] One possible explanation of the relationship among body roll, head position and shoulder pain is as follows: an excessive body roll away from the breathing side may be coupled with an incomplete body roll away from the nonbreathing side. This scenario may result in an increased mechanical impingement on the nonbreathing side.

With a thorough understanding of both the com-

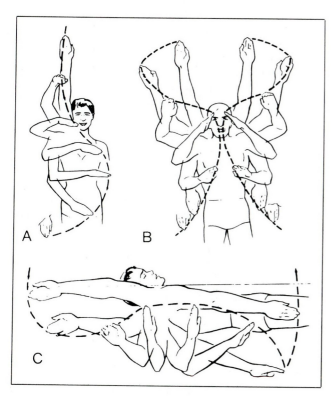

Figure 25-5. Phases of pull for the freestyle **(A)**, butterfly **(B)**, and backstroke **(C)**. *(From Counsilman JE.* Competitive Swimming Manual. *Bloomington, Ind: Counsilman Inc; 1977, with permission.)*

MECHANISM OF SHOULDER OVERUSE INJURIES IN SWIMMING

It has been estimated that more than 60% of all competitive swimmers at the high school and collegiate level have experienced shoulder pain in the anterior or lateral aspects of the shoulder, due in part to overuse or improper biomechanics of the swimming stroke, primarily freestyle.[3–5] The majority of competitive swimmers routinely train an average of 7000 yd per workout, 10 to 13 workouts per week and 40 to 45 weeks per year.[4,5,17] An additional stress to the swimmer's shoulder has been the advent of swim paddle training, which serves to increase the power of the stroke. Figure 25–7 shows the design of the hand paddle. Although many swimmers have increased their power and speed by using hand paddles during various components of the training season, the paddles may also place an increased force on the shoulder and cause the swimmer to employ faulty stroke mechanics. This may further generate abnormal biomechanical stress.[18] When faulty stroke mechanics are combined with excessive use and long training sessions, as well as abnormal stresses from hand paddles and other training devices, the result many times is an overuse syndrome commonly referred to as "swimmer's shoulder." The primary diagnosis of swimmer's shoulder is a suprahumeral impingement of the supraspinatus near its insertion onto the greater tuberosity of the humerus.[4,5] The tendon of the long head of the biceps may also be an associated or isolated impinged structure. Other structures, such as damage to the glenoid labrum,[5] may result in shoulder pain as the result of swimming. This topic is addressed after the discussion of suprahumeral impingement in swimmers, and its management.

ponents and biomechanics of the freestyle, the sports medicine professional should be able to analyze and recognize potential problems. If there is early intervention by the sports medicine professional with the swimming coach, many of these problems are preventable.

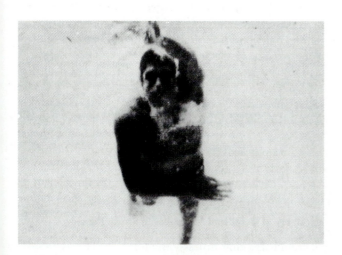

Figure 25-6. Example of hand crossing midline as result of faulty stroke mechanics. *(From Counsilman JE.* Competitive Swimming Manual. *Bloomington, Ind: Counsilman Inc; 1977, with permission.)*

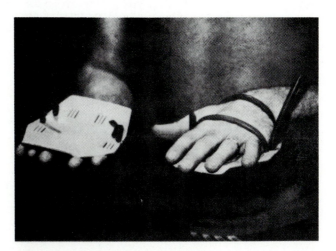

Figure 25-7. Hand paddles are frequently used to increase resistance during the pull in freestyle. Use of hand paddles may result in improper stroke mechanics. *(From Falkel JE, Murphy TC.* Shoulder Injuries. *Baltimore, Md: Williams & Wilkins Co; 1988, with permission.)*

The primary mechanism of impingement in the suprahumeral space is by the approximation of the greater tuberosity of the humerus to the coracoacromial arch during the recovery, and, to a lesser extent, during the early pull-through.[13] If there is a sufficient degree of external rotation during the recovery, there will be a minimal amount of impingement, and the shoulder will be in the optimal position at hand entry, which will be less likely to develop an impingement in the early phase of pull-through.

One mechanism that might account for the two potential stroke faults that lead to impingement may be fatigue of the external rotators.[9,13,19,20] In the first situation, there is a slight decrease in the degree of external rotation as the shoulder completes the recovery phase. As the recovery phase proceeds, the shoulder is effectively in an internally rotated position, and this would result in excessive impingement forces. This position of internal rotation at the end of the recovery will not allow for the proper hand position at the catch. The resultant stroke fault yields the elbow in a dropped position, and even further stresses and increases the impingement. Figure 25–8 shows the dropped elbow position that results from a recovery that has an insufficient amount of external rotation. The second situation involves the achievement of full external rotation only at the latter stages of the recovery. The optimal degree of external rotation should occur by the mid point of the recovery. When there is late external rotation, there is an increased impingement stress on the shoulder. During long workouts, as the external rotators fatigue, the efficiency of the stroke becomes reduced, resulting in a recovery that has a greater degree of internal rotation. This results in the further breakdown of the stroke biomechanics. In these swimmers, who already have faulty stroke mechanics, the only way to compensate for the inefficiency of their stroke is to take additional strokes to cover the distance of the workout. These additional strokes are also done improperly, and thus the vicious cycle of overuse impingement continues.

Rathbun and Macnab[15] have provided the classic research that describes the mechanism of the avascular impingement of the shoulder in the swimmer with faulty stroke mechanics. Their data suggest that when the shoulder is abducted, there is a complete filling of the microvasculature in the blood vessels that supply the supraspinatus tendon. When the shoulder is adducted, however, and the arm is at the side, there is an area approximately 1 cm proximal to the insertion of the supraspinatus tendon that becomes poorly supplied with blood. This is due to the "wringing out" of the tendon as it passes over the head of the humerus.[15] There is a similar response seen if the arm is flexed and horizontally adducted, a position that occurs during the pull-through phase of the stroke. Figure 25–9 shows the blood flow through microvasculature in the abducted position, and the avascular "wringing out" response seen when the arm is adducted.[15] In the swimmer whose faulty stroke mechanics results in a midline crossover pattern, there will be additional vascular impingement, particularly as a long workout progresses. The faulty mechanics of a dropped elbow at the catch will result in a similar vascular impingement of the supraspinatus tendon. Not only does the supraspinatus tendon show this avascular impingement, but there is a similar response and avascular zone in the tendon of the long head of the biceps as it passes over the humerus. In summary, the "swimmer's shoulder" impingement is the result of both a mechanical impingement of the supraspinatus tendon by the greater tuberosity of the humerus against the coracoacromial arch and the avascular impingement of blood flow to the supraspinatus and biceps long head tendons due to the improper position of the shoulder during the pull-through phase of the stroke.

MANAGEMENT OF SWIMMING SHOULDER PAIN—IN-SEASON

The sports physical therapist frequently faces the difficult situation of treating an overuse injury during the course of the competitive season. This becomes even a larger problem when neither the coach nor the athlete is willing to stop swimming practices all together. The conflict for the sports physical therapist lies in his or her knowledge that unless some form of intervention is introduced, the overuse injury will only become worse. If the injury is left untreated, it will more than likely reduce the potential of the swimmer in that particular season and may even permanently impair his or her

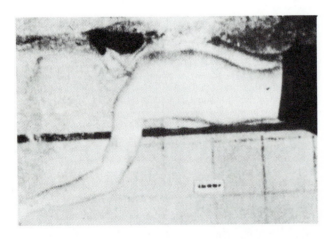

Figure 25-8. Dropped elbow during pull phase of freestyle. This position exaggerates the degree of mechanical and avascular impingement on the shoulder. *(From Counsilman JE. Competitive Swimming Manual. Bloomington, Ind: Counsilman Inc; 1977, with permission.)*

The first component of the in-season management of swimmers consisted of 3 weeks of reduced swim training (i.e., 3000 as opposed to 6000 to 8000 yd/day). Before each of the reduced training workouts, the swimmer received 20 minutes of moist heat hydrocollator treatments. The shoulder was positioned in approximately 30 degrees of abduction in an attempt to achieve maximal blood flow to the supraspinatus tendon, as suggested by Rathbun and Macnab.[15] Ultrasound phonophoresis treatments with 10% hydrocortisone cream were given using continuous ultrasound at 0.7 W/cm^2 for 5 to 7 minutes over the suprahumeral space with the shoulder placed in internal rotation and adduction (with the dorsum of the hand against the lumbar spine). This position improves the exposure of the distal portion of the supraspinatus tendon.[13,21] The third component of the in-season management consisted of two forms of exercise to improve the strength and endurance of the external rotators of the shoulder. Subjects sat on the Cybex U.B.X.T. (Cybex, Ronkonkoma, NY) and were positioned such that the shoulder was in approximately 30 degrees of abduction to minimize impingement stress on the supraspinatus tendon. The subjects exercised the external and internal rotators using two to five sets of 20 to 50 repetitions at a velocity of 240 degrees per second on the Cybex II Isokinetic Dynamometer, using the testing position seen in Figure 25–10.[13,21] The number of sets and repetitions progressed each week based on their individual tolerance to the exercise stress. The other type of exercise consisted of Lifeline Pull Cord exercises. Figure 25–11 shows the six external rotation exercises that were performed using three sets of 30 to 40 seconds of effort in each exercise position. All of the above procedures and exercises were performed daily prior to the actual reduced swimming training session.

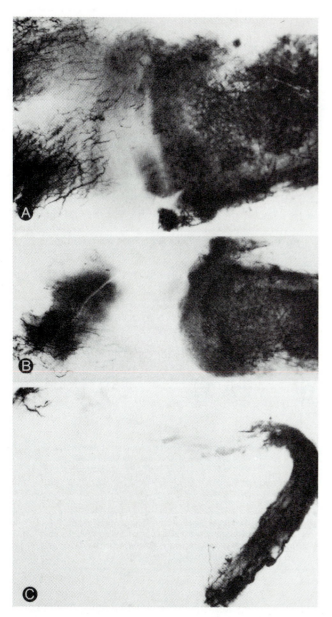

Figure 25–9. Injection study demonstrating rotator cuff vascularity: supraspinatus tendon in shoulder abduction **(A)** and supraspinatus tendon in adduction **(B).** Note the incomplete filling. Similar pattern is demonstrated by the biceps long head as it passes over the humerus **(C).** *(From Rathbun JB, Macnab I. The microvascular pattern of the rotator cuff.* J Bone Joint Surg. *1970; 52B:540–553, with permission.)*

ability to swim painfree ever again. It has been the experience of this sports medicine professional that both coaches and athletes alike are more receptive to a program that consists of reduced training, therapeutic modality intervention, and sport- and injury-specific exercises designed to improve the faulty stroke mechanics.[21] The following program for in-season management of the swimmer with shoulder pain has proven very successful and it is recommended as a possible therapeutic regime.[21]

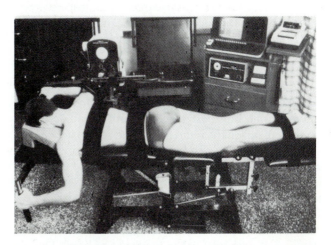

Figure 25–10. Prone positioning for testing and training the internal and external rotators of the shoulder in swimmers. *(From Falkel JE, Murphy TC. Shoulder Injuries. Baltimore, Md: Williams & Wilkins Co; 1988, with permission.)*

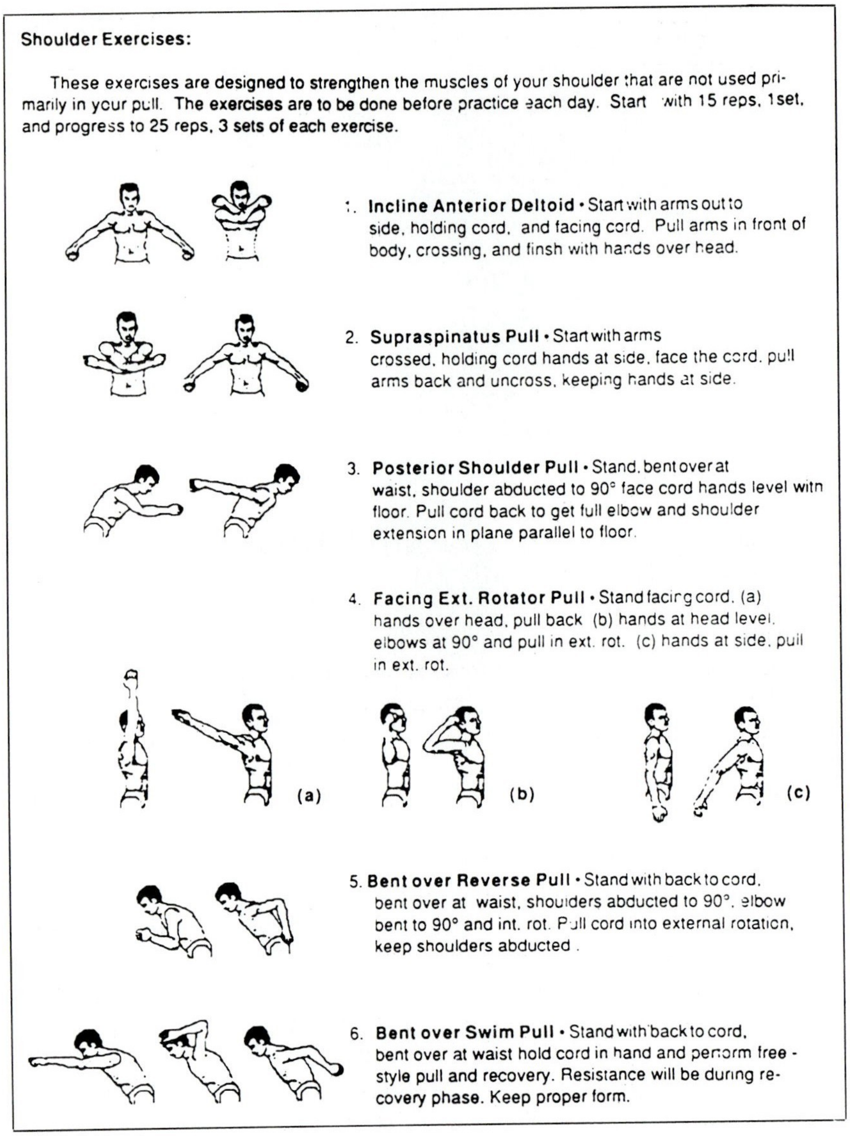

Shoulder Exercises:

These exercises are designed to strengthen the muscles of your shoulder that are not used primarily in your pull. The exercises are to be done before practice each day. Start with 15 reps, 1 set, and progress to 25 reps, 3 sets of each exercise.

1. **Incline Anterior Deltoid** • Start with arms out to side, holding cord, and facing cord. Pull arms in front of body, crossing, and finish with hands over head.

2. **Supraspinatus Pull** • Start with arms crossed, holding cord hands at side, face the cord, pull arms back and uncross, keeping hands at side.

3. **Posterior Shoulder Pull** • Stand, bent over at waist, shoulder abducted to 90° face cord hands level with floor. Pull cord back to get full elbow and shoulder extension in plane parallel to floor.

4. **Facing Ext. Rotator Pull** • Stand facing cord. (a) hands over head, pull back (b) hands at head level, elbows at 90° and pull in ext. rot. (c) hands at side, pull in ext. rot.

(a)   (b)   (c)

5. **Bent over Reverse Pull** • Stand with back to cord, bent over at waist, shoulders abducted to 90°, elbow bent to 90° and int. rot. Pull cord into external rotation, keep shoulders abducted.

6. **Bent over Swim Pull** • Stand with back to cord, bent over at waist hold cord in hand and perform freestyle pull and recovery. Resistance will be during recovery phase. Keep proper form.

Figure 25-11. Exercises designed to enhance external rotation endurance and strength. *(From Falkel JE, Murphy TC. Shoulder Injuries. Baltimore, Md: Williams & Wilkins Co; 1988, with permission.)*

After the swim training workout, subjects received ice massage to the suprahumeral region for 15 minutes after practice. In addition, cross-friction massage was performed over the supraspinatus tendon in the same position used for the phonophoresis.[22]

The results of this investigation have shown that this particular regime of reduced training, modality intervention, and sport-specific exercises had dramatic improvements in the reduction of shoulder pain and the return to relatively painfree swimming. There was also a significant improvement in the endurance of the external rotators. Table 25–2 shows the results of the isokinetic endurance tests before and after 3 weeks of the in-season management routine. The swimmers were able to return to the regular daily yardage within a 10-day period without further incidence of pain. The reduced training of 3000 yd daily seemed to provide enough of a training stimulus to maintain an adequate fitness level. This amount of training seems to have en-

abled the swimmers to return to the regular workout yardage within a relatively short period of time. The principles employed in this program for the management of swimmer's shoulder pain can be modified to fit the individual needs of any given swimmer or other athlete.

PREVENTION OF SWIMMING SHOULDER COMPLICATIONS

The sports medicine professional frequently does not see the athlete until he or she has already sustained an injury like swimmer's shoulder, and it has become a chronic problem. Yet one of the major goals of the sports medicine professional has always been prevention of injury. It would appear that the complications of impingement and the causes of swimmer's shoulder pain may be preventable in many swimmers if early

TABLE 25-2. SHOULDER EXTERNAL AND INTERNAL ROTATION ENDURANCE BEFORE AND AFTER THE IN-SEASON MANAGEMENT OF SHOULDER PAIN[a]

	IR Initial (1–3)	IR Final (48–50)	IR End %	ER Initial (1–3)	ER Final (48–50)	ER End %	ER/IR Ratio
Pretraining	53.4	50.1	93.8	30.8	11.3	36.6	39.1
	1.1	0.4	2.0	1.4	1.6	0.3	1.0
Week 1 training	55.6[b]	52.1[b]	93.7	34.5[b]	17.9[b]	51.8[b]	55.2[b]
	1.4	0.7	1.8	1.1	0.9	1.2	1.4
Week 2 training	59.2[b]	52.9[b]	88.9	36.8[b]	20.8[b]	56.5[b]	63.5[b]
	1.1	0.8	2.1	1.5	0.8	1.5	1.3
Week 3 training	62.3[b]	55.5[b]	89.1	40.9[b]	23.3[a]	56.9[b]	63.8[b]
	2.1	1.0	1.6	1.1	0.9	1.3	1.0

[a]All values are reported as average torque in ft-lbs (X + SE).
[b]$p < 0.05$.

detection of predisposing conditions can be achieved by the sports medicine professional.

Muscular Strength and Endurance Factors

The functional ability of the external rotators of the shoulder has been shown to be a factor in both the mechanical and avascular impingement of the swimmer's shoulder complications. It would seem logical that an improvement of the muscular strength, and perhaps more importantly the muscular endurance of these shoulder external rotators, may result in both the prevention as well as the rehabilitation of this problem. The objective goal in designing a strengthening and endurance program should be to attempt to achieve a more optimal balance or ratio between the internal and external rotators of the shoulder by incorporating exercises for both movements. Recent investigations have shown that swimmers with shoulder pain present with significantly lower absolute external rotation endurance, and lower external-to-internal rotation endurance ratios than do swimmers without pain or nonswimmers.[23,24] Table 25–3 presents isokinetic muscular strength data comparing the shoulder internal and external rotators in nonswimmers, swimmers without shoulder pain, and swimmers with shoulder pain.[23] There does not appear to be any difference in muscular

strength between swimmers with or without shoulder pain for either internal or external rotation strength. Table 25–4, however, shows the difference in isokinetic endurance of the shoulder external and internal rotators in these same three populations.[23] Although the absolute external rotation endurance is significantly ($p < 0.05$) lower for the swimmers with pain, the ratio of external-to-internal rotation endurance (which might reflect the balance between these two muscle groups more accurately) was only 42.0%, as compared to 56.1% for the swimmers without pain and 67.8% for the nonswimmers. It would appear that once the imbalance of the external rotation to internal rotation endurance falls below 50%, the swimmer no longer has a sufficient external rotation muscular endurance capacity to allow for the proper maintenance of the correct stroke biomechanics in the recovery period. These faulty mechanics due to the fatigue of the external rotators over the course of a long workout, after days, weeks, and months of swimming training, may subject the swimmer to the cascade of events previously described that result in shoulder impingement and pain.[13,23]

If the swimmer can be screened prior to the season, and a deficit in the ratio of external to internal rotation can be detected, preventative exercises might

TABLE 25-3. ISOKINETIC STRENGTH OF THE INTERNAL AND EXTERNAL ROTATORS OF THE SHOULDER IN NONSWIMMERS, SWIMMERS WITHOUT PAIN, AND SWIMMERS WITH SHOULDER PAIN[a]

	IR 120 (sec^{-1})	ER 120 (sec^{-1})	ER/IR (%)	IR 180 (sec^{-1})	ER 180 (sec^{-1})	ER/IR (%)
Nonswimmers	24.9	17.1	68.9	20.6	14.3	69.4
	2.6	1.9	3.3	2.9	2.0	3.3
Swimmers—no pain	40.8[b]	29.1[b]	71.3	39.1[b]	27.7[b]	70.8
	2.4	2.1	2.1	2.5	2.5	2.3
Swimmers—pain	40.1[b]	28.2[b]	70.3	39.1[b]	26.3[b]	67.2
	2.1	2.7	2.6	2.0	2.8	2.6

[a]All values are expressed as the mean of right and left shoulder peak torque in ft-lb (X + SE).
[b]$p < 0.05$.

TABLE 25-4. ISOKINETIC ENDURANCE OF THE INTERNAL AND EXTERNAL ROTATORS OF THE SHOULDER IN NONSWIMMERS, SWIMMERS WITHOUT PAIN, AND SWIMMERS WITH PAIN[a]

	IR Initial (1–3)	IR Final (48–50)	IR End %	ER Initial (1–3)	ER Final (48–50)	ER End %	ER/IR Ratio
Nonswimmers	59.0	22.9	37.9	41.7[b]	10.7	25.7	67.8[b]
	4.5	3.3	3.2	4.1	2.1	3.6	3.6
Swimmers—no pain	61.0	55.6[b]	94.0[b]	43.0[b]	22.7[b]	52.8[b]	56.1[b]
	3.2	5.1	4.6	2.1	1.8	2.2	2.5
Swimmers—pain	60.4	55.5[b]	91.9[b]	32.9	12.6	38.5	42.0
	3.1	2.9	2.4	2.9	1.2	2.0	2.3

[a] all values are expressed as the average peak torque in ft·lb (X + SE).
[b] $p < 0.05$.

be able to reduce the incidence of shoulder pain in these swimmers. To test this hypothesis, two investigations were undertaken with a group of swimmers who presented with external-to-internal-rotation endurance ratios that would suggest that they either already had shoulder pain, or would be prone to developing impingement problems.[9,25] In the first study, we had swimmers with these low external-to-internal-rotation ratios train on a Cybex Isokinetic Dynamometer in a position similar to that achieved while swimming in the water.[19] Figure 25–10 shows the testing position used to assess shoulder internal and external rotation endurance, and also used for training the shoulder external rotators in this group. The results of this investigation showed clearly that once the ratio of external to internal rotation endurance reached greater than 50%, the pain became significantly reduced, and in many of the swimmers, disappeared completely. Table 25–5 presents the improvement of isokinetic muscular endurance after 10 weeks of isokinetic training of the external rotators of the shoulder in swimmers who had or were prone to develop impingement pain.

The second investigation[25] used the Lifeline Cord exercises seen in Fig 25–11 as the training stimulus for improving the external rotation endurance in a second group of swimmers who had complaints of shoulder pain. The results were very similar to the isokinetically trained group: Table 25–6 presents the increased endurance ratios and concomitant decreased pain in these swimmers after 10 weeks of external rotation endurance training in only 15 minutes prior to each practice session. It should be noted that in both of these groups of swimmers, any faulty stroke mechanics that were present were addressed by both the coaches and the investigators, and every effort was made to improve the faulty mechanical conditions during the course of the training program. In conclusion, it would seem that when swimmers who have shoulder pain, or present with sufficiently low external-to-internal ratios that may predispose them to shoulder impingement in the future, are placed on training programs designed to improve their muscular endurance of the external rotators, once they obtained a ratio of greater than 50% between the external and internal rotators, they became significantly less painful or painfree in several instances.[9,21,25]

In addition to the training of the external rotation endurance, specific exercises for the biceps and shoulder musculature are also very important to include in a sport-specific resistance training program to prevent shoulder injuries. Biceps training has been eliminated from many competitive swimming resistance training programs, presumably to avoid becoming "muscle bound" and having a limited range of motion. The emphasis has been on training the triceps that are used in the propulsion phase of the pull-through. The biceps

TABLE 25-5. EFFECT OF CYBEX ISOKINETIC TRAINING ON THE ISOKINETIC ENDURANCE IN THE INTERNAL AND EXTERNAL ROTATORS OF THE SHOULDER IN SWIMMERS[a]

	IR Initial (1–3)	IR Final (48–50)	IR End %	ER Initial (1–3)	ER Final (48–50)	ER End %	ER/IR Ratio
Pretraining	60.42	45.47	75.13	32.72	9.96	30.45	40.41
	4.21	3.25	3.01	2.96	2.76	2.41	2.47
Posttraining	69.90	58.17[b]	83.11[b]	39.33[b]	23.04[b]	58.56[b]	70.43[b]
	5.34	4.57	2.88	2.51	1.96	2.70	2.91

[a] All values are expressed as average peak torque at 240 sec^{-1} (X + SE).
[b] $p < 0.05$.

TABLE 25-6. EFFECT OF LIFELINE PULL CORD TRAINING ON THE ISOKINETIC ENDURANCE OF THE INTERNAL AND EXTERNAL ROTATORS OF THE SHOULDER IN SWIMMERS[a]

	IR Initial (1–3)	IR Final (48–50)	IR End %	ER Initial (1–3)	ER Final (48–50)	ER End %	ER/IR Ratio
Pretraining	56.90	44.54	78.12	28.72	9.62	33.88	43.21
	4.11	3.47	2.18	2.90	1.10	2.45	2.91
Posttraining	60.12	51.03[b]	84.88[b]	35.21[b]	18.79[b]	53.36[b]	62.86[b]
	3.78	4.09	1.66	2.90	1.98	2.63	2.33

[a]All values are expressed as average peak torque at 240 sec^{-1} (X + SE).
[b]$p < 0.05$.

long head is an important mover in the early pull-through and ignoring its need for strengthening and endurance may leave the swimmer open for injury and overuse problems.[13,26,27] It is important in swimming as it is in every sporting activity to design specific training exercises that most closely duplicate the strengths, endurance, and skills involved in the sport. In competitive swimming, almost all competitive swimmers perform the majority of each training workout in the freestyle stroke. For example, a butterfly swimmer may spend as little as 800 to 1500 yd of a 7000-yd workout actually swimming the butterfly stroke.[13] Therefore, when ever possible, training should be done in a position that most closely matches the specifics of the sporting skill, and creativity and imagination on the part of the sports medicine professional and swim coach can provide the swimmer with a resistance training program that will best suit his or her needs and result in optimal performances.

Flexibility Training

More often than not, swimmers are "too flexible" rather than insufficiently flexible (Fig 25–12). For this reason, a clinical judgment is required by both the coaches and sports physical therapist prior to placing a swimmer on an aggressive flexibility training program. In most swimmers, the flexibility of the anterior shoulder is not a major concern. It is appropriate to stretch the rotator cuff and biceps prior to swimming, and again after practice is over. Some earlier studies of the management of shoulder pain and complications in swimmers suggested that anterior capsule tightness and inflexibility of the anterior shoulder muscles were responsible for impingement complications because of restricted external rotation during recovery.[28] It was also felt that swimmers who breathed to only one side were more likely to develop impingement problems.[13] Subsequent studies of detailed flexibility programs and bilateral breathing patterns have been unable to provide an adequate explanation as to how or why flexibility problems result in the complications of swimmer's shoulder.[13,27]

Stroke Mechanics Corrections

Videotape analysis has revealed that it is not only the degree and timing of external rotation that has a significant impact on degree or severity of the impingement complications. Recent analyses have provided evidence that external rotation is usually complete by the halfway point in the recovery in swimmers who have no complaints of shoulder pain.[11,29] Swimmers who have pain have shown subsequent breakdown of the recovery mechanics as the workout progresses. Slow motion analysis of fluoroscopic videotapes have revealed that the impingement contact between the greater tuberosity and the coracoacromial arch occurs at about 90 degrees of abduction when the shoulder is internally rotated, whereas external rotation during the first 90 degrees allows the tuberosity to roll posteriorly and clear

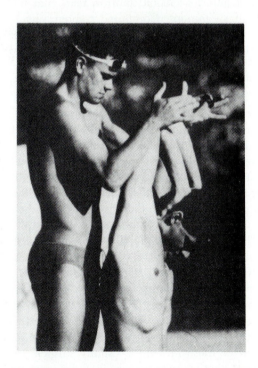

Figure 25-12. Excessive flexibility of shoulders in swimmers. (From Falkel JE, Murphy TC. Shoulder Injuries. Baltimore, Md: Williams & Wilkins Co; 1988, with permission.)

the arch.[11,29] Proper coaching is, first and foremost, the most effective tool in the identification of the breakdown of stroke mechanics, and the restoration of proper swimming form. Maintenance of the proper mechanics throughout the workout is the responsibility of not only the coach but the athlete as well. Many of the swimmers that have been tested in our laboratory have revealed that they were aware of the breakdown in stroke mechanics as they began to fatigue. With proper coaching and video analysis, the swimmer may be able to modify the workout at the point of stroke failure, and reduce the potential for impingement stresses. The addition of supplemental exercises to enhance external rotation endurance will also result in the decreased incidence of shoulder complications in swimmers. Finally, coaches and swimmers alike need to beware of progressing too far, too fast, or too soon with regard to intensity and duration of swimming training sessions. A careful analysis of the overall training program needs to be performed to examine the "quality versus quantity" issues of swim training, and whether or not quantity of training may indeed be hindering the quality of the swimmer's performance.

ANTERIOR GLENOID LABRUM DAMAGE

One of the other causes of shoulder pain in swimmers is now thought to be due to damage to the anterior glenoid labrum. McMaster[30] presents arthroscopic evidence of anterior glenoid labrum tears that have occured in swimmers. Computed tomography arthroscopy has also been useful in the diagnosis of this condition in the painful shoulder of some swimmers.[30,31]

The clinical presentation of these swimmers has been described by McMaster[30] as a painful shoulder that occurs at the catch and becomes maximal as the arm arrives at the level of the shoulder in mid pullthrough. The swimmer will also complain of a click with certain motions, and may report the shoulder "going out" at certain times. One possible explanation for this is an anterior subluxation rather than dislocation of the glenohumeral joint.[30] The "click" can be reproduced by adducting and internally rotating the shoulder. The Clunk Test[32] may also be positive in patients with an anterior glenoid labrum injury. The arthroscopic findings in these patients reveal damage to the anterior glenoid labrum with normal looking rotator cuff and biceps tendons.[30] The damage may range from a frayed section of the labrum to actual rupture and separation of the labrum from the glenoid. The management of these injuries is usually surgical, in that most conservative management including rest does not correct the lesion.[30] The current surgical procedures found to be most successful with these lesions can most

often be handled using an arthroscopic surgical approach.[30,32] If there are any loose fragments, or other debris in the region, they are removed. If the glenoid labrum is still attached, the roughened edges are smoothed. A full-thickness tear in the labrum requires debridement to prevent the lateral edge from catching and snapping as the humeral head glides across the labrum during swimming movements.

A surgical approach like arthroscopic management seems to have enjoyed the greatest success in returning the swimmer to a competitive level after surgical repair. There are numerous reports in the literature, and in personal observations, that surgical management of swimmers often results in the athlete failing to attain their previous level of competition.[30,33] McMaster[30] concludes that the poor results of shoulder surgery in swimmers may have resulted from improper diagnosis and a consequent incorrect surgical correction. This would result in persistent pain and symptoms, thus compromising the swimmer's ability to return to competitive training. As with any injury, correct diagnosis, proper surgical management, and complete postsurgical rehabilitation are necessary if the swimmer is to be able to return to competition.[30] Arthroscopic shoulder procedures can be a tremendous diagnostic tool in determining the etiology of the swimmer's shoulder pain and may be all that is necessary to correct the lesion, and return the athlete to painfree training.

The vast majority of injuries to swimmers occur at the shoulder, with incidence reports of anywhere from 42% to 67%.[23,34,35] Of these complications, however, many can be prevented through (1) proper coaching and stroke technique, (2) sensible training distances and intensities, and (3) supplemental resistance training programs that provide a balance of strength and endurance to the primary muscles of the shoulder that are involved in all phases of the swimming stroke.

COMPLICATIONS AT THE KNEE— BREASTSTROKER'S KNEE

It has been estimated that more than 25% of the orthopaedic complications seen in swimmers occur at the knee in breaststroke swimmers.[36] As was seen in the swimming shoulder, there may be several mechanisms of injury that result in the breaststroker's knee pain. One specific injury that occurs as the result of the whipkick performed during the breaststroke is an injury or sprain of the medial collateral ligament of the knee.[36-38] Another possible pathological condition that causes pain in these particular swimmers may be patellofemoral joint problems.[37] This section identifies the normal mechanics of the whipkick, the etiology and pathology of the breaststroker's knee, and the treatment and cor-

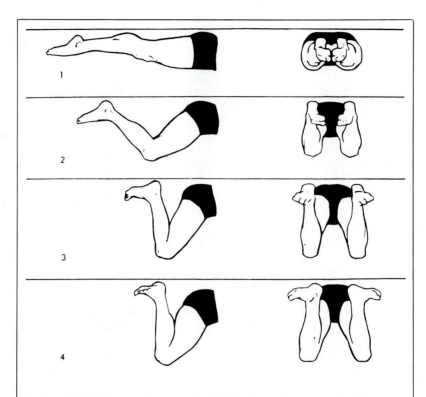

1. When the feet are not engaged in the kicking motion, they should be held in a fully extended, streamlined position close to the surface of the water. The feet should be plantar-flexed.

2. The leg recovery begins with a flexion of the legs at the hips and at the knees. Most coaches, including myself, attempt to have the swimmers keep their heels together as they are brought upward. The better kickers keep their heels close together as shown here, but very few of them touch heels at this point.

3. As the heels approach the buttocks, the feet begin to dorsi-flex and the heels and the knees to separate slightly.

4. The knees and hips reach their maximum flexion as the toes are turned outward and the ankles dorsi-flexed. The angle formed between the trunk and the upper leg is 125°.

Figure 25-13. This sequence of drawings depicts the correct mechanics of the breaststroke whip kick, as it should be done when performing kicking drills on the kick board. When actually using the kick in the whole stroke, the feet will drop lower under the surface of the water at other times in the stroke than shown here. This is due to the reaction from the pull and the head lift. (*continues*)

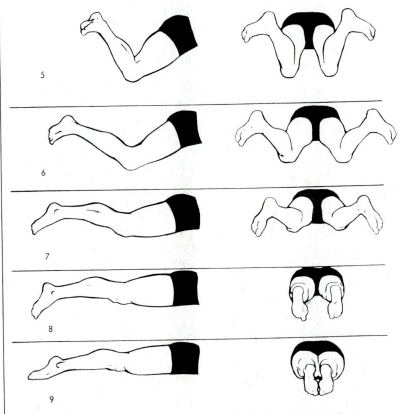

Figure 25-13. Sequencing of the breaststroke whipkick. *(From Counsilman JE.* The Science of Swimming. *Englewood Cliffs, NJ: Prentice-Hall; 1968, with permission.)*

5. The first few inches of the backward leg thrust are non-propulsive and are used for the legs to accelerate and to permit the feet to position themselves for a good backward thrust with the sides and the bottoms of the feet. At this point, the feet have engaged the water and are becoming effective.

6. The feet are pushed outward and backward as the knees extend. The upper legs are driven upward toward the surface of the water through the action of the strong hip extensor muscles. The feet, still dorsi-flexed, engage the water with the soles of the feet.

7. As the legs continue to extend at the knees, they are also brought together. The upper leg continues to be driven upward.

8. The knees almost reach full extension when the feet are only a few inches apart.

9. As the kick finishes, the feet are plantar-flexed. The swimmer will hold this glide position for a short time during which his feet will rise a few inches until his heels almost break the surface.

Figure 25-13. Continued

TABLE 25-7. BIOMECHANICAL DESCRIPTION OF THE BREASTSTROKE WHIPKICK

Stroke Phase	Description
Catch phase	Knees fully flexed with feet above the buttocks; feet dorsiflexed and everted; thigh, knee, and ankle begin slight abduction
Downsweep phase	Knee extension causing feet to travel downward and outward until they reach their widest point; feet then begin to move inward and downward after this point; feet position becomes inverted and plantar flexion begins; hip adduction and hip extension also occur during this phase; this is considered the "whip" part of the whip kick
Insweep phase	Feet continue into inversion and plantar flexion; knee extension finishes; this position is held for the glide component for a short time during which the feet will rise and the heels will come close to the surface of the water
Recovery phase	Knees begin to flex to bring the feet up toward the buttocks; hip flexion accompanies knee flexion to keep the feet below the surface of the water; the recovery phase occurs simultaneously with the propulsion phase of the arm stroke to prevent any absence of forward movement during the complete stroke

Adapted from Rodeo S. Swimming the breaststroke—A kinesiological analysis and considerations for strength training. NSCA J. 1984; 4:4–6; and Counsilman JE. The Science of Swimming. Englewood Cliffs, NJ: Prentice-Hall; 1968, with permission.

rection of the biomechanical problems associated with this swimming injury.

Figure 25–13 is a schematic diagram of the biomechanical sequence of the whipkick used in the breaststroke.[1] This is an extremely propulsive kick and contributes to most of the speed of this particular swimming stroke.[1,2,37,39] Rodeo[39] provides an excellent kinesiological analysis of the breaststroke, and he describes four phases to the legstroke of the whipkick: (1) catch, (2) downsweep, (3) insweep, and (4) recovery. Table 25–7 presents the biomechanical stages and kinesiological analysis of the whipkick.[1,39]

MECHANISMS OF KNEE PAIN IN BREASTSTROKE SWIMMERS

It would appear that there are two mechanisms responsible for the knee pain that occurs in breaststroke swimmers: (1) injury to the medial collateral ligament, and (2) patellofemoral pain.[36,37] Figure 25–14 shows the excessive tension placed on the medial collateral ligament during the movement of the whipkick.[40] The tension on the medial collateral ligament is increased as the knee moves from extension into flexion. Then, as a valgus stress is placed on the knee during the external rotation of the tibia to place the foot in position for the downsweep, the tension is further increased.[39,40] Patients complain of point tenderness at the origin of the medial collateral ligament on the adductor tubercle, as well as along the course of the ligament.[37,40] Another specific test that may elicit pain is forced abduction and external rotation of the knee with the knee in 20 to 30 degrees of flexion.[40] In this group of swimmers with knee pain, it appears that the adduction of the leg with marked knee flexion places an excessive valgus stress on the medial collateral ligament. If the swimmer extends

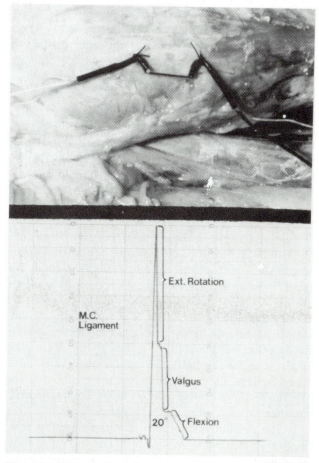

Figure 25–14. A small strain gauge is sutured to the tibial collateral ligament, and the constant buildup in tension is recorded. (From Schneider RC, Kennedy JC, Plant ML. Sports Injuries: Mechanisms, Prevention, and Treatment. Baltimore. Md: Williams & Wilkins Co; 1985, with permission.)

the leg first and then initiates the adduction, the valgus stress does not become excessive, and these swimmers are asymptomatic. Stulberg et al[37] also found asymptomatic swimmers who (1) keep the legs adducted together as the knee and hip flexes, (2) keep the thighs together as the feet are thrust backward and the hip and knee extends, and (3) bring the knees into full extension with the feet together. These are some of the constituents of the proper stroke mechanics described earlier. Counsilman[1] and others[2,37,40] have found that the proper execution of the whipkick does not cause knee discomfort, and that if swimmers can modify their stroke mechanics once the pain first begins, there is a much greater probability of swimming the breaststroke without knee pain.[34,38,40]

The other more debated cause of knee pain in breaststroke swimmers is patellofemoral complications. Kennedy and colleagues[36,38,40] have addressed various orthopaedic complications in swimmers but have not identified a problem with patellofemoral pain in their population of swimmers. They also make reference to studies done in Sweden by Eriksson that examined all swimmers with breaststroke knee pain under arthroscopy and found no evidence of chondromalacia.[40] Stulberg et al,[37] however, have found patellofemoral joint pain associated with the whipkick in a group of younger swimmers. Although they conclude that the mechanism of patellofemoral pain is unknown, their hypothesis (which is based on underwater videotape analysis of the whipkick in swimmers with and without pain) is as follows: The patella is pulled proximally and medially as the knee is forcefully extended with the legs abducted and the tibia and feet externally rotated. This causes the medial facet of the patella to abut against the intercondylar ridge. The legs must also move into a position of wide abduction, and this requires the medial portion of the quadriceps to be most active during the downsweep or thrust phase of the kick. Therefore, the patella will be forcefully pulled in a medial direction as the knee is extended and the tibia externally rotated.[37] Swimmers are also likely to have patellofemoral pain if they suffer the following stroke mechanic defects: (1) abduct the thigh as the hip and knee are flexed; (2) accentuate the amount of hip flexion, external rotation, and foot dorsiflexion at the end of the catch or recovery phase; (3) rapidly extend the knees with the legs abducted, the tibia externally rotated, and the feet dorsiflexed; and (4) allow the legs to drift together.[37]

The patellofemoral knee pain described by Stulberg et al[37] has not been seen in older, and more elite, swimmers.[1,2,38,40] This may be due to several factors such as proper technique, which would eliminate the mechanism for knee discomfort, and also a self-selection of older swimmers who can successfully accomplish the whipkick without undue stress on the knee. As was seen in the complications of swimming

shoulder pain, the most important preventative mechanism is proper stroke technique and coaching. If the whipkick is done correctly, there should be no reason for any type of knee pain associated with swimming this stroke. There are supplemental strength training exercises that should be done by breaststroke swimmers to provide better muscular power and stability at the knee, and these have been outlined by Rodeo.[39] It cannot be overemphasized, however, that proper technique, proper coaching, and sensible training are the cornerstones of prevention of knee discomfort in breaststroke swimmers. The sports medicine professional needs to understand the mechanisms of injury, and the normal biomechanics involved in the execution of the stroke, but must work closely with the coach and athlete to prevent the injury from occurring in the first place.

One final observation on knee discomfort in breaststroke swimmers. It has been observed in our laboratory (unpublished data) that previous knee pathology, or surgical correction of knee lesions, may predispose the athlete to knee pain even with the execution of the proper biomechanics of the whipkick. In fact, in several of these individuals, knee pain is experienced within the first 25 yd of swimming the breaststroke. The stresses placed on the medial collateral ligament of the knee in the motion of the whipkick (Fig 25–14) are excessive, and this type of kicking motion may be best done by swimmers who have no history of knee complications.

SUMMARY AND CONCLUSIONS

This chapter has focused on the two primary sources of injury to swimmers—impingement and overuse syndromes at the shoulder and breaststroker's knee pathology. With both of these conditions, most swimmers could swim painfree if they use proper technique. The proper technique will frequently fall apart with fatigue, however, and can predispose the athlete to overuse types of injuries. The sports physical therapist can only do so much in regards to preventative exercises, screening for potential problems, and treatment and rehabilitation of minor injuries to the shoulder and knee. One of the major goals of the sports physical therapist is to work closely with the coaching staff and the swimmer to help them understand the necessity of proper technique, proper training, and the role of preventative exercises in the overall preparation of the swimmer.

REFERENCES

1. Counsilman JE. *The Science of Swimming.* Englewood Cliffs, NJ: Prentice-Hall; 1968.
2. Maglischo EW. *Swimming Faster.* Palo Alto, Calif: Mayfield Publishing; 1982.

3. Dominguez RH. Coracoacromial ligament resection for severe swimmer's shoulder. In: Eriksson B, Furburg B, eds. *Swimming Medicine IV.* Baltimore, Md: University Park Press; 1978.

4. MaGee D. Care and prevention of injuries. Coaching the Championship Swimmer: Level III—National Coaching Certification Program. Canadian Amateur Swimming Association, 1982.

5. McMaster WC. Painful shoulder in swimmer: A diagnostic challenge. *Physician Sportsmed.* 1986; 14:108–122.

6. Counsilman JE. *Competitive Swimming Manual.* Bloomington, Ind: Counsilman Inc; 1977.

7. Ciullo JV, ed. *Clin Sports Med.* 1986; 5(1).

8. Nuber GW, Jobe FW, Perry J, et al. Fine wire electromyography analysis of muscle of the shoulder during swimming. *Am J Sports Med.* 1986; 14:7–11.

9. Falkel JE, Murphy TC, Trotta SJ, et al. Effect of resistive exercise on shoulder external and internal rotation strength and endurance in swimmers. *J Ortho Sports Phys Ther.* Submitted.

10. Booth RE, Marvel JP. Differential diagnosis of shoulder pain. *Ortho Clin N Am.* 1975; 6:353–376.

11. Murphy TC, Falkel JE. Videotape analysis of swimmers. Unpublished data: 1986.

12. Cailliet R. *Shoulder Pain.* Philadelphia, Pa: F A Davis; 1986.

13. Falkel JE, Murphy TC. *Shoulder Injuries.* Baltimore, Md: Williams & Wilkins Co; 1988.

14. Lewillie L. Graphic and electromyographic analysis of various styles of swimming. *Med Sport Biomech.* 1971; 11:253–257.

15. Rathbun JB, Macnab I. The microvascular pattern of the rotator cuff. *J Bone Joint Surg.* 1970; 52B:540–553.

16. MaGee DJ. *Orthopaedic Physical Assessment.* Philadelphia, Pa: W B Saunders; 1987.

17. McMaster WC. Diagnosing swimmer's shoulder. *Swimming Techn.* 1987; 23:17–23.

18. Hall G. Hand paddles may cause shoulder pain. *Swimming World.* 1980; 21:9–11.

19. Falkel JE, Murphy TC, Murray TF. Prone positioning for testing shoulder internal and external rotation on the Cybex II Isokinetic Dynamometer. *J Orthop Sports Phys Ther.* 1987; 8:368–370.

20. Hawkins RJ, Kennedy JC. Impingement syndrome in athletes. *Am J Sports Med.* 1980; 8:151–158.

21. Murphy TC, Falkel JE. Management of shoulder pain in swimmers: A case presentation. *J Orthop Sports Phys Ther.* Submitted.

22. Engin AE. On the biomechanics of the shoulder complex. *J Biomech.* 1980; 13:575–590.

23. Falkel JE, Murphy TC. Relationship between internal and external rotation strength and endurance in swimmers. *Am J Sport Med.* Submitted.

24. Fowler P. Rotation strength about the shoulder—Establishment of internal to external strength ratios. *NZ J Sports Med.* 1985; 13:88–89.

25. Falkel JE, Murphy TC, Murray TF. Effect of pull cord exercise on external rotation endurance in swimmers. *J Sport Sci Rev.* Submitted.

26. Penny JN, Smith C. The prevention and treatment of swimmer's shoulder. *Can J Appl Sport Sci.* 1980; 5:195–202.

27. Fowler P. Swimmers problems. *Am J Sports Med.* 1979; 7:141–142.

28. Greipp JF. Swimmer's shoulder: The influence of flexibility and weight training. *Physician Sportsmed.* 1985; 13:92–105.

29. Kapandji IA. *The Physiology of Joints.* New York, NY: Churchill Livingston; 1982.

30. McMaster WC. Anterior glenoid labrum damage: A painful lesion in swimmers. *Am J Sports Med.* 1986; 14:383–387.

31. Pappas AM, Gross TP, Kleinman DK. Symptomatic shoulder instability due to lesions of the glenoid labrum. *Am J Sports Med.* 1983; 11:279–288.

32. Andrews JR, Gillogly S. Physical examination of the shoulder in throwing athletes. In: Zarins B, Andrews JR, Carson W, eds. *Injuries to the Throwing Arm.* Philadelphia, Pa: W B Saunders; 1985.

33. Tibone JE, Jobe FW, Kerian RK, et al. Shoulder impingement syndrome in athletes treated by anterior acromioplasty. *Clin Orthop.* 1985; 198:134–140.

34. Dominguez RH. Shoulder pain in age group swimmers. In: Eriksson B, Furburg B, eds. *Swimming Medicine IV.* Baltimore, Md: University Park Press; 1978.

35. Richardson AB, Jobe FW, Collins HR. The shoulder in competitive swimming. *Am J Sports Med.* 1980; 8:159–163.

36. Kennedy JC, Hawkins RJ. Breast stroker's knee. *Physician Sportmed.* 1974; 2:33–38.

37. Stulberg SD, Shulman K, Stuart S, Culp P. Breaststroker's knee: pathology, etiology and treatment. *Am J Sports Med.* 1980; 8:164–171.

38. Kennedy JC, Hawkins RJ Krissoff WB. Orthopaedic manifestations of swimming. *Am J Sports Med.* 1978; 6:309–322.

39. Rodeo S. Swimming the breaststroke—A kinesiological analysis and considerations for strength training. *NSCA J.* 1984; 4:4–6, 74–80.

40. Kennedy JC, Craig AB, Schneider RC. Swimming. In: Schneider RC, Kennedy JC, Plant ML, eds. *Sports Injuries.* Baltimore, Md: Williams & Wilkins Co; 1985.

26

Throwing Injuries

Walt Jenkins and Sam Kegerreis

INTRODUCTION

The throwing mechanism is probably second only to running as an essential movement pattern in athletic endeavors.[1] Repeated force adequate to hurl a baseball in excess of 90 miles per hour or serve a tennis ball over 140 miles per hour must be imparted from the axial skeleton to the hand or racquet in milliseconds.[2] The upper extremity functions as an open kinetic chain, sequentially transmitting force from the slow moving trunk to rapidly accelerating distal segments.[3] Although the osseous components of this chain accept considerable stress, the soft tissue links at the elbow and shoulder appear most vulnerable to injury (Fig 26–1). Perry[4] reports peak torques of 17,000 kg/cm as the anterior capsule of the shoulder recoils from external to internal rotation. Pappas et al[2] have measured peak angular velocity of internal rotation at 9198 degrees per second and peak angular elbow extension velocities of 6933 degrees per second.

The burden of the throwing motion is further illuminated when one considers that the only anatomic joint attaching the upper extremity to the axial skeleton is the sternoclavicular joint. The shoulder girdle, and hence the entire throwing arm, is united with the trunk by a myofascial matrix that is in itself vulnerable to length–tension abnormalities as well as macrotrauma and microtrauma. A fragile balance of mobility and stability is critical in producing desirable speed and direction of a thrown object.

The throwing motion requires a violent antagonistic contraction as the shoulder explodes from external to internal rotation, loading joints from the vertebral column to the forearm.[5] Mechanical inefficiencies multiplied by frequency of repetition serve to further predispose the thrower to traumatic or insidious injury. Broer[6] and Toyoshima et al[7] indicate that only 50% of throwing speed is a result of the upper extremity. Numerous attempts to correlate strength with throwing speed have revealed disagreement among investigators,

further emphasizing the complexity of the throwing maneuver and the critical nature of mechanical competence. McCue et al[8] report the following biomechanical requirements for successful throwing:

1. Forces exerted in proper direction
2. Forces exerted in the proper time
3. Forces exerted in the proper sequence
4. Forces exerted over the greatest possible range
5. Ground contact maintained until ball release

The detailed analysis of throwing mechanics has yielded valuable insight as to the nature of throwing injuries in recent years.[2,3,5,9–14] An overview of throwing mechanics is presented later in this chapter.

In 1981, there were 4,500,000 amateur baseball players in the United States.[15] Although a majority of throwing injuries involve overhand pitching, the popularity of slow-pitch softball among a growing population of older athletes represents a further source of throwing injury victims. Brewer[16] notes the naturally occurring degenerative progression of the rotator cuff, which may be reflected in an increasing number of shoulder complaints among active, but aging, athletes. Injuries associated with the throwing mechanism are obviously not limited to baseball and softball players, although the nature of an object being thrown may dictate modification of specific techniques. A javelin requires a similar throwing mechanism as a baseball. Because of its weight and potential damage to the elbow, however, coaches encourage athletes to keep their elbows forward, and not lateral, to reduce stress.[17] A pumping action is involved in throwing a football accompanied by a shorter windup and weaker follow-through. Ground strokes in tennis are similar to batting and hockey in that the major propelling force is across the body.[8] The tennis serve possesses many stresses common to throwing mechanics. Priest[18] and Priest and Nagel[19] examined 84 expert tennis players, finding that greater than 50% had suffered "shoulder symptoms at some time during their careers." The service and over-

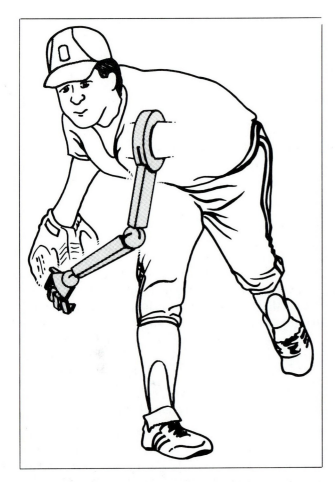

Figure 26-1. Upper Extremity as an open kinetic chain.

head smash were the most commonly involved strokes. Competitive swimmers reveal mechanics that are very similar to those of throwers, with the degree of external rotation and the velocity of internal rotation lessened. Richardson[20] has calculated that the average male swimmer will perform approximately 50,000 strokes per arm per year, further magnifying the potential for overuse injury. Swimming injuries are investigated in greater depth in chapter 25.

PHYSICAL CHANGES IN THE THROWING ARM

Wolff's law specifies that connective tissue architecturally adapts to functional stresses placed upon it. A retrospective analysis of physical changes in the upper extremity of throwing athletes permits us to further appreciate the forces of the throwing mechanism. King et al[12] examined 50 major and minor league pitchers observing the following:

1. An increase in cortical size and density of the humerus including the olecranon fossa and the olecranon

2. A decrease in volume of the olecranon fossa
3. Hypertrophy of upper extremity musculature extending proximally to the level of the shoulder, but most notably in the forearm flexor group
4. Elbow flexion contractures in 50%
5. Valgus elbow deformities in 30%
6. A uniform increase in shoulder external rotation accompanied by a decrease in internal rotation
7. Traction spurs on the medial aspect of the ulnar notch in 44%
8. Loose bodies in the radiohumeral joint space in 8%

Brown et al[21] goniometrically measured 41 professional baseball players, examining dominant to nondominant arm range of motion, comparing range of motion between pitchers and nonpitchers. Pitchers revealed increases in dominant side external rotation (with the arm at 90 degrees abduction) of 9 and 5 degrees more forearm pronation when compared with the dominant arm of position players. Position players revealed 9 degrees more shoulder extension on the dominant arm when compared with the dominant arm of pitchers. Priest and Nagle[19] cite unilateral depression or "droop" in the dominant arm of highly skilled tennis players, associated with an apparent scoliosis. They theorized that the overhead service motion may repeatedly stretch the trapezius, levator scapular, and rhomboids, contributing to an eventual elongation deformity. It was also proposed that osseous and muscular hypertrophy contributed to the dominant upper extremity of tennis players and may depress the shoulder via gravitational pull. Kendall et al[22] report a basic handedness pattern involving lowering of shoulder and elevation of the dominant hip in normal populations. Speculatively, one could note the disproportionate mass of the scapula protractors and humeral internal rotators versus the muscles responsible for scapular retraction and external rotation and make a case for "drooping" secondary to muscular imbalance. The neural bias and myofascial shortening of a throwing athlete may reflect a unilateral enhancement of a naturally occurring postural pattern. In 1968, Michele and Eisenberg[23] cited similar distress of the levator scapula secondary to a lack of scapular control.

Retrospective examination leads one to believe that despite its marvelous functional adaptations, the human arm was not designed to bear the repetitive burden of the throwing mechanism without complaint.

THROWING BIOMECHANICS

Pitching a baseball should be a smooth, natural motion, free of accessory motion that can lead to injury.

This simplicity of motion makes the pitching act similar to an outfielder's throwing mechanics when returning a fielded ball. Wasted motion leads to improper sequencing and timing and losses of balance and power. Overuse injuries of the throwing arm can occur within a short period of time in those individuals who display a loss of this economy in motion.

The biomechanics of pitching can be broken down into various phases. There are a number of classification systems, with McLeod's[13] being used in this chapter.

Windup

The initial phase in the pitching motion is the windup (Fig 26–2). This is primarily a preparatory phase that is relatively slow when compared to the other phases. Windup begins with the hands together and both feet on the ground.[24] Motion is initiated by movement of the hands, with the contralateral lower extremity coming off the ground soon thereafter. There is great variation in the magnitude of arm and lower extremity motion during this phase. Windup ends with the hands moving apart and the throwing hand beginning to reach backward. Upper extremity prime movers for

this motion include the posterior and middle deltoid. There are very few injuries that occur during this time.

Cocking

The cocking phase is designed to place the muscles of acceleration, the prime movers in the next phase, on stretch to allow for maximal tension production and ball velocity.[10] Upper extremity motion during cocking begins as the hands move apart and ends with maximal external rotation of the shoulder. Terminal position of the throwing arm is 90 degrees of abduction at the shoulder, 10 to 32 degrees of horizontal abduction, and in excess of 120 degrees of shoulder external rotation (Fig 26–3).[2,10,13] The elbow is more variable, with 90 degrees of flexion being most common.[3] During cocking, the contralateral lower extremity moves forward with the foot planting and pointing at the target.[13] The ipsilateral lower extremity is placed behind the trunk and continues to bear the majority of body weight. Concentric action of the shoulder musculature includes the posterior deltoid and the external rotators with the biceps acting late in cocking.[10,11] There is also an eccentric contraction of the latissimus dorsi and the pectoralis major.[11]

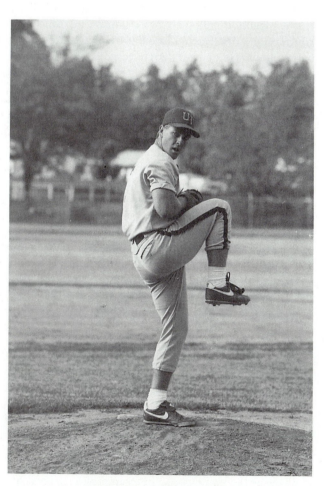

Figure 26–2. Wind-up phase.

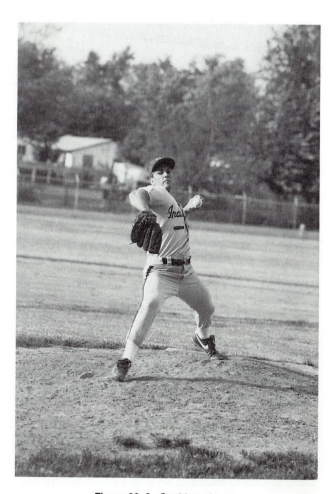

Figure 26–3. Cocking phase.

Pathomechanical considerations include poor foot placement in the contralateral lower extremity and a failure of the shoulder to achieve full range of motion.[9,13,25] Improper foot placement can increase the shoulder stress during later phases by causing an imbalance in the length–tension relationship of the shoulder musculature. Failure to achieve full shoulder range of motion will change the sequencing of the lower extremity with the upper extremity and shorten the time frame for the acceleration occurring in the next phase.

Acceleration

Acceleration is the period of time in which the athlete must achieve the proper power and speed in order to propel the ball forward at fast velocities (Fig 26–4). There is maximal tension placed on the anterior shoulder musculature during the beginning of this phase, which can lead to injury if proper timing and sequencing in the upper and lower extremities are absent.[13,25]

A lower-extremity weight shift from the ipsilateral to contralateral side initiates movement during this phase.[13] The trunk then rotates forward so as to face the target, leaving the throwing arm behind for a short time period. When the trunk squares up to the target

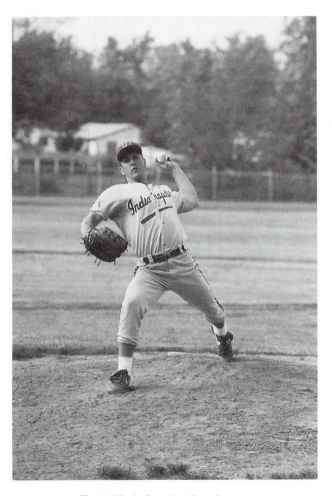

Figure 26-4. Acceleration phase.

the arm is passively propelled forward by the combined action of the trunk and lower extremities.[10,13] The shoulder is then forcefully moved into internal rotation and horizontal adduction. The elbow may range from 120 degrees of flexion to nearly full extension, with overhand pitchers exhibiting more flexion than pitchers who use a sidearm delivery.[2,24] Valgus stress on the elbow is maximal during this period, with the sidearm delivery having more valgus stress than the overhand delivery.[2,13]

Shoulder movement during this phase is by a combination of methods. Most authors feel that this phase is primarily a passive movement in the upper extremity, with the necessary power and speed for ball movement achieved by the trunk and lower extremity.[10,26,27] The shoulder girdle musculature along with the triceps muscle appear to be very active electromyographically during the later stages of this phase.[11] Concentric muscle action includes the latissimus dorsi, pectoralis major, subscapularis, triceps, and serratus anterior.[11] The pectoralis major and the latissimus dorsi muscles are the same muscles that were asked to eccentrically contract during the cocking phase. This is another example of the stretch-shortening cycle described by Komi.[28] The stretch-shortening cycle exists in most efficient body movements and is marked by a stretching/eccentric contraction followed by a shortening concentric contraction of the same musculature. The series elastic components are at least partly responsible for the increase in power achieved during this stretch-shortening movement. The eccentric component stretches the series elastic components, with the concentric component benefiting from the stored energy in the muscle tendon unit.[28]

During the acceleration phase, muscular injury can result from excessive stress placed on the anterior shoulder musculature. The anterior musculature is placed on maximal stretch early in this phase. This is a position in which the muscle–tendon unit is easily injured if proper mechanics are not followed. The trunk and lower extremity opening up too soon during this phase can increase the stretching of the anterior musculature, causing an increase in the stress about these muscles.

Atwater[3] states that the method of delivery for baseball pitchers is dependent upon the angle of trunk sidebending. The overhand thrower has a very upright posture during the acceleration phase whereas the sidearm pitcher has a trunk that is sidebent towards the dominant side. It follows that the position of the shoulder is fixed at a 90 degree angle regardless of the method of delivery.

Release (Deceleration)

Ball release occurs at different positions depending upon the individual athlete and the pitch delivered.[13] Optimal release point is at the time of maximal accel-

eration of the upper extremity (Fig 26–5).[13] Following the release of the ball, the throwing arm must decelerate at the shoulder and the elbow (Fig 26–6).[13] The shoulder continues to move into internal rotation and horizontal adduction, and begins to extend relative to the flexed position that the shoulder assumed during acceleration. The elbow will extend if the pitcher is an overhand thrower, and the forearm will pronate. The contralateral lower extremity now bears the majority of body weight for the first time during the pitching movement.[13]

The shoulder musculature is most active during this phase of the pitching cycle. The anterior shoulder musculature is concentrically contracting while the posterior musculature is eccentrically contracting.[10] The external rotators must act as the prime decelerators of the shoulder during this phase. Failure to do so will allow the humeral head to move anteriorly during the later stage of this phase, which will increase the incidence of injury.[9] Elbow deceleration into extension takes place due to an eccentric contraction of the long head of the biceps.[11,13] The biceps are further stressed when being asked to decelerate the forearm in pronation during this phase.

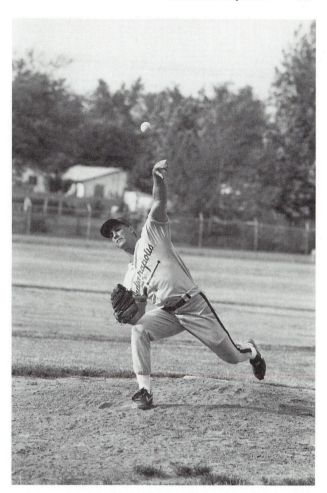

Figure 26–6. Deceleration phase.

Potential for injury is quite high during this phase secondary to the high amount of muscular activity particularly the eccentric component. Again imbalances in the upper- and lower-extremity sequencing and timing of movements can increase the potential for injury.

Follow-Through

The follow-through phase completes the pitching motion (Fig 26–7). It is a period of minimal risk to the throwing arm due to smaller amounts of tension produced in the musculature.[13] The shoulder motion is marked by forward movement, with the arm crossing the midline as it moves in front of the body.[29] The shoulder continues to internally rotate and extend with adduction of the arm also noted. The elbow is now fully extended and the forearm is in maximal pronation. The trunk must sidebend and rotate away from the pitching side to complete this phase. Body weight is now on the forward lower extremity, which is responsible for maintenance of proper balance and gross body movement. Many pitchers are unable to fully control their movements at the completion of this follow-through phase, leading to an inability to field a batted

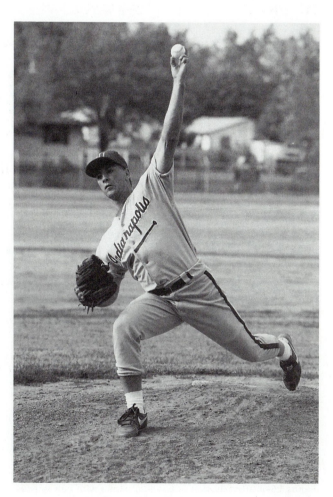

Figure 26–5. Ball release.

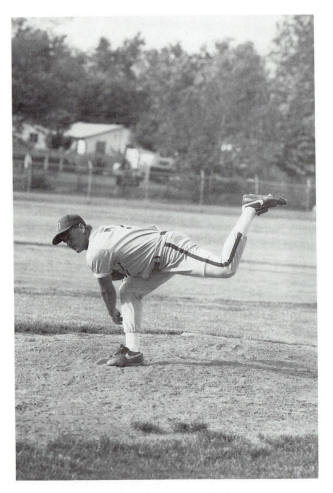

Figure 26-7. Follow-through phase.

ball. Improper positioning or lack of control can lead to injury as a result of being hit by a batted ball.

TENNIS SERVE MECHANICS

Although forehand and backhand strokes represent common upper extremity patterns, the tennis serve most closely resembles the mechanics of overhand throwing. The most obvious distinction one observes when comparing pitching to serving a tennis ball is an extended link to the existing kinetic chain in the form of a racquet. The additional leverage provided by a racquet significantly augments angular momentum and power. Authors differ, however, regarding the potential role of the racquet in contributing to injury. Richardson[20] Ryu et al[30] speculate that the greater force generated by the racquet may contribute to increased shoulder stress during acceleration and especially during the deceleration phase of follow through. Leach[31] contends that tennis players do not throw their shoulders away from their body in the manner that pitchers do, but rather control the racquet as it hits the ball. He

adds that this "element of control seems to render less strain of muscle tendon units controlling the shoulder," and although "stress is delivered to the elbow and wrist there is less deceleration force around the shoulder."

The tennis serve can be broken down into four stages analogous to the pitching motion.[30]

Windup
Windup represents the preparatory period from the start of the service motion until ball release by the contralateral hand (Fig 26-8). Although multiple variations exist, trunk hyperextension and rotation often exceed that of the baseball pitcher. This stage is dominated by shoulder abduction, extension, and early external rotation.

Cocking (Back Scratch)
Cocking is initiated with the ball toss from the nondominant hand and ends with maximum external shoulder rotation (Fig 26-9). The ball toss is seldom analyzed from a biomechanical perspective but remains an important clinical phenomenon in that errant releases may disrupt an otherwise fluid serving mecha-

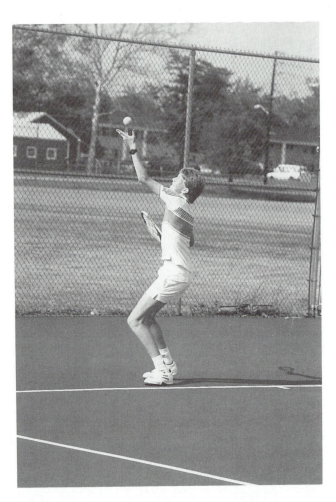

Figure 26-8. Termination of wind-up phase with ball release.

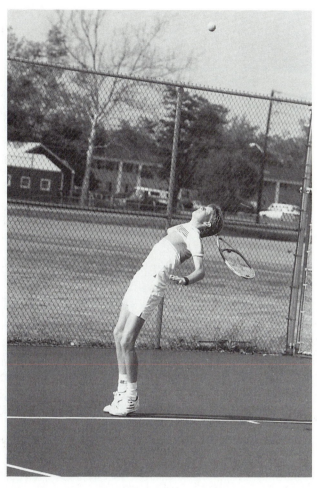

Figure 26-9. Back scratch.

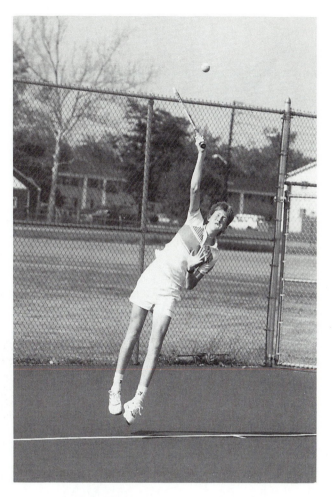

Figure 26-10. Acceleration—impact.

nism. Athletes may, furthermore, unconsciously modify their service motion to accommodate a habitual poor ball toss, resulting in inefficient biomechanics and increased potential for injury. The ball should be placed in front of and lateral to the dominant shoulder and just slightly higher than the extended racquet.[32] Increased scapular rotation enhances the motions initiated in the windup phase. Leach[31] contends that external rotation during this phase is significantly less than that of the baseball pitcher, in that wrist extension significantly contributes to the back scratch position.

Acceleration—Impact

Rapid internal rotation initiates the acceleration phase, which concludes with ball impact (Fig 26–10). Trunk flexion and rotation precede the shoulder into internal rotation and adduction, although to a lesser degree than in the pitching motion.[31] An important distinction between pitching and serving may be noted during this phase. Dulany[32] states that the tennis serving motion differs from the throwing of a baseball in that the predominant direction of force during acceleration is upward. He points out that if a server with a racquet used

the same motion as that of a pitcher, every serve would go into the net! Nirschl[33] encourages high arm elevation during the acceleration phase to diminish medial elbow force load and reduce rotator cuff shear forces (Fig 26–11). Poppen and Walker[34] concur in reporting that joint compression at 90 degrees abduction is equivalent to 89% of body weight, as compared to 40% with the arm at 150 degrees. Atwater[3] reports, however, that the position of the arm relative to the trunk is "far more determined by lateral trunk flexion than by shoulder joint motion." She concludes that the position of the arm near release in most throwing skills approximates a 90 degree angle with the trunk. Acceleration is dominated by the action of the brachial internal rotators, the subscapularis, the pectoralis major, and the latissimus dorsi.

Follow-Through

The follow-through phase involves a gradual decline of firing by the shoulder adductors and internal rotators as the external rotators decelerate the arm and racquet (Fig 26–12). The athlete should be encouraged during this phase to rotate the trunk so that the arm crosses

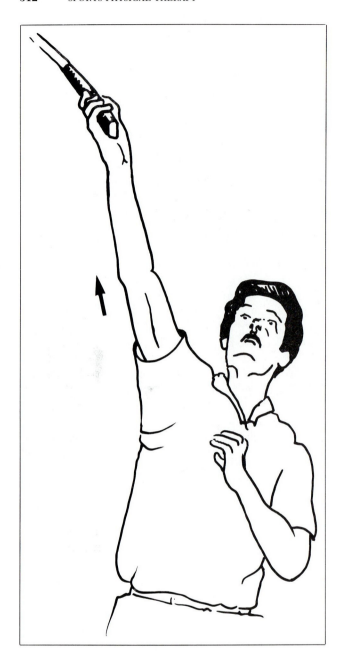

Figure 26-11. Arm elevation during acceleration of tennis serve.

the body to avoid undue compression of the shoulder suprahumeral space (Fig 26–13). Ryu et al[30] reinforced the need for proximal stability by observing that serratus anterior firing is significant during follow-through in all phases of the serving motion.

PATHOLOGY

Shoulder

Injuries to the shoulder are very common in throwing sports.[10] The large amount of stress placed upon the

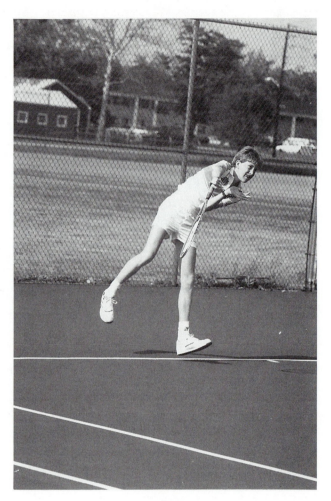

Figure 26-12. Follow-through.

shoulder during the act of throwing has been well documented and, when combined with the delicate balance that must exist in the shoulder for normal movement, it makes for an easily injured joint.[2,10,35] Long-term participation in athletics as a throwing athlete requires a dedication to detail in conditioning for both the upper and lower extremity and a thorough knowledge of the specific mechanics of that sport. Even small flaws in mechanics or a change in routine can manifest themselves in injury if left unrecognized. Macrotrauma and microtrauma can be a result of either of these phenomena. Coaches, athletic trainers, physical therapists, and physicians who are working with throwing athletes on a regular basis should have a good working knowledge of these areas in order to recognize and advise the athlete regarding the potential for injury, the injury itself, and the proper return to competition.

The prime anatomic consideration for the shoulder in throwing sports is the delicate balance between the joint capsule, the glenohumeral bony articulation, and the musculoskeletal component. Weakness or imbalance in the rotator cuff musculature, the biceps

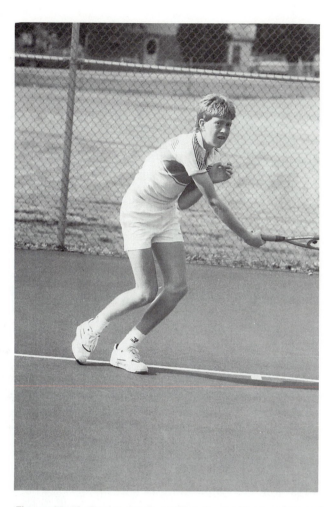

Figure 26-13. Proper trunk rotation to avoid suprahumeral compression during follow-through.

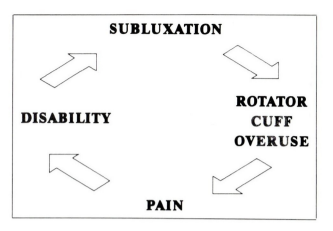

Figure 26-14. Overuse disability cycle.

mechanism, and the scapular musculature are common in both the normal population and the throwing athlete.[25,36] These weaknesses are commonly seen in athletes who have problems with subluxation or impingement. Subluxation is important to recognize in that the rotator cuff and biceps must work very hard to keep the humerus in the proper position for articulation with the glenoid fossa in individuals who have a weakness in the joint capsule.[25] Throwing athletes may continue to wear down these muscles with the constant repetitive trauma of throwing over a long season and career. This leads to further weakness and with that weakness more subluxation. Therefore, the subluxation and rotator cuff/biceps weakness become part of a vicious cycle of pain and disability (Fig 26–14). The scapular musculature may also become involved in that it must stabilize the shoulder complex during the pitching act.[25] Poor scapular stability results in an increased amount of stress to be placed on the glenohumeral joint musculature, leading to further subluxation and then overuse injuries.[25]

Impingement injuries are common in individuals who have tightness in the glenohumeral joint. The bony anatomy, joint capsule, and associated ligaments, fascia, and musculature may all be involved in this process. The coracoacromial arch, comprised of the acromion and the coracoacromial ligament, forms a hard and unyielding roof over the head of the humerus. Directly under the coracoacromial arch lies the long head of the biceps tendon and the rotator cuff muscles. The latter are attached via their tendons on the greater and lesser tuberosity of the humerus whereas the long head of the biceps runs across the superior portion of the humeral head and attaches to the superior glenoid tubercle. When a throwing athlete has a loss of the normal elasticity of the glenohumeral joint capsule or the fascia of the upper extremity the coracoacromial arch can impinge upon the rotator cuff and biceps during elevated tasks.[37,38] The acceleration and deceleration phases of the throwing motion or tennis serve are such that the greater tuberosity and coracoacromial arch may come into contact in those individuals who have this loss of elasticity. The repetitive motion of throwing in an individual who has this type of problem will result in an inflammatory condition in the tendons of these muscles or a subacromial bursitis. A gradual wearing down of the rotator cuff or the biceps ensues, possibly resulting in macrotrauma or microtrauma in the muscle or tendons. The physical changes of increased joint motion on the dominant side and muscle hypertrophy in the scapular musculature make it extremely unlikely that impingement is a likely problem in a throwing athlete who has participated for a number of years in his or her sport. A younger individual who is just beginning to take up throwing sports or someone who has not participated for a number of years is more likely to have the impingement phenomenon.

Lesions of the anterior shoulder normally occur during the acceleration phases of the tennis serve and the pitching motion.[25,38] During this period of time, the

anterior musculotendinous structures are placed on a maximum stretch while simultaneously being asked to contract. This results in large forces being placed on these structures, which can result in injury. The subscapularis, pectoralis major, the long head of the biceps, and the anterior deltoid muscles can be injured during the acceleration phases of movement. Additionally, the subdeltoid and subacromial bursae and the anterior joint capsule are at risk during this phase.[39]

Poor mechanics, such as "opening up too soon," have long been implicated in increasing stress on the anterior shoulder musculature.[39] Opening up too soon refers to the athlete rotating so that the trunk is facing the target more quickly than it should. It is natural for the trunk to rotate towards the target during the acceleration phase. The athlete who opens up too soon, however, will rotate far too early in the acceleration phase or even during the cocking phase of throwing. This places undue stress on the anterior shoulder musculature, causing an abnormal amount of stretch and resulting in a poor length–tension relationship in these muscles. Any and all of the above mentioned muscles can be injured with this mechanism. The long head of the biceps can also dislocate during the acceleration phase of throwing in individuals who have excessive joint range of motion or problems with the transverse humeral ligament.[9,39]

Instability of the anterior portion of the shoulder can also occur during the acceleration phase. Those individuals who have excessive capsular laxity are susceptible to glenohumeral joint subluxation and possibly even dislocation at the initiation of this phase. The anterior/inferior joint capsule is placed on maximal stretch with full external rotation, 90 degrees of abduction, and full horizontal abduction in this position. As described by Rowe and Zarins,[40] the "dead arm syndrome," or the recurrent transient subluxation of the shoulder, provides a clear picture of what can happen with this type of injury.[40] According to Rowe and Zarins, the athlete will subluxate the shoulder at the initiation of the acceleration phase during the period of maximal external rotation, abduction, and horizontal abduction. The subluxation will cause a sudden pain in the upper extremity, with the limb going "dead," resulting in a loss of control in the entire upper extremity. A classic "Bankart" lesion is normally found with the anterior joint capsule, the inferior glenohumeral ligament, and the anterior glenoid labrum being injured. Frank dislocations of the glenohumeral joint are less common at this joint with throwers.

McLeod and Andrews[35] describe how the subluxation phenomenon can also lead to tears of the glenoid labrum via the biceps mechanism. The biceps mechanism works to decelerate the humerus and the forearm during the deceleration phase of throwing. If an individual has excessive joint laxity, the biceps mechanism has to work harder than normal to keep the proper articulation. The origin of the biceps on the superior glenoid tubercle and the superior glenoid labrum appears to be the weak link in this chain and is, therefore, injured with this type of mechanism.

Bursitis in the subdeltoid and subacromia bursae is less common, but may also occur during the acceleration phase.[9,39] During this phase, the subdeltoid and subacromial bursae are compressed in an athlete who has impingement type problems. When functioning properly, the subdeltoid and subacromial bursae act to allow for a smooth gliding mechanism between the coracoacromial arch and the rotator cuff and biceps. An increase in friction in this area during the throwing act due to tight anterior structures may be the cause of this problem. Norwood et al[39] have also described the subdeltoid area as being susceptible to adhesions in the bursae that can effectively limit range of motion and cause pain during the cocking or acceleration phase of throwing.

Throwing athletes may suffer from a variety of posterior shoulder disorders.[26,27] Problems with subluxation and musculoskeletal injuries are the most common in this area. Norwood[27] states that the shoulder is susceptible to posterior subluxation during the deceleration phase of throwing due to the humerus being placed in a position of adduction and internal rotation. The internally rotated position places tension on the posterior joint capsule and posterior portion of the glenoid labrum. The humeral head glides posteriorly during internal rotation of the shoulder, which places further tension on the posterior capsule and glenoid labrum. If an individual is predisposed to joint laxity prior to becoming a thrower or if there are abnormal mechanics in throwing, the posterior subluxation may occur.

Lesions of the posterior rotator cuff musculature are also seen in throwing athletes.[25,35] The primary muscles for deceleration are the biceps, the teres minor, and the infraspinatus.[2,10,11,25] The teres minor and infraspinatus function to decelerate the arm into internal rotation during this phase. These muscles are asked to accept large tension forces with a relatively small muscle mass, leading to injury if proper mechanics and conditioning programs are not followed. The posterior rotator cuff also tends to be weaker when compared to the more powerful hypertonic anterior musculature.[21,41] Off-season and in-season conditioning programs must address this tendency towards weakness in the posterior rotator cuff or the athlete will be predisposed to injury in this area. Tendonitis and muscle strains are the most common forms of injury in the posterior musculature.

Vascular injuries to the throwing arm have been documented in the literature during the last several years.[42] Both the anterior and posterior shoulder have

problems with this type of injury. Anterior lesions normally involve the axillary artery or the subclavian vein. The abducted, externally rotated, and horizontally abducted positions may result in compression of the axillary artery by the overlying pectoralis minor muscle during the acceleration phase. Effort thrombosis of the subclavian vein has also been noted, with the etiology being uncertain at this time. The posterior humeral circumflex artery is the most commonly injured vascular structure in the posterior shoulder. Compression of this artery occurs in the quadrilateral space posteriorly due to fibrous bands found within this space, restricting the normal motion during the late cocking or early acceleration. The axillary nerve may also be injured in conjunction with the posterior humeral circumflex artery in the quadrilateral space. Vascular injury symptoms include generalized pain in the shoulder, arm, or forearm, and the acute onset of diffuse swelling and distension of the superficial veins of the arm and forearm. A venogram is helpful in the diagnosis of the vascular lesion in the anterior or posterior shoulder.

The suprascapular nerve can become impinged in the pitchers as it travels through the suprascapular notch in the spine of the scapula.[43] Traction on this nerve is commonly a product of poor posture, improper biomechanics, and overuse. The suprascapular nerve innervates the supraspinatus and infraspinatus, with the infraspinatus innervation more commonly compromised after the suprascapular nerve passes through the notch. The suprascapular nerve is a motor nerve only and, therefore, is silently pathological. The infraspinatus and supraspinatus muscles can atrophy with little warning when injured in this manner, resulting in weakness and loss of motion in the throwing athlete.

humeral joints represent concave surfaces moving on their proximal convex counterparts and producing flexion and extension. The proximal and distal radioulnar joints contribute to forearm pronation and supination. The trochlear surface of the humerus is angulated such that elbow extension is accompanied by an accentuated valgus bias, rendering the joint vulnerable to medial traction stresses. The lateral collateral ligament is essentially nonfunctional, originating from the lateral epicondyle and inserting into the annular ligament. It is minimally reinforced by the anconeus. Varus-producing forces are, fortunately, rarely encountered, and lateral stability is seldom a problem.[45] Medial stability represents a significant difficulty, however, necessitating greater functional support. The medial collateral ligament consists of three parts: the anterior oblique, posterior oblique, and the transverse ligament (Fig 26–15). The transverse ligament appears to be of little significance. The posterior oblique is broad and fan shaped, inserting into the posterior medial aspect of the olecranon.[46] It is lax in extension and taut in flexion. The anterior oblique ligament represents the primary static stabilizer of the medial elbow. Divided into two functional components, the anterior oblique ligament is taut throughout both flexion and extension. Cadaveric sectioning reveals that this ligament is also the primary guard against posterior instability.[45] Valgus stability is dynamically reinforced by the flexor forearm mass and osseously by compression of the radial articulation.[45] The origin of the common extensor tendon is noted on the lateral epicondyle, which is commonly involved in the "tennis elbow" syndrome.[33] The ulnar nerve, lying within the ulnar groove of the humerus, is another important medial structure vulnerable to valgus stress.

THROWING ELBOW

The deteriorative effect of repetitive throwing on the elbow has been well documented.[12] The elbow is reportedly second only to the knee as a site of overuse injury. Overuse injuries are observed as physiological changes in bone and soft tissue that occur when healing lags behind the microtrauma of repetitive activity. Bennett was perhaps the first to focus on the effect of repetitive pitching on the elbow.[44] Concern for the welfare of young throwing athletes further created the nonspecific diagnosis of "Little League Elbow" that is discussed later in this chapter.

Functional Elbow Anatomy

Anatomically, the elbow consists of three articulations (humeroulnar, radiohumeral, and proximal radioulnar) contained within a common synovial and fibrous capsule. Functionally, the humeroulnar and radio-

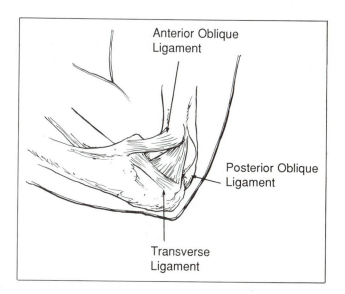

Figure 26–15. Medial collateral ligament complex.

Pathophysiology

During the overhead throwing motion, the elbow rapidly progresses from flexion to extension, with the forearm exhibiting strong pronation. Valgus stresses increase in proportion to velocity as the forearm lags behind the humerus at ball release.[47] Repetition of valgus stress and forced extension represent the major pathological mechanisms of injury to the throwing elbow.[48] Attenuation of the anterior oblique ligament can contribute to biomechanical dysfunction, precipitating medial traction, lateral compression, and valgus extension overload (Fig 26–16).

Albright et al[49] have strongly implicated sidearm throwing in elbow injuries, especially if a "whipping or snapping motion is used to obtain more speed." They add that a three-quarter arm or overhand delivery decreases valgus stress, therefore decreasing the incidence of injury. Empirically based assumptions have further associated medial elbow pathology with muscle activity during the throwing of a curve ball. Sisto et al[14] refute this concept based on EMG analysis of the forearm flexor musculature. Atwater[3] adds, "Thus, there appears to be no evidence directly linking the curve ball pitch with a specific site of injury or with a unique movement that is part of the curve ball throwing motion."

Elbow Injuries

Slocum[50] divides throwing injuries of the elbow into three categories: medial tension overload, extensor overload, and lateral compression injuries.

Medial Tension Overload Injuries

Of 50 baseball players complaining of elbow symptomatology, Barnes and Tullos[51] diagnosed 41 as suffering from some component of medial elbow stress syndrome. Flexion contractures and bony hypertrophy, including enlargement of the medial condyl, with "fragmentation, breaking, and possibly separation," may be symptomatic or asymptomatic. It has been theorized that fixed flexion contractures may actually prevent

olecranon impingement.[12] Acute overuse syndrome of the forearm musculature is clinically manifested by pain and point tenderness and is often accompanied by a loss of complete elbow extension. Accurate palpation and pain on resisted wrist flexed delineate forearm musculature strains from other medial elbow lesions. The vast majority of flexor musculature injuries respond to rest, ice, and active range of motion exercises, as complete rupture in adults is rare.[52]

Bennett[44,53] described a forearm compression syndrome involving medial elbow pain, hypertrophy of the flexor musculature, and enlargement of localized edema. He reported that pain from this lesion could force a pitcher to discontinue throwing after two to three innings. Rest and modification of throwing patterns was suggested, with fasciotomy used only as a last resort.

The integrity of the anterior oblique portion of the medial collateral ligament is critical to throwing mechanics. Jobe and Nuber[52] report four stages of medial collateral ligament pathology resulting from repetitive valgus stress: (1) edema, (2) scarring and disassociation of ligament fibers, (3) calcification, and (4) ossification. Roentgenographic examination may reveal loose bodies or spurring. In addition to insidious attenuation, traumatic valgus stress may be experienced as a pitcher reports an audible "pop" when throwing a baseball. The elbow abduction stress test (at 20 degrees of flexion) may be augmented radiographically by a gravity stress test in assessing medial integrity. Nonthrowing individuals may function adequately following disruption of an ulnar collateral ligament, but Jobe and Nuber[52] encourage immediate exploration for throwers exhibiting valgus instability. Medial reconstruction is completed, when necessary, using the palmaris longus (or short toe extensor in the absence of a palmaris longus). Conservative care consists of rest, ice, and anti-inflammatory medication, in addition to strengthening and gentle range of motion techniques. Throwing should only be resumed in the absence of tenderness. Pitching mechanics should be evaluated to decrease excessive valgus stress whenever possible.

Traction ulnar neuritis commonly accompanies the valgus instability resulting from medial collateral attenuation.[47] Degenerative spurring and calcium deposits create further peril for the ulnar nerve, which is often transferred during medial elbow reconstructions. Throwers complaining of primary symptoms of ulnar neuritis should be examined closely for medial instability. Decompression procedures in such circumstances may prove insufficient if valgus insufficiency exists as the athlete returns to pitching.[54] Hypermobility of the ulnar nerve from congenital or developmental laxity may contribute to friction neuritis. Childress[55] reports that approximately 16% of the population demonstrate dislocation of the ulnar nerve as the elbow is flexed

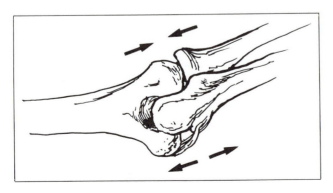

Figure 26-16. Medial traction and lateral compression overload.

from a position of full extension. Throwers exhibiting this characteristic may suffer from ulnar neuritis in the absence of valgus instability. Ulnar nerve entrapment is also noted beneath a thickened arcuate ligament (Osborne lesion).[47] Ulnar nerve compromise is associated with numbness and tingling in the ring and little fingers. Radiating pain in the ulnar distribution is often accompanied by a positive Tinel's sign. Conservative care consists of rest, anti-inflammatory agents, and, occasionally, immobilization. Symptoms resume, however, upon a return to throwing. Anterior transposition is advocated in this instance, accompanied by reconstruction in the presence of medial instability.

Extensor Overload Injuries

Extensor overload injuries range from triceps tendonitis through chronic osseous changes. Treatment of triceps lesions involves ice, rest, and, when necessary, immobilization. Transverse friction massage and progressive eccentric exercise are often excellent treatment adjuncts. Osteophyte formation on the tip of the olecranon and posterior loose bodies have traditionally been associated with the extension block during the follow-through phase of throwing. Wilson et al[56] describe an osteophyte often accompanied by local chondromalacia of the olecranon against the medial olecranon fossa, which is commonly missed by traditional radiographic technique. They suggest that this posterior lesion is produced during the early acceleration phase of pitching as valgus stress wedges the medial olecranon into the olecranon fossa. Pitchers with this malady commonly lose control after two or three innings as they apparently begin to throw high secondary to a premature release. They recommend a balanced program of strengthening and stretching about the elbow as a conservative measure to be followed by resection of the offending structure, if necessary.

Lateral Compression Injuries

Indelicato et al[57] and others[48,58] consider lateral compression injuries to have a poor prognosis in comparison to medial and posterior lesions. Throwing subjects the capitellum and radial head to compressive and rotational forces with respect to valgus overload that can be accentuated by medial laxity. Repeated trauma can lead to capitellar fractures, osteochondritis, and, ultimately, traumatic arthritis.[59] Osteochondritis is cited as the leading cause of permanent disability in throwing athletes.[48] The dilemma of osteochondritis in the young athlete will be addressed later in this chapter. Surgical removal of loose bodies, hypertrophic marginal spurs, and osteocartilaginous fragments is recommended.[59] Andrews[48] encourages early mobilization of the elbow to re-establish or increase range of motion in adult patients. As the prognosis for a return to high-level throwing is dismal for patients suffering from significant lateral compression lesions, prevention remains the preferred mode of treatment.

THE YOUNG THROWING ATHLETE

Overview

Pappas[58] identifies the termination of childhood with the appearance of all secondary centers of ossification and the termination of adolescence with the fusion of all secondary centers of ossification. He adds that in young throwers complaints are most frequently elicited from pitchers and, in descending order, from infielders, catchers, and outfielders.[58] The elbow is the most frequent area of involvement in children and adolescent baseball players[60] and has represented a considerable source of disagreement among notable authors[60-64] Adams's[61] classic article in 1965 radiographically studied the elbows of 80 9- to 14-year-old pitchers reporting "some degree of accelerated growth, separation, and fragmentation of the medial epicondylar epiphyses" in 95%. Similar changes were present in 15% of 47 nonpitching little leaguers and in 8% of 35 active children of the same age who did not play baseball. Other authors[60,63-65] have disagreed as to the importance of "Little League Elbow," citing a significantly lower incidence of pathological changes. It has also been observed that many radiographic findings are not accompanied by symptoms, but perhaps reflect normal bodily adaptation to overuse. Among the important distinctions to be made, however, is the fact that Adams's[61] study involved throwers in year-round competition (secondary to climatic conditions), and also included athletes ranging in age from 9 to 14 years, whereas most other studies limited their populations to participants of little league age. It is theorized that asymptomatic throwers possessing radiographic changes in little league may actually reveal lesions that will become disabling at a later date. Despite the aforementioned disagreements, it is generally accepted that excessive throwing during childhood and adolescence can lead to pathological changes to the elbow.

Little League Elbow

The term "Little League Elbow" was first coined by Brogdon and Cross[66] in 1960 relating to "an avulsion of the ossification center of the medial epicondylar epiphysis." This term has evolved to include a plethora of complaints, with the common denominator involving a pathological process in the elbow of a young thrower. The most common diagnoses associated with "Little League Elbow" include variations of medial traction syndrome and less common, but more serious, compression of the lateral side. The majority of medial elbow injuries in young throwers include delayed closure of the medial epicondylar growth plate, traction apophy-

sitis producing fragmentation, and widening of the medial epicondylar apophysis. Symptoms commonly include tenderness and swelling, often accompanied by a loss of range of motion. Treatment in these instances should be aggressive, in the form of *complete rest* until full painfree motion is restored. Athletes revealing the aforementioned symptoms should be counseled, along with their parents and coaches, as to proper technique and appropriate throwing restrictions. Avulsion fractures of the medial epicondyle can occur and are reported by Gugenheim et al[60] and Tullos and King[64,67] to be the most commonly observed throwing lesion among growing children. Fragment separation in excess of 5 mm is reportedly best treated surgically.[68] The significance of lateral compression injuries in the throwing athlete has been alluded to previously.[48,57] The exact etiology of osteochondritis in the young thrower remains an enigma. Several authors[52,69] suggest that osteochondritis dissecans represents a delayed reflection of osteochondrosis of the capitellum (Panner's disease), whereas others insist that the two processes are distinctly unique.[70]

Osteochondrosis of the elbow is an uncommon finding. The etiology of this affliction is believed to be one of vascular insufficiency, similar to Calvé–Perthes disease. It is commonly associated with fragmentation of the entire capitellum ossific nucleus, but normally responds to conservative care without loose body formation. Osteochondrosis has been diagnosed in the nondominant arm as well as in youngsters not involved with throwing. A strong link to little league participants has been made, however.[52,60,64,67,70]

Osteochondrosis is most commonly witnessed as a preteen phenomena, whereas osteochondritis dissecans is associated with throwers in the 13- to 14-year-old group.[60] Proponents associating osteochondrosis and osteochondritis dissecans note that vascular predisposition in combination with repetitive stresses may lead to asymptomatic changes during little league participation that become significant if throwing is maintained in subsequent seasons. Larson et al[62] reported that 5% of little league pitchers in Eugene, Oregon, revealed radiographic changes in the lateral compartment (capitellum and radial head) and Adams[61] cited similar findings in 8% of little league pitchers. When one considers the prognosis of advanced lateral compression syndrome in a young thrower, prevention, early diagnosis, and conservative care take precedence over academic dispute. Although many disagreements exist, the following observations are universally accepted pertaining to the young thrower:

1. The elbow is the most frequent area of complaint among young throwers.
2. Pitchers, infielders, catchers, and outfielders, in respective order, complain of elbow pain.

3. The mechanism of medial traction and lateral compression can contribute to pathological changes in the young thrower.
4. The most vulnerable areas to injury of the young thrower include the medial epicondylar growth plate and the medial epicondylar apophysis.
5. Medial lesions occur more frequently than lateral injuries.
6. Lateral compression lesions occur with less frequency than medial traction injuries and are more common among older adolescents (14 to 15 years old).
7. The prognosis of advanced lateral compression injuries with respect to a return to throwing sports is poor.
8. Why some youngsters develop pathology, while others at similar competitive levels do not is not known.
9. "Overwhelming" adult supervision can result in youngsters attempting to perform beyond their inherent capabilities, increasing the likelihood of injury.
10. Prevention is preferable to treatment. Controlling the number of pitches thrown in competition is beneficial. The adolescent arm, however, cannot distinguish between competition and backyard practice. The education of coaches and parents is of paramount importance.

REHABILITATION

Rehabilitation of the injured throwing arm must restore the proper balance to the musculature in both length and strength. The rotator cuff, biceps, scapular musculature, and the forearm musculature need to have painfree flexibility and strength for the throwing athlete to return to competition safely. The physical therapist must take into consideration the physical changes of increased range of motion, and muscle hypertrophy that are normally seen in the arm of the throwing athlete prior to restoration of normal function.[3,21,72] As with all rehabilitation, the return of painfree range of motion is the first priority in the initial phases of rehabilitation. Traditional passive range of motion, mobilization techniques, proprioceptive neuromuscular facilitation, and myofascial release techniques can all be used very effectively during this phase of rehabilitation. Low levels of strengthening are initiated as soon as the patient can tolerate resisted exercise followed by gradual progression of strength.

The injured rotator cuff musculature must be treated in a very delicate manner so as to minimize any negative effects during the early phases of rehabilita-

tion. Passive forced range of motion into the end range of forward flexion will adversely affect the rotator cuff by reproducing the impingement phenomenon, whereas excessive stretching into internal rotation has the potential to disrupt the infraspinatus and teres minor muscles. Once the rotator cuff muscles have become inflamed, it can take a long period of time to restore proper length and strength to them. Active range of motion within the painfree limits of movement is effective in helping to decrease inflammation without aggravating the symptoms early in rehabilitation. Internal and external rotation within the painfree limits can be performed quite easily in patients without increasing their pain and disability (Fig 26–17).

Once the inflammation has subsided in the rotator cuff, the use of hand-held weights, surgical tubing, manual resistance, or the impulse exercise unit can be initiated (Fig 26–18). Light hand-held weights can be used effectively within a painfree limited motion in abduction, flexion, and extension.

Additionally, the supraspinatus muscle may be specifically exercised by having a standing athlete internally rotate the shoulder and then elevate the arm from a point midway between flexion and abduction (Fig 26–19). Jobe[73] also advocates the use of hand-held weights for internal and external rotation in a sidelying position. Surgical tubing may also be used in a variety of planes of motion (Fig 26–20). The eccentric component is effectively exercised with surgical tubing, making this form of exercise very attractive in the treatment of tendonitis.[74] Maximal eccentric muscle contractions have been held largely responsible for the onset of tendonitis. Curwin and Stanish, however, advocate the use of low levels of eccentric contraction to specifically treat the injured structure.[74] The rationale behind ther-

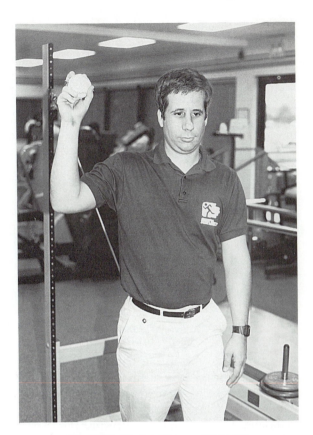

Figure 26–18. Impulse exercise unit.

apy of this type is that it is necessary to reach the tendon and strengthen it with submaximal exercise in order to cause significant change. Curwin and Stanish caution against the use of eccentrics with the supraspinatus muscle due to the possibility of an impingement syndrome. Manual resistance in cardinal planes of mo-

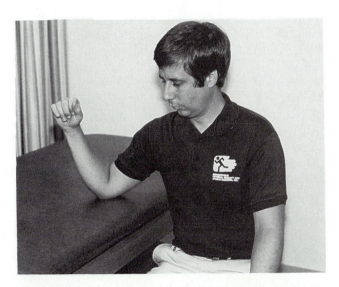

Figure 26–17. Active internal and external glenohumeral rotation.

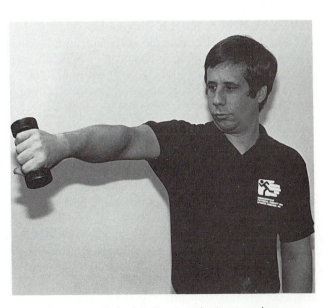

Figure 26–19. Isolated supraspinatus exercise.

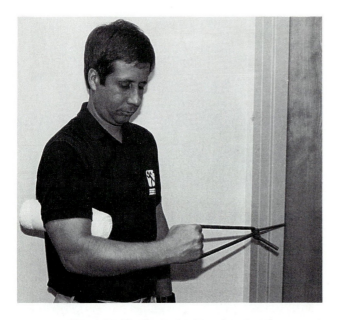

Figure 26–20. Surgical tubing exercises.

tion or in proprioceptive neuromuscular facilitation patterns is very useful in the strengthening of the entire upper extremity. Specific stabilization patterns for the scapula and distal mobility patterns for the arm and shoulder are effective both early and late in the rehabilitation process.

The impulse exercise unit is also quite effective for strengthening in the eccentric mode. This unit works both the concentric and eccentric phases of muscle contraction, emphasizing the transition between the two types of contraction. The impulse exercise unit uses low weight with functional speeds and can be performed at any number of specific planes of motion similar to surgical tubing.

Isokinetic testing and exercise are also important in the treatment of the throwing athlete. Davies[41] has developed a set of norms for both men and women when testing the shoulder isokinetically whereas Brown et al[21] have published a more recent study of both range of motion and strength in major league baseball players. Isokinetic strength training has been advocated for the throwing athlete because of the ability to train at functional speeds with accommodating resistance.

Scapular motion, scapulohumeral rhythm, and scapular strength must also be addressed in a comprehensive rehabilitation program. Proper scapular function is necessary for the glenohumeral joint to be in the right position for the throwing act. A scapula that is moving too freely or one that has lost the normal range of motion will prevent the glenoid fossa from facing in the right direction, resulting in an abnormal length–tension relationship in the glenohumeral musculature. Scapular mobilization and myofascial techniques are most effective in increasing scapular mobility. Manual resistance techniques including PNF patterns and iso-

metric exercises can be very helpful in improving scapular stability. Scapulohumeral rhythm can be improved with bilateral activities in the upper extremity such as cane or rifle exercises and wall pushups.

The forearm musculature may be strengthened by use of manual resistance, hand-held weights, surgical tubing, or the impulse exercise unit. The use of a hand gripping implement such as a rubber or sponge ball can be helpful with grip strength and elbow function as well. Myofascial techniques can help with trigger points and adhesions in this area.

The use of a functional progression such as the long toss–short toss program has been advocated and implemented by Blackburn.[9] The long-toss–short-toss program is helpful in increasing functional strength, range of motion, and endurance postinjury, in a maintenance program during the season, and in an off-season program. Additionally, any athlete returning to throwing is encouraged to go through a program of this nature in order to decrease the incidence of injury. Prior to beginning this program the athlete should have good range of motion and strength and perform an adequate warmup consisting of elevation of body temperature and specific stretching for the dominant upper extremity. The athlete should allow for rest periods by only throwing for 3 to 4 days a week with this program.

The long-toss–short-toss program is initiated by lobbing the ball for 30 ft or so in order to warmup, progressing to 60 ft or more as the athlete becomes comfortable. It is important to emphasize that the athlete should not attempt to throw the ball on a line parallel to the ground in the early phase of this program. As time passes, the athlete may go into the outfield and simply toss the ball into the infield, allowing it to bounce several times and roll into second base. This long tossing from the outfield will allow the athlete to work on functional strengthening and range of motion. Throwing from distances of 120 ft or more can begin later, initially with a lobbing motion and then with a flatter trajectory as strength and range of motion increase.

A short-toss program can be instituted simultaneously with the long-toss program, using approximately half speed at the initiation of the program and progressing to full speed. The use of a pitcher's mound should be contraindicated until the pitcher is able to demonstrate good strength and range of motion and perform short throws at full speed for consistent periods with a recurrence of symptoms. Table 26–1 describes the long-toss–short-toss program.

ARM CARE AND PREVENTION OF INJURY

The throwing arm is asked to perform at a high level of function for extended periods of time during the season. The delicate balance between the proper range of

TABLE 26-1. LONG-TOSS-SHORT-TOSS PROGRAM

I.	Warmup	Distance	Intensity	Time
	A. Short toss	30 ft	Lob	5 min
	B. Long toss	60 ft	Lob	5 min
II.	**Long Toss**	**Distance**	**Intensity**	**Time**
	A. Long toss	90 ft	Lob	5 min
	B. Long toss	120 ft	Lob	5 min
	C. Long toss	90 ft	Flat Trajectory	5 min
	D. Long toos	120 ft	Flat Trajectory	5 min
III.	**Short Toss**	**Distance**	**Intensity**	**Time**
	A. Short toss	60 ft	Lob	5 min
	B. Short toss	60 ft	1/2 speed	5 min
	C. Short toss	60 ft	3/4 speed	5 min
	D. Short toss	60 ft	Full speed	5 min
IV.	**Mound Work**	**Distance**	**Intensity**	**Time**
	A. Fast ball	60 ft, 6 in full speed		5–10 min
	B. Other pitches	60 ft, 6 in full speed		5–10 min
V.		**Game Simulation**		
	A. 15–25 pitches per inning using a variety of pitches			
	B. 7–10-minute rest between innings			

motion and strength must be maintained for the athlete to continue to perform for long periods free of injury during the season.[9] Likewise, the off season must be used to allow the athlete to improve his or her conditioning level and rehabilitate any injuries that are sustained during the season. A holistic approach to the throwing athlete must be adhered to for best results both during and following the season. All elements of conditioning, including the cardiopulmonary system, muscular strength, muscular endurance, and specific conditioning for the throwing arm, should be included. All too often one of these elements is emphasized at the expense of others, upsetting the balance that one must strive to achieve in conditioning. The sports physical therapist must also consider the normal physical changes that occur in the throwing athlete when developing and evaluating conditioning programs for these individuals.

The off-season conditioning and arm care must start with an evaluation of the throwing arm for injuries. A thorough history should be taken to determine if there are any lingering symptoms from the recently completed competitive season. Any injuries should be treated as soon as possible to allow for a more thorough and complete healing to occur. The cardiovascular program may be initiated whenever the athlete can begin a regular routine of aerobic training. Aerobic training will provide the essential baseline of cardiovascular endurance for the next competitive season. Cardiovascular endurance is a necessary component for throwers due to the fact that competition lasts for several hours

in both tennis and baseball. A running program of three to four times a week for 20 to 30 minutes is very helpful in improving the aerobic fitness level of the athlete. As the season nears, there should also be an effort to include an anaerobic type of workout several times a week. Sprint training can be helpful in improving the explosive qualities in the lower extremity so necessary in the throwing act.

Muscular strength and endurance training should encompass the lower extremity, spine, trunk, and the upper extremity. Upper extremity exercises for the shoulder girdle, shoulder, arm, forearm, and wrist should all be included in weight training. As with rehabilitation, these exercises should work towards good muscular balance in both the flexor and extensor groups. Care should be taken to maintain proper flexibility in all muscle groups, with emphasis on the shoulder, arm, and forearm musculature. Performing resistance exercise in a limited range of motion will reinforce problems with flexibility in the throwing athlete, resulting in poor performances the following season. The initial emphasis for the off-season weight training program is in endurance, with muscle strength being emphasized only after a good endurance base has been established.

The use of hand held weights has been advocated by Jobe et al[78] in their conditioning of the throwing athlete. These exercises use a low amount of weight with many repetitions and are primarily designed to exercise the rotator cuff musculature and the long head of the biceps (Fig 26–21). Special attention should be given to

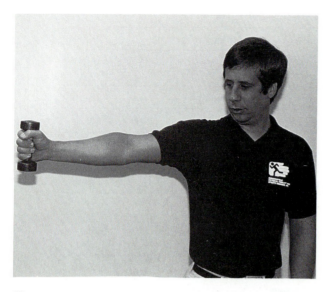

Figure 26-21. Shoulder exercises utilizing hand-held weights.

the infraspinatus and teres minor muscles, as they are of great importance in the deceleration phase of throwing. The eccentric contractions required of these muscles result in excessive wear and tear during the competitive season and are, therefore, critical to the maintenance of an injury-free throwing athlete. The impulse exercise unit and surgical tubing may also be used to improve eccentric strength.

The musculature of the spine and trunk are very important in stabilization for the throwing act. These muscles need both strength and endurance in order for the athlete to function properly. Special attention should be paid to the abdominal musculature and spinae erectors. The abdominals work to pull the trunk forward during the acceleration and ball-release phase whereas the spinae erectors must function eccentrically and isometrically during these same phases of throwing.

The major source of power in the throwing act for pitchers is in the lower extremity.[24,36] The hip, pelvis, knee, and lower leg should all be considered in a comprehensive conditioning program. The gluteus maximus and hamstrings are powerful hip extensors, providing a great drive forward with the ipsilateral lower extremity during the acceleration phase of throwing, and are, therefore, important to providing velocity to the pitched ball. The quadriceps muscles on the contralateral lower extremity accept the majority of body weight during acceleration and ball release, and must control the weight shift of the body forward during the deceleration phase of throwing. Exercises for the gluteus maximus, hamstrings, and quadriceps should take into account the specific functions of each of these muscles in a conditioning program. The squat rack, leg press, or the hip sled are commonly and effectively used in strengthening of hip extension and knee extension,

whereas hamstring curls and heel raises are indicated for strengthening the hamstrings and gastroc-soleus complex. Hip abduction and adduction should not be neglected and can be strengthened by the use of surgical tubing or cuff weights.

A proper in-season program should include all the same components as the off-season program, with emphasis on maintenance of conditioning levels rather than increasing specific elements.[36] Cardiovascular conditioning, muscular endurance, and flexibility for the trunk, upper, and lower extremity should be maintained during the competitive season. The aerobic and anaerobic components of cardiovascular fitness should be addressed in a running program three or four days a week to help prevent fatigue and injury. Jobe and colleagues[74] strongly believe that a proper in-season program must include muscular endurance for the entire upper extremity.[36,74] Light hand-held weights are effectively employed in the various planes of motion for the upper extremity, with several sets of a large number of repetitions used.[36,74] The flexibility program for the trunk, upper extremity, and lower extremity is necessary to maintain good pitching velocity, pitching control, and to prevent injury. This holistic approach to the stretching program will allow a smooth pitching delivery that is economical from a biomechanical and musculoskeletal point of view.

CONCLUSION

Injuries to the throwing arm are numerous, with the upper extremity being injured most frequently. A thorough knowledge of applied anatomy, biomechanics of the various throwing motions, and the conditioning process can be helpful in prevention of injury. Once injury has occurred, a review of pathomechanics with the athlete and the coach is of primary importance to help prevent further injury. Prior to treatment, it is also necessary to have a good understanding of the physical changes that occur with the long-term use/abuse of the throwing arm. Treatment and rehabilitation must take into consideration the enormous stress placed on the throwing arm during competition and successfully return the athlete to pre-injury levels of strength, endurance, and range of motion.

REFERENCES

1. Cofield RH, Simonet WT. The shoulder in sports. *Mayo Clin Proc.* 1984; 59:157–164.
2. Pappas AM, Sawacki RM, Sullivan TJ. Biomechanics of baseball pitching. *Am J Sports Med.* 1985; 13:216–222.
3. Atwater AE. Biomechanics of overarm throwing movements and of throwing injuries. *Exerc Sport Sci Rev.* 1979; 7:43.

4. Perry J. Anatomy and biomechanics of the shoulder in throwing, swimming, gymnastics and tennis. *Clin Sports Med.* 1983; 2:247–270.

5. Braatz KJ, Gogia PP. The mechanics of pitching. *J Orthop Sports Phys Ther.* 1988; 16:577–585.

6. Broer MD. *Efficiency of Human Movement.* Philadelphia, Pa: W B Saunders; 1969.

7. Toyoshima S, Hoshikawa T, Miyashita M, et al. Contribution of the body parts to throwing performance. In: Nelson RC, Morehouse CA, eds. *Biomechanics IV.* Baltimore, Md: University Park Press; 1974:169–174.

8. McCue FC, Gieck JH, West JO. Throwing injuries of the shoulder. *Athlete Train.* 1977; 4:202–211.

9. Blackburn TA. Throwing injuries to the shoulder. In: Donatelli R, ed. *Clinics in Physical Therapy, Physical Therapy of the Shoulder.* New York, NY: Churchill Livingstone; 1987:209–240.

10. Jobe FW, Tibone JE, Perry J, Moynes D. An EMG analysis of the throwing shoulder in throwing and pitching. *Am J Sports Med.* 1983; 11:3–5.

11. Jobe FW, Tibone JE, Perry J, Moynes D. An EMG analysis of the shoulder in throwing and pitching: A second report. *Am J Sports Med.* 1984; 12:218–220.

12. King JW, Brelsford HJ, Tullos HS. Analysis of the pitching arm of the professional baseball pitcher. *Clin Orthop.* 1969; 67:116–123.

13. McLeod WD. The pitching mechanism. In: Zarins B, Andrews JR, Carson WG, eds. *Injuries to the Throwing Arm.* Philadelphia, Pa: W B Saunders Co; 1985.

14. Sisto DJ, Jobe FW, Moynes DR, Antonelli DJ. An electromyographic analysis of the elbow in pitching. *Am J Sports Med.* 1987; 15:260–263.

15. Collins HR, Lund D. Baseball injuries. In: Schneider RC, Kennedy JC, Plant ML, eds. *Sports Injuries: Mechanisms, Prevention, and Treatment.* Baltimore, Md: Williams & Wilkins; 1985.

16. Brewer DB. Aging of the rotator cuff. *Am J Sports Med.* 1979; 7:102–110.

17. Waris W. Elbow injuries in javelin throwers. *Acta Chir Scand.* 1946; 93:563.

18. Priest JD. The shoulder of the tennis player. *Clin Sports Med.* 1988; 7:387–401.

19. Priest JD, Nagel DA. Tennis shoulder. *Am J Sports Med.* 1976; 4:23–42.

20. Richardson AB. Overuse syndromes in baseball, tennis, gymnastics and swimming. *Clin Sports Med* 1983; 2:379–390.

21. Brown LP, Niehues SL, Harrah A, et al. Upper extremity range of motion and isokinetic strength of the internal and external shoulder rotators in major league baseball players. *Am J Sports Med.* 1988; 16:577–585.

22. Kendall HO, Kendall FP. Wadsworth GE. *Muscles: Testing and Function.* Baltimore, Md: Williams & Wilkins; 1971.

23. Michele AA, Eisenberg J. Scapulocostal syndrome. *Arch Phys Med Rehabil.* 1968; 49:383.

24. Sain J, Andrews JR. In: Zarins B, Andrews JR, Carson WG, eds. *Proper Pitching Techniques in Injuries to the Throwing Arm.* Philadelphia, Pa: W B Saunders Co; 1985.

25. Pappas AM, Zawacki RM, McCarthy CF. Rehabilitation of the pitching shoulder. *Am J Sports Med.* 1985; 13:223–235.

26. Lombardo SF, Jobe FW, Kerlan RK, et al. Posterior shoulder lesions in throwing athletes. *Am J Sports Med.* 1977; 5:106–110.

27. Norwood LA. Posterior shoulder instability. In: Zarins B, Andrews JR, Carson WG, eds. *Injuries to the throwing arm*, Philadelphia, Pa: W B Saunders Co; 1985.

28. Komi PV. The stretch-shortening cycle and human power output in human muscle power. In: Jones NL, McCartney N, McComas AJ, eds., *Human Power Muscle* Champaign, Ill. Human Kinetics Publishers Inc.; 1986.

29. Hageman CF, Lehman RC. Stretching, strengthening, and conditioning for the competitive tennis player. *Clin Sports Med.* 1988; 2:211–228.

30. Ryu RK, McCormack J, Jobe FW, et al. An electromyographic analysis of shoulder function in tennis players. *Am J Sports Med.* 1988; 10:481–485.

31. Leach R. Tennis serving compared with baseball pitching. In: Zarins B, Andrews JR, Larson WG, eds. *Injuries to the Throwing Arm.* Philadelphia, Pa: W B Saunders Co; 1985:307–311.

32. Dulany R. Tennis strokes. In: Pettrone FA, ed. *American Academy of Orthopaedic Surgeons Symposium on Upper Extremity Injuries in Athletes.* St. Louis, Mo: C V Mosby Co; 1986:47–58.

33. Nirschl RP. Prevention and treatment of elbow and shoulder injuries in the tennis player. *Clin Sports Med.* 1988; 7:289–327.

34. Poppen NK, Walker PS. Forces at the glenohumeral joint in abduction. *Clin Orthop.* 1978; 136:165–170.

35. McLeod WD, Andrews JR. Mechanisms of shoulder injuries. *Phys Ther.* 1986; 66:1901–1904.

36. Boscardin JB, Johnson P, Schneider H. The wind-up, the pitch, and pre-season conditioning. *Sports Care Fit.* Jan/Feb 1989:30–35.

37. Andrews JR, Gillogly SD: Shoulder examination and diagnosis in the throwing athlete. In: Pettrone FA, ed. *American Academy of Orthopaedic Surgeons Symposium on Upper Extremity Injuries in Athletes.* St. Louis, Mo: C V Mosby Co., 1986:306–321.

38. Lehman RC. Shoulder pain in the competitive tennis player. *Clin Sports Med.* 1988; 7:309–328.

39. Norwood LA, DelPizzo W, Jobe FW, Kerlan RK. Anterior shoulder pain in baseball pitchers. *Am J Sports Med.* 1978; 6:103–106.

40. Rowe CR, Zarins B. Recurrent transient subluxation of the shoulder. *J Bone Joint Surg.* 1981; 63A:863–871.

41. Davies GJ. *A Compendium of Isokinetics in Clinical Usage.* 3rd ed. Onalaska, Wisc: S & S Publishers; 1987.

42. Baker CL, Thornberry R. Neurovascular Syndromes. In: Zarins B, Andrews JR, Carson WD, eds. *Injuries to the Throwing Arm.* Philadelphia, Pa: W B Saunders Co; 1985.

43. Wells R. Suprascapular nerve entrapment. In: Zarins B, Andrews JR, Carson WD, eds. *Injuries to the Throwing Arm.* Philadelphia, Pa: W B Saunders Co; 1985.

44. Bennett GE. Shoulder and elbow lesions of the professional baseball pitcher. *JAMA.* 1941; 117:510–514.

45. Schwab GH, Bennett JB, Woods GW, Tullos HS. Bio-

mechanics of elbow instability: The role of the medial collateral ligament. *Clin Orthop Relat Res.* 1980; 146:42–51.

46. Warwick R, Williams PL, eds. *Gray's Anatomy, British Ed.* Philadelphia, Pa: W B Saunders Co; 1973.

47. Jobe FW, Fanton GS. Ulnar neuritis at the elbow in athletes. In: Morrey BF, ed. *The Elbow in Its Disorders,* Philadelphia, Pa: W B Saunders; 1985.

48. Andrews JR. Bony injuries about the elbow in the throwing athlete. In: Pettrone FA, ed. *American Academy of Orthopaedic Surgeons Symposium on Upper Extremity Injuries in Athletes.* St. Louis, Mo: C V Mosby Co; 1986:221–232.

49. Albright JA, Jokl P, Shaw R, et al. Clinical study of baseball pitchers: correlation of injury to the throwing arm with method of delivery. *Am J Sports Med.* 1978; 6:15–21.

50. Slocum DB. Classification of elbow injuries from baseball pitching. *Texas Med.* 1968; 64:48–53.

51. Barnes DA, Tullos HS. An analysis of one hundred symptomatic baseball players. *Am J Sports Med.* 1978; 6:62–67.

52. Jobe FW, Nuber G. Throwing injuries of the elbow. *Clin Sports Med.* 1986; 5:621–636.

53. Bennett GE. Elbow and shoulder lesions of baseball players. *Am J Surg.* 1959; 98:484–492.

54. Rettig A. Personal communication.

55. Childress HM. Recurrent ulnar nerve dislocation at the elbow. *Clin Orthop.* 1975; 108:168–173.

56. Wilson FD, Andrews JR, Blackburn TA, McCluskey G: Valgus extension overload in the pitching elbow. *Am J Sports Med.* 1983; 11:83–88.

57. Indelicato PA, Jobe FW, Kerlin RK, et al. "Correctible elbow lesions in professional baseball players." *Am J Sports Med.* 1979; 7:72.

58. Pappas AM. Elbow problems associated with baseball during childhood and adolescence. *Clin Orthop Relat Res.* 1982; 164:30–41.

59. DeHaven KE, Evarts CM. Throwing injuries of the elbow in athletes. *Orthop Clin N Am.* 1:801, 1973.

60. Gugenheim JJ, Stanley RF, Woods GW, et al. Little league survey: The Houston study. *Am J Sports Med.* 1976; 4:189–199.

61. Adams JE. Injury of the throwing arm: A study of traumatic changes in the elbow joints of boy baseball players. *Calif Med.* 1965; 102:127.

62. Larson RL, Singer KM, Bergstrom R, Thomas S. Little league survey: The Eugene study. *Am J Sports Med.* 1976; 4:204–209.

63. Torg JS, Pollack H, Sweterlitsch P. The effect of competitive pitching on the shoulders and elbows of pre-adolescent baseball players. *Pediatrics.* 1972; 49:267–272.

64. Tullos HS, King JW. Lesions of the pitching arm in adolescents. *JAMA.* 1972; 220:264–271.

65. Francis R, Bunch T, Chandler B. Little league elbow: A decade later. *Physician Sportsmed.* 1978; 6:88–94.

66. Brogdon BG, Cross NW. Little leaguer's elbow. *Am J Roentgenol.* 1960; 83:671.

67. Tullos HS, King JW. Throwing mechanism in sports. *Orthop Clin Am.* 1973; 4:709–720.

68. Pettrone FA. The adolescent elbow. In: Pettrone FA, ed. *American Academy of Orthopaedic Surgeons Symposium in Upper Extremity Injuries in Athletes.* St. Louis, Mo: C V Mosby Co; 1986:211–220.

69. Singer KM, Roy SP. Osteochondritis of the humeral capitellum. *Am J Sports Med.* 1985; 12:351–360.

70. Bennett JB, Tullos HS. Ligamentous and articular injuries in the athlete. In: Morrey BF, ed. *The Elbow and Its Disorders.* Philadelphia, Pa: W B Saunders; 1985.

71. Ellman H. Unusual affections of the pre-adolescent elbow. *J Bone Joint Surg.* 1967; 49A:203.

72. Sobel J. Shoulder rehabilitation: Rotator cuff tendonitis, strength training, and return to play. In Pettrone FA, ed. *American Academy of Orthopaedic Surgeons Symposium on Upper Extremity Injuries in Athletes.* St. Louis, Mo: C V Mosby Co; 1986:338–347.

73. Jobe FW, Moynes DR, Brewster CE. Rehabilitation of shoulder joint instabilities. *Orthop Clin N Am.* 1987; 18:473–482.

74. Curwin S, Stanish WD. *Tendinitis: Its Etiology and Treatment.* Lexington, Mass: D C Heath & Co; 1984.

Index

Page numbers followed by *t* refer to tables.
Page numbers followed by *f* refer to figures.

Page numbers followed by *t* refer to tables.
Page numbers followed by *f* refer to figures.

Page numbers followed by *t* refer to tables.
Page numbers followed by *f* refer to figures.

Page numbers followed by *t* refer to tables.
Page numbers followed by *f* refer to figures.

Page numbers followed by *t* refer to tables.
Page numbers followed by *f* refer to figures.

Page numbers followed by *t* refer to tables.
Page numbers followed by *f* refer to figures.

Page numbers followed by *t* refer to tables.
Page numbers followed by *f* refer to figures.

Page numbers followed by t refer to tables.
Page numbers followed by f refer to figures.

Page numbers followed by *t* refer to tables.
Page numbers followed by *f* refer to figures.

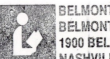